W9-CUU-969

THIRD EDITION

PEDIATRIC

PRIMARY CARE

Practice Guidelines for Nurses

Edited by

Beth Richardson, PhD, RN, CPNP, FAANP

Associate Professor Emeritus
School of Nursing
Indiana University
Pediatric Nurse Practitioner
HealthNet, Inc.
Indianapolis, Indiana

JONES & BARTLETT
L E A R N I N G

World Headquarters
Jones & Bartlett Learning
5 Wall Street
Burlington, MA 01803
978-443-5000
info@jblearning.com
www.jblearning.com

Jones & Bartlett Learning books and products are available through most bookstores and online booksellers. To contact Jones & Bartlett Learning directly, call 800-832-0034, fax 978-443-8000, or visit our website, www.jblearning.com.

Substantial discounts on bulk quantities of Jones & Bartlett Learning publications are available to corporations, professional associations, and other qualified organizations. For details and specific discount information, contact the special sales department at Jones & Bartlett Learning via the above contact information or send an email to specialsales@jblearning.com.

Copyright © 2017 by Jones & Bartlett Learning, LLC, an Ascend Learning Company

All rights reserved. No part of the material protected by this copyright may be reproduced or utilized in any form, electronic or mechanical, including photocopying, recording, or by any information storage and retrieval system, without written permission from the copyright owner.

The content, statements, views, and opinions herein are the sole expression of the respective authors and not that of Jones & Bartlett Learning, LLC. Reference herein to any specific commercial product, process, or service by trade name, trademark, manufacturer, or otherwise does not constitute or imply its endorsement or recommendation by Jones & Bartlett Learning, LLC and such reference shall not be used for advertising or product endorsement purposes. All trademarks displayed are the trademarks of the parties noted herein. *Pediatric Primary Care: Practice Guidelines for Nurses, Third Edition* is an independent publication and has not been authorized, sponsored, or otherwise approved by the owners of the trademarks or service marks referenced in this product.

There may be images in this book that feature models; these models do not necessarily endorse, represent, or participate in the activities represented in the images. Any screenshots in this product are for educational and instructive purposes only. Any individuals and scenarios featured in the case studies throughout this product may be real or fictitious, but are used for instructional purposes only.

The authors, editor, and publisher have made every effort to provide accurate information. However, they are not responsible for errors, omissions, or for any outcomes related to the use of the contents of this book and take no responsibility for the use of the products and procedures described. Treatments and side effects described in this book may not be applicable to all people; likewise, some people may require a dose or experience a side effect that is not described herein. Drugs and medical devices are discussed that may have limited availability controlled by the Food and Drug Administration (FDA) for use only in a research study or clinical trial. Research, clinical practice, and government regulations often change the accepted standard in this field. When consideration is being given to use of any drug in the clinical setting, the health care provider or reader is responsible for determining FDA status of the drug, reading the package insert, and reviewing prescribing information for the most up-to-date recommendations on dose, precautions, and contraindications, and determining the appropriate usage for the product. This is especially important in the case of drugs that are new or seldom used.

Production Credits
VP, Executive Publisher: David D. Cella
Executive Editor: Amanda Martin
Associate Acquisitions Editor: Rebecca Myrick
Editorial Assistant: Lauren Vaughn
Production Editor: Vanessa Richards
Senior Marketing Manager: Jennifer Scherzay
VP, Manufacturing and Inventory Control: Therese Connell
Composition: S4Carlisle Publishing Services
Cover Design: Kristin E. Parker
Rights & Media Specialist: Wes DeShano

Media Development Editor: Shannon Sheehan
Cover Images: Background: © antishock/Shutterstock;
Bubbles: © Marish/Shutterstock; Male doctor at bedside:
© Monkey Business Images/Shutterstock; Female
pediatrician with baby: © Monkey Business Images/
Shutterstock; Male pediatrician using stethoscope:
© michaeljung/Shutterstock
Printing and Binding: Edwards Brothers Malloy
Cover Printing: Edwards Brothers Malloy

Library of Congress Cataloging-in-Publication Data
Pediatric primary care (Richardson)
Pediatric primary care : practice guidelines for nurses / [edited by] Beth Richardson.—Third edition.
  p. ; cm.
Includes bibliographical references and index.
ISBN 978-1-284-09310-0 (spiral)
I. Richardson, Beth, 1944- , editor, author. II. Title.
[DNLM: 1. Pediatric Nursing—methods. 2. Primary Care Nursing. 3. Child. 4. Infant. 5. Nurse Practitioners. WY 159]
RJ245
618.92'00231—dc23
2015026978

6048

Printed in the United States of America
20 19 18 17 16   10 9 8 7 6 5 4 3 2 1

Contents

CHAPTER 18
Seven- to Ten-Year Visit (School Age)   143
Elizabeth Godfrey Terry

CHAPTER 19
Eleven- to Thirteen-Year Visit (Preadolescent)   159
Mary J. Alvarado

APPENDIX J

Preface

Pediatric Primary Care: Practice Guidelines for Nurses, Third Edition can be used as a resource for a variety of diagnoses, including differential diagnoses and treatment strategies. It is divided into three sections. The first section includes taking a medical history with a family seen for the first time, taking an interval history, newborn rounding, and breastfeeding. Well-child visits are included, along with information about nutrition, elimination, sleep patterns, growth and development, and injury prevention. The second section is organized by body system and is written in outline format, making it easy to read and find information quickly. Common medical conditions are presented with information about etiology, occurrence, clinical manifestations, physical findings, diagnostic tests, differential diagnosis, treatment, follow-up, complications, and patient/family education. The third section (Appendices A–J) provides additional essential resources, including growth charts, a BMI reference table, asthma guidelines, and fluoride dosing. The charts are to be used to locate needed information quickly. This section also includes common medications used in pediatrics, as well as information about their common uses, availability, adverse effects, and nursing implications.

—BETH RICHARDSON

Acknowledgments

I would like to thank my children, Jason, Sarah, and Walker; my grandchildren, Caroline and Darren; Sadie, Sam, and my friends; and all the students I have had the privilege of knowing. Thank you for teaching me.

To students, friends, and colleagues—thank you for all you do in caring for children.

Contributors

Mary J. Alvarado, MSN, RN, CPNP
Pediatric Nurse Practitioner
HealthNet, Inc.
Indianapolis, Indiana

Samantha Casselman, DNP, RN, CPNP-PC
Pediatric Dermatology
Phoenix Children's Hospital
Phoenix, Arizona

Patricia Clinton, PhD, ARNP, PNP, FAANP
Clinical Professor Emeritus
University of Iowa College of Nursing
Iowa City, Iowa

Karen M. Corlett, RN, CPNP-AC/PC
Pediatric Nurse Practitioner
Cardiac Intensive Care Unit
Children's Medical Hospital
Dallas, Texas

Mary Jo Eoff, MSN, RN, CPNP
Clinical Associate Professor
School of Nursing
Indiana University
Indianapolis, Indiana

Amy L. Feldman, RN, MSN, CPNP, IBCLC, CIMI
International Board Certified Lactation Consultant
Nurse Consultant
Bradenton, Florida

Jane A. Fox, EdD, PNP-BC
Professor
School of Nursing
University of North Carolina
Wilmington, North Carolina

Terea Giannetta, MSN, RN, CPNP
Professor
School of Nursing
California State University
Fresno, California

Linda S. Gilman, EdD, RN, CPNP
Pediatric Nurse Practitioner
HealthNet, Inc.
Associate Professor Emeritus
School of Nursing
Indiana University
Indianapolis, Indiana

Donna Hallas, PhD, PNP-BC, CPNP, FAANP
Clinical Associate Professor
Director of PNP Program
College of Nursing
New York University
New York, New York

Betsy Atkinson Joyce, EdD, MSN, CPNP
Pediatric Nurse Practitioner
Northpoint Pediatrics
Associate Professor Emeritus
School of Nursing
Indiana University
Indianapolis, Indiana

Susan J. Kersey, PMHCNS-BC
Child/Adolescent/Mental Health Clinical Nurse Specialist
Wabash Valley Alliance
Lafayette, Indiana
Lecturer
School of Nursing
Purdue University
West Lafayette, Indiana

Shelly J. King, MSN, RN, CPNP
Pediatric Nurse Practitioner
Director of Children's Continence Center and Pediatric Urology
Riley Hospital for Children
Indianapolis, Indiana

Julie LaMothe, RN, MSN, CPNP
Childhood Obesity
Riley Hospital for Children
Indianapolis, Indiana

Tracy Magee, PhD, RN, CPNP
Assistant Clinical Professor
Director of the PNP Program
School of Nursing
Indiana University
Indianapolis, Indiana

Kristin Miller, MSN, RN, CPNP
Pediatric Neurology
Peyton Manning Children's Hospital at St. Vincent Hospital
Indianapolis, Indiana

Meg Moorman, RNC, MSN, WHNP
Assistant Clinical Professor
School of Nursing
Indiana University
Indianapolis, Indiana

Judith O'Haver, PhD, RN, CPNP-PC
Pediatric Nurse Practitioner
Pediatric Dermatology
Phoenix Children's Hospital
Phoenix, AZ

Miki M. Patterson, PhD, PNP, ONP
Director of Clinical Solutions
Stryker Performance Solutions
Assistant Professor Nursing
University of Massachusetts, Lowell
Lowell, Massachusetts

Frances K. Porcher, EdD, RN, CPNP
Pediatric Nurse Practitioner
Pediatric Emergency Department
Medical University of South Carolina
Charleston, South Carolina

Susan G. Rains, BSN, MA, CPNP
Pediatric Nurse Practitioner
HealthNet, Inc.
Indianapolis, Indiana

Beth Richardson, PhD, RN, CPNP, FAANP
Pediatric Nurse Practitioner
HealthNet, Inc.
Associate Professor Emeritus
School of Nursing
Indiana University Indianapolis, Indiana

Megan Reynolds, MSN, RN, CPNP-PC
Pediatric Dermatology
Ann and Robert H. Lurie Children's Hospital
Chicago, Illinois

Mary Lou C. Rosenblatt, MS, RN, CPNP
Senior Pediatric Nurse Practitioner
Harriet Lane Primary Care Center for Children and Adolescents
Johns Hopkins Hospital
Baltimore, Maryland

Robin Shannon, MS, RN, CPNP
Pediatric Nurse Practitioner
Pediatric Gastroenterology, Hepatology, and Nutrition
University of Minnesota Amplatz Children's Hospital
Minneapolis, Minnesota

Elizabeth Godfrey Terry, MSN, RN, CPNP
Adjunct Professor
School of Nursing
Indiana University
Indianapolis, Indiana

Nancy Valentine, RN, MSN, CPNP
Pediatric Pulmonolgy
Riley Outpatient Center
Riley Children's Hospital
Indianapolis, Indiana

Kim Walton, MSN, RN, CPNP
Director Youth Services
Community Health Network
Indianapolis, Indiana

Candace F. Zickler, RN, MSN, CPNP, NCSN
School Nurse
MSD Wayne Township Schools
Marion County, Indiana

Child Health Care

Obtaining an Initial History

Beth Richardson

I. INTRODUCTION

A. The complete health history taken at the first visit is an opportunity for the practitioner to establish a relationship with the child and family, gain insight into family relationships, and obtain pertinent health information.

II. INITIAL INFORMATION

A. Parent(s).
   1. Name(s).
   2. Age(s).
   3. Health status.
B. Sibling(s).
   1. Age(s).
   2. Health status.

III. REASON FOR CURRENT VISIT

A. Current problem or illness.
   1. Background information.
      a. When did it start?
      b. What are the symptoms?
      c. Are others in family ill with similar symptoms?
      d. What has been done to treat symptoms?

IV. PAST HISTORY

A. Prenatal history and care if child younger than 5 years.
  1. Was pregnancy planned?
  2. Did the mother smoke? Drink alcohol? Take any medications or drugs?
  3. Any problems such as:
     a. Vaginal infection?
     b. Kidney infection?
     c. High blood pressure?
     d. Diabetes?
     e. Edema?
     f. Bleeding?
     g. Any accidents during pregnancy?
B. Natal history and care.
  1. Labor and delivery.
     a. Where was infant born?
     b. Type of delivery?
     c. Length of labor?
     d. Anesthesia used during labor?
     e. Any problems with mother or infant after birth?
     f. Infant's birth weight? Length? Head circumference? Gestational age?
     g. Did infant go home with the mother?
  2. Feeding.
     a. Baby fed by bottle or breast?
     b. Type of formula used?
     c. Frequency of feedings?
     d. Pattern of weight gain?
  3. Childhood illness.
     a. Rheumatic fever, chickenpox, number of ear infections, strep throat, respiratory syncytial virus (RSV), whooping cough, mononucleosis, sexually transmitted infections (STIs).
  4. Hospitalizations.
     a. Dates, names of hospitals, diagnoses.
  5. Surgeries.
     a. Dates, names of hospitals, diagnoses, complications.
  6. Immunizations (see Appendix A).
     a. Dates, reactions.
  7. Screening tests.
     a. Vision, hearing, speech, hemoglobin, urine, tuberculosis skin test, X-rays, other laboratory tests.

8. Allergies.
   a. Medications, environment, foods.
9. Transfusions.
   a. Dates, number of units transfused, reactions.
10. Medications.
    a. Prescription; over the counter; herbal; current/recent medications including dosage, length of time taking medication, adverse reactions/side effects.

V. REVIEW OF SYSTEMS

A. History.
   1. Head, eyes, ears, nose, throat.
      a. Head: Headaches or head injuries?
      b. Eyes: Tearing, strabismus? Has child had vision test? Does child wear glasses/contacts?
      c. Ears: Ear infections? Drainage? Has child had a hearing test?
      d. Nose: Allergies? Frequency of colds? Does child snore, have nosebleeds, or have postnasal drip?
      e. Throat: Sore throat, dental hygiene, lymph glands, hoarseness?
   2. Cardiovascular.
      a. Heart murmur.
      b. Congenital heart disease.
      c. Cyanosis.
      d. Edema.
      e. Activity tolerance, shortness of breath, syncope.
   3. Respiratory.
      a. Pneumonia, bronchitis.
      b. Asthma.
      c. Cystic fibrosis.
      d. Croup, cough.
   4. Gastrointestinal.
      a. Diarrhea, constipation.
      b. Vomiting, reflux, upset stomach, abdominal pain.
      c. Bloody stools, rectal bleeding.
      d. Fissures, ulcer.
      e. Jaundice.
   5. Genitourinary.
      a. When did child achieve night dryness?
      b. Frequency of urination, urinary tract infections, dysuria, polyuria.

      c. Hematuria.

      d. Menstrual history (pain, flow), vaginal drainage.

      e. Penis or testes abnormalities, STIs, sexual activity.

  6. Musculoskeletal.

      a. Painful joints, swelling, strains, sprains, fractures.

      b. Deformities.

      c. Activity tolerance.

  7. Neurologic.

      a. Headaches.

      b. Seizures, epilepsy.

      c. Fainting, dizziness, tremors.

      d. Clumsy, uncoordinated.

      e. ADD/ADHD, learning disability, developmental delay.

  8. Endocrine.

      a. Sexual maturation.

      b. Diabetes.

      c. Thyroid or adrenal diseases.

  9. Skin.

      a. Rashes, birth marks.

VI. FAMILY HISTORY

  A. History of any of following in family members:

    1. High blood pressure.

    2. Heart disease, stroke.

    3. Diabetes.

    4. Cataracts, glaucoma.

    5. Anemia.

    6. High cholesterol levels.

    7. Asthma, allergies.

    8. Kidney infections.

    9. Colitis, ulcers.

    10. Cancer.

    11. Thyroid problems.

    12. Epilepsy.

    13. Dysplasia of hip.

    14. Mental retardation.

    15. Alcoholism or substance abuse.

VII. DISEASE HISTORY

   A. Disease/problem.
      1. When was patient diagnosed?
      2. How was patient treated? Response to treatment?
      3. How have symptoms changed? How is patient doing now?
      4. Is patient taking medications to treat problem?

VIII. SOCIAL HISTORY

   A. Parents'/guardians' employment site(s) and hours worked.
   B. Child care.
      1. Daycare or sitter?
      2. Preschool or after-school programs?
   C. Family relationships: How do family members get along?
   D. Home life.
      1. Does home have a yard where child can play?
      2. Stairs in house?
      3. City, well, or bottled water?
      4. Is home in safe neighborhood?
   E. School life.
      1. How is child's progress?
          a. What are child's grades?
          b. What are child's strengths and weaknesses in learning? Does child need extra help in learning?
          c. What type of classroom (advanced, regular, learning disability)?
      2. Behavior.
          a. Does this child bully others or is child a victim of bullying?
          b. What is child's behavior in learning situations?
          c. History of absenteeism or truancy?
      3. Classmates/friends.
          a. How does child relate to and play with those in classroom, daycare, or preschool?
          b. Does child have a best friend?
          c. What does child like to play?

IX. DEVELOPMENT

   A. For child younger than 2 years ask when first:
      1. Smiled.
      2. Rolled.
      3. Sat without assistance.
      4. Crawled.
      5. Walked without assistance.
      6. Said 2 words.
      7. Fed self.
      8. Said 10 words.
   B. Behavior.
      1. Temper tantrums, whining.
      2. Thumb sucking.
      3. Sleep patterns.
      4. Temperament.

BIBLIOGRAPHY

Bickley LS. *Bates' Guide to Physical Examination and History Taking.* 11th ed. Philadelphia, PA: Lippincott; 2013.

Duderstadt KG. *Pediatric Physical Examination: An Illustrated Handbook.* 2nd ed. St. Louis, MO: Mosby; 2014.

Obtaining an Interval History

Donna Hallas

I. THE INTERVAL HISTORY

A. Definition.
   1. Interval history: Data collection that occurs at subsequent visits to one in which comprehensive history and physical examination were completed.
   2. Amount of information reviewed and collected for interval history depends on child's age and length of time since comprehensive history was obtained and/or prior appointments in which interval history was updated.
   3. General guideline for obtaining interval history: Review and update data every 6 months for infants, toddlers, preschool-age children, and every year for school-age children, adolescents.
B. Significance of interval history.
   1. Although comprehensive history is used to establish initial health promotion plan, analysis of data collected during interval history is often used in one of four ways:
      a. To continue established health promotion plan.
      b. To identify new healthcare problems.
      c. To make changes to health promotion plan based on new data.
      d. To establish new health promotion plan.
C. Preparation for obtaining interval history.
   1. Prior to beginning data collection for interval history, review comprehensive history and any prior interval histories available on medical record.
      a. Helps nurse practitioner focus questions that will elicit data needed to complete interval history.
      b. Sample data contained in comprehensive history that may need further exploration during interval history is listed in **Table 2-1**.

Table 2-1 Focusing the Interval History from Details in the Comprehensive History

Comprehensive History	Interval History
Past medical history	Any data in past medical history that is significant and requires further clarification. Consider previous acute illnesses including hospitalizations, injuries, accidents, surgeries, chronic illnesses.
Review problem list	If all prior problems are listed as resolved, then no further data should be elicited at this visit. If problems still exist, then ask questions specific to identified problem.
Allergies	Always obtain update on allergies to foods, medications, environmental pollutants.
Developmental history	Review results of prior DDST or the Ages and Stages Questionnaires. Note achievement of developmental milestones at each interval visit. If delays are noted, question status of intervention services (early intervention for children at 5 years old, OT, PT, speech, special education services for all children).
Social history	Exercise and activity, wellness behaviors, behavior issues at home or at school.
Family history	Review family structure and family support systems. If data contained in comprehensive history suggests dysfunctional family, ask about present family structure and function. Review genogram and review significant family history prior to interview. Pay particular attention to strong family history of conditions in which family lifestyle modifications can have significant impact (e.g., cardiovascular conditions, hypertension, diabetes, obesity). Implementing lifestyle modifications in early childhood years may significantly affect health throughout lifetime.
Medication history	Prescription, over the counter, homeopathic remedies.
Nutritional history	Timing and frequency of meals, ethnic and cultural considerations in food choices.
Immunization history	Immunization records should be reviewed at each visit.
Mental health	Assess mental health status for school age and adolescence at each interval visit. Anxiety and depression frequently occur in these populations.

D. Elements of an interval history.
  1. Elements included in interval history should be related to the age of the child.
  2. Major focus for interval history for each child and adolescent should include questions concerning eating, sleeping, bladder and bowel patterns, and any unusual behaviors or changes in behaviors. Additional questions are then age related.
  3. Infant, toddler, and preschool-age children.
     a. Ask questions related to achievement of developmental milestones.
     b. Denver Developmental Screening Test (DDST) may be used as a guide for questioning patterns concerning achievement of developmental milestones.
     c. Toddlers and preschoolers: Assess information regarding speech and language development and development of social skills.
     d. Use the Surveillance and Screening Algorithm: Autistic Spectrum Disorders for toddlers at the 18-, 21-, and/or 24-month-old episodic visit if it has not been completed at a maintenance health visit.
  4. School-age children.
     a. Should also include questions related to sociobehavioral development with peers and progress in school.
     b. If female school-age child has secondary sex characteristics, ask about menstrual cycle: Age of onset, frequency, length of cycle, any discomfort prior to or during menstruations.
     c. Children older than 10 years of age should be asked: Have they or their friends tried alcohol or drugs? Use a brief alcohol/drug screening tool at each episodic visit.
        • What is their diet?
        • Happy with appearance/weight?
        • Thought about harming themselves or others?
        • Sexually active?
  5. Adolescents.
     a. Use the HEADSSS assessment (home, education/employment, activity, drugs/alcohol, sexuality, suicide/depression, safety and exposure to violence).
     b. Adolescent female: Ask questions related to menstrual cycle.
     c. Ask about high-risk social behaviors: Smoking; alcohol/drug use; sexual activity, including diagnosis and treatment of sexually transmitted infections [STIs]; driving motor vehicle in reckless manner; use of guns; etc.
E. Review of systems (ROS).
  1. Age-appropriate ROS: Conduct in head-to-toe manner as identified in comprehensive physical examination (**Table 2-2**).

Table 2-2 Review of System (ROS) in an Interval History

System	ROS—Gathering the Interval History[a]
On a regular basis, do you have problems with:	
Head and neck	Headaches
	Blurred vision or any vision problems
	Earaches
	Nosebleeds
	Sore throats
	Difficulty swallowing
	Any lumps in head or neck area
Chest and lungs	Chest pain
	Heart beating fast in chest (palpitations)
	Shortness of breath
	Fainting
	Frequent cough
Abdomen	Nausea
	Vomiting
	Diarrhea
	Urinating or bowels
	Menstruation
	Testicular pain
Musculoskeletal	Leg pain or cramps
	Stiffness, swelling, bone deformities
	Skin, hair, and nails
	Rashes
	Moles
	Darkened or discolored areas
	Abnormal hair growth
	Clubbing of nails
	Bruising easily
Sexual history	History of sexually transmitted infections

[a] This information is gathered in addition to the details related to eating, sleeping, bladder, and bowel patterns.

Table 2-3 Red Flags: The Interval History for the Athletic Child or Adolescent

Interval History Questions That May Elicit Red Flag Data	System	Red Flag Data
Any relatives < 50 years of age die as result of sudden unexpected cardiac death?	Cardiovascular	Change in family history Sudden death of relative < 50 years of age
Does the child report chest pain or palpitations, syncope during or after exercise?		Chief complaint from child: Chest pain, palpitations, syncope
Does the child report any breathing problems during or after exercise?	Respiratory	Chief complaint from child: Dyspnea, wheezing
Child had any episodes of dizziness, syncope, fainting, concussion?	Neurologic	Chief complaint from child: Syncope, loss of consciousness

II. INTERVAL HISTORY FOR ATHLETIC CHILD OR ADOLESCENT

    A. Pre-participation sports history and physical have well-established guidelines; follow explicitly.

    B. Interval history is integral part of assessment.

        1. Question parent and child about significant family history changes (e.g., sudden death of relative who was 50 years old from cardiovascular condition). Include questions that elicit information about significant episodes (red flags) of chest pain, dyspnea, syncope, palpitations, loss of consciousness, history of concussions (**Table 2-3**).

III. FOCUSED HISTORY

    A. Focused history: Used to collect data about a specific problem, usually chief complaint identified by parent/child (**Table 2-4** and **Table 2-5**).

    B. Focus all questions on eliciting data about chief complaint.

    C. Focused history usually limited to one or two systems.

Table 2-4 Sample Focused History: Medical

Subjective Data	Questions to Focus the History
"My child has a chronic cough."	What do you mean by a chronic cough?
"My child begins coughing each night. I cannot remember the last time he didn't cough at night."	Does child cough during day or just at night?
	What time of night does child begin coughing?
	Describe the cough.
	Is the cough productive or nonproductive?
	Does the cough affect child's sleeping pattern?
	Any products currently being used in household that weren't being used before child began having this "chronic" cough?
	Pets in your household?
	Did you change the pillow your child uses?
	Did you use any over-the-counter or prescription medications to treat this cough?
	Has the child been evaluated for asthma or allergies?
	Anything make cough better or worse?

Table 2-5 Sample Focused History: Mental Health

Subjective Data	Questions to Focus the History
"My child's behavior has become so difficult at home."	Describe what you mean by "difficult behavior."
	Does anything trigger these behaviors?
	What do you do when this behavior becomes "so difficult"?
	What is your child's response?
	Does this behavior pattern occur at school or outside the home, such as at a friend's house or relative's home?
	Has there been a change in your family lifestyle, such as parents arguing at home, parental separation, new family member living in the home?
	Has there been any change in your child's physical abilities, such as change in cognitive or psychomotor skills?
	Does your child complain of headaches?

IV. APPLYING DATA OBTAINED IN INTERVAL HISTORY TO CLINICAL PRACTICE

A. After completing interval history and physical examination, compare findings in comprehensive history to data obtained in interval history.

1. If no significant changes found in interval history, advise parent, infant/child to continue to follow established health promotion plan.

2. If significant changes are found in interval history, revise health promotion plan.

   a. Example: If interval family history reveals family members have diabetes mellitus, evaluate and modify family/child exercise and dietary patterns.

3. If significant changes are found in interval history in relation to child's health, establish new health promotion plan with parent and child/adolescent active participation.

   a. Example: If interval history reveals significant change in frequency of coughing and upper respiratory symptoms, complete a detailed focused history and establish a new health promotion plan.

BIBLIOGRAPHY

Bickley LS. *Bates' Guide to Physical Assessment and History Taking*. 11th ed. Philadelphia, PA: Lippincott; 2013.

Burns CE, Dunn AM, Brady MA, Starr NB, Blosser CG. *Pediatric Primary Care*. 5th ed. Philadelphia, PA: Saunders; 2013.

Duderstadt KG. *Pediatric Physical Examination: An Illustrated Handbook*. 2nd ed. St. Louis, MO: Mosby; 2014.

Johnson CP, Myers SA, Council on Children with Disabilities. Identification and evaluation of children with autistic spectrum disorders. *Pediatrics*. 2007;120(5):1183-1215.

Performing a Physical Examination

Mary Jo Eoff and Beth Richardson

I. INTRODUCTION

A. Pediatric physical assessment is a continual process that includes interviews, inspection, observation of children.

B. Physical growth, motor skills, and cognitive and social development change as the child matures.

C. The assessment of the pediatric patient must include what is considered to be normal within the child's age limits.

D. Children will differ among themselves at various stages of development.

E. The following is an outline that can be used as a guide in doing a comprehensive physical assessment.

II. PEDIATRIC PHYSICAL EXAMINATION

A. Growth measurements.
 1. Length/height.
  a. Recumbent (2 years).
  b. Standing height.
 2. Weight.
 3. Head circumference (occipital frontal circumference [OFC]).
 4. Chest circumference (up to 1 year).
 5. Skinfold thickness.
B. Vital signs.
 1. Temperature, heart rate, respirations, blood pressure.
C. General appearance.
 1. Cleanliness, posture, hygiene.
 2. Nutrition.

      3. Behavior, ability to cooperate.

      4. Development.

      5. Alertness.

D. Skin.

      1. Color: Pallor, cyanosis, erythema, ecchymosis, petechiae, jaundice.

      2. Texture.

      3. Temperature.

      4. Turgor.

      5. Describe size, shape, and location of rashes, eruptions, and lesions.

      6. Sweating.

E. Hair.

      1. Color, texture, quantity, distribution, infestations (nits).

F. Nails.

      1. Inspect color, texture, quality, distribution, hygiene.

      2. Observe for nail biting.

G. Hands and feet.

      1. Observe flexion crease on palm.

      2. Assess for foot and ankle deformities.

H. Lymph nodes.

      1. Palpate for nodes in following areas:

         a. Submaxillary.

         b. Cervical.

         c. Axillary.

         d. Inguinal.

      2. Note size, mobility, or tenderness of any enlarged node.

I. Head.

      1. Assess shape and symmetry.

      2. Assess head control; should be well established by 6 months of age.

      3. Palpate skull.

         a. Fontanels (2 years of age).

         b. Suture ridges and grooves (up to 6 months of age).

         c. Nodes.

         d. Any swelling.

      4. Examine scalp for hygiene, lesions, signs of trauma, loss of hair, or discoloration.

      5. Percuss frontal sinuses (children 7 years of age).

J. Neck.

      1. Palpate trachea for deviation.

      2. Palpate thyroid, noting size, shape, symmetry, tenderness, or nodules.

      3. Palpate carotid arteries.

    4. Palpate neck structure.
       a. Pain or tenderness.
       b. Enlargement of parotid gland.
       c. Weblike tissue.

K. Eyes.
    1. Check peripheral vision.
    2. Check visual acuity.
       a. Snellen E chart.
       b. Allen test.
    3. Note whether eyelashes curl away from eye.
    4. Note whether eyebrows are above eye and do not meet at midline.
    5. Test for any strabismus. *(crossed eye)*
       a. Hirschberg test. *(deviation of 1 eye)*
       b. Cover–uncover test. → *repetative uncontrolled movements*
    6. Observe for nystagmus or ptosis. → *drooping of eye lid*
    7. Inspect conjunctiva for drainage, redness, swelling, pain.
    8. Inspect sclera, cornea, iris.
    9. Check: Pupils equal, round, react to light.
    10. Examine with ophthalmoscope.
       a. Optic disk, macula, arteriole/vein, fovea centralis, red reflex.
    11. Inspect lachrymal ducts: Tears, drainage.
    12. Inspect placement, alignment of outer eye: Palpebral slant, epicanthus, lids.

L. Ears.
    1. Inspect placement and alignment of pinna.
    2. Inspect auditory canal: Color, cerumen, patency.
    3. Observe for skin tags and hygiene.
    4. Examine middle ear with otoscope.
       a. Color of tympanic membrane, light reflex, bony landmarks.
    5. Check hearing.
       a. Rinne test. – *strike fork, place on Mastoid bone, tell when can no longer hear*
       b. Weber test. – *strike fork, place on top of head, can hear better on one side or other*

M. Nose.
    1. Observe mucosal lining for color, discharge, patency.
    2. Observe color of the turbinates and meatus.
    3. Note if septum is midline.

N. Mouth and throat.
    1. Observe internal structures.
       a. Hard and soft palate, palatoglossal arch, palatine tonsil, tongue, oropharynx, palatopharyngeal arch, uvula.

2. Palpate ethmoid, frontal, and maxillary sinuses.
3. Observe lip edges.
4. Observe eruption of teeth.
    a. Number appropriate for age.
    b. Color and hygiene.
    c. Occlusion of upper and lower jaw.
5. Check salivation.
6. Check drooling.
7. Check swallowing reflex.
8. Note color, texture, or any lesions of the lips.
9. Observe gingiva and mucous membranes for color, texture, moistness.

O. Tongue.
    1. Observe for smoothness, fissuring, coating, or redness.
    2. Tongue able to extend forward to lips?
    3. Tongue interfere with speech?

P. Chest.
    1. Observe shape of thorax.
    2. Check costal angles; should be between 45° and 50°.
    3. Check that points of attachments between ribs and costal cartilage are smooth.
    4. Check movement.
        a. Inspiration: Chest expands, costal angle increases, diaphragm descends.
        b. Expiration: Reverse occurs.

Q. Lungs.
    1. Evaluate respiratory movement: Rate, rhythm, depth, quality, character.
    2. Auscultate breath sounds.
        a. Vesicular breath sounds.
        b. Bronchovesicular breath sounds.
        c. Bronchial breath sounds.
    3. Note adventitious breath sounds.
        a. Crackles, wheezes, stridor, pleural friction rub.
    4. Check for cough.
        a. Productive/nonproductive.
        b. Color of secretions.
    5. Check retractions.
    6. Check abdominal breathing.
    7. Check thoracic expansion.
    8. Palpate tactile fremitus.

R. Heart.

Right 2nd ICS *Left 3rd ICS* *← LG, medial to Mid-Clavicular line* *Left 5th*

1. Auscultate heart sounds.
   a. Aortic area, pulmonic area, Erb's point, tricuspid area, mitral or apical area.

Left 2nd ICS

2. Check S1–S2.
3. Palpate for thrill.
4. Record murmurs.

Lower left sternal border 4th ICS

   a. Area best heard.
   b. Timing within S1–S2 cycle.
   c. Change with position.
   d. Loudness and quality.
   e. Grade intensity of murmur.

S. Vascular.
1. Assess capillary refill; should occur in 1–2 seconds.
2. Assess circulation.
   a. Color and texture of skin.
   b. Nail and hair distribution.
3. Assess perfusion.
   a. Edema.
   b. Pulses (4–0).
4. Assess collateral circulation.

T. Abdomen.
1. Inspect contour and size of abdomen.
2. Note condition of skin.
3. Inspect umbilicus for hernias, fistula, discharge.
4. Auscultate bowel sounds.
5. Auscultate for any aortic pulsations.
6. Percuss abdomen.
7. Palpate outer edge of liver.
8. Palpate spleen.
9. Elicit abdominal reflux.
10. Palpate femoral pulses.

U. Neurologic.
1. Observe behavior, mood, affect, interaction with environment, level of activity, positioning, level of consciousness, orientation to surroundings.
2. Check reflexes of the infant.

Turn face toward

   a. Rooting (present birth to 6 months of age). — *stimulus & makes sucking motion*
   b. Sucking (present birth to 10 months of age).
   c. Palmar grasp (present birth to 4 months of age).

suckon fingers toes

↳ Put object in babies palm → baby will make a fist

   d. Tonic neck (present at 6–8 weeks of age and lasts until 6 months).
   e. Stepping (present birth to 3 months of age).
   f. Plantar grasp (present birth to 8 months of age).
   g. Moro (present birth to 4–6 months of age).
   h. Babinski (child 15–18 months of age normally fans toes outward and dorsiflexes greater toe).
   i. Galant (present birth to 1–2 months of age).
   j. Placing (lack of response is abnormal).
   k. Landau (present 3 months to 2 years of age).
3. Test cranial nerves.
   a. I: Olfactory.
   b. II: Optic.
   c. III: Oculomotor.
   d. IV: Trochlear.
   e. V: Trigeminal.
   f. VI: Abducens.
   g. VII: Facial.
   h. VIII: Acoustic.
   i. IX: Glossopharyngeal.
   j. X: Vagus.
   k. XI: Spinal accessory.
   l. XII: Hypoglossal.
4. Test cerebellar functioning: Finger-to-nose test, heel-to-shin test, Romberg.
5. Test deep tendon reflexes (grading 4–0): Biceps, triceps, brachioradialis, patellar, Achilles.
6. Check sensory functioning: Pain, temperature, touch.

V. Musculoskeletal.
1. Inspect curvature and symmetry of spine.
2. Test for scoliosis.
3. Inspect all joints for size, temperature, color, tenderness, mobility.
4. Test for developmental dysplasia of the hips (DDH).
   a. Ortolani maneuver (evaluate up to 12 months of age).
   b. Barlow's maneuver.
   c. Trendelenburg's test (used after child is walking).
5. Examine tibiofemoral bones: Knock knee, bow legs.
6. Inspect gait: Waddling gait (DDH), scissor (cerebral palsy [CP]), toeing-in.
7. Note flexibility and range of motion of joints.
8. Elicit planter reflex.
9. Test motor strength of arms, legs, hands, feet (grading 4–0).

W. Breast.
  1. Pigmentation.
  2. Location.
  3. Tanner stages (sexual maturity rating).
X. Genitalia.
  1. Male.
      a. Inspect size of penis.
      b. Inspect glands and shaft for swelling, skin lesions, inflammation.
      c. Inspect uncircumcised male: Prepuce.
      d. Inspect location of urethral meatus, note any discharge.
      e. Inspect scrotum for size, location, skin, and hair distribution.
      f. Palpate each scrotal sac for testes.
      g. Tanner stages (sexual maturing rating).
  2. Female.
      a. Palpate genitalia for any masses, cysts.
      b. Observe for any venereal warts.
      c. Inspect for location of urethral meatus, Skene glands, mons pubis, Bartholin gland, clitoris, labia majora, labia minora.
      d. Note any discharge: Color and odor.
      e. Tanner stages (sexual maturity rating).
Y. Anus.
  1. Inspect anal area for firmness and condition of skin.
  2. Elicit anal reflex.

BIBLIOGRAPHY

Bickley LS. *Bates' Guide to Physical Examination and History Taking.* 11th ed. Philadelphia, PA: Lippincott; 2013.

Duderstadt KG. *Pediatric Physical Examination: An Illustrated Handbook.* 2nd ed. St. Louis, MO: Mosby; 2014.

Making Newborn Rounds

Candace F. Zickler

Asthma, J45

Accessory nipple, Q83.3

Caput succedaneum, P12.81

Cardiac murmur, unspecified, R01.1

Choanal atresia, Q30.0

Coarctation of aorta, Q25.1

Cyanotic attacks of newborn, P28.2

Congenital non-neoplastic nevus, Q82.5

Constipation, K59.0

Convulsions of newborn, P90

Cytomegaloviral disease, unspecified, B25.9

Diabetes mellitus arising in
 pregnancy, O24.4

Dyspnea, unspecified, R06.00

Epispadias, Q64.0

Feeding problems of newborn, P92

Female infertility, unspecified, N97.9

Galactosemia, E74.21

Gestational [pregnancy-induced]
 hypertension, O13

Gonococcal infection, A54

Hemangioma of skin and subcutaneous
 tissue, D18.01

Herpesviral infection, unspecified, B00.9

Human immunodeficiency virus [HIV]
 disease, B20–B24

Hypospadias, Q54

Irritability and anger, R45.4

Lymphangioma, any site, D18.1

Meconium plug syndrome, P76.0

Neonatal cutaneous hemorrhage, P54.5

Neonatal jaundice, unspecified, P.59.9

Other diseases of tongue, K14.8

Other specified disorders of
 pigmentation, L81.8

Pallor, R23.1

Rash and other nonspecific skin
 eruption, R21

Rubella without complication, B06.9

Sickle-cell disorders, D57

Spontaneous abortion, O03

Stillbirth, P95

Streptococcus, group B, as the cause
 of diseases classified elsewhere, B95.1

Toxoplasmosis, unspecified, B58.9

Umbilical hernia without obstruction
 or gangrene, K42.9

Vomiting, unspecified, R11.10

I. MAKING NEWBORN ROUNDS

    A. Determine number of newborns delivered in last 24 hours.

    B. Prioritize assessments by birth time and concerns of nurses.

    C. Evaluate each infant within 12–24 hours of age and daily until discharge.

II. REVIEW OF THE INDIVIDUAL RECORDS

    A. Mother.

        1. Past obstetric history: Infertility, spontaneous abortions, stillbirths/perinatal deaths, parity, gravity, length of pregnancy, congenital anomalies in other infants, assistive reproductive technology (ART) used, isoimmune disease (Rh, ABO), pregnancy-induced hypertension (PIH), cesarean births, vaginal birth after cesarean, gestational diabetes. Current pregnancy history: Maternal age, overall health (asthma, sickle cell disease), estimated date of confinement (EDC), prenatal care, number of previous pregnancies, multiple or single fetus, presentation/position of fetus, amount of amniotic fluid, fetal growth/size (small, appropriate, or large for gestational age), nationality, public assistance.

        2. Results of prenatal lab work: Blood type; rubella IgG level; hepatitis B immunization status; serologic tests; HIV status (elective); gonorrhea and chlamydia cultures; maternal alpha fetal protein; urinalysis (bacteria, blood, protein); glucose screen; exposure to drugs, alcohol, tobacco, or teratogenic medications (valproate, tetracycline); exposure to viruses (TORCH: Toxoplasmosis, rubella, cytomegalovirus, herpes simplex virus); sexually transmitted infections; Group B streptococcus status.

    B. Newborn.

        1. Prenatal history: Vaginal or cesarean delivery; length of labor and delivery; tocolytics used during labor; narcotics, anesthesia, or analgesics mother received; presentation; placental abnormalities (three-vessel cord); amniotic fluid color/volume; Apgar scores (heart rate, respirations, muscle tone, reflex irritability, color) with 5-minute Apgar > 7.

        2. At birth: Gender delivery weight/length/occipital frontal circumference (OFC), temperature, blood pressure, pulse, respirations, feeding/nursing with breast or bottle, voiding spontaneously, passage of meconium, infant contact with mother/parents.

III. PHYSICAL ASSESSMENT OF THE NEWBORN

A. General appearance.
1. Gender, current weight, length, OFC, color, heart rate, respirations, temperature, blood glucose at birth, response to stimuli, posture, determination of gestational age from the New Ballard Score (physical maturity and neuromuscular maturity).
2. Full-term infant > 37 weeks but < 42 weeks.
3. Premature infant < 37 weeks, late preterm infant > 34 weeks to 36 weeks and 6 days.
4. Post-term infant > 42 weeks.
B. Late preterm infants at greater risk for airway instability when upright, respiratory distress, apnea/bradycardia, excessive lethargy and floppiness, > 7% birth weight loss during hospitalization, poor feeding, hyperbilirubinemia, hypoglycemia, hypothermia, sepsis, weak suck, and rehospitalization.
1. At risk for persistent, severe, or progressive tachypnea: Retractions, nasal flaring, grunting. Monitor with pulse oximeter and blood gases, chest X-ray, and frequent reexamination.
2. At risk for ability to regulate body temperature due to immature epidermis, large body surface area, and inability to regulate temperature. Goal is axillary temperature of 97.7–99.3°F (36.5–37.4°C).
3. At risk for hypoglycemia due to low glycogen stores, decreased enzymes, depressed hormone responses, and slower than average increase in newborn's blood glucose level. Assess for maternal risks (gestational diabetes, PIH, maternal obesity, tocolytics, difficult or prolonged delivery, late antepartum IV glucose or fetal decellerations), as well as neonatal risks (preterm delivery, intrauterine growth retardation [IUGR], twins, Apgars at < 7 at minutes, temperature instability, respiratory distress, polycythemia) for abnormalities. Infants whose mothers had diet-controlled or insulin-controlled gestational diabetes have significant fetal hyperinsulinism and slow adaptation of the neonatal pancreas.
4. At risk for sepsis due to transfer of maternal Immunoglobulin G (IgG) antibodies from the mother. Monitor for maternal risk factors for sepsis (prolonged rupture of membranes, intra-amniotic infection, intrapartum fever of 100.4°F, young maternal age, black race, Hispanic ethnicity, prior history of Group B strep disease, low antibody levels) and for neonatal risk factors (preterm delivery, male gender, multiple births, birth weight under 2500 grams [GMs], congenital anomalies, difficult delivery, and black race). Repeat physical assessment frequently, looking for signs of sepsis.

5. At risk for hyperbilirubinemia due to deficient UDP glucuronyl transferase in most newborns the first few days of life, decreased gastrointestinal motility, greater resorption of bilirubin, less than needed lactation, and poor feeding. Assess serum total bilirubins and utilize the Bhutani nomogram to assess levels by hour of age. Assess total bilirubin prior to discharge and repeat physical assessment and history.

6. At risk for feeding difficulties due to oromotor sucking and swallowing incoordination, neurobehavioral disorganization, and immature gastric system (coordination for infants is achieved at 36–38 weeks of gestational age). Preterm infants are sleepier, tire easily, and have difficulty latching on and sucking vigorously. Monitor for weight loss > 3% per day or 7% of birth weight loss prior to discharge.

7. At risk for readmission to the hospital after discharge due to any or all of the above. Infants born over 40 weeks' gestation are at risk for hypoglycemia, failure to grow proportionally, and dry and flaky skin since placenta starts to atrophy after 40 weeks, which slows fetal growth and results in difficulty with hypoxia and increased fetal swallowing. Fetus may try to breathe and is at risk for aspiration of meconium and slowed fetal growth. Plan to monitor blood sugars, quality of nursing/eating and total intake, plus quality/rate of respirations.

IV. ABNORMAL PHYSICAL FINDINGS (CONSULT WITH STAFF PHYSICIAN AND/OR REFER FOR EVALUATION, AS INDICATED)

A. Dysmorphic facies hyper- or hypotelorism, epicanthal folds, symmetrical facies and extremities.
   1. Skin and scalp with plethora, pallor, jaundice, cyanosis, bruising, abrasions, petechiae, hemangioma, port wine stain, café au lait spots.
   2. Shape of skull, molding.
   3. Bruising, hematoma/caput succedaneum.
   4. Size and tone of anterior and posterior fontanels.
B. Pupils without red reflex and unequal pupillary sizes, nares patent (choanal atresia), mouth with teeth, hypoglossia/macroglossia, palate high arched or missing, external ears with tags or pinhole openings, neck short/masses (cystic hygroma) or webbing.
C. More/fewer than five fingers/toes on each hand/foot.
D. Check clavicles for fractures/dislocations/pain. Chest shape with pectus excavatum/carinatum, and supernumerary nipples. Breath sounds that

are moist and grunting/retractions after 4 hours of age, apnea/respirations < 30 or > 60 per minute.

E. Heart rate with murmur (soft III/IV systolic murmur normal for first 12–24 hours since patent ductus may not be closed), or an irregular rate/rhythm < 100 or > 180 bpm, a cuff blood pressure < 65 or > 95 mm Hg of systolic pressure, and diastolic < 30 or > 60 mm Hg. Absent or decreased femoral pulses (coarctation of aorta), slow capillary refill is indicative of poor perfusion.

F. Temperature instability < 97.7°F (36.5°C) after 4 hours of age.

G. Abdominal skin thin or missing, asymmetrical, distended, umbilicus with hernia, discharge, redness, odor. Missing or overactive bowel sounds. Lower liver edge 3 cm below costal margin (heart disease), infection, hemolysis, palpable spleen (infection or hemopoiesis), enlarged bladder (1–4 cm above symphysis pubis).

H. Female.
   1. Masses in labia (hernia, enlarged Bartholin gland, vesicles).

I. Male.
   1. Meatal opening on penis placed abnormally (hypospadias or epispadius), absence of testes in either inguinal canals or scrotal sac, hydrocele, bifid scrotum, discoloration, or bruising.

J. Anus absent or not patent.

K. Absent or missing extremities, bands, masses, imperforate anus, dimples or asymmetry of the buttocks, abnormal Ortolani or Barlow sign, bowing of extremities, abnormal foot positions, flaccid upper extremity, lesions or dimpling of lower spine.

L. Abnormal posturing, floppy or very jittery, abnormal cry. Exaggerated tonic neck, Moro reflex, poor sucking, or poor rooting.

V. LABORATORY ASSESSMENT OF NEWBORN

A. Glucose screening (normal 40–90 mg/dL), venous hematocrit (normal 45–65%), cord blood (ABO, Rh). If baby is Rh–, maternal RhoGAM status should be Rh+.

B. Bilirubin: Determine etiology of any jaundice, i.e., physiologic or pathologic. Obtain baseline total serum bilirubin, plus a direct and indirect level.
   1. In the first week of life, 60% of all term newborns and 80% of preterm infants will have some jaundice.
   2. Any jaundice within the first 24 hours after birth is considered pathologic. If the total serum bilirubin (TSB) rises more than 5 mg/dL/day or is higher than 12 mg/dL in full-term infants or 10–14 mg/dL for preterm, further evaluation and treatment is indicated. If the infant has signs of

sepsis, irritability, or lethargy, this needs further evaluation. In infants 25–48 hours old, a TSB level above 15 mg/dL is indicative of rapid rise, and infant needs further evaluation. Infants 49–72 hours old with a TSB above 18 mg/dL or any infants more than 72 hours old with a TcB of 20 mg/dL need further evaluation and treatment.

    3. When obtaining serial bilirubins, utilize noninvasive transcutaneous (TcB) bilirubinometer and nomogram.

  C. Newborn hearing screening. To be done no later than 1 month of age. Most hospitals offer this screening for newborns prior to discharge. Risk factors for infants include family history of sensorineural hearing loss, in utero infections (TORCH), craniofacial anomalies, hyperbilirubinemia, postnatal bacterial meningitis, findings indicative of a syndrome with hearing loss, neurodegenerative disorders, sensorimotor neuropathies, parental concerns for hearing, head trauma, and recurrent/persistent otitis media. If infant fails the hearing screening, an audiologic evaluation needs to be done as follow-up by 3 months of age.

VI. MEETING WITH THE PARENT

  A. Introduce self, sit by bedside. Describe your role. Answer parents' questions, describe the general process of how you will be working with them over the next day or so.

  B. Praise parents, compliment baby.

  C. Call baby by name.

  D. Determine mother's health/wellness/contact with infant so far.

  E. Review your findings, briefly.

  F. If male, determine if baby is to be circumcised. Discuss pros and cons.

  G. Ask about method of feeding, car seat, help when home, concerns.

VII. NUTRITION

  A. Breastfeeding is encouraged for all newborns (see Chapter 5). Late preterm infants may not be as vigorous an eater as expected and may need close monitoring of weight. Obtain a breastfeeding consult and encourage nursing every 2 hours around the clock until infant is nursing at least 20 minutes during feedings.

    1. No breastfeeding if HIV infected, active herpes of breast, untreated tuberculosis, maternal debilitating disease (cancer), illicit drug use by mother, infant galactosemia.

B. If bottle-feeding, reassure that baby will grow and thrive on formula.
1. Only commercially prepared, iron-fortified formulas should be used: Powder, concentrate, ready-to-feed. Do not dilute ready-to-feed; do not reuse if > 4 hours since opened.
2. Mix formulas with bottled water for first month, continue if on well or unsure of water quality. Store in refrigerator if open no longer than 24 hours.
3. Specialized formulas have similar preparation directions. Goat's milk, whole cow's milk, rice milk have inadequate amounts of vitamins and minerals.
4. Serve formula at room temperature. Do not microwave to heat. Do not let formula sit out at room temperature to warm for more than 15–20 minutes.
C. Clean technique is sufficient for mixing formulas. Clean off cans with soap and water before opening. Use hot soapy water and bottlebrush to clean nipples and bottles or clean in dishwasher.
D. Hold during feedings; burp every 1–2 oz.
E. Hold in upright, semireclined position for feedings. No bottle propping.
F. Newborn will suckle 0.5–1 oz of formula/feeding every 2–3 hours for first 24 hours (60–100 mL/kg/day). Volume increases to 12–24 oz/day and interval between feedings > 3–4 hours in first month. May be days when baby takes more or less, depending on sleep pattern. Baby should take in 90% of feeding in first 20 minutes.

VIII. ELIMINATION

A. Meconium stools in first 48 hours, transition stools green-brown, change to yellow pasty after 2–3 days of oral feeding.
B. Infant should have 1–6 yellow pasty stools for 24 hours.
C. Breastfed baby may have upper range of frequency, bottle-fed may have less.
D. Void every 1–3 hours or with each feeding and diaper change.

IX. SLEEP

A. Awake for feedings; feed every 2–4 hours. Should be alert, nurse vigorously for 15–20 minutes, then fall back to sleep. Respirations may be slightly irregular.
B. Babies should sleep on back in their crib. No pillows/toys in the crib that baby could get face against and be smothered.
C. Babies should sleep in own cribs, not with parents, to minimize potential for rollovers, suffocation, and falls.

X. GROWTH AND DEVELOPMENT

A. Newborn can lose up to 10% of body weight in first 10 days of life. Should regain birth weight by 2 weeks of age.
B. Infant grows 1 in., on average, per month for first 6 months.
C. Head circumference increases 9 cm in first year.
D. Has minimal head control.
E. Looks at person during feeding.
F. Tracks 45°.

XI. SOCIAL DEVELOPMENT

A. Babies have different cries, will fuss/cry 1 to 2 hours/day.
    1. Similar time/pattern daily.
    2. Provide for infant's needs and crying should cease.
    3. Cry gradually decreases by 3 months of age.
B. Refer all high-risk infants/mothers to social worker before release. High-risk situations include:
    1. Adolescent pregnancy.
    2. No prenatal care.
    3. Consideration about giving up the baby for adoption.
    4. Unwanted pregnancy.
    5. Insufficient support from those at home.
    6. Physical limitations of parent.
    7. Inadequate housing/finances.
    8. Domestic violence.
    9. Positive toxicology.
    10. Incarcerated parent.
    11. Emotional disorders.
    12. Parent with mental retardation.
    13. Multiple small children in home.

XII. IMMUNIZATIONS

A. Only monovalent hepatitis B can be used for birth dose. If mother is hepatitis B surface antigen (HBsAg)–positive, administer hepatitis B vaccine and 0.5 mL of hepatitis B immune globulin (HBIG) within 12 hours of birth. If mother's HBsAg status is unknown, administer hepatitis B vaccine within 12 hours of birth and determine mother's HBsAg status as soon as possible. If she is then

positive, the newborn should receive HBIG within 1 week of life. Monovalent hepatitis B should be given if second dose is given less than 6 weeks of age. Monovalent or combination vaccine can be used to complete series.
   B. See Appendix A.

XIII. SAFETY/ANTICIPATORY GUIDANCE

   A. Sleep position "back to sleep."
   B. Not safe for baby to sleep in adult bed; must discuss with parents.
   C. Use federal motor vehicle safety standards (FMVSS)–tested and –approved car seat; install properly in backseat, facing backward in automobile. Contact local hospital, fire department, or March of Dimes chapter for car seat rental program. Infants should ride in the rear-facing position in either an infant seat or a convertible car seat until they are at least 2 years of age or they reach highest weight and height mandated by car seat manufacturer.
   D. No smoking around infant.
   E. One-piece pacifiers only.
   F. No corn syrup (Karo) for constipation, but may give 1 oz of sterile water/24 hours.
   G. No solids, only breastmilk or formula fed to infant.
   H. When to call healthcare provider:
      1. Breathing difficulties: Too fast or too slow or color changes; seizures; irritability; poor feeding; vomiting; no urine in 12 hours; black or decreased bowel movements; reddened, draining umbilical site; jaundice; rash or pustules not present on discharge; concerns.
   I. Give office phone number, explain how to use system.

XIV. DISCHARGE TO HOME

   A. Review all records/progress.
   B. Repeat complete physical examination.
   C. Identify abnormal findings that require ongoing monitoring.
   D. Review hearing screening results and if not done, schedule before discharge.
   E. Collect newborn blood screen.
   F. Administer hepatitis B immunization.
   G. Complete all consults.
   H. Staff nurses will have covered discharge instructions of bathing, cord care, bulb syringe, diapering, dressing, fingernail care, holding, feeding.
   I. If concerns, infants should be scheduled for office visit within 2 days, otherwise parents need a 2-week follow-up appointment assigned before discharge. Make them comfortable knowing they can call with any concerns.

BIBLIOGRAPHY

Ballard JL, Khoury JC, Wedig K, Eilers-Walsman BL, Lipp R. New Ballard Score expanded to include extremely premature infants. *J Pediatr.* 1991;119(3):417-423.

Centers for Disease Control and Prevention. Recommended immunization schedules for persons aged 0 through 18 years–United States, 2015. http://www.cdc.gov/vaccines/schedules/downloads/child/0-18yrs -child-combined-schedule.pdf. Accessed June 15, 2015.

Delaney AM. Newborn hearing screening. Medscape Reference. http://emedicine.medscape.com/ article/836646. Updated September 11, 2014. Accessed June 15, 2015.

Fouzas S, Mantagou L, Skylogianni E, Mantagos S, Varvarigou A. Transcutaneous bilirubin levels for the first 120 postnatal hours in healthy neonates. *Pediatrics.* 2010;125(1):e52-e57.

Hagan JF, Shaw JS, Duncan P, eds. *Bright Futures: Guidelines for Health Supervision of Infants, Children, and Adolescents.* 3rd ed. Elk Grove Village, IL: American Academy of Pediatrics; 2008.

HealthyChildren.org. Car safety seats: information for families for 2015. https://www.healthychildren.org /English/safety-prevention/on-the-go/Pages/Car-Safety-Seats-Information-for-Families.aspx. Accessed June 15, 2015.

Porter ML, Dennis BL. Hyperbilirubinemia in the term newborn. *Am Fam Physician.* 2002;65(4):599-607.

Thureen PJ, Hall D, Deacon J, Hernandez J. Obstetric considerations in the management of the well newborn. In: Thureen PJ, Hall D, Deacon J, Hernandez J, eds. *Assessment and Care of the Well Newborn.* 2nd ed. Philadelphia, PA: W.B. Saunders; 2005:3-20.

Wolf A, Hubbard E, Stellwagen LM. The late preterm infant: A little baby with big needs. *Contemp Pediatr.* 2007;24(11):51-59.

Guidelines for Breastfeeding

Amy L. Feldman

Abnormal weight gain, R63.5	Methicillin susceptible *Staphylococcus aureus*
Candidiasis, unspecified, B37.9	infection as the cause of diseases classified
Galactosemia, E74.21	elsewhere, B95.61
Induration of breast, N64.51	Neonatal candidiasis, P37.5
Jaundice, unspecified R17	Neonatal jaundice, unspecified, P59.9

I. INTRODUCTION

A. Breastfeeding provides optimal nutrition for newborns and infants, protecting against many diseases and infections and improving maternal and infant health. Exclusive breastfeeding is recommended by numerous public health, professional, and governmental organizations for the first 6 months of life, with continued breastfeeding throughout the first year and beyond with the addition of appropriate complementary foods. If there is a contraindication to breastfeeding or for preterm infants, using pasteurized donor human milk with fortification as needed is recommended by the AAP.

II. PHYSIOLOGY OF LACTATION

A. Mammary glands are complex organs that function independently in response to an intricate combination of hormones and stimulation to produce milk. After expulsion of the placenta following delivery, a significant drop in progesterone readies the body for milk production (**Figure 5-1**).

B. Oxytocin and prolactin are two of many important hormones in controlling lactation.

Figure 5-1 Physiology of lactation.

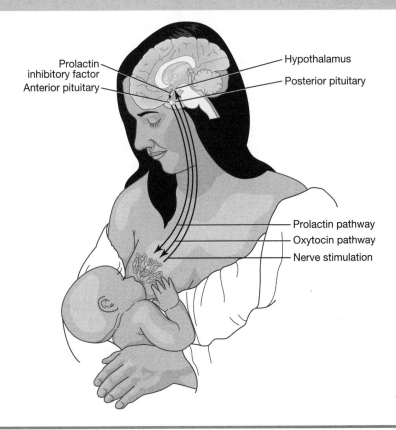

C. Optimal milk production depends on several factors, including release of lactation hormones, frequent and effective milk removal, and adequate breast stimulation.

D. Full lactation can be produced by breasts from 16 weeks of pregnancy.

E. Important to understand balance of supply and demand to optimize successful lactation.

F. Lactation begins as a result of hormonal control (endocrine) but changes to autocrine (frequent emptying of breasts) over time.

III. HUMAN MILK

A. Human milk is exceptional in its ability to sustain appropriate growth and development for infants.

B. "Liquid gold," as human milk is often referred to, is living tissue, which encompasses fats, proteins, carbohydrates, antibodies, and hundreds of components.

C. Composition of human milk changes to provide optimal nutrition as infant grows.

1. Colostrum, the first milk, is produced during pregnancy and is considered the infant's first immunization; is rich in antibodies and provides protection to the newborn from many viruses and bacteria. The volume is small in the first three days. Colostrum has fewer calories than mature milk but is rich in immunoglobulins, especially sIgA. The protein in colostrum helps to stabilize blood glucose levels in baby.

2. Transitional milk is produced after colostrum and has less total protein and immunoglobulins; however, it has an increase in fat, lactose, and calories.

3. Mature milk is produced as lactogenesis stage II begins. By day 5, a mother produces approximately 500 ml/day.

IV. CONTRAINDICATIONS FOR BREASTFEEDING

A. Occasionally there are circumstances that preclude mothers from breastfeeding.

1. Maternal contraindications include:
   a. HIV-positive mother (in the United States).
   b. Maternal drug abuse.
   c. Maternal chemotherapy.
   d. Herpetic lesions on mother's nipple, areola. Expressed milk can be used from the unaffected side. Do not allow infant to come into direct contact with HSV lesions. Encourage excellent handwashing technique by mother.
   e. Untreated, active tuberculosis. Expressed breastmilk can be used.
   f. Varicella in mother developed 5 days prior to delivery to 2 days after delivery requires mother and baby to be separated, but expressed breastmilk can be used.
   g. Certain radioactive compounds and few medications may require temporary cessation of breastfeeding. It is unusual for the amount of medication transferred into breastmilk to cause a problem in the infant. Drugs that are problematic for breastfeeding can frequently be substituted with drugs that are compatible with breastfeeding.
   h. Positive HTLV-I and HTLV-II (human T-cell lymphotropic virus).

2. Infant contraindications include:
   a. Classic galactosemia.

V. MATERNAL ASSESSMENT

A. Assess both mother and baby for all factors that may affect the ability to successfully initiate and maintain breastfeeding.
   1. Breastfeeding goals and family support.
   2. Previous breastfeeding experience.
   3. General health and nutritional status.
   4. History of breast, nipple, or thoracic surgery.
   5. Medications, prescriptions, supplements, and OTC.
   6. Pregnancy, labor, birth history.
   7. Inverted or flat nipples.
   8. Breast assessment.

VI. INFANT ASSESSMENT

A. General health, including gestational age.
B. Congenital anomalies.
C. Birth history.
D. Medications received and procedures experienced.
E. Initial feeding attempts, and frequency of feedings and ability to latch at breast.
F. Has infant roomed in with the mother 24/7 to successfully breastfeed in response to hunger cues?
G. Oral facial assessment.

VII. BREASTFEEDING IN THE EARLY DAYS

A. Initial feedings.
   1. Facilitate skin-to-skin contact immediately after birth and as often as possible.
   2. Encourage breastfeeding within first hour after birth during quiet alert phase. Do not restrict length or frequency of feedings.
   3. Promote rooming in 24 hours a day.
   4. Encourage exclusive breastfeeding; this helps to establish and maintain a sufficient milk supply.
   5. Instruct parents and support persons in correct latch-on techniques.

6. Educate parents and support persons regarding initial feedings of colostrum: Quantity is very small, but sufficient nutrition as baby is learning to breastfeed.
7. Discourage use of any supplements unless medically indicated.
8. Avoid use of bottles and pacifiers until breastfeeding is well established.
9. Teach parents and support persons how to breastfeed in response to infant feeding cues (rooting, increased alertness, fists in mouth), at least 8–12 times/day. Crying is a late sign of hunger.
10. Baby should finish feeding on one breast, then be offered second if he/she will take more. Fat content of milk is higher at end of feeding than at beginning. Forcing baby to switch breasts too soon may decrease amount of higher calorie milk consumed.
11. Babies who sleep for long periods of time without eating or feed only for few minutes should be awakened and encouraged to nurse (i.e., unwrap, rub feet).

B. Positioning and latch.
1. Mother and infant should be comfortable with infant on his/her side at nipple height supported by pillows or blankets.
2. Support infant's head so he/she can easily reach areola without turning neck.
3. Infant's ear, shoulder, hips should be in alignment.
4. Mother can align her nipple with infant's nose, quickly bringing infant to breast only when his mouth opens widely, getting more of the areola on the bottom than top into his mouth, creating an asymmetrical latch (see **Figure 5-2**).
5. Infant's lips should be flanged outward with chin touching breast. When latched properly, the tongue is drawn back to the junction of the hard and soft palate (see **Figure 5-3**).
6. Infant's tongue will protrude over gum ridge and "cup" breast.
7. If baby latches incorrectly, the mother should insert her clean finger to break the suction, and repeat latch-on attempts until baby is latched correctly. Mother's nails should be short to avoid injuring the baby's mouth.
8. Common breastfeeding positions are cradle position (see **Figure 5-4**), cross cradle and football holds (see **Figure 5-5**), and side-lying position (see **Figure 5-6**).
9. Trained practitioners should observe latch-on, milk transfer, and feeding at least once every 8 hours throughout postpartum hospitalization. Observations should be documented in the medical record.
10. The mother's nipple should not be pinched, bruised, or creased at the end of a feeding or show any signs of damage (see **Figure 5-7**).

Figure 5-2 Positioning the baby nipple to nose.

Source: Printed with permission of Catherine Watson Genna, BS, IBCLC.

Figure 5-3 Sucking action (breast and bottle).

Source: Reproduced from Lauwers J, Swisher A. *Counseling the Nursing Mother: A Lactation Consultant's Guide*. 6th ed. Burlington, MA: Jones & Bartlett Learning; 2016. Courtesy of Rebecca Glover, RN, RM, IBCLC.

Figure 5-4 Madonna (cradle) position: A) front view, B) side view.

A

B

Figure 5-5 A) Cross-cradle hold, B) football hold.

A

B

Figure 5-6 Side-lying position.

C. Signs of milk transfer in infant.
   1. Observe sustained, rhythmic suck/swallow pattern with intermittent pauses.
   2. Listen for audible swallowing.
   3. Baby's arms and hands should be relaxed at the end of the feeding.
   4. Baby's oral mucous membranes should be moist after feedings.
   5. Baby should appear satisfied after feedings.
D. Signs of milk transfer in mother.
   1. Mother feels strong tugging sensation when baby is sucking, which is not painful.
   2. Mother feels uterine contractions and increased lochia flow during initial days postpartum.
   3. Milk may leak from opposite breast during feedings.
   4. Mother may feel relaxed or drowsy during feedings.
   5. Breast softens after feeding (after milk supply is established).
   6. Nipples are elongated but not pinched or bruised after release of latch.
E. Assessing infant weight gain.
   1. Parents should be aware of baby's birth and discharge weight.

Figure 5-7 Normal nipple postfeed and creased nipple postfeed.

Source: Courtesy of Linda Smith, BSE, FACCE, IBCLC.

2. Encourage parents to keep a daily journal of first week to track feedings, output.

3. Healthy, breastfeeding infants may lose 3–7% of birth weight in initial days.

4. After mother's milk is in, infant should gain 0.5–1 oz/day (4–7 oz/week).

5. Babies often regain birth weight by 10 days of age, double birth weight by 6 months, triple it by 1 year.

6. Exclusively breastfed infants tend to be leaner than bottle-fed infants in second 6 months of life.

F. Assessing infant output.

1. Colostrum acts as laxative, encouraging expulsion of meconium in first days.

2. Effective and regular breastfeeding helps to prevent jaundice in early days.

3. Infants showing signs of jaundice should be assessed carefully for ineffective breastfeeding.

4. Babies who are breastfeeding well should have 3 or more stools/day by day 3.

5. Bowel movements become lighter in color, then turn to a mustard color and are seedy in consistency by day 4 or 5.

6. Inadequate stools are a red flag for ineffective breastfeeding.

7. Stool output may decrease to one stool every few days after first few weeks.

8. Urine output is less helpful than stool output in assessing adequate milk intake.

9. Exclusively breastfed baby should produce 1 wet diaper on day 1, 2 on day 2, 3 on day 3, and so on, for first week.

10. By end of first week, baby should have 6 soaking wet, pale yellow diapers/day.

VIII. SEPARATION OF MOTHER AND INFANT

A. Pumping.

1. All mothers should be taught how to hand express their milk after birth.

2. If a small number of feedings must be missed, the mother can hand express or, if she prefers, use a battery-operated pump to express milk from both breasts every few hours.

3. Lengthy separation warrants use of hospital-grade, piston-style pump with double hookup system to establish, maintain, or increase her milk supply. Mothers should be instructed to pump at least 8 times/24 hours for approximately 15 minutes each session.

4. Pumping should begin within 6 hours of birth if the infant is not able to go to breast or if there is a contraindication to breastfeeding. Hand expression is often preferred during the first 24 hours when the quantity of colostrum is small.

5. Even the smallest quantity of expressed colostrum or milk can be fed to infant via eyedropper, syringe, or cup.

B. Milk collection and storage.

1. Recommendations for collection and storage of mother's milk for hospitalized infant differ from those of the following instructions for the well child at home.

2. Mothers should wash hands thoroughly prior to pumping and keep nails short.

3. Follow manufacturer's instructions for cleaning of pump parts.

4. Glass containers or BPA-free hard plastic containers with well-fitting lids are a good choice for storing milk.

5. Mother can encourage milk let down by looking at picture of baby, smelling piece of baby's clothing.

6. Warm, wet washcloths on breast combined with breast massage may be helpful in starting milk flow.

7. Breastfeeding on one breast while pumping from other breast is an option.

8. All pumps are different. Encourage mother to find one that creates comfortable seal that provides appropriate suction. Pumping should not be painful.

9. For specific information on storing milk for home use for full-term infants, see the Academy of Breastfeeding Medicine Revised Protocol #8 March 2010.

IX. SUPPORTING BREASTFEEDING PAST THE EARLY DAYS

A. Follow-up.

1. Breastfeeding infants should be seen by an appropriate healthcare professional within 48–72 hours after discharge and again at 2 weeks of age for successful feeding and appropriate weight gain assessment. Infants should always be evaluated in between scheduled visits for any concerns.

2. Breastfeeding mothers should be referred to a breastfeeding support group and local breastfeeding resources following hospital discharge.

B. Maternal diet.

1. Encourage mother to eat a wide variety of healthy foods, eating when hungry and drinking to quench her thirst. Breastfeeding mothers should consume an additional 450–500 calories/day.

   a. Forcing large quantities of fluids will not increase milk production.

   b. No specific foods must be avoided by all breastfeeding mothers.

    c. Most foods do not bother most babies.

    d. If a particular food seems to bother baby, decrease/eliminate for a week to 10 days.

    e. Many healthcare providers recommend continuing prenatal vitamins during breastfeeding.

2. It is recommended that all breastfed babies be supplemented with vitamin D 400 IU starting soon after birth. All infants, children, and adolescents should be receiving 400 IU/day of vitamin D.

3. Families with significant allergies should receive knowledgeable dietary counseling regarding possible need to eliminate certain foods while breastfeeding.

C. Growth spurts.

1. Regardless of culture, women frequently worry about ability to provide enough milk for their baby.

2. Teach parents that growth spurts (periods when babies want to nurse more frequently to meet rapid growth) usually occur around 2–3 weeks, 6 weeks, 3 months.

3. Feed as often as baby wants to nurse to increase, then maintain, adequate milk supply.

4. Reinforce concept of supply and demand.

5. Supplementing with formula is strongly discouraged; mother's milk supply will not increase without adequate stimulation to meet baby's growing demand for more milk.

    a. Breastfed infants have a more acidic intestinal environment than formula-fed babies early in life, which is beneficial. Bifidobacterium is the predominant intestinal bacteria in breastfed infants that has significant health benefits on the infant's immune and digestive systems. Supplementing an infant in the early days with even small amounts of formula changes the gut environment.

D. Medications and breastfeeding.

1. It is imperative that healthcare providers give information to mothers who breastfeed on the safety of medications based on appropriate, current research, citing the source. Each infant's individual situation must be assessed prior to determining the appropriate use of any medication during breastfeeding. An excellent reference guide such as Hale (2014) should be available in every clinical setting that deals with breastfeeding mothers. LactMed, published by the National Library of Medicine/National Institutes of Health, is available online as a comprehensive

source of information on medications and their risks when used by breastfeeding mothers.

2. Many of the medications likely to be prescribed to breastfeeding mothers should not affect maternal milk supply or infant's safety. Ibuprofen is a commonly used analgesic postpartum and is considered compatible with breastfeeding. Penicillins and cephalosporins, along with several of the selective serotonin reuptake inhibitors (SSRIs) often used for depression, are also generally considered compatible.

3. Dose of medication transferred through breastmilk is almost always too low to be clinically significant or is poorly bioavailable to infant.

4. It is preferable for mothers to avoid using medication whenever possible.

5. Extensive benefits of breastfeeding far outweigh any potential risks in majority of cases.

   a. Medications should be safe for infants to consume.

   b. Choose drugs with breastfeeding information whenever possible.

   c. Choose shortest acting form of medication.

   d. Encourage feeding when maternal drug level is lowest.

   e. Educate parents as to potential side effects to observe in infant, and effect on milk supply.

   f. Be extra cautious with preterm, low-birth-weight, or sick infants.

   g. Certain herbal substances may be harmful to infants.

   h. Drugs of abuse are contraindicated in breastfeeding.

   i. Temporary cessation of breastfeeding is necessary with certain radioactive compounds. Consult appropriate resources for detailed information.

E. Maternal employment.

1. Returning to the workplace while continuing to provide breastmilk for baby may initially seem overwhelming to some mothers. Strong encouragement, praise, and continuous support can make the difference between a mother being successful and giving up.

2. Women need a private, clean place to pump every few hours while separated from their infant. Encourage mothers to rent or purchase a pump that is comfortable and that is efficient for their particular needs.

3. The Patient Protection and Affordable Care Act, signed into law on March 23, 2010, requires employers with greater than 50 employees to provide break times for nursing mothers. Lactation supplies and counseling are also covered by private insurance companies but not Medicaid. Encourage patients to check with their individual policy for their specific benefits.

4. Expressed milk can be kept at room temperature (77°F) for 6–8 hours, in a cooler with an ice pack (39°F) for 24 hours, in a refrigerator (40°F) for 5 days, in the freezer compartment of the refrigerator (5°F) for 2 weeks, and in a deep freezer (–4°F) for 6–12 months.

5. Provide information on how to introduce a bottle to the infant, as well as suggestions for the caregiver that will promote extended breastfeeding (i.e., not bottle feeding immediately before mother will pick up infant, proper handling and storage of breastmilk).

X. COMMON PROBLEMS

A. Mothers can complain about pain even when damage is not visible on the breast or nipple. Determine that baby is positioned properly at breast height with adequate support and is latching on correctly. Mothers often describe the feeling of their baby feeding as a strong tugging sensation. Breastfeeding should not be painful. Nipples do not "toughen up" as breastfeeding proceeds. Assess for other causes of sore nipples such as trauma, improper latch and release, thrush, milk plugs on nipple, incorrect use of breastfeeding devices, or a tight frenulum in the infant (see **Figure 5-8**). Paget's disease, an uncommon

Figure 5-8 Tight frenulum.

type of breast cancer, must also be ruled out. Breastfeeding issues that do not resolve quickly should promptly be referred to pediatric or maternal experts for further management.

B. Sore nipple management includes:
1. Assess for correct positioning and latch-on.
2. Teach mothers how to express colostrum/hindmilk to apply to nipples after each feeding.
3. Allow nipples to dry before putting bra back on.
4. Offer use of breast shells to prevent clothing from rubbing against sore nipples. Instruct in proper cleaning of shells.
5. Breastfeed from least sore side first.
6. Change positions at each feeding to decrease pressure on sore area.
7. Suggest moist wound healing methods (i.e., modified lanolin or hydrogel dressings).
8. Analgesics as needed.

C. Flat or inverted nipples.
1. Can initially make breastfeeding more of a challenge. May be difficult for baby to latch on and breastfeed well. Provide adequate support to ensure successful feedings.
2. "Pinch test": Determines if nipple is flat or inverted upon compression. With thumb behind nipple and first two fingers underneath, grasp about 1 in. back from base of nipple and compress skin.
   a. Normal nipple will evert.
   b. Flat nipple remains flat with compression.
   c. Inverted nipple looks sunken in.
   d. Nipples can look flat or inverted, but evert on compression.
3. Flat or inverted management includes:
   a. Encouraging deepest possible latch onto breast.
   b. Make sure infant is at breast height and well supported to prevent sliding to base of nipple.
   c. Release latch and repeat attempts until proper latch is obtained. Allowing baby to suck at base of nipple prevents stimulating milk supply and will cause sore nipples.
   d. Encourage offering flat/inverted breast first when baby is hungriest and sucking is strongest.
   e. Teach mother to evert nipple with gentle pulling/rolling immediately prior to latch.
   f. Hand express a few drops of colostrum to entice baby to latch on.
   g. Use hand/electric pump for a few minutes immediately prior to latch.

   h. If supplement is medically indicated, use expressed milk first using an eyedropper, syringe, cup, or feeding tube at the breast.

   i. Avoid pacifiers and bottle nipples until breastfeeding is well established.

 D. Severe engorgement.

  1. Milk stasis caused by inefficient, infrequent removal of milk results in extremely full, swollen, lumpy, painful breasts.

  2. Result is different from transient breast fullness associated with milk "coming in" 2–4 days after birth.

  3. Breastfeeding emergency: Milk stasis can cause damage to tissue, decrease milk supply, and make it difficult to impossible for infant to compress areola and remove milk.

  4. Severe engorgement management includes:

   a. Analgesics as necessary.

   b. Warm, wet compresses to breast prior to feedings to help increase milk flow.

   c. Reverse pressure softening; soften areola using hand expression so baby can latch properly.

   d. Use breast compression during feedings to improve milk flow. Using thumb on top of breast and fingers underneath, the mother brings her fingers together, which compresses breast.

   e. Use of cold compresses may help to decrease engorgement after feeding. Some mothers like to use this prior to feeding as well.

   f. Use of clean, chilled green cabbage leaves left on breast for a short period several times/day can be helpful to some mothers. Stop using this as soon as engorgement decreases.

   g. Express milk after feeding as needed for comfort. Any expressed milk can be fed to baby using alternative feeding methods.

 E. Mastitis.

  1. Infection of breast, usually caused by *Staphylococcus aureus*.

  2. Frequently occurs in upper outer quadrant of breast, often by 2–3 weeks postpartum.

  3. Symptoms commonly include hard, swollen, reddened area on breast accompanied by flulike symptoms.

  4. Difficult to differentiate between engorgement, plugged duct, mastitis (**Table 5-1**).

  5. Mastitis management includes:

   a. Rest (decrease stress and fatigue by enlisting support from friends, family).

Table 5-1 Comparison of Findings of Engorgement, Plugged Duct, and Mastitis

Characteristics	Engorgement	Plugged Duct	Mastitis
Onset	Gradual, immediately postpartum	Gradual, after feedings	Sudden, after 10 days
Site	Bilateral	Unilateral	Unusually unilateral
Swelling and heat	Generalized	May shift; a little or no heat	Localized, red, hot, and swollen
Pain	Generalized	Mild but localized	Intense but localized
Body temperature	$< 38.4°C$	$< 38.4°C$	$> 38.4°C$ (101°F)
Systemic symptoms	Feels well	Feels well	Flulike symptoms

Source: Lawrence RA, Lawrence RM. *Breastfeeding: A Guide for the Medical Profession.* 7th ed. St Louis, MO: Mosby; 2011, with permission from Elsevier.

    b. Antibiotics; encourage completing full course as prescribed.

    c. Increase maternal fluid intake.

    d. Frequent, effective emptying of breasts (important to continue breastfeeding, milk is not infected, fine for baby).

    e. Abrupt weaning can predispose to an abscess.

    f. Analgesics as needed.

    g. Correct latch to prevent further nipple trauma (cracked, bleeding nipples allow bacteria to enter milk ducts).

    h. Mother's preference of warm or cool packs for comfort.

F. Jaundice.

    1. Rarely requires cessation of breastfeeding.

    2. Pathologic jaundice, with onset in first 24 hours of life, warrants medical evaluation in addition to lactation support.

    3. Encourage early initiation of breastfeeding, then frequent, effective, unrestricted feedings to minimize jaundice.

    4. Colostrum acts as laxative, eliminating bilirubin through meconium expulsion.

    5. Physiologic jaundice, which begins 48–72 hours after birth and peaks on day 3–5, is seen in thriving infants with normal weight gain and output.

6. Observe for effective breastfeeding and continue assessment for normal weight gain and output. Onset and peak of breastfeeding associated with jaundice is similar to physiologic jaundice, but infant is fussy/sleepy with poor feeding and inadequate weight gain, output.
7. Assist with frequent, unrestricted, effective breastfeeding.
8. Teach parents to watch for signs of milk transfer during feedings. If necessary, express milk in addition to feedings, use alternate feeding methods to give baby milk.

G. Thrush.
1. Often described as burning, itching, stinging lasting throughout feeding and beyond, radiating from nipple and breast to shoulder and back.
2. Nipple or areolar skin is often red and shiny.
3. May have period of pain-free nursing, then have sudden onset of pain.
4. Pain from poor latch is often described as feeling like a knife or being stabbed, dissipates as feeding progresses, frequently limited to nipple and areola.
5. Regardless of nipple pain, poor latch must be corrected immediately.
6. Broken skin is perfect environment for organisms to invade.
7. Signs in infant may range from nothing to white patches on buccal mucosa, tongue, and palate, which may bleed when scraped with tongue blade. Fiery red diaper rash with shiny red patches and pustules may also be present.
8. Both mother and baby should be treated simultaneously with appropriate antifungal medications to prevent reinfection from one to the other.
9. All objects (pumping supplies, pacifiers, bottles) coming in contact with baby's mouth should be boiled daily.
10. Mothers should be encouraged to continue breastfeeding while treating infection.
11. *Candida albicans* thrives in warm, moist, dark areas. Nipples can be rinsed with clear water or vinegar solution of 1 tablespoon vinegar in 1 cup of water after each feeding, exposing to air after each feeding.
12. Bed linens, sheets, bras can be rinsed in vinegar solution after hot wash cycle. Breast pads should be disposable and changed as soon as wet.
13. Sexual contact between mother and partner can spread infection. Partner should be treated appropriately.

H. Weight-gain concerns.
1. Breastfed infants gaining less than appropriate amount for age should be carefully evaluated. Often, correcting latch and positioning is enough to facilitate efficient breastfeeding and improve weight gain.

2. Do not recommend formula supplementation without evaluating breast-feeding. If extra calories are needed, have mother hand express or pump in addition to breastfeeding and use alternative feeding methods to give baby breastmilk.
3. Allowing baby to finish feeding on one breast before feeding on second allows sufficient amounts of higher calorie breastmilk.
4. Review with parents appropriate signs of infant hunger, encourage frequent (8–12 or more/24 hours) unrestricted feedings.
5. Keeping written log of feedings and output is also helpful. Imperative that infant have adequate caloric intake.
6. If after evaluation and management with skilled breastfeeding consultant breastfeeding is not going well, formula supplementation may be appropriate. Plan for maintaining/increasing mother's milk supply must be implemented.
7. Return office visit within 24–48 hours to monitor situation should be scheduled. Frequent phone follow-up, support are necessary.
8. Global growth charts released by the World Health Organization (WHO) in 2006 reflect standards on how children should grow based on breastfeeding as the norm.

XI. HELPFUL BREASTFEEDING RESOURCES

A. Locating a board-certified lactation consultant:
International Lactation Consultant Association, 1-919-861-5577, www.ilca.org
International Board of Lactation Consultant Examiners, 1-703-560-7330, www.iblce.org
B. Internet resources:
Academy of Breastfeeding Medicine, www.bfmed.org
American Academy of Pediatrics Breastfeeding Initiatives Health Professionals Resource Guide, www2.aap.org/breastfeeding/healthprofessionais resourceguide.html
Baby-Friendly Hospital Initiative, USA, www.babyfriendlyusa.org
Breastfeeding Benefits under the Affordable Care Act, www.healthcare .gov/coverage/breast-feeding-benefits/
CDC Guide to Strategies to Support Breastfeeding Mothers and Babies, www.cdc.gov/breastfeeding/resources/guide.htm
Human Milk Banking Association of North America, www.hmbana.com
Infant Risk Center, 1-806-352-2519, www.infantrisk.org

LactMed, http://toxnet.nlm.nih.gov/newtoxnet/lactmed.htm

La Leche League International, www.lalecheleague.org

The Surgeon General's Call to Action to Support Breastfeeding, www .surgeongeneral.gov/library/calls/breastfeeding/calltoactiontosupport breastfeeding.pdf

United States Breastfeeding Committee's Core Competencies in Breastfeeding Care and Services for All Health Professionals, http://www.usbreastfeed ing.org/p/cm/ld/fid=170

U.S. Department of Labor. Wage and Hour Division (WHD). Fact sheet #73: Break Time for Nursing Mothers Under the FLSA, www.dol.gov/whd /regs/compliance/whdfs73.htm

WomensHealth.gov, womenshealth.gov/breastfeeding/

C. Book resources:

Cadwell K, Turner-Maffei C. *Breastfeeding A–Z: Terminology and Telephone Triage.* 2nd ed. Burlington, MA: Jones & Bartlett Learning; 2014.

Hale TW, Rowe HE. *Medications and Mother's Milk.* 16th ed. Amarillo, TX: Hale Publishing, L.P.; 2014.

Lauwers J, Swisher A. *Counseling the Nursing Mother: A Lactation Consultant's Guide.* 6th ed. Burlington, MA: Jones & Bartlett Learning; 2016.

Lawrence RA, Lawrence RM. *Breastfeeding: A Guide for the Medical Profession.* 7th ed. St. Louis, MO: Elsevier Mosby; 2011.

Newman J, Pitman T. *Dr. Jack Newman's Guide to Breastfeeding.* Revised edition. New York, NY: Harper Collins; 2014.

Walker M. *Breastfeeding Management for the Clinician: Using the Evidence.* 3rd ed. Burlington, MA: Jones & Bartlett Learning; 2014.

Wambach K, Riordan J. *Breastfeeding and Human Lactation.* 5th ed. Burlington, MA: Jones & Bartlett Learning; 2016.

Wilson-Clay B, Hoover K. *The Breastfeeding Atlas.* 5th ed. Manchaca, TX: LactNews Press; 2013.

BIBLIOGRAPHY

American Academy of Family Physicians Breastfeeding Advisory Committee. Breastfeeding, family physicians supporting (position paper). http://www.aafp.org/about/policies/all/breastfeeding-support.html. Accessed February 13, 2015.

Eglash A. ABM Clinical Protocol #8: human milk storage information for home use for full-term infants (Original Protocol March 2004 Revision #1 March 2010). *Breastfeed Med.* 2010;5(3):127-130. http:// www.bfmed.org/Media/Files/Protocols/Protocol%208%20-%20English%20revised%202010.pdf. Accessed February 13, 2015.

Eidelman AI, Schanler RJ. Breastfeeding and the use of human milk. *Pediatrics.* 2012;129(3):e827-e841.

Hale TW, Rowe HE. *Medications and Mother's Milk.* 16th ed. Amarillo, TX: Hale Publishing, L.P.; 2014.

International Lactation Consultant Association. *Clinical Guidelines for the Establishment of Exclusive Breastfeeding.* Morrisville, NC: International Lactation Consultant Association; 2014.

Lauwers J, Swisher A. *Counseling the Nursing Mother: A Lactation Consultant's Guide.* 6th ed. Burlington, MA: Jones & Bartlett Learning; 2016.

Lawrence RA, Lawrence RM. *Breastfeeding: A Guide for the Medical Profession.* 7th ed. St. Louis, MO: Elsevier Mosby; 2011.

Lu MC, Lange L, Slusser W, Hamilton J, Halfon N. Provider encouragement of breast-feeding: evidence from a national survey. *Obstet Gynecol.* 2001;97(2):290-295.

Marks JM, Spatz DL. Medications and lactation: what PNPs need to know. *J Pediatr Health Care.* 2003;17(6):311-319.

National Association of Pediatric Nurse Practitioners' Executive Board. NAPNAP position statement on breastfeeding. http://www.jpedhc.org/article/S0891-5245(12)00187-3/fulltext. Published 2013. Accessed May 15, 2015.

Newman J, Pitman T. *Dr. Jack Newman's Guide to Breastfeeding.* Revised edition. New York, NY: HarperCollins; 2014.

Sachs HC; Committee On Drugs. The transfer of drugs and therapeutics into human breast milk: an update on selected topics. *Pediatrics.* 2013;132(3):e796-809.

U.S. Department of Health and Human Services. *HHS Blueprint for Action on Breastfeeding.* Washington, DC: U.S. Department of Health and Human Services, Office on Women's Health; 2000.

U.S. Department of Labor Wage and Hour Division (WHD). Fact sheet #73: break time for nursing mothers under the FLSA. http://www.dol.gov/whd/regs/compliance/whdfs73.htm. Revised August 2013. Accessed February 13, 2015.

Wagner CL, Greer FR; American Academy of Pediatrics Section on Breastfeeding; American Academy of Pediatrics Committee on Nutrition. Prevention of rickets and vitamin D deficiency in infants, children, and adolescents. *Pediatrics.* 2008;122(5):1142-1152.

Walker M. Formula supplementation of the breastfed infant: assault on the gut microbiome. *Clinical Lactation.* 2014;5(4):128-132.

Wambach K, Riordan J. *Breastfeeding and Human Lactation.* 5th ed. Burlington, MA: Jones & Bartlett Learning; 2016.

World Health Organization. The launch of the WHO Child Growth Standards. http://www.who.int/childgrowth/launch/en/index.html. Accessed February 13, 2015.

Common Genetic Disorders

Tracy Magee

I. OROFACIAL CLEFTS

Cleft lip, Q36

Cleft palate, Q35

Cleft soft palate, Q35.3

A. Etiology.
   1. The causes of isolated orofacial clefts are unknown. However, more than 300 syndromes have clefts associated.
B. Occurrence.
   1. Cleft lip with or without cleft palate affects approximately 1 in 1000 births in the United States.
   2. Racial differences have been noted, with Asian decent having the highest incidence and African American decent having the lowest incidence.
   3. Risk factors include family history and some medications, including phenytoin, isotretinion, and diazepam.
C. Clinical manifestations.
   1. Infant: Feeding including a week suck and lengthy feeds.
   2. Childhood: May have articulation difficulties, dental issues and can have increase in ear infections
D. Physical findings.
   1. Cleft lip: Fissure of the upper lip usually along the frenulum that often includes the bones of the upper jaw and/or gum.
   2. Cleft palate: Fissure in either the hard palate and/or soft palate.
   3. Submucous cleft palate: The cleft of the muscles and/or bone for the palate is covered by a mucous membrane, making it difficult to see the presence of the cleft when looking in the mouth.

    4. Can occur unilaterally or bilaterally and is possible to have a cleft lip, a cleft palate, or both.

E. Diagnostic tests.

    1. Can be diagnosed during pregnancy by a routine ultrasound by 13–16 weeks' gestation.

    2. Most cleft lip and palate are found on clinical exam during the newborn period.

F. Differential diagnoses.

    1. Treacher Collins syndrome.

    2. Velocardiofacial syndrome.

    3. Pierre Robin sequence.

    4. Down syndrome.

G. Treatment.

    1. Phase 1: In the first hours of life, management is concerned with airway management and establishing safe feeding, which may include the use of specialized bottles or significant help from lactation consultant.

    2. Phase 2: Concerns evaluations by otolaryngology for possible middle ear involvement, audiology for hearing evaluation, and possibly orthodontia.

    3. Phase 3: Surgical repair; repair of the cleft lip is recommended the third of fourth month of life and surgical repair of a cleft palate is recommended within the first 18 months, usually within the first 12 months of life.

H. Follow-up.

    1. Based on extent and severity of the cleft.

    2. Continued throughout childhood and into adolescence and sometimes adulthood.

I. Complications.

    1. Related to the severity and extent of the cleft.

    2. May include feeding difficulties latching onto the breast or bottle nipple and sucking, ear infections and hearing loss, dental problems, speech problems, psychological problems.

J. Education.

    1. Related to the type and severity of the orofacial cleft as well as the complications involved.

    2. Special awareness of risk for ear infections, hearing loss.

    3. Visible clefts high risk for bullying.

    4. Families should be aware of the American Cleft Palate Craniofacial Association.

II. SPINA BIFIDA

Lumbar spina bifida without hydrocephalus, Q05.7

A. Etiology.
1. Unknown but low levels of folic acid are thought to play a role.
2. Four types of spina bifida: Occulta, closed neural tube defects, meningocele, and myelomeningocele.
3. Occulta: A layer of skin covers the malformation, present in 10–20% of the general population, rarely causes disability or symptoms.
4. Closed neural tube defects: Malformation of fat, bone, or meninges.
5. Meningocele: Spinal fluid and meninges protrude through an abnormal vertebral opening.
6. Myelomeningocele: Spinal cord/neural elements are exposed.
B. Occurrence.
1. 3.40 per 10,000 births.
2. Racial differences noted; Hispanic women (4.17 per 10,000) have the highest incidence compared with non-Hispanic white women, 3.22 per 10,000, and non-Hispanic black women, 2.64 per 10,000.
C. Clinical manifestations.
1. Infants.
a. Lethargy.
b. Poor feeding.
c. Irritability.
d. Stridor.
e. Ocular motor incoordination.
f. Development delay.
2. Older children may present with the following:
a. Cognitive or behavioral changes.
b. Decreased strength.
c. Increased spasticity.
d. Changes in bowel or bladder function.
e. Lower cranial nerve dysfunction.
f. Back pain.
g. Worsening spinal or lower extremity orthopedic deformities.
D. Physical findings.
1. Abnormal tuft or clump of hair.
2. Small dimple or birthmark on the skin at the site of the spinal malformation.
3. Visible fluid-filled sac protruding from the spinal canal.

E. Diagnostic tests.
 1. Prenatal diagnosis: Fetal ultrasound at 16–18 weeks' gestation.
 2. Postnatal diagnosis: Plain film X-ray, CT/MRI of the spine.
F. Differential diagnoses.
 1. Tethered spinal cord.
 2. Mass lesions of the cord.
 3. Diastematomyelia.
 4. Cord cavitation and narrowing.
 5. Adhesions.
 6. Dural bands.
 7. Uncontrolled hydrocephalus.
 8. Chiari II malformation.
G. Treatment.
 1. Depends on the type and severity of the disorder as well as complications.
 2. Children with the mildest form need no treatment.
 3. Some children will need subsequent surgeries to manage problems with the feet, hips, or spine.
 4. May require assistive device, such as crutches, leg braces, walkers, or wheelchair.
 5. Treatment for bladder and bowel problems typically begins soon after birth, and may include bladder catheterizations and bowel management regimens.
H. Follow-up.
 1. Every 6 months in a specialized multidisciplinary clinic throughout childhood and annually thereafter.
 2. Depending on medical and surgical issues, more frequent visits with certain specialists may be necessary.
I. Complications.
 1. Meningitis, in newborn period.
 2. Chiari II malformation.
 3. Hydrocephalus.
 4. Intellectual disabilities and learning disabilities.
 5. Latex allergies.
 6. Bowel and bladder issues.
 7. Depression during adolescence.
J. Education.
 1. Need for multidisciplinary team.
 2. High risk for latex allergy.
 3. Special education issues.
 4. Social-emotional issues in adolescence.

III. TURNER SYNDROME

Turner syndrome, unspecified, Q96.9

A. Etiology.
   1. One normal X chromosome is present, the other sex chromosome is missing or structurally altered (45 X).
B. Occurrence.
   1. 1 in 2500 newborn girls worldwide.
C. Clinical manifestations.
   1. Short stature, which becomes evident by about age 5.
   2. Ovarian hypofunction or premature ovarian failure.
   3. Developmental delays, nonverbal learning disabilities, and behavioral problems are possible.
D. Physical findings.
   1. Webbed neck.
   2. Low-set ears.
   3. A low hairline at the back of the neck.
   4. Lymphedema of the hands and feet.
   5. Skeletal abnormalities.
   6. Short stature.
   7. Kidney abnormalities.
   8. Coarctation of the aorta.
   9. Abnormalities of the aortic valve.
E. Diagnostic test.
   1. Conventional cytogenetic studies.
F. Differential diagnoses.
   1. Noonan syndrome.
G. Treatment.
   1. Based on associated conditions and complications.
H. Follow-up.
   1. Based on associated conditions and complications.
I. Complications.
   1. Cardiac disease.
   2. Hypertension.
   3. Delayed puberty.
   4. Amenorrhea.
   5. Infertility.
   6. Hashimoto thyroiditis.
   7. Celiac disease.

      8. Inflammatory bowel disease.

      9. Juvenile rheumatoid arthritis.

    10. Hypothyroidism.

    11. Dental issues.

    12. Obesity.

    13. Hearing loss.

J. Education.

    1. Related to the presenting issues as well as the complications involved.

    2. Special awareness of risk for:

      a. Osteoporosis related to lack of estrogen.

      b. Hypertension.

      c. Hyperthyroidism.

      d. Obesity.

    3. Families should be aware of:

      a. Use of growth hormone for short stature.

      b. Use of estrogen replacement therapy.

IV. DOWN SYNDROME

Down syndrome, unspecified, Q90.9

A. Etiology.

    1. Extra copy of the proximal part of 21q22.3.

B. Occurrence.

    1. Maternal age under 30: 1 in 1000 births.

    2. Incidence increases substantially with maternal age.

C. Clinical manifestations.

    1. Phenotypical dysmorphic facial feature.

      a. Slanting palpebral fissures.

      b. Bilateral epicanthal folds.

      c. Flat nasal bridge.

      d. Open mouth with tendency of tongue protrusion.

      e. Small ear with overfolded helix.

    2. Developmental delays.

    3. Hypertonia.

D. Physical findings.

    1. Decreased muscle tone at birth.

    2. Excess skin at nape of neck.

      3. Congenital heart defects.

      4. Dysmorphic features.

      5. Simian creases.

E. Diagnostic tests.

      1. Conventional cytogenetic studies.

F. Treatment.

      1. No specific treatment.

      2. Ongoing cardiac assessment.

      3. Supportive therapies for developmental issues.

      4. X-rays of the upper or cervical spine between the ages of 3 and 5 years.

G. Follow-up.

      1. Ongoing evaluations of the child's physical and neurological status.

      2. Genetic counseling for future pregnancies.

H. Complications.

      1. Obesity.

      2. Constipation.

      3. Sleep apnea.

      4. Hypothyroidism.

      5. Gastroesophageal reflux.

      6. Atlantoaxial instabilities.

      7. Leukemias.

      8. Cardiac disease.

      9. Refractive eye disorders.

      10. Recurrent otitis media.

      11. Diabetes mellitus.

      12. Immunoglobulin deficiencies.

      13. Psychiatric disorders including depression and obsessive compulsive disorders.

      14. Autism.

      15. Early-onset Alzheimer disease.

I. Differential diagnoses.

      1. Trisomy 18.

J. Education.

      1. Encourage sports participation due to trend toward obesity (i.e., Special Olympics).

      2. No contact sports due to atlantoaxial instabilities.

      3. Special education.

      4. Vocational training and career planning.

V. FETAL ALCOHOL SPECTRUM DISORDERS

Fetal alcohol syndrome (dysmorphic), Q86.0

A. Etiology.
   1. Spectrum of disorders caused by maternal ingestion of alcohol during pregnancy. The amount of alcohol ingested to cause impairment is not known. Habitual drinking and binge drinking during any point in pregnancy may have adverse effects. Alcohol is thought to affect every organ system.
B. Occurrence.
   1. Estimates vary by geographic location, ranging from 0.2 to 1.5 in 1000 live births.
C. Clinical manifestations.
   1. Stereotypical facial features.
   2. Cognitive disabilities.
   3. Growth issues.
   4. Behavior issues.
   5. Cardiac issues.
   6. Kidney issues.
   7. Hearing problems.
   8. Orthopedic issues.
D. Physical findings.
   1. Contingent on placement on spectrum.
   2. Stereotypical facial features: Smooth philtrum, thin vermillion border, small palpebral fissures.
   3. Microcephaly.
   4. Poor coordination.
   5. Vision and hearing problems.
E. Diagnostic tests.
   1. Four areas:
      a. Prenatal alcohol exposure (confirmed or unconfirmed).
      b. Growth retardation.
      c. Facial characteristics.
      d. Central nervous system (CNS) abnormalities.
F. Differential diagnoses.
   1. Autism.
   2. Conduct disorder.
   3. Facial dysmorphia.
   4. Growth retardation.

G. Treatment.
 1. Treatment for the CNS damage caused by fetal alcohol syndrome (FAS) is treated on an individual basis using a multimodel approach.
H. Follow-up.
 1. Follow-up is done on a case-by-case basis, with regard to socialization and behavioral issues, CNS symptoms, and treatment for other specific physical ailments.
 I. Complications.
 1. Attention deficit hyperactivity disorder.
 2. Conduct disorder.
 3. Depression.
 4. Addiction.
 J. Education.
 1. Local resources for support of families and children with FASD.
 2. Behavioral therapy.
 3. Special education services.

VI. PRADER-WILLI SYNDROME

Congenital malformation syndromes predominantly associated with short stature, Q87.1

A. Etiology.
 1. Deletion or disruption of genes in the proximal arm of chromosome 15 or by maternal disomy in the proximal arm of chromosome 15.
B. Occurrence.
 1. Approximately 1 in 25,000 live births.
C. Clinical manifestations.
 1. Infant hypotonia.
 2. Poor suck in infancy.
 3. Hypogonadotropic hypogonadism.
 4. Sleep disturbances (from central apnea to narcolepsy).
 5. Hyperphasia.
 6. Obesity.
 7. Delayed puberty.
 8. Developmental delay/cognitive disability.
 9. Growth hormone deficiency.
D. Physical findings.
 1. Failure to thrive in infancy.
 2. Obesity later in childhood.

      3. Strabismus.

      4. Small hands and feet.

      5. Short stature.

      6. Hypotonia.

  E. Diagnostic tests.

      1. Conventional cytogenic studies.

  F. Differential diagnoses.

      1. Anxiety disorder.

      2. Obsessive compulsive disorder.

      3. Fragile X.

      4. Growth hormone deficiency.

      5. Hypogonadism.

      6. Obesity.

      7. Obesity-hypoventilation syndrome.

      8. Pulmonary consequences of obesity.

      9. Angelman syndrome.

    10. Hypotonia.

  G. Treatment.

      1. Good infant nutrition usually requiring enteral feedings.

      2. Hormonal therapy: Growth hormone and estrogen or testosterone.

      3. Behavioral therapy.

      4. Physical therapy for hypotonia.

  H. Follow-up.

      1. Follow-up is done on an individual basis for symptoms/complications present.

  I. Complications.

      1. Complication of obesity.

      2. Cardiac disease.

      3. Type 2 diabetes mellitus.

      4. Behavioral problems.

  J. Education.

      1. Nutritional counseling and education for parents.

      2. Special education issues.

VII. FRAGILE X SYNDROME

Fragile X chromosome, Q99.2

  A. Etiology.

      1. Constriction and thin string that extends the long arm of the Xq27.3 (FMR1 gene), which gives the appearance of fragility to the X chromosome.

B. Occurrence.
   1. Conservatively, 1 in 4000 males and 1 in 8000 females.
   2. Female carrier status has been estimated to be as high as 1 in 130–250 of the population.
   3. Male carrier status is estimated to be 1 in 250–800 of the population.

C. Clinical manifestations.
   1. Developmental delays in infancy.
   2. Cognitive delays, particularly in language, memory, and problem solving.
   3. IQ can range from mild (70) to severe (20).
   4. Autistic-like behaviors, particularly poor eye contact and hand biting and flapping.

D. Physical findings.
   1. No phenotypical physical findings prepuberty, though may have larger head.
   2. Pectus excavatum, cardiac murmurs, and scoliosis are frequent findings, though not phenotypical.
   3. Postpuberty physical finding may include:
      a. Presence of a hallucal crease (a single crease between the first and second toes).
      b. Sensitivity to touch.
      c. The inability to touch the tongue to the lips.

E. Diagnostic tests.
   1. Conventional cytogenic testing.

F. Differential diagnoses.
   1. Autism.
   2. Attention deficit-hyperactivity disorder.
   3. Cognitive disabilities/low IQ.
   4. Epilepsy.
   5. Obsessive-compulsive disorder.
   6. Sensory integration issues.

G. Treatment.
   1. Treatment is individualized according to needs, usually special education and developmental therapies (speech, physical, and occupational therapies).

H. Follow-up.
   1. Follow-up is done on an individual basis for symptoms/complications present.

I. Complications.
   1. Serious complications are unusual, but cardiac, vision, and orthopedic problems do occur.

J. Education.
1. Parents need counseling around special education services.
2. Be aware of need for early career counseling/vocational training.

BIBLIOGRAPHY

American Cleft Palate Craniofacial Association [homepage]. http://www.acpa-cpf.org. Accessed June 15, 2015.

Center for Disease Control and Prevention. Facts about Down syndrome. http://www.cdc.gov/ncbddd/birthdefects/DownSyndrome.htm. Accessed June 15, 2015.

Centers for Disease Control and Protection. Fetal alcohol spectrum disorders (FASDs). http://www.cdc.gov/ncbddd/fasd/index.html. Accessed June 15, 2015.

Centers for Disease Control and Prevention. Fragile X syndrome. http://www.cdc.gov/ncbddd/single_gene/fragilex.htm. Accessed June 15, 2015.

Doswell BH, Visootsak J, Brady AN, Graham JM Jr. Turner syndrome: an update and review for the primary pediatrician. *Clin Pediatr (Phila)*. 2006;45(4):301-313.

Eunice Kennedy National Institute Child Health and Human Development. Down syndrome: overview. http://www.nichd.nih.gov/health/topics/down/Pages/default.aspx. Updated April 9, 2014. Accessed June 15, 2015.

Eunice Kennedy National Institute Child Health and Human Development. Fragile X syndrome: overview. https://www.nichd.nih.gov/health/topics/fragilex/Pages/default.aspx. Updated April 3, 2014. Accessed June 15, 2015.

Eunice Kennedy National Institute of Child Health and Human Development. Prader-Willi syndrome: overview. http://www.nichd.nih.gov/health/topics/prader-willi/Pages/default.aspx. Updated January 30, 2014. Accessed June 15, 2015.

Fetal Alcohol Spectrum Disorders Center for Excellence [homepage]. http://www.fasdcenter.samhsa.gov. Accessed June 15, 2015.

Foundation for Prader Willi Research [homepage]. http://www.fpwr.org. Accessed June 15, 2015.

Genetics Home Reference. Prader-Willi syndrome. http://ghr.nlm.nih.gov/condition/prader-willisyndrome. Accessed June 15, 2015.

Hartzell LD, Kilpatrick LA. Diagnosis and management of patients with clefts: a comprehensive and interdisciplinary approach. *Otolaryngol Clin North Am*. 2014;47(5):821-852.

National Down Syndrome Society [homepage]. http://www.ndss.org. Accessed June 15, 2015.

National Fragile X Foundation [homepage]. https://fragilex.org. Accessed June 15, 2015.

National Institute of Neurological Disorders and Stroke [homepage]. http:// www.ninds.nih.gov. Accessed June 15, 2015.

National Organization on Fetal Alcohol Syndrome [homepage]. http://www.nofas.org. Accessed June 15, 2015.

Prader-Willi Syndrome Association [homepage]. http://www.pwsausa.org. Accessed June 15, 2015.

Spina Bifida Association [homepage]. http://www.spinabifidaassociation.org. Accessed June 15, 2015.

U.S. National Library of Medicine. Down syndrome. http://www.nlm.nih.gov/medlineplus/downsyndrome.html. Accessed June 15, 2015.

Two-Week Visit

Candace F. Zickler

Dyspnea, unspecified, R06.00	Neonatal jaundice, unspecified, P59.9
Constipation, K59.0	Other specified symptoms and signs involving
Convulsions, unspecified, R56.9	the digestive system and abdomen, R19.8
Feeding difficulties, R63.3	Rash and other nonspecific skin eruption, R21
Irritability and anger, R45.4	Retention of urine, unspecified, R33.9
Jaundice, unspecified R17	Vomiting, unspecified, R11.10

I. GENERAL IMPRESSION

A. Parents are settling in with 2-week-old, each getting acquainted with other. If infant was still losing weight at discharge, the bilirubin was above 10 mg/dL, or the infant had a heart murmur at discharge, he/she needs to be seen in the office within 2 days.

B. Infant should have a naked weight, length on length board, and head circumference performed at each visit. Compare the birth weight and the discharge weight with the weight obtained today. Determine daily weight gain since discharge.

C. A brief exam noting muscle tone, symmetry, and heart sounds and murmurs should be performed. Check for hip clicks by doing the Orolani and Barlow tests.

D. At 2 weeks of age, the infant's cord should have fallen off or be dry or looking like it will likely fall off soon, but not moist and smelly.

E. Jaundice should be resolved except in some breastfed infants. If unresolved, do a transcutaneous bilirubin.

F. Newborn screen results should be reviewed and be negative. Share report with parents.

G. Review the newborn hearing screen. If hearing is within normal limits, share with the parents. If abnormal, schedule baby for an auditory brainstem response (ABR) or an otoacoustic emissions test (OAE) before leaving the office.

H. Reflexes present should be rooting, Galant (trunk incurvation), placing and stepping, Landau (infant lifts head when suspended in prone position), asymmetric tonic neck.

II. NUTRITION

A. Breastfeeding is encouraged for all newborns. If mother is breastfeeding, ask specific questions:
    1. Does the baby latch on well?
    2. How long does the baby nurse at one time?
    3. How frequently are you nursing the baby?
    4. How many wet diapers?
    5. How many stools?
    6. Are you having any irritation or pain from your nipples?

B. Review all medications that mother may be taking (see Chapter 5). If mother expresses concerns about the nursing, observe a nursing session, give suggestions, and obtain a lactation consult from the hospital lactation resource.

C. If baby is bottle fed, review preparation and number of feedings, how much the baby is taking each time, number of wet diapers, and number of stools per day. Commercially prepared, iron-fortified formulas come in powder, concentrate, and ready-to-feed formulas. Remind parent to not dilute ready-to-feed. Follow directions for mixing concentrate and powder.
    1. Do not reuse bottle/formula if more than 4 hours since opened.
    2. Mix formulas with bottled water for first month; continue to use bottled water if house is on well/unsure of water quality. Store mixed and open formula in refrigerator; do not feed formula that has been premixed and in the refrigerator longer than 24 hours. Specialized formulas have similar preparation directions; read labels. Goat's milk, whole cow's milk, and rice milk have inadequate amounts of vitamins and minerals.
    3. Serve formula at room temperature. Do not microwave to heat. Do not let formula sit out to warm for more than 15–20 minutes.
    4. Clean technique is sufficient for mixing formulas. Clean off cans with soap and water before opening. Use hot soapy water and bottlebrush to clean nipples and bottles or clean in dishwasher.
    5. Hold infant in upright, semireclined position; burp every 1–2 oz. No bottle propping. Babies will suck and then rest during the entire feeding.

Encourage mother to let her husband/partner feed the baby at least once during the day.

6. No smoking or drinking hot beverages while holding baby. Limit noise in the immediate area when doing feeding, and focus on baby. Talk or sing to the baby.

7. Infant should take in 90 cc of feeding in first 20 minutes. Two-week-old infant takes 3–5 oz/feeding, 5–6 feedings/24 hours (90–120 cal/kg/day). Remind parents that they should not be feeding the baby for more than 20–25 minutes at a time as this tires the baby out, and baby has no time to rest between feedings.

III. ELIMINATION

A. Bowel movements should be formed or soft with no green color. Infant should have 1–6 yellow pasty stools/24 hours. Breastfed infant may have upper range of frequency with less formed texture. Void every 1–3 hours or with each feeding and diaper change.

IV. SLEEP

A. Awake and alert for feedings, every 2–4 hours. Should nurse vigorously for 15–20 minutes, then fall back to sleep.

B. Babies should sleep in own cribs to decrease smothering or injury. Babies should sleep on their back in cribs to decrease incidence of sudden infant death syndrome (SIDS).

V. GROWTH AND DEVELOPMENT

A. Growth.
   1. Should regain birth weight by 2 weeks. Should gain 0.5–1 oz/day or approximately 2 lbs/month for next 5 months.
   2. Infant grows, on average, 1 in./month for first 6 months.
   3. Head circumference increases 0.5 cm/month in first year.

B. Development.
   1. Moves all 4 extremities, keep hands fisted, and has flexed posture.
   2. Has startle response to noises.
   3. May have a smile. May begin to look for "who is talking."

4. May have "fussy" time of 1–2 hours/day, often in evening.

5. Should have some supervised, "tummy" play time (15–20 minutes/session).

6. Ask about behavior after feedings to determine any colic or reflux.

VI. SOCIAL DEVELOPMENT

A. Babies have specific sounds/cries for specific needs. They will fuss/cry 1–2 hours/day. Providing for infant's needs should stop the crying. Crying gradually decreases by 3 months of age.

B. Infant needs holding; touching; feeding; dry, clean diaper; warm, yet comfortable environment.

C. Discourage taking baby to public places or visiting relatives since infant has not been immunized. Sick adults should stay away from infant.

D. Encourage mother to rest when baby rests/sleeps. Determine if night times are "awake times for the pair" and the mother is not getting her sleep.

VII. IMMUNIZATIONS

A. If mother is HBsAg–, infant may not have received first hepatitis B vaccine in newborn nursery and will need to get it today or before 2 months of age. If infant received hepatitis B immunization in the nursery, he/she will need to get four hepatitis B immunizations.

B. Infant should not have fever or fussiness from the immunization.

C. Discuss importance of getting immunizations. Many parents are concerned about risks. One in eight parents in the United States refused at least one recommended vaccine for their child. The AAP has resources on the importance of vaccines that can be shared with parents.

D. See Appendix A.

VIII. SAFETY/ANTICIPATORY GUIDANCE

A. Sleep position "back to sleep."

1. Not safe for baby to sleep in adult bed.

2. Discuss room temperature (comfortable), amount of clothing to put on baby (not to overdress infant).

3. No pillows/toys in the crib that could potentially smother child.

4. Federal motor vehicle safety tested and approved car seat: Installed properly in backseat, facing backward in automobile. Contact local hospital, fire department, or local March of Dimes for car seat rental programs.

B. No smoking around infant.

C. Reassure parents they cannot spoil infant at this age. Encourage responding to the infant's needs and learning the baby's temperament.

D. Discuss sibling jealousy and possible regression of toddler. Encourage parent to spend "special time" with older sibling.

E. Discuss pet safety: Do not leave infant unattended near pet.

F. Discuss toys.

G. Discuss what to look for when choosing babysitter or daycare (e.g., handwashing, number of children, sick policy, feeding techniques).

H. One-piece pacifiers only, discuss appropriate use of pacifiers. Should not pin them on a string to baby's clothing, wash with soap and water if they fall out of the baby's mouth, do not lick or moisten it prior to giving to baby.

I. May give 1 oz of sterile water in 24 hours if stools are very hard. No corn syrup (Karo) for constipation.

J. No solids.

K. Remind parents of when and how to call healthcare provider. Review call-in phone policy and explain hours that are best to call office.

1. Breathing difficulties.
2. Seizures.
3. Irritability.
4. Poor feeding, vomiting.
5. No urine in 12 hours, black or decreased bowel movements.
6. Reddened, draining umbilical site.
7. Jaundice.
8. Rash or pustules not present on discharge.
9. Concerns.

BIBLIOGRAPHY

Centers for Disease Control and Prevention. Recommended immunization schedules for persons aged 0 through 18 years–United States, 2015. http://www.cdc.gov/vaccines/schedules/downloads/child /0-18yrs-child-combined-schedule.pdf. Accessed February 28, 2015.

De Michele AM, Ruth RA. Newborn hearing screening. Medscape Reference; 2010. http://emedicine .medscape.com/article/836646. Accessed June 2, 2011.

Delaney, AM. Newborn hearing screening. Medscape Reference. http://emedicine.medscape.com/article /836646-overview#showall. Updated September 11, 2014. Accessed June 1, 2015.

Diekema DS, American Academy of Pediatrics Committee on Bioethics. Responding to parental refusals of immunization of children. *Pediatrics*. 2005;115(5):1428-1431.

Fouzas S, Mantagou L, Skylogianni E, Mantagos S, Varvarigou A. Transcutaneous bilirubin levels for the first 120 postnatal hours in healthy neonates. *Pediatrics*. 2010;125(1):e52-e57.

Hagan JF, Shaw JS, Duncan P, eds. *Bright Futures: Guidelines for Health Supervision of Infants, Children, and Adolescents*. 3rd ed. Elk Grove Village, IL: American Academy of Pediatrics; 2008.

HealthyChildren.org. Car safety seats: information for families 2015. https://www.healthychildren.org /English/safety-prevention/on-the-go/Pages/Car-Safety-Seats-Information-for-Families.aspx. Accessed February 27, 2015.

Kaneshiro NK. Neonatal weight gain and nutrition. MedlinePlus. http://www.nlm.nih.gov/medlineplus /ency/article/007302.htm. Updated May 10, 2013. Accessed June 15, 2015.

March of Dimes. National standard for newborn screening is announced. *redOrbit*. http://www.redorbit.com /news/health/1869169/national_standard_for_newborn_screening_is_announced/. Accessed June 2, 2011.

March of Dimes. Newborn screening tests for your baby. http://www.marchofdimes.org/baby/newborn -screening-tests-for-your-baby.aspx. Accessed June 15, 2015.

Medoff-Cooper B, Bakewell-Sachs S, Buus-Frank ME, Santa-Donato A. Near-Term Infant Advisory Panel. The AWHONN Near-Term Infant Initiative: a conceptual framework for optimizing health for near-term infants. *J Obstet Gynecol Neonatal Nurs*. 2005;34(6):666-671.

National Center for Immunization and Respiratory Diseases. Provider resources for vaccine conversations with parents. Centers for Disease Control and Prevention. http://www.cdc.gov/vaccines/hcp/patient-ed /conversations/index.html. Updated December 17, 2014. Accessed February 28, 2015.

One-Month Visit

Candace F. Zickler

Constipation, K59.0	Feeding difficulties, R63.3
Convulsions, unspecified, R56.9	Irritability and anger, R45.4
Dyspnea, unspecified, R06.00	Vomiting, unspecified, R11.10

I. GENERAL IMPRESSION

A. Parents and infant should be settling into routine and more comfortable with each other. Parent should be very attentive to the infant and have lots of questions. There should also be a sense that parent is comfortable with the infant. Parent is able to describe characteristics of infant's temperament. Mother should have someone identified that she can leave baby with for brief periods of time.

II. NUTRITION

A. Breastfeeding is to be encouraged. Determine if baby is satisfied after feedings, how frequently baby is nursing, how long a feeding takes, and any concerns mom has about continuing nursing. Ask about plans/arrangements to return to work.

B. Formula.

1. Mix formula with bottled water for first month, continue to use bottled water if house is on well/unsure of water quality. Have well water tested at local health department for small fee.

2. Store ready-to-feed and open formula bottles in refrigerator. Refrigerate no longer than 24–36 hours.

3. Specialized formulas have similar preparation directions; read labels. Goat's milk, whole cow's milk, rice milk have inadequate amounts of vitamins and minerals.
4. Serve formula at room temperature. Do not microwave to heat. Do not let formula sit out to warm for more than 15–20 minutes.
5. Clean technique is sufficient for mixing formulas.
   a. Clean off cans with soap and water before opening.
   b. Use hot soapy water and bottlebrush to clean nipples and bottles or clean in dishwasher.
6. Hold infant in upright, semireclined position; burp every 1–2 oz.
   a. No bottle propping.
   b. No smoking or drinking hot beverages while holding baby.
7. One-month-old infant will take 4–6 oz/feeding and 5–6 feedings/24 hours (90–120 cal/kg/day).

III. ELIMINATION

A. Should have 1–6 yellow pasty stools/24 hours.
B. With each feeding, breastfed infant may have softer, formed/seedy stools.
C. Void every 1–3 hours or with each feeding.

IV. SLEEP

A. Awake and alert for feedings, every 2–4 hours. Baby will suck vigorously for 15–20 minutes, then fall back to sleep.
B. Babies should sleep in own cribs, not with parents, to decrease risk of smothering or injury.
C. Babies should sleep on back or side in cribs to decrease risk of sudden infant death syndrome (SIDS).
D. No pillows/toys that baby could get face against and smother.

V. GROWTH AND DEVELOPMENT

A. Growth. Weigh infant naked on infant scales. Compare weight to last visit. Calculate rate of gain since last visit. Measure length on length board and head circumference. Plot values on National Center for Health Statistics (NCHS) growth chart. Discuss your findings from the growth charts.

1. Should gain 0.5–1 oz/day or approximately 2 lbs/month for next 4 months.
2. Infant grows, on average, 1 in./month for first 6 months.
3. Head circumference increases 0.5 cm/month in first year.

B. Development. Responds to human face and follows briefly with eyes. Is attentive to sound of parent's voice.

1. May be able to lift head off bed if on tummy.
2. May have a smile.
3. Has positive red reflexes bilaterally and blinks to light. Tear ducts may have tears appear; tear ducts should be patent.
4. Assess scalp for cradle cap and diaper area for dermatitis. Review how to care for baby's skin.
5. Examine baby's mouth for teeth, intact palate, and presence of thrush. If bottle feeding and thrush is found, discuss cleaning of pacifiers, nipples. If breastfeeding, review washing nipples before feedings and applying antifungal (prescription) after feedings.
6. Gently palpate abdomen looking for masses, and location of the liver.
7. Observe movement of all 4 extremities, usually simultaneously. Has a flexed posture and keeps hands fisted.
8. May cry but parents are learning what each cry means; crying ceases with needs being met. Cry gradually decreases by 3 months of age.
9. May have "fussy" time of 1–2 hours/day, often in evening. Use "fussy" time as interaction time, not extra feeding.
10. Baby may have symptoms of "colic" start around 2–3 weeks of age. Infant cries for prolonged periods, no specific cause or pathology identified. Infant requires additional comfort measures to quiet and settle.

VI. SOCIAL DEVELOPMENT

A. Parent should be assessed for sadness, depression, fatigue. Parent should show attentive, animated behavior toward baby. Listen carefully for frustration, potential for abuse/neglect.

B. Parents should hold, cuddle, and talk to infant when awake. Infant should have 15–20 minutes of "tummy time" with supervision, daily.

C. Discourage taking baby to public places or visiting relatives because no immunizations as yet.

D. Encourage mother to rest when baby rests/sleeps.

E. Baby is learning to "trust" parent and caretakers.

VII. IMMUNIZATIONS

A. If mother is HBsAg–, infant may not have received hepatitis B #1 in newborn nursery or at 2-week visit. Will need to get it today.

B. Discuss need for immunizations at next visit. Parents hear many negative remarks from friends and family and the Internet. But they do listen to a trusted healthcare provider.

C. Infants should not have fever or fussiness from immunization.

D. See Appendix A.

VIII. SAFETY/ANTICIPATORY GUIDANCE

A. Sleep position "back to sleep."

B. Protect baby from direct sunlight. Skin is very sensitive and babies burn easily.

C. Not safe for baby to sleep in adult bed.

D. Temperature of room comfortable. Discuss type of clothing needed to dress infant for inside, outside, and for bed.

E. A Federal Motor Vehicle Safety Standards seat (FMVSS) should be installed properly in backseat, facing backward in their automobile. Contact local hospital, fire department, or March of Dimes chapter for car seat rental program.

F. No smoking around infant. Do not drink hot beverages when holding baby.

G. One-piece pacifiers only. Do not pin it to clothing. Clean and dry it thoroughly frequently.

H. No corn syrup (Karo) for constipation. May give 1–2 oz of sterile water daily for infrequent or hard stools.

I. Infant still not old enough to be fed solid foods. Diet should be breastmilk or formula.

J. Obtain CPR training. Make sure smoke alarms are working and functional in the home.

K. Remind parents of when and how to call the healthcare provider.

1. Breathing difficulties.

2. Seizures.

3. Irritability, lethargy.

4. Poor feeding, vomiting, diarrhea (describe how stools would be if diarrhea).

5. No urine in 12 hours, black or decreased bowel movements.

6. Fever or rash that lasts more than 24 hours.

BIBLIOGRAPHY

American Academy of Pediatrics Task Force on Sudden Infant Death Syndrome. The changing concept of sudden infant death syndrome: diagnostic coding shifts, controversies regarding the sleeping environment, and new variables to consider in reducing risk. *Pediatrics.* 2005;116(5):1245-1255.

Centers for Disease Control and Prevention. Recommended immunization schedules for persons aged 0 through 18 years–United States, 2015. http://www.cdc.gov/vaccines/schedules/downloads/child /0-18yrs-child-combined-schedule.pdf. Accessed February 28, 2015.

Centers for Disease Control and Prevention. Growth charts for birth through 36 months. http://www.cdc.gov /growthcharts/clinical_charts.htm. Accessed June 2, 2011.

Centers for Disease Control and Prevention. Provider resources for vaccine conversations with parents. http://www.cdc.gov/vaccines/hcp/patient-ed/conversations/index.html. Accessed February 28, 2015.

Diekema DS, American Academy of Pediatrics Committee on Bioethics. Responding to parental refusals of immunization of children. *Pediatrics.* 2005;115(5):1428-1431.

Hagan JF, Shaw JS, Duncan P, eds. *Bright Futures: Guidelines for Health Supervision of Infants, Children, and Adolescents.* 3rd ed. Elk Grove Village, IL: American Academy of Pediatrics; 2008.

HealthyChildren.org. Car seats: information for families for 2015. http://www.healthychildren.org/English /safety-prevention/on-the-go/Pages/Car-Safety-Seats-Information-for-Families.aspx. Accessed June 15, 2015

HealthyChildren.org. Safety for your child; birth to 6 months. http://www.healthychildren.org/English /ages-stages/baby/Pages/Safety-for-Your-Child-Birth-to-6-Months.aspx. Accessed September 1, 2015.

Two-Month Visit

Candace F. Zickler

Constipation, K59.0	Feeding difficulties, R63.3
Convulsions, unspecified, R56.9	Fever of other and unknown origin, R50
Dyspnea, unspecified, R06.00	Vomiting, unspecified, R11.10

I. GENERAL IMPRESSION

A. Parents should be enjoying their infant and taking joy from infant's accomplishments.

B. Infant is more responsive with smiling and cooing.

C. Parents should have many questions and be able to share stories of babies' activities.

II. NUTRITION

A. Two-month-old infant will take 6–8 oz/feeding, 4–6 feedings/24 hours (94–130 cal/kg/day). Feedings should be more predictable, and infant should have periods when he/she sleeps for 3–4 hours at a time.

B. Baby should take in 90 cc of feeding in first 20 minutes of the feeding. Prolonging feedings for more than half an hour at a time tires the baby and the mother and tends to make feedings stressful.

C. Hold infant in semireclined position; burp every 1–2 oz.

D. Specialized formulas have similar preparation directions; read labels. Goat's milk, whole cow's milk, and rice milk have inadequate amounts of vitamins and minerals.

E. Serve formula at room temperature. Do not microwave to heat. Do not let formula sit out to warm for more than 15–20 minutes.

F. Clean technique is sufficient for mixing formulas.
    1. Clean off cans with soap and water before opening.
    2. Use hot soapy water and bottlebrush to clean nipples and bottles or clean in dishwasher.
G. No bottle propping. Pacifiers are used for nonnutritive sucking. Breastfeeding should be well established before starting infant on a pacifier, but babies who suck pacifiers are at decreased incidence of sudden infant death.
H. No smoking or drinking hot beverages while holding baby.

III. ELIMINATION

A. Should have 1–5 yellow pasty but formed stools/24 hours.
B. Breastfed babies may have more stools than bottle-fed babies.
C. Void every 1–3 hours or with each feeding and diaper change.

IV. SLEEP

A. Babies sleep 16–18 hours/24 hours. Infant is developing sleep pattern. May sleep through night. May have longer awake periods during day.
B. Sleep cycles have both active and quiet sleep periods in equal proportions. Each sleep cycle lasts 50–60 minutes. Infants are less efficient with sleep and easily interrupted with noise. Should be alert for feedings, nurse vigorously for 15–20 minutes, and fall back to sleep/stay awake for short periods.
C. Babies should sleep in own cribs, not with parents, to decrease smothering injury to infant.
    1. Babies should sleep on back in their cribs and not in the parents' bed.
    2. No pillows/toys that baby could get face against and smother.

V. GROWTH AND DEVELOPMENT

A. Growth. Plot length, weight, head circumference, and weight-for-height on the National Center for Health Statistics (NCHS) growth grids. Compare to last visit growth plots.
    1. Babies should gain 0.5–0.75 oz/day or approximately 2 lbs/month for the first 4–5 months.
    2. Infant grows, on average, 1 in./month for first 6 months.
    3. Head circumference increases 0.5 cm/month in first year.
B. Development.
    1. Holds head upright for short periods. Follows people and looks for voice.

2. Responds to smiling with return smile.
3. Babbles and makes sounds with prompt of verbal cue.
4. Shows interest in what is happening in room.
5. Moves all 4 extremities, simultaneously.
6. May cry but parents are learning what each cry means. Crying ceases when needs are met.

VI. SOCIAL DEVELOPMENT

A. Baby learning to "trust" parent and caretakers to meet needs.
B. Family is settling into routines with infant.
C. Listen carefully for frustration, potential for abuse/neglect. Discuss child's unique temperament characteristics, relate to parents' feelings.
D. Parent should be assessed for sadness, depression, fatigue.
   1. Encourage mother to rest when baby rests/sleeps.
   2. Encourage mother to take breaks away from baby to do self-nurturing (needs designated sitter).
E. Take baby on selective, limited outings because infant is not fully immunized; will only receive first set today.
F. Ask about plans for returning to work. Discuss guidelines for selecting sitter/daycare.
G. May have "fussy" time of 1–2 hours/day, often in evening. Use "fussy" time as interaction time, not extra feeding. Cry gradually decreases by 3 months of age. Baby may have symptoms of "colic" (starts 2–3 weeks of age, ceases by 12 weeks). Infant cries for prolonged periods, no specific cause or etiology identified. Infant continues to grow well. Infant is alert and playful at other times. Infant may require additional comfort measures to quiet and settle and should be accepted as expected for age.
H. Should have some supervised, "tummy" play time while awake during each day. This helps infant develop strength and coordination, and minimizes flattening of the skull.
I. Encourage parent to actively talk, play with infant. Select age-appropriate toys.

VII. IMMUNIZATIONS

A. Infant will receive first set of immunizations today. Combinations are available that decrease number of injections. Parents trust providers to guide them in their decision to immunize their children. Need to discuss risks and benefits of immunizations and have parent sign consent. The following immunizations are best practice for 2-month-old infants: 2nd hepatitis B (HBV), rotovirus (RV), diphtheria-acellular pertussis tetanus (DTaP), hemophilus influenza b (Hib), pneumococcal conjugate (PCV13), inactivated poliovirus (IPV).

B. Giving acetaminophen prophylactically after immunizations may decrease the response to the vaccine. Only a few infants tend to have fevers after immunizations.

C. See Appendix A.

VIII. SAFETY/ANTICIPATORY GUIDANCE

A. Needs safe sleep position "back to sleep."
   1. Not safe for baby to sleep in adult bed.
   2. Discuss temperature of room, temperature of water, bathing safety guidelines.
   3. Discuss appropriate amount of clothing to keep baby comfortable in varied environments.
B. Never leave baby unattended near pet or sibling.
C. Keep hand on baby when on changing tables and sofas to avoid risk of falling.
D. Review need for proper installation and use of infant car seat. Seat should be Federal Motor Vehicle Safety tested and approved, installed properly in backseat, facing backward in automobile.
E. No smoking around infant.
F. To treat constipation, advise giving extra water (no more than 1 oz/day).
G. No solids should be offered. Offer pacifier if acting "hungry" or going to nap.
H. Make sure smoke detectors are installed and functioning in home. Home should have working fire detectors, a fire evacuation plan, and periodic drills to ensure preparedness.
I. Limit sun exposure, use sunscreen with SPF rating of at least 15 if out for even 15 minutes of direct sun exposure. Protect babies by using hats and long-sleeved shirts and pants.
J. Baby will be seen for regular appointment again at 4 months. Discuss skills infant will acquire and how to work with baby to learn them: Babbling, cooing, trying to roll over, and more. Discuss second set of immunizations, similar to what baby had at this visit.
K. Remind parents of when and how to call the healthcare provider.
   1. Breathing difficulties.
   2. Seizures.
   3. Irritability.

4. Poor feeding, vomiting.
5. No urine output in 12 hours, black/decreased bowel movements.
6. Any fever.
7. Praise the parents for all that they are doing for the infant.

BIBLIOGRAPHY

American Academy of Pediatrics. Protecting All Children's Teeth (PACT): Oral health. In: *Protecting All Children's Teeth (PACT): A Pediatric Oral Health Training Program.* American Academy of Pediatrics; 2010. http://www2.aap.org/oralhealth/pact/ch8_intro.cfm. Accessed June 15, 2015.

American Academy of Pediatrics Task Force on Sudden Infant Death Syndrome. The changing concept of sudden infant death syndrome: diagnostic coding shifts, controversies regarding the sleeping environment, and new variables to consider in reducing risk. *Pediatrics.* 2005;116(5):1245-1255.

Centers for Disease Control and Prevention. Growth charts for birth through 36 months. http://www.cdc.gov/growthcharts/clinical_charts.htm. Accessed June 15, 2015.

Centers for Disease Control and Prevention. Recommended immunization schedules for persons aged 0 through 18 years—United States 2015. http://www.cdc.gov/vaccines/schedules/downloads/child/0-18yrs-child-combined-schedule.pdf. Accessed March 29, 2015.

Dowshen S. Choosing childcare. KidsHealth from Nemours; 2007. http://kidshealth.org/parent/positive/amily/child_care.html. Accessed June 15, 2015.

Hagan JF, Shaw JS, Duncan P, eds. *Bright Futures: Guidelines for Health Supervision of Infants, Children, and Adolescents.* 3rd ed. Elk Grove Village, IL: American Academy of Pediatrics; 2008.

Healthy Child Care America. *Back to Sleep, Tummy to Play.* American Academy of Pediatrics; 2008: http://www.healthychildcare.org/pdf/SIDStummytime.pdf. Accessed June 15, 2015.

HealthyChildren.org. Car seats: information for families for 2015. http://www.healthychildren.org/English/safety-prevention/on-the-go/Pages/Car-Safety-Seats-Information-for-Families.aspx. Accessed June 15, 2015.

HealthyChildren.org. Safety for your child; birth to 6 months. https://www.healthychildren.org/English/ages-stages/baby/Pages/Safety-for-Your-Child-Birth-to-6-Months.aspx. Accessed September 1, 2015.

Port Washington Fire Department. E.D.I.T.H.: exit drills in the home. http://www.pwfd.com/content/850_fs3.html. Accessed June 15, 2015.

Soloway B. Prophylactic acetaminophen could lower response to childhood immunizations. Medscape Today. http://www.medscape.com/viewarticle/712540. Accessed June 2, 2011.

White J. Overview of infant colic. AboutHealth. http://baby.about.com/od/healthandsafety/p/infant_colic.htm. Updated November 24, 2014. Accessed June 15, 2015.

Four-Month Visit

Patricia Clinton

Diarrhea, unspecified, R19.7	Volume depletion, E86
Fever of other and unknown origin, R50	Vomiting, unspecified, R11.10

I. GENERAL IMPRESSION

A. Four-month-old infant is generally well integrated into family unit, interacts with family members, is beginning to actively explore environment by making more purposeful movements.

B. Patterns of sleeping, eating, elimination are fairly well established.

II. NUTRITION

A. Caloric needs: 98–108 kcal/kg/day.

B. Breastfeeding.
   1. Recommended as sole source of nutrition; Minimum 6 months, preferably first year.
   2. Infant easily distractible.
   3. Support mother in continuing to nurse throughout first year; discuss strategies for continuing to breastfeed if mother is returning to work.
   4. Vitamin D supplementation recommended at 400 IU/day.
   5. If exclusively breastfed, supplement with iron 1 mg/kg/day until iron-rich foods incorporated in diet.

C. Formula feeding.
   1. Iron-fortified only; prepare with fluoridated water.
   2. No cow's milk of any kind.
   3. Will consume 26–36 oz/day.

D. Introduction of solids.
1. May begin after 4-month visit.
2. Preference is to postpone until 6 months to minimize allergies.
3. Introduce solids when tongue thrust diminishes, infant has good head control (see Chapter 11).

III. ELIMINATION

A. Voiding pattern.
1. Average 6–8 wet diapers/day; may have as many as 15–20 small voids per day.
2. Illness (fever, vomiting, diarrhea) associated with decreased voiding and concerns of dehydration.
B. Stooling pattern.
1. Breastfed infants generally have 1 stool/day to 1 stool every 7–10 days.
2. Consistency more important than frequency.
3. Stools should be soft, semiformed, odor not offensive.
4. Formula-fed infants generally have 1 or more stools/day, color varies by formula, may be more odoriferous.

IV. SLEEP

A. Requirements.
1. Total sleep recommended 12–15 hours per day; range 10–18 hours.
2. Nighttime 9–12 hours; may still wake for nighttime feedings.
3. Naps 2–4 times/day; 30 minutes to 2 hours.
B. Environment.
1. Begin to establish consistent bedtime routine.
2. Put to bed drowsy but awake.
3. Room temperature should be temperate and not excessively warm.
4. Transitional object such as blanket may be comforting.
5. Room dim, may use night-light.
6. Cosleeping is family/culturally determined; encourage discussion, avoid being judgmental; safety should be focus.
7. Avoid bottles in bed.
C. Safety.
1. Put to bed on back. Once he/she rolls over, infant determines position during sleep.
2. Sleeping surface should be firm; avoid pillows, comforters. Slats 2⅜ in. apart; corner posts $\frac{1}{16}$ in. high.

3. Smoke-free environment.
4. Remove mobiles, Venetian blind cords, other hanging toys before infant learns to pull up in crib.

V. GROWTH AND DEVELOPMENT

A. Growth.
　1. Infants should gain 0.5–1 oz/day or about 2 lbs/month; doubles birth weight between 4 and 6 months.
　2. Infants grow, on average, 0.8 in./month.
　3. Head circumference increases 0.4 cm/month.
B. Development.
　1. Grasps objects, begins with raking motion.
　2. Brings hands together.
　3. Follows objects with eyes to 180°.
　4. Good head control, lifts head and chest when prone.
　5. Bears weight on legs.
　6. Rolls from front to back with sufficient tummy time.
　7. Rooting and palmar grasp disappear.
　8. Moro, Babinski, and tonic neck no longer as prominent, may disappear by 4 months.
　9. Begins to link event with action, such as quieting when put in nursing position.
　10. Ability to wait begins to develop as infant learns to anticipate response from caregiver.
　11. Drooling begins.
　12. Cooing, laughing, squealing. Vocalizes in variety of ways to initiate and sustain interaction.
　13. Beginning to listen when others speak.

VI. SOCIAL DEVELOPMENT

A. Relationships.
　1. Recognizes primary caregiver.
　2. Variety of facial expressions such as smiling, surprise, fear.
　3. Enjoys being cuddled.
B. Environment: Conditions that foster trust, positive psychosocial feelings, development.
　1. Learning to trust caretakers.

2. Responsiveness to infant's needs and cues reinforces trust and does not result in spoiling.
3. Smiles are purposeful.

VII. IMMUNIZATIONS

A. See Appendix A. Review immunization schedule: DTaP #2, Hib #2, IPV #2, PCV13 #2, RV #2, hepatitis B if not previously started.
B. Review immunization reactions.

VIII. SAFETY/ANTICIPATORY GUIDANCE

A. Always check bathwater temperature.
B. Never leave infant alone in tub or on changing table.
C. Use sunscreen of at least SPF 15 and avoid prolonged sun exposure.
D. Use car seat consistently. Never leave infant alone in car.
E. Avoid use of walkers.
F. Begin "baby proofing": Outlet covers, door and drawer latches, safety gates. Remove cords, wires, string, plastic bags from baby's environment.
G. Maintain smoke-free environment.
H. If mother is returning to work, plan strategies for breastfeeding.
I. No honey or corn syrup (Karo).
J. Do not prop bottles. Do not put cereal in bottles.
K. Allow infant to self-regulate amount eaten: Watch for cues, such as turning head away.
L. Secure infant in highchair. Never leave infant alone in highchair.
M. Encourage floor "tummy" time so infant can begin to explore surroundings.
N. Talk, read, sing to infant.
O. Use variety of toys/other household objects to stimulate infant. Introduce infant to different textures in toys, objects.
P. Discuss infant's temperament and how it relates to sleep/wake activities.
Q. Begin exploring parental ideas about discipline.
R. Cleanse gums with soft cloth after feeding.
S. Increased drooling indicates functional salivary glands, not teething.
T. Stress handwashing by all caregivers.
U. Use of cool mist vaporizers for upper respiratory illness.
V. Review guidelines for calling healthcare provider, illness signs (i.e., fever, vomiting, diarrhea).

BIBLIOGRAPHY

American Academy of Pediatric Dentistry. Guideline on fluoride therapy. *Reference Manual: Clinical Guidelines.* 2013;36(6):171-174.

Burns CE, Dunn AM, Brady MA, Starr NB, Blosser CG. *Pediatric Primary Care.* 5th ed. Philadelphia, PA: Saunders; 2013.

Centers for Disease Control and Prevention. Recommended immunization schedules for persons aged 0 through 18 years–United States, 2015. http://www.cdc.gov/vaccines/schedules/downloads/child/0 -18yrs-child-combined-schedule.pdf. Accessed February 3, 2015.

Consolini DM. Nutrition in infants. In: *The Merck Manual Professional Edition.* http://www.merckmanuals.com /professional/pediatrics/care-of-newborns-and-infants/nutrition-in-infants?qt=nutrition%20in%20 infants&alt=sh%202013#

Hagan JF, Shaw JS, Duncan P, eds. *Bright Futures: Guidelines for Health Supervision of Infants, Children, and Adolescents.* 3rd ed. Elk Grove Village, IL: American Academy of Pediatrics; 2008.

Hirshkowitz M, Whiton K, Albert SM, et al. National Sleep Foundation's sleep time duration recommendations: methodology and results summary. *Sleep Health.* 2015;1(1):40-43.

Holt K, Wooldridge MS, Story M, Sofka D, eds. *Bright Futures: Nutrition.* 3rd ed. Elk Grove Village, IL: American Academy of Pediatrics; 2011.

Mannheim JK. Infant–newborn development. http://www.nlm.nih.gov/medlineplus/ency/article/002004 .htm. Updated January 27, 2013. Accessed May 15, 2015.

United States Department of Agriculture Food and Nutrition Service. *Infant Nutrition and Feeding: A Guide for Use in the WIC and CSF Programs.* Alexandria, VA: United States Department of Agriculture; 2009.

Six-Month Visit

Patricia Clinton

Convulsions, unspecified, R56.9   Rash and other nonspecific skin eruption, R21
Dyspnea, unspecified, R06.00

I. GENERAL IMPRESSION

A. Six-month-old infant is active, social person in family and with others, although new people may be cause for some anxiety.

B. Parents are comfortable in their role, look forward to infant's new achievements.

II. NUTRITION

A. Caloric and nutrient needs.
   1. 95–105 kcal/kg/day.
   2. Iron stores may not meet needs; encourage iron-fortified cereals, foods, and formulas.
   3. Nutrient needs generally cannot be met from breastmilk or formula alone.

B. Breastfeeding.
   1. Continue to encourage breastfeeding through first year.
   2. Continue vitamin D supplementation.

C. Formula feeding.
   1. Continue with iron-fortified formula using fluoridated water.
   2. Average intake 24–32 oz/day.
   3. No cow's milk until after first birthday.

D. Solid foods.
1. Should be offering solid foods by 6 months 2–3 times/day.
2. Goal is to accustom infant to new textures and tastes.
3. Introduce solids with spoon; do not put cereal in bottle.
4. May begin with iron-fortified rice cereal; prepare with either breastmilk or formula.
5. Choice of foods is arbitrary and may be related to cultural and/or typical family diet.
6. Add new foods one at a time (fruits, vegetables, pureed meat) and start with 1–2 teaspoons, waiting 2–5 days between introduction of new food.
7. Limit juices to 4–6 oz/day or avoid altogether; only offer in cup.
8. Avoid feeding as a comfort measure.
9. Use fluoridated water; bottled water should have fluoride at 0.8 to 1.0 mg/L (ppm) concentration.
E. Eating habits/safety.
1. No bottles in bed.
2. Infants with strong family history of allergies should avoid foods with high allergy potential (strawberries, eggs, etc.) until end of first year.
3. No honey until after first year.
4. Vary textures from pureed to fine grind.
5. Eating is social time; include infant in family meals. Introduce cup. As infant's pincer grasp develops, may offer finger foods.
6. Position infant in highchair or infant seat to eat.

III. ELIMINATION

A. Continues to have 6 wet diapers/day.
B. Stool consistency and color change with intake of solid foods.

IV. SLEEP

A. Should be sleeping through night; 9–12 hours.
B. Naps in morning and afternoon from 30 minutes to 2 hours.
C. Regular patterns are established, although there may be occasional lapses.
D. Continue to put to bed drowsy but awake. Encourage consistent bedtime rituals.

E. Transitional objects continue to be important.

F. Night feedings not needed.

V. GROWTH AND DEVELOPMENT

A. Doubles birth weight between 5 and 6 months. Length increases 0.5 in./month; weight about 1 lb/month. Growth may occur in spurts; always plot.

B. Anterior fontanel still open, no overriding sutures palpated. Head circumference increases about 0.5–1 cm/month.

C. Rakes objects. Grasps objects with hands. Transfers objects between hands.

D. "Plays" with objects: Drops, shakes, bangs.

E. Sits alone or with minimal support and no head lag.

F. Rolls over both directions.

G. May begin to crawl

H. Bears weight on legs.

I. Moro and tonic neck reflexes have disappeared.

J. Parachute reflex emerges.

K. Responds to name.

L. Babbles ("ba," "ga," "da"), laughs, squeals.

VI. SOCIAL DEVELOPMENT

A. Enjoys interacting with parents.

B. Expects that needs will be met and expresses frustration when they are not.

C. Separation anxiety begins to emerge.

D. Begins to differentiate angry or friendly tone of others and respond accordingly.

E. Uses gestures to gain attention (pointing, reaching).

VII. IMMUNIZATIONS

A. DTaP #3.

B. Hib (depending on which vaccine used).

C. IPV #3 (3rd dose anytime between 6 and 18 months).

D. PCV #3.

E. RV (not necessary if Rotarix administered at 2 and 4 months); if RotaTeq (RV5) used, need 3rd dose.

F. Influenza annually.

G. See Appendix A.

VIII. SAFETY/ANTICIPATORY GUIDANCE

A. Always check bathwater temperature. Never leave infant alone in tub or on changing table.

B. Use sunscreen of at least SPF 15 and avoid prolonged sun exposure.

C. Use rear-facing car seat consistently, always in the back seat. Never leave infant alone in car.

D. Avoid use of walkers.

E. Baby proof environment with outlet covers, door and drawer latches, safety gates. Remove cords, wires, string, or plastic bags from baby's environment. Avoid tablecloths; remove heavy/hot objects from tables that have tablecloths.

F. Maintain smoke-free environment, ensure smoke alarms in baby's home.

G. Do not leave alone in room with pets or siblings.

H. Monitor for small objects or toys, especially if other young children present.

I. Keep bathroom door closed, toilet lid down, remove buckets with water.

J. Use protective enclosures or barriers around swimming pools, hot tubs, other water sites (ponds, fountains); also around space heaters, wood stoves, kerosene heaters.

K. Provide poison control number to be placed by telephone; syrup of ipecac no longer recommended.

L. Play games such as "peek-a-boo." Encourage reading activities with picture books, infant board books.

M. Treat teething discomfort with oral massage, frozen wet washcloths, other cold hard objects for chewing, acetaminophen, or ibuprofen. Discourage use of numbing gels because of likelihood of numbing entire oral cavity, suppressing gag reflex.

N. Assess fluoride source, supplement as necessary (see Appendix B).

O. Illness prevention.
   1. Review illness symptoms and interventions.
   2. Reinforce handwashing.
   3. Use of cool mist vaporizers for upper respiratory illness.

P. When to call healthcare provider:
   1. Breathing difficulties.
   2. Irritability.
   3. No urine output in 12 hours.
   4. Seizures.
   5. Rash.
   6. Concerns.

BIBLIOGRAPHY

American Academy of Pediatric Dentistry. Guideline on fluoride therapy. *Reference Manual: Clinical Guidelines.* 2013;36(6):171-174.

Burns CE, Dunn AM, Brady MA, Starr NB, Blosser CG. *Pediatric Primary Care.* 5th ed. Philadelphia, PA: Saunders; 2013.

Centers for Disease Control and Prevention. Recommended immunization schedules for persons aged 0 through 18 years–United States, 2015. http://www.cdc.gov/vaccines/schedules/downloads/child/0-18yrs-child-combined-schedule.pdf. Accessed February 3, 2015.

Consolini, DM. Nutrition in infants. In: *The Merck Manual Professional Edition.* http://www.merckmanuals.com/professional/pediatrics/care-of-newborns-and-infants/nutrition-in-infants?qt=nutrition%20in%20infants&alt=sh%202013#. Accessed February 5, 2015.

Hagan JF, Shaw JS, Duncan P, eds. *Bright Futures: Guidelines for Health Supervision of Infants, Children, and Adolescents.* 3rd ed. Elk Grove Village, IL: American Academy of Pediatrics; 2008.

Hirshkowitz M, Whiton K, Albert SM, et al. National Sleep Foundation's sleep time duration recommendations: methodology and results summary. *Sleep Health.* 2015;1(1):40-43.

Holt K, Wooldridge MS, Story M, Sofka D, eds. *Bright Futures: Nutrition.* 3rd ed. Elk Grove Village, IL: American Academy of Pediatrics; 2011.

Mannheim JK. Infant–newborn development. http://www.nlm.nih.gov/medlineplus/ency/article/002004.htm. Updated January 27, 2013. Accessed February 5, 2015.

United States Department of Agriculture Food and Nutrition Service. *Infant Nutrition and Feeding: A Guide for Use in the WIC and CSF Programs.* Alexandria, VA: United States Department of Agriculture; 2009.

Nine-Month Visit

Patricia Clinton

Convulsions, unspecified, R56.9	Rash and other nonspecific skin eruption, R21
Dyspnea, unspecified, R06.00	Separation anxiety disorder of childhood, F93.0

I. GENERAL IMPRESSION

    A. On the move! Need to explore critical for cognitive development.

    B. Rapidly gaining new motor/cognitive skills; 9-month-olds present new challenges to parents.

    C. Separating from parents is difficult.

II. NUTRITION

    A. Caloric needs: 98–100 kcal/kg/day.

    B. Breastfeeding/formula feeding.

       1. Infant receiving most nutrients from solid foods.

       2. Continue to encourage breastfeeding through first year.

       3. If using formula, continue with iron-fortified product.

       4. Avoid cow's milk until after first year.

    C. Assess for risk factors, screen for iron-deficiency anemia if necessary.

       1. Watch for use of cow's milk, low-iron formulas, low intake of iron-rich foods.

       2. Supplement as necessary (see Chapter 33 for more on iron-deficiency anemia).

    D. Solids.

       1. Infant should be eating table food with family.

       2. Finely chopped meats may be introduced.

3. Finger foods appropriate at this time as fine pincer grasp has developed.
4. May take up to 10 offerings before infant accepts new food.

E. Eating habits/safety.
   1. Offer liquids from cup.
   2. Limit juice to 4–6 oz/day.
   3. No honey or corn syrup (Karo) until after first year.
   4. Offer solids 3–4 times/day.
   5. Atmosphere should be relaxed, pleasant. Expect a mess!
   6. Avoid foods that may cause choking: Grapes, raisins, peanuts/peanut butter, popcorn, hard candy, carrots, celery, other hard vegetables/fruits.
   7. Encourage infant to self-feed; provide infant with spoon.
   8. Eating slows down; watch for infant cues to signal satiation, such as pushing food away.

III. ELIMINATION

A. Voiding pattern.
   1. Stays dry for longer periods.
   2. Usually voids after naps.
B. Stooling pattern.
   1. Stools usually firm, dark.
   2. Individual pattern established between 9 and 12 months.
   3. Generally 1–2 stools/day (but may vary considerably between infants).

IV. SLEEP

A. Requirements.
   1. Total sleep in 24 hours between 11 and 13 hours.
   2. Night awakenings common but should be able to put self back to sleep.
   3. Continues to nap in morning and afternoon.
B. Environment.
   1. Bedtime rituals well established.
   2. Room should remain dim and not overly warm.
C. Safety.
   1. Avoid bottles in bed.
   2. Lower crib mattress.
   3. Remind parents about removing blind or drapery cords, hanging objects (especially mobiles), small objects in cribs.

V. GROWTH AND DEVELOPMENT

A. Physical.
1. Growth is slower in second half of first year.
2. Weight gains average 1 lb/month and length 1 in./month.
3. Growth should be steady but pattern may vary from early infancy; growth spurts more common.
B. Motor.
1. Fine.
a. Pincer grasp developed. Able to pick up small objects.
b. Begins to poke with index finger.
c. Can drop, bang, throw objects.
d. Can self-feed.
2. Gross.
a. Sits well.
b. Creeping/crawling.
c. May begin to pull up on furniture.
d. Weight bearing when pulled to stand.
3. Infant reflexes.
a. Primitive reflexes should be absent.
b. Parachute reflex present and never disappears.
C. Cognitive.
1. Object permanence more prominently developed.
2. May look for objects and go after them.
D. Language.
1. Combines syllables.
2. Imitates speech sounds. Uses intonations.
3. "Dada" and "mama" are nonspecific.
4. Responds to name.
5. Responds to simple commands; understands "no."

VI. SOCIAL DEVELOPMENT

A. Relationships.
1. Beginning to indicate wants.
2. May begin to wave "bye-bye."
B. Environment: Conditions that foster trust and development of positive psycho-social feelings. Separation anxiety emerges; stranger anxiety apparent. May be fearful in new situations.

VII. IMMUNIZATIONS

A. See Appendix A: Make up for missed immunizations.

B. Influenza annually.

VIII. SAFETY

A. Infant care activities.
   1. Always check bathwater temperature.
   2. Never leave infant alone in tub, changing table, highchair.
   3. Use sunscreen; avoid prolonged sun exposure.

B. Environment.
   1. Use car seat consistently.
   2. Never leave infant alone in car.
   3. Avoid use of walkers.
   4. Reinforce "baby proofing": Outlet covers, door/drawer latches, safety gates. Remove cords, wires, string, small objects, plastic bags from baby's environment.
   5. Keep sharp objects out of reach.
   6. Maintain smoke-free environment; use smoke alarms.
   7. Do not leave alone in room with pets or young children. Keep litter boxes away from infant's environment. Feed pets in area away from infant; do not allow infant near pet when eating.
   8. Avoid tablecloths or remove heavy/hot objects from tables with tablecloths.
   9. Keep toilet lid down, remove buckets with water.
   10. Use protective enclosures around swimming pools, hot tubs, other water sites (ponds, fountains).
   11. Provide poison control number (to be placed by telephone); syrup of ipecac no longer recommended.
   12. Keep houseplants out of reach; remove any poisonous plants.

IX. ANTICIPATORY GUIDANCE

A. Parent–infant interaction.
   1. Continue to encourage floor time for infant to provide opportunities to explore.
   2. Talk with infant while engaging in other activities (e.g., grocery shopping).

3. Continue singing and movement activities with infant. Play games such as "peek-a-boo."

4. Encourage reading activities with picture books, infant board books.

5. Foster infant's ability to self-soothe with transitional objects such as blanket, stuffed toy.

B. Discipline.

1. Discuss appropriate discipline measures aimed primarily at protecting infant from injury, such as physical removal from danger.

2. Distraction most effective to redirect behavior.

3. Limited use of word "no."

4. Begin to think about rules: Keep them few and simple.

5. Consistency is key to discipline.

C. Oral hygiene.

1. No bottles in bed.

2. Use soft toothbrush without toothpaste to clean teeth. Assess fluoride source and supplement as necessary (see Appendix B).

D. Illness prevention.

1. Review illness symptoms/interventions.

2. Reinforce importance of handwashing.

3. Use cool mist vaporizer for upper respiratory illness.

E. When to call healthcare provider:

1. Breathing difficulties.

2. Seizures.

3. Irritability.

4. No urine output in 12 hours.

5. Rash.

6. Concerns.

BIBLIOGRAPHY

American Academy of Pediatric Dentistry. Guideline on fluoride therapy. *Reference Manual: Clinical Guidelines*. 2013;36(6):171-174.

Burns CE, Dunn AM, Brady MA, Starr NB, Blosser CG. *Pediatric Primary Care*. 5th ed. Philadelphia, PA: Saunders; 2013.

Centers for Disease Control and Prevention. Recommended immunization schedules for persons aged 0 through 18 years–United States, 2015. http://www.cdc.gov/vaccines/schedules/downloads/child/0-18yrs -child-combined-schedule.pdf. Accessed February 3, 2015.

Consolini DM. Nutrition in infants. In: *The Merck Manual Professional Edition*. http://www.merckmanuals.com /professional/pediatrics/care-of-newborns-and-infants/nutrition-in-infants?qt=nutrition%20in%20 infants&alt=sh%202013#. Accessed February 3, 2015.

Hagan JF, Shaw JS, Duncan P, eds. *Bright Futures: Guidelines for Health Supervision of Infants, Children, and Adolescents.* 3rd ed. Elk Grove Village, IL: American Academy of Pediatrics; 2008.

Hirshkowitz M, Whiton K, Albert SM, et al. National Sleep Foundation's sleep time duration recommendations: methodology and results summary. *Sleep Health.* 2015;1(1):40-43.

Holt K, Wooldridge MS, Story M, Sofka D, eds. *Bright Futures: Nutrition.* 3rd ed. Elk Grove Village, IL: American Academy of Pediatrics; 2011.

Mannheim JK. Infant–newborn development. http://www.nlm.nih.gov/medlineplus/ency/article/002004 .htm. Updated January 27, 2013. Accessed February 5, 2015.

United States Department of Agriculture Food and Nutrition Service. *Infant Nutrition and Feeding: A Guide for Use in the WIC and CSF Programs.* Alexandria, VA: United States Department of Agriculture; 2009.

Twelve-Month Visit

Patricia Clinton

Convulsions, unspecified, R56.9	Iron deficiency anemia, unspecified, D50.9
Dyspnea, unspecified, R06.00	Rash and other nonspecific skin eruption, R21

I. GENERAL IMPRESSION

A. Twelve-month visit heralds onset of toddlerhood.

B. Toddler's increasing mobility opens new worlds to explore and requires close supervision to prevent injuries.

II. NUTRITION

A. Caloric needs: 95–100 kcal/kg/day.

B. Breastfeeding/formula feeding.
   1. Breastfeeding may continue, but toddler is getting majority of nutrients from table food.
   2. If formula feeding, discuss switching to whole cow's milk. May use goat or soy milk.

C. Assess for risk factors, screen for iron-deficiency anemia if necessary.
   1. Birth weight $<$ 1500 grams, result of use of cow's milk or low-iron formulas during first year, low intake of iron-rich foods, low socioeconomic status.
   2. Supplement as necessary (see Chapter 33 for more on iron-deficiency anemia).

D. Solids.
   1. Offer infant variety of foods from all food groups. Typical serving size is 1 tablespoon per year of age.

      2. Offer liquids from cup.

      3. Limit juice to 4–6 oz/day. Limit whole milk to 16–24 oz/day.

  E. Eating habits/safety.

      1. Reinforce mealtime as family time.

      2. 3 meals and 2 snacks/day appropriate; be consistent with meal/snack time to avoid constant eating or grazing.

      3. Toddler's attention span limits ability to sit for long periods.

      4. Foods should be chopped into small pieces. Avoid foods that may cause choking: Grapes, raisins, peanuts, popcorn, raw vegetables.

      5. Encourage toddler to self-feed with spoon, cup.

      6. If breastfeeding, discuss interest in weaning to cup.

      7. If bottle feeding, weaning to cup should be started.

      8. Reassure parents that toddlers' eating patterns are inconsistent from meal to meal; think in terms of several days when reviewing recommended servings of foods.

III. ELIMINATION

  A. Voiding and stooling pattern.

      1. Regular patterns may be established, but these continue to be involuntary.

      2. Discourage toilet training until closer to 24 months; toilet training dependent on complete myelinization of pyramidal tracts in spinal cord.

IV. SLEEP

  A. Requirements.

      1. 11–14 hours total/day recommended; may vary from 9–10 to 15–16 hours/day.

      2. 1–2 naps/day.

  B. Environment.

      1. Put to bed in cool, quiet, dark room.

      2. Continue bedtime rituals; consistency is key.

      3. Transitional objects continue to be important.

      4. Bedtime resistance and night wakings are common.

      5. Avoid naps late in day that may interfere with nighttime sleeping.

  C. Safety.

      1. Mattress should be in lowest position to prevent climbing out of crib.

    2. No bottles in bed.

    3. All cords, small objects, plastic bags, latex balloons removed.

V. GROWTH AND DEVELOPMENT

  A. Physical.

    1. Most toddlers will have tripled birth weight.

    2. Overall growth slows; typically will gain 3–3.5 kg (6–8 lbs) in next year and gain about 12 cm (5 in.) in length.

    3. Head circumference averages about 47 cm (18 in.); brain weight doubles its birth weight in first year.

  B. Motor.

    1. Fine.

      a. Pincer grasp well developed.

      b. Puts block in cup.

      c. Can hold crayon/pencil and make marks on paper.

    2. Gross.

      a. Stands alone for a few seconds. May take some free steps.

      b. Cruising around furniture.

  C. Cognitive.

    1. Continues in Piaget's sensorimotor stage; actions more intentional.

    2. Increasing mobility fosters exploration of environment.

    3. Toddler observes other's actions, listens, touches/mouths objects.

    4. Play more spontaneous and self-initiated.

  D. Language.

    1. Expressive language is 3–4 words.

    2. "Dada" and "mama" specific.

    3. Imitates sounds.

    4. Begins to respond to simple commands.

    5. Understands "no," "hot."

    6. When an object is named, will look for it.

    7. Can follow simple one-step requests.

VI. SOCIAL DEVELOPMENT

  A. Relationships.

    1. Anxious around strangers or new/strange environments.

    2. Emotions emerge such as anger, affection.

B. Environment: Conditions that foster trust and development of positive psychosocial feelings.
1. Waves "bye-bye."
2. Plays games such as "pat-a-cake."
3. Indicates wants.
4. Imitates activity of others.

VII. IMMUNIZATIONS

A. Hepatitis B #3 if necessary.
B. Hib #4 between 12 and 18 months.
C. IPV #3 if necessary.
D. MMR between 12 and 15 months.
E. Varicella at 12 months or after.
F. PCV 12–15 months.
G. Influenza annually.
H. See Appendix A.

VIII. SAFETY

A. Toddler care activities.
1. Always check bathwater temperature; make sure hot water thermostat < 120°F (48.9°C).
2. Never leave toddler alone in tub, changing table, highchair.
3. Use sunscreen, avoid prolonged sun exposure.
B. Environment.
1. Switch to toddler car seat. Never leave toddler alone in car.
2. Never leave toddler alone outside.
3. Reexamine "baby proofing" from toddler walking perspective: Outlet covers, door/drawer latches, safety gates. Remove cords, wires, string, small objects, plastic bags from toddler's environment.
4. Climbing follows walking; anticipate dangers on counters, tables, stairs.
5. Keep sharp objects out of reach.
6. Maintain smoke-free environment; use smoke alarms.
7. Do not leave alone in room with pets or young children. Feed pets in area away from toddler. Do not allow infant near pet when eating. Keep litter boxes away from toddler's environment.
8. Avoid tablecloths or remove heavy or hot objects from tables with tablecloths.

9. Keep toilet lid down, remove buckets with water.
10. Protective enclosures around swimming pools, hot tubs, other water sites (ponds, fountains).
11. Provide poison control number (to be placed by telephone). Syrup of ipecac no longer recommended.
12. Keep houseplants out of reach; remove any poisonous plants.

IX. ANTICIPATORY GUIDANCE

A. Parent–toddler interaction.
   1. Continue to talk, sing, tell stories to toddler.
   2. Parent should make it a habit to describe what she/he is doing with toddler (e.g., "this is how we put on socks").
   3. Play games such as naming things, body parts, people.
   4. Encourage reading activities with picture books, infant board books.
   5. Limit TV to 1 hour or preferably less per day.
   6. Toddlers explore; this includes genital area.
B. Discipline.
   1. Consistency reinforces trust.
   2. Discuss appropriate discipline measures aimed primarily at protecting infant from injury; cognitively, infant cannot appreciate danger or intent.
   3. Positive reinforcement to support appropriate behavior; distraction continues to be effective.
   4. Limit use of word "no."
   5. Spanking never appropriate.
   6. Occasionally gentle physical restraint (holding toddler) may be necessary to prevent injury.
   7. Decide on a few important rules and be consistent about enforcing them.
C. Oral hygiene.
   1. No bottles in bed.
   2. Assess for bottle mouth caries.
   3. Use soft toothbrush, small pea-sized amount of fluoridated toothpaste. Assess fluoride source, supplement as necessary (see Appendix B).
   4. Make appointment for first dental visit.
D. Illness prevention.
   1. Review illness symptoms and interventions.
   2. Reinforce importance of immunizations.
   3. Reinforce importance of handwashing.
   4. Use cool mist vaporizer for upper respiratory illness.

E. When to call healthcare provider:
   1. Breathing difficulties.
   2. Seizures.
   3. Irritability.
   4. No urine output in 12 hours.
   5. Rash.
   6. Concerns.

BIBLIOGRAPHY

American Academy of Pediatric Dentistry. Guideline on fluoride therapy. *Reference Manual: Clinical Guidelines.* 2013;36(6):171-174.

Burns CE, Dunn AM, Brady MA, Starr NB, Blosser CG. *Pediatric Primary Care.* 5th ed. Philadelphia, PA: Saunders; 2013.

Centers for Disease Control and Prevention. Recommended immunization schedules for persons aged 0 through 18 years–United States, 2015. http://www.cdc.gov/vaccines/schedules/downloads/child /0-18yrs-child-combined-schedule.pdf. Accessed February 3, 2015.

Consolini DM. Nutrition in infants. In: *The Merck Manual Professional Edition.* http://www.merckmanuals.com /professional/pediatrics/care-of-newborns-and-infants/nutrition-in-infants?qt=nutrition%20in%20 infants&alt=sh%202013#. Accessed February 5, 2015.

Hagan JF, Shaw JS, Duncan P, eds. *Bright Futures: Guidelines for Health Supervision of Infants, Children, and Adolescents.* 3rd ed. Elk Grove Village, IL: American Academy of Pediatrics; 2008.

Hirshkowitz M, Whiton K, Albert SM, et al. National Sleep Foundation's sleep time duration recommendations: methodology and results summary. *Sleep Health.* 2015;1(1):40-43.

Holt K, Wooldridge MS, Story M, Sofka D, eds. *Bright Futures: Nutrition.* 3rd ed. Elk Grove Village, IL: American Academy of Pediatrics; 2011.

Mannheim JK. Infant—newborn development. http://www.nlm.nih.gov/medlineplus/ency/article/002004 .htm. Updated January 27, 2013. Accessed February 5, 2015.

United States Department of Agriculture Food and Nutrition Service. *Infant Nutrition and Feeding: A Guide for Use in the WIC and CSF Programs.* Alexandria, VA: United States Department of Agriculture; 2009.

Fifteen- to Eighteen-Month Visit

Susan G. Rains

Disorder of binocular movement, unspecified, H51.9	Separation anxiety disorder of childhood, F93.0
Rash and other nonspecific skin eruption, R21	Varus deformity, not elsewhere classified, unspecified knee, M21.169

The toddler is no longer an infant. The world is forever changed by the new ability to *move*, explore, and *control* the environment.

I. NUTRITION

A. Requirements: Growth slows in toddlerhood, decreasing energy needs to 102 kcal/kg/day (approximately 1000–1400/day), 1.23 g of protein/kg/day, fluids to 115 mL/kg/day; growth may average only 4.5 lbs/year.
   1. Servings should be 1–2 tablespoons of each food for each year of life, or about ¼–⅓ of adult servings.
   2. Milk (whole until age 2) should be limited to < 24 oz/day (16 oz is adequate) due to lack of iron and interference with intake of other nutrients. Calcium requirements are 700 mg/day and vitamin D 600 IU/day.
   3. Limit fat to < 30% of diet; protein 15–20%, carbohydrates to 55%.
   4. Screen for anemia if appropriate: Large amounts of cow's milk/day, if still on the bottle; diet deficient in other iron-rich foods.
B. Eating habits.
   1. Understanding toddlers.
      a. Lifelong eating habits, food preferences, and activity level have roots in the early self-feeding experiences of toddlers.
      b. They are able to recognize themselves as separate from others and need to explore independence by testing limits, including feeding limits.

    c. They recognize the newness and difference of foods and also crave the comfort of rituals.

    d. Toddlers often have appetite slumps or are sporadic eaters. If at daycare, they may only eat well at midday with the other children, so the parent rarely sees them eat. Or they may need 2 days to get all of the food groups in.

2. Promoting good habits: Now is the time to help your child develop healthy eating habits and make good choices. As they become more independent:

    a. Be a good role model. Eat meals as a family, without TV, at regularly scheduled times.

    b. Provide nutritious snacks 2–3 times/day in between meals, not as a reward; limit sugar. Ideas for healthy snacks including amounts: ½ cup low-sugar breakfast cereal; ½ banana; ½ cup cut-up, other soft fruit; ⅓ cup yogurt; ½ cup soft cheeses; 3–4 whole grain crackers.

    c. Allow choices and experimentation; do not force. Offer new foods several times in order to give the child an opportunity to learn to accept and like it.

    d. Allow toddler to self-feed with hands or utensils. Use cup, not bottle.

    e. Limit fruit juice to 4–6 oz/day.

    f. Serve appropriately sized portions; examples:
- ½ piece of fresh or ¼ cup canned (preferably in its own juice) fruit.
- 2 tablespoons cooked vegetables.
- 1 tablespoon smooth peanut butter (thinly spread on cracker or bread).
- ½ egg, 2 tablespoons ground meat.
- ⅓ cup yogurt, ½ cup milk.
- 1–2 crackers, ¼–½ slice of bread.

3. Safe eating.

    a. Sit when eating; avoid eating in the car.

    b. Avoid screaming, fighting, tickling while eating.

    c. Avoid foods that can cause choking:
- Popcorn.
- Hot dogs, chunks of meat.
- Globs of peanut butter with or without bread.
- Large seeds, nuts, especially peanuts (or foods containing nuts).
- Hard candy, jelly beans.
- Large chunks of raw vegetables or fruits.
- Whole grapes.
- Chewing gum.
- Carrot sticks.

4. Preventing obesity.
   a. Obesity rates in children aged 2–5 have actually gone down from 13.9% in 2004 to 8.4% in 2012, though the overall rate of obesity in children and adolescents is at an all-time high.
   b. Develop healthy eating habits at an early age, such as not overfeeding, limiting sugary foods, encouraging healthful snacks, limiting amounts, and cultivating a toddler's natural tendency to eat only when hungry.

II. ELIMINATION: TOILET TRAINING

A. Attempting to toilet train a child younger than 24 months of age is generally inadvisable; however, developmental readiness and success rates are somewhat dependent on gender, ethnicity, and even childcare settings. Most children do begin to show some interest in elimination, though perhaps not in training, between the ages of 18 and 24 months.
   1. Parents are encouraged to watch the child for signs of readiness:
      a. Child is dry at least 2 hours at a time during the day or is dry after naps.
      b. Bowel movements become regular and predictable.
      c. Facial expressions, posture, or words reveal that the child is about to urinate or have a bowel movement. This is one of the most crucial signs—to be able to tell *prior to the incident*, not just after the event, which is an earlier skill.
      d. Child asks to wear grown-up underwear.
      e. Child asks to use the potty chair or toilet.
      f. Child seems uncomfortable with soiled diapers and wants to be changed.
      g. Child is able to follow simple directions.
      h. Child is able to walk to and from the bathroom and help undress.
   2. Parents are encouraged to introduce children to the "business" of toileting by allowing children to observe older children/parents when appropriate, obtain a potty chair and sit on it, and flush the toilet.
   3. Discourage parents from considering toilet training if the child is under stress; they should not suppress their desire to use the potty, but should not pressure them in any way to train, nor be surprised if they regress. Stress factors can include:
      a. New sibling arriving.
      b. Moving houses.
      c. Family crisis such as death, major illness.

4. Encourage use of proper names for body parts and for products of elimination. Without making bowel movements sound "dirty" or "nasty," teach children that we do not play with feces.

5. Pick a potty chair that offers foot support either in the chair itself or because it is low to the floor. Some children may prefer to use the adult toilet with a "ring," making it an appropriate fit.

6. Read books about pottying together with the child.

7. Try to make pottying routine. Everyone generally goes first thing in the morning, before bed, before bath, after meals. Try for a few minutes, but don't fight about it as that undoubtedly will hinder the process.

8. Be sensitive to the child's fears concerning toileting such as "loud" toilets, spilling potties, using public restrooms, differences over having bowel movements and urinating.

9. Positive reinforcement and sensing the child's readiness and pace of learning are essential for success.

III. SLEEP

A. Requirements.
   1. Averages 12 hours total/day.
   2. One to two naps/day; may have difficulty combining morning and afternoon naps.

B. Difficulty with sleep.
   1. Common, especially going to sleep and falling asleep.
   2. May be due to separation anxiety and independence issues.

C. Strategies to assist sleep.
   1. Bedtime rituals: Standard sleep time, snack, quiet activity.
   2. Utilizing transitional objects such as special toy, blanket.
   3. Place child in bed while *awake*.
   4. Check on child at progressively longer intervals.
   5. Comfort, but do not feed, rock, or place child in bed with parent.
   6. Ideally, institute above strategies prior to child being able to climb out of crib.

IV. GROWTH AND DEVELOPMENT

A. Physical growth slows.
   1. Average increases in second year of life: 5 lbs, height 3", OFC 1".
   2. Anterior fontanel closes by 18 months.

3. Head is in smaller proportion to the body.
4. Physique ducklike: Lordotic, pot-bellied, bow-legged.
5. Vision binocular (true strabismus should be referred).
6. 14 teeth averaged by 18 months.
7. Immune system much better developed, but passive immunities from mother gone (especially if not breastfed) and just beginning increased exposure to antigens in environment.

B. Development.
1. Physical: Utilizing newly developed locomotion skills and wanting to control the environment. Toddlers push and carry large objects; put themselves into spaces such as boxes, cabinets, and under tables; delight in repetitive throwing and retrieving; scribbling. Handedness is established.
2. Speech: By 18 months, understands much of language spoken to him but commands relatively few words (has good receptive skills). Largest jump in language is in second half of second year. The "big talkers" tend to be first-born girls.
3. Emotional/social: Toddlers strive for independence, autonomy, and are looking for admiration and positive reinforcement of newly found skills. They still experience dependency needs (separation anxiety) during this quest. Beginning body image development. Negativism is a part of individualization. May be becoming aware of gender.
4. Cognitive (intellectual): Toddlers are beginning to work on causality with an increase in physical abilities and memory development. Starting to see objects symbolically. Imagination begins.
   Note: Early signs of autism spectrum disorder (ASD), including atypical development in socialization and communication, are now detected by pediatric providers in children as young as toddlerhood. The American Academy of Pediatrics recommends screening all children for ASD at ages 18 and 24 months using a standardized questionnaire. Most pediatric practices use the Modified Checklist for Autism in Toddlers Revised (M-CHAT-R). Broadly, early signs of autism behaviors include decreases in frequency of gaze to the examiner's face, social smiles, and vocalizations to others.

C. Developmental milestones.
1. By 15 months: Says 3–6 words; can point to a body part; understands simple commands; walks well; stoops; climbs stairs; stacks two blocks; feeds self with fingers; drinks from a cup; listens to a story; tells what he wants by pulling, pointing, or grunting.
2. By 18 months: Walks backward; throws ball; says 15–20 words; imitates words; uses two-word phrases; pulls a toy along the ground; stacks three

blocks; uses a spoon and cup; listens to a story, looking at pictures and naming objects; shows affection; kisses; follows simple directions; points to some body parts; scribbles.

D. Developmental delay: Possible referral if not present by 18 months:
   1. Walks upstairs with assistance.
   2. Self-feeds, with spoon at times.
   3. Mimics actions of others.
   4. Uses at least 6 words.

V. SOCIAL

A. Growth, development, and socialization of the child are demonstrated in play activities. The toddler progresses from the sensorimotor play of infancy to parallel play, incorporating imitation, fine and gross motor skills, and new language.

B. Appropriate toys for the toddler are: Swing sets, sandboxes, play kitchens, play tools, musical and "talking" toys (especially interactive ones), riding toys (especially without pedals), push toys, balls, containers, telephones, mirrors, dolls and puppets, large crayons, and books. (Contact Reach Out and Read for information in setting up a literacy promotion program in clinics and offices: www.reachoutandread.org.)

C. The toddler's new mobility and drive for autonomy make discipline a new challenge for the parent and caregiver. Appropriate discipline guidelines for the toddler include offering choices when available, including following a "no" with a "yes"; keeping rules simple and few; removing objects about which there is constant disagreement; "catching the child being good"; and rewarding positive behaviors with verbal praise and physical affection. Time-out is not appropriate until 2.5–3 years.

D. Parents should be encouraged to help the child learn to express emotions such as joy, fear, anger, sadness, and frustration.

E. Dealing with temper tantrums.
   1. Tantrums are a frequent occurrence in toddlers as the young child begins to establish independence and easily becomes frustrated in doing so. He also often does not have his every need met immediately (hunger and fatigue) and is even told "no" on occasion.
   2. Parents should: Attend to hunger and sleep needs if possible to help allay underlying causes; stay calm, firm, and consistent; help allay frustrations by helping the child do/learn whatever it is that is frustrating him/her; distract the child by offering an alternate activity; quietly walk away.

3. Time out can be used with a toddler. One minute per year of age is recommended for time out. This may be too long for a toddler, however, and the adult may need to help the child physically (and calmly) stay in time out, again, keeping all conversation to a minimum, to avoid reinforcing negative behavior by giving it attention. Many children quickly learn that they are able to acquire a parent's one-on-one attention with negative behavior and often do not care if it is negative attention.

4. Praise and give reinforcement for positive behaviors such as tantrums ceasing. Give choices if possible.

5. Spanking has no place in the discipline (which means teaching) of children. When spanking and hitting are used by parents, children often learn to use physical force to express anger and deal with conflict.

6. Signs of abnormal behaviors may include: Self-injurious behavior during a tantrum, consistent aggressive behavior toward others or destructive behavior toward objects > 50% of the time during a tantrum, high frequency of tantrums (> 5/day or > 10–20/month), tantrums > 25 minutes.

VI. SAFETY

A. Toddlers are at increased risk for injury due to increased locomotion and primitive cognition. Leading causes of death and injury and prevention strategies are listed.

B. Motor vehicles.
   1. Use federally approved car seat in backseat of vehicle. Previous guidelines said that the child could face forward if older than 1 year and > 20 lbs but now it is recommended that a child be rear-facing until 2 years of age. Use 1-866-SEAT-CHECK or www.seatcheck.org for child safety seat inspection.
   2. Use bike helmet.
   3. Teach children pedestrian/vehicle safety.
   4. Never allow toddlers to play alone outside.

C. Poisoning.
   1. Use child-proof caps on medications; keep medications and household poisons (including plants) out of reach or better locked.
   2. Have poison control number readily available for all caregivers, 1-800-222-1222. Never tell children medication is candy.
   3. Screen for lead risk. See screening guidelines.

D. Burns.
   1. Use caution in kitchen with young children present.
   2. Turn handles of cooking utensils away from outer edge of stove.

      3. Adjust hot water to 120°F.

      4. Keep matches/candles out of reach.

      5. Use sunscreen when children are exposed to sunlight.

      6. Keep sockets covered and cords out of sight.

      7. Have working smoke detector on every floor of the house.

E. Drowning.

      1. Supervise closely near any water, including buckets.

      2. Fence swimming pools.

      3. Close bathroom doors and put lid down on toilet.

      4. Utilize life preservers in addition to above.

F. Choking and suffocation.

      1. Do not give danger foods listed in nutrition section (including nuts, hot dogs, gum, hard candy).

      2. Only allow play with age-appropriate items (no small pieces).

      3. Discard old appliances/furniture or remove doors.

      4. Keep automatic garage door opener inaccessible.

      5. Select safe toy chests without heavy, hinged lid.

G. Falls.

      1. Confine play in fenced areas.

      2. Supervise all climbing play.

      3. Place gates at top and bottom of stairs.

      4. Lock windows, screens, doors.

      5. Keep crib rails up and mattress at lowest level.

      6. Keep bumper pads and large stuffed animals out of crib or playpen (child may climb on top).

      7. Dress in safe clothing that will not catch or drag.

H. Other injuries.

      1. Never leave children alone in a car or at home.

      2. Do not allow play near any machinery.

      3. Do not allow running with sharp objects or with anything in the mouth.

      4. Teach children to avoid strange animals, especially ones that are eating.

      5. Avoid personalized clothing in a public place.

      6. Use safety glass and decals on large windows/doors.

      7. Remove guns from house.

VII. IMMUNIZATIONS

A. HIB #4 if not previously given.

B. PCV #4.

C. IPV #3.

D. DTaP #4.

E. Hepatitis B #3 if not previously given.

F. MMR #1 if not previously given.

G. Varivax if not previously given.

H. Hepatitis A if not previously given. Often given at 12 months and at least 6 months later.

I. Influenza seasonally.

J. See Appendix A.

VIII. OTHER SCREENINGS IF RISK ASSESSMENT INDICATES

A. Dental (ensure fluoride source).

B. B/P: If high risk history.

C. Vision: Prematurity < 32 weeks, family history of ophthalmologic problems (other than acuity).

D. Hearing: Caregiver concern, postnatal infection, head trauma, family history, certain syndromes associated with hearing loss.

E. TB: Exposure, born outside United States, HIV associated.

F. Lead screening: Recommendations vary by state as incidence has decreased in young children due to surveillance efforts. States are charged with identifying geographic areas at risk and children at risk due to exposure. WIC centers generally facilitate lead screening. Children should be screened at 9–12 months and again at about 2 years by a questionnaire and/or lab if found to be at risk.

IX. ANTICIPATORY GUIDANCE

A. Primary responsibility of the PNP is to assist the parent in understanding and parenting this emerging person—the toddler—and his thoughts, behaviors, and needs, as well as attending to the parent's needs.

B. Social competence.

1. Give individual attention, create opportunities for exploration and physical action.

2. Encourage self-care, self-expression, choices.

3. Limit number of rules but consistently enforce them.

4. Suggest acceptable alternatives.

5. Keep discipline brief.

6. Allow assertiveness within limits, but no hitting, biting, or aggressive behavior.

7. Reassure once negative behavior has stopped.

8. Delay toilet training.
9. Expect genital curiosity.

C. Family relationships.
1. Parent needs to take time for himself or herself and with partner.
2. Pick up toddler, hold, cuddle, show affection.
3. Listen, show respect and interest in activities.
4. Encourage all family members to spend time playing with toddler.
5. Help child express emotions.
6. Keep family outings short.
7. Do not expect child to share all toys.
8. Help siblings resolve conflicts. Allow older children own space/things.
9. Serve as role model for healthy habits and care.

D. Health promotion.
1. Nutrition.
   a. Eat meals as family.
   b. Allow toddler to self-feed with hands and utensils and drink from cup, not bottle.
   c. Provide healthy choices, allow experimentation, and do not force eating.
   d. Give two to three snacks/day, not as a reward; limit sugar.
   e. Avoid choking foods.
2. Oral health.
   a. Never put to bed with a bottle.
   b. Brush teeth (allow imitation, but parent must do the job well).
   c. Investigate level of fluoride in child's water.
   d. Encourage making appointment with dentist.
3. Injury prevention (expanded list in safety section).
   a. Maintain smoke-free environment.
   b. Check smoke and carbon monoxide detectors.
   c. Check car seat use.
   d. Reexamine home to ensure it is child-proof.
   e. Supervise toddler closely, especially near dogs, lawnmowers, streets, and driveways.
   f. Ensure water safety.
   g. Use sunscreen.
   h. Discuss first-aid procedures.

E. Community interaction.
1. Assess needs of the family for appropriate referrals: Financial assistance, Medicaid, housing, transportation.
2. Refer child for appropriate developmental, physical, behavioral problems.
3. Refer parent to support group if appropriate.

4. Review childcare.
5. Maintain community involvement by attending local activities.

BIBLIOGRAPHY

American Academy of Pediatrics. *Red Book: Report of the Committee on Infectious Diseases.* http://www .aapredbook.org

American Academy of Pediatrics Committee on Infectious Diseases. Recommended childhood and adolescent immunization schedule–United States, 2015. *Pediatrics.* 2015;135(2):396-397.

American Academy of Pediatrics Committee on Injury, Violence, and Poison Prevention. Poison treatment in the home. *Pediatrics.* 2003;112(5):1182-1185.

Belden AC, Thomas NR, Luby JL. Temper tantrums in healthy versus depressed and disruptive preschoolers: defining tantrum behaviors associated with clinical problems. *J Pediatrics.* 2008;152(1):117-122.

Burns CE, Dunn AM, Brady MA, Starr NB, Blosser CG. *Pediatric Primary Care: A Handbook for Nurse Practitioners.* 5th ed. Philadelphia, PA: Saunders; 2013.

Centers for Disease Control and Prevention. Vaccines and immunizations. http://www.cdc.gov/vaccines

Children's Medicine. HEAT: healthy eating and activity together. Early childhood parent tips. http://www .childrensmedicine.net/nutrition/heat-early-childhood.html. Accessed March 7, 2015.

Food Nutrition and Information Center. Toddler nutrition and health resource list. http://www.nal.usda.gov /fnic/pubs/toddler.pdf

Gabrielsen TP, Farley M, Speer L, Villalobos M, Baker CN, Miller J. Identifying autism in a brief observation. *Pediatrics.* 2015;135(2):e330-e338.

Gidding SS, Dennison BA, Birch LL, et al. Dietary recommendations for children and adolescents: a guide for practitioners. *Pediatrics.* 2006;117(2):544-559.

Glascoe FP, Marks KP. Developmental-behavioral screening and surveillance. In: Kliegman RM, Stanton BF, St. Geme J, Schor N, Behrman RE, eds. *Nelson Textbook of Pediatrics.* 19th ed. Philadelphia, PA: WB Saunders; 2011:39-44.

Gottesman MM. Nurturing the social and emotional development of children, a.k.a. discipline. *J Pediatr Health Care.* 2000;14(2):81-84.

Gottesman MM. Helping toddlers eat well. *J Pediatr Health Care.* 2002;16:92-96.

Hagan JF, Shaw JS, Duncan P, eds. *Bright Futures: Guidelines for Health Supervision of Infants, Children, and Adolescents.* 3rd ed. Elk Grove Village, IL: American Academy of Pediatrics; 2008.

Howell DM, Wysocki K, Steiner MJ. Toilet training. *Pediatr Rev.* 2010;31(6):262-263.

Liu J, Liu X, Wang W, et al. Blood lead concentrations and children's behavioral and emotional problems: a cohort study. *JAMA Pediatr.* 2014;168(8):737-745.

Ozonoff S, Iosif AM, Baguio F, et al. A prospective study of the emergence of early behavioral signs of autism. *J Am Acad Child Adolesc Psychiatry.* 2010;49(3):256-266.

Peterson S, Sigman-Grant M. Impact of adopting lower-fat food choices on nutrient intake of American children. *Pediatrics.* 1997;100(3):e4.

Reach Out and Read [homepage]. http://www.reachoutandread.org

Slade EP, Wissow LS. Spanking in early childhood and later behavior problems: a prospective study of infants and young toddlers. *Pediatrics.* 2004;113(5):1321-1330.

United States Department of Agriculture. Choose MyPlate. http://www.choosemyplate.gov

United States Department of Agriculture. National nutrient database for standard reference. http://ndb.nal .usda.gov

Vazquez M, LaRussa P, Gershon AA, et al. Effectiveness over time of varicella vaccine. *JAMA.* 2004;291(7):851-855.

Wardle J, Guthrie C, Sanderson S, Birch L, Plomin R. Food and activity preferences in children of lean and obese parents. *Int J Obes Relat Metab Disord.* 2001;25(7):971-977.

Two-Year Visit

Frances K. Porcher

Consulsions, unspecified, R56.9	Fever of other and unknown origin, R50
Dyspnea, unspecified, R06.00	Rash and other nonspecific skin eruption, R21

I. GENERAL IMPRESSION

   A. Two-year old is very active, has good vocabulary, and is integral part of family.

II. NUTRITION

   A. Quadruples birth weight by age 2 years.
   B. Average 2-year-old weighs 12.5–13.5 kg (26–28 lbs), is 85–90 cm (34–35 in.) tall, has head circumference of 48–50 cm (19–19.5 in.).
   C. Requires approximately 102 kcal/kg.
   D. Needs approximately 1.2 g/kg of protein, 500–800 mg of calcium, 10 mg iron.
   E. Fluoride supplement is necessary if water supply contains < 0.3 ppm fluoridation (see Appendix B).
   F. Requires 2–3 servings of protein, 2–4 servings of fruit, 3–5 servings of vegetables, 6–11 servings of grains, and 2 servings of milk each day.
   G. Limit juice to 4–6 oz/day. Offer skim, 1%, 2% milk versus whole milk.
   H. Offer 5–6 smaller nutritious meals or snacks each day.
   I. Start limiting fat intake to ≈30% of daily calories.
   J. Child's serving is about ⅔ of a standard adult serving.
   K. Needs structured mealtime environment.
   L. Has unpredictable eating habits (likes one food one day but not next day).

M. Usually eats only 1–2 foods at meal.

N. Feeds self, loves finger foods.

O. Complete set of 20 primary teeth (second molars may not erupt until age 3 years).

P. Assess child's risk for hyperlipidemia.

III. ELIMINATION

A. Regular elimination pattern is usually established with soft, formed stool daily or every other day and several urinations/day.

B. Toilet training is major developmental task between ages 2 ½ and 3 ½ years.

C. Ready for toilet training if bowel movements are regular, child interested in toileting.

IV. SLEEP

A. Should be able to sleep all night and maintain one nap/day.

B. Important to have pleasant bedtime routine.

C. Not uncommon to experience nighttime sleep awakenings, bedtime difficulties.

D. May sleep in crib or small bed depending on child's size, climbing skills.

V. GROWTH AND DEVELOPMENT

A. Age of autonomy, egocentrism, negativism.

B. Gains 4.5–6.6 lbs and 2.5–3.5 in./year from ages 2–5 years.

C. Gross motor: Runs without falling; kicks large ball; jumps; walks up/down stairs one step at a time.

D. Fine motor: Stacks 5–6 blocks; makes/imitates horizontal/circular strokes with crayon/large pencil; manipulates/solves single-piece puzzle; can unravel, undo, untie.

E. Language: 50% of speech is understandable by stranger; has at least a 20-word vocabulary; uses 2-word phrases; understands more than says; understands and uses "I" and "you"; clearly verbalizes wants; follows 2-step commands.

F. Fears bodily harm (limit intrusive procedures, soften approaches).

G. Increasingly independent, loves to explore.

H. Negativity, temper tantrums often become an issue (hence, the "terrible twos").

I. Empower child by offering acceptable choices to limit frustrations and tantrums.

J. Time-out measures (no longer than 2 minutes/episode) recommended rather than hitting or spanking for discipline.

K. Consistency with discipline by all persons involved with child measures important (discipline for same behavior tomorrow as today).

L. Lots of love, reassurance needed.

VI. SOCIAL DEVELOPMENT

A. Increasingly independent, curious (exploring, climbing, hiding).

B. Active and delightful but testy and frustrating at times as child learns to become social.

C. Frustration manifested as temper tantrums.

D. Differentiates self from others but still needs frequent parental reassurance.

E. Common to experience stranger anxiety (will hide head in parent's arms/ behind legs).

F. Engages in parallel play (plays alongside peers, not with them).

G. Imitates adult activities/tasks (e.g., sweeping, dusting, shaving, combing hair).

H. Often develops fears (e.g., fear of going down toilet with flushing).

I. Needs positive behavior reinforced frequently (praise good behaviors).

VII. IMMUNIZATIONS

A. Bring up to date.

B. Consider varicella vaccine if no reliable history of disease or if not previously given.

C. Consider hepatitis A vaccine if indicated by geographical area of residence.

D. Consider tuberculin skin test (PPD) if meets risk criteria.

E. See Appendix A.

VIII. SAFETY

A. Install and periodically check smoke alarms.

B. Ensure crib slats are no more than 2⅜ in. apart.

C. Avoid crib mobiles due to risk of strangulation or choking.

D. With small bed, ensure mattress is close to floor to minimize injury if child falls out of bed.

E. Encourage use of potty chair that sits directly on floor rather than toilet.

F. Remove dangling objects such as blind cords, curtain draws.

G. Supervise play and do not allow toys with small or sharp parts.

H. Supervise eating: Do not allow foods that may lead to choking (popcorn, peanuts, marshmallows, wieners, raw vegetables).

I. Use child-proof lids on all medications; store medications in locked cabinet.

J. Keep household cleaning products out of reach.

K. Use gates and fences where appropriate to prevent falls.

L. Supervise in kitchen (turn pot handles away from edge of stove, store knives out of sight).

M. Supervise around water; set hot water thermostat to $< 120°F$ (48.9°C).

N. Use child-approved sunscreen with at least SPF 15.

O. Use child safety seats approved for child's weight at all times in motor vehicles. If weighs at least 20 lbs, use forward-facing car seat in middle of backseat; never place car seat in front seat of vehicle with a passenger airbag.

P. Teach stranger safety.

IX. ANTICIPATORY GUIDANCE

A. Nutrition.
1. Will eat variety of all food groups. Will eat larger servings.
2. Still likes finger foods but can use child-sized fork, spoon.
3. Continues to drink skim, 1%, 2% milk (no more than 2–3 cups/day). Avoid flavored milk and soda.
4. Encourage to drink water, especially if playing outside in heat.
5. Encourage to wash hands before eating.
6. Brushes teeth with fluoridated toothpaste and parents' assistance.
7. Needs dental check-up.

B. Elimination.
1. Daytime and nighttime bowel movement control established by age 3 years.
2. Daytime urine control established by age 3 years. May still experience nighttime urination.
3. Needs to be encouraged to wash hands after toileting and blowing nose.

C. Sleep.
1. Continues to need regular bedtime routine.
2. Needs 10–12 hours of sleep at night (does usually awaken).
3. Usually continues to have one daytime nap.

      4. Should sleep in own bed alone.

      5. May experience nightmares.

D. Growth and development.

      1. Rate of growth slowing down.

      2. Gross motor: Jumps in place, kicks ball, throws ball overhand, rides tricycle, climbs everything.

      3. Fine motor: Copies circle and cross, dresses self, feeds self using small fork, washes and dries hands, can put on T-shirt, may be able to dress self without help.

      4. Language: At least 50% of speech is understandable, uses sentences, can carry on a conversation of 2–3 sentences, uses prepositions, may use adjectives, may be able to identify 4 colors, identifies friend by naming, identifies 4 pictures by naming, knows own name, age, gender.

E. Social.

      1. Parallel play still prevails; unlikely to share toys.

      2. Should not view more than 1 hour television/video/computer per day.

      3. Needs daily physical activities (outdoors if possible).

      4. Curious about body parts, may start exploring (use correct terms for body parts).

      5. Needs positive reinforcement of good behaviors.

F. Safety.

      1. Needs supervision while playing, eating, when around water.

      2. Continues to need child safety seat or restraint appropriate to child's weight.

      3. May be able to learn own telephone number.

G. Immunizations: If current, should not need any until age 4 years.

H. When to call healthcare provider:

      1. Breathing difficulties.

      2. Seizures.

      3. No urine output in 12 hours.

      4. Rashes.

      5. Fever.

      6. Concerns.

I. Sibling rivalry.

      1. Defined as jealousy that develops between brothers and sisters as they compete for parental time, attention, love, and approval.

      2. Often occurs following arrival of second child in family.

      3. Older child often becomes aggressive, acts out, or regresses.

4. Prevention is key. Discuss new baby during pregnancy, allow firstborn to help make decisions, including preparations for new baby, move older child to new bed months before arrival of new baby.

5. After baby arrives, spend one-on-one time with older child, listen to how older child feels, let child know he/she is special, try not to compare two siblings, and do not play favorites.

6. Passive noninterventions recommended for minor squabbles between older siblings, such as ignoring the conflict or allowing children to resolve the conflict themselves.

7. Encouraging articulation of disagreements recommended for more significant conflicts in older children, such as allowing siblings to express emotions and problem solve with parental support.

8. Parental intervention recommended in situations involving physical or verbal abuse—do not allow older sibling to hit new baby; avoid yelling; separate children if necessary and discuss actions after everyone has calmed down.

BIBLIOGRAPHY

Anderson JE. Sibling rivalry: when the family circle becomes a boxing ring. *Contemp Pediatr.* 2006;23(2):72-84.

Burns CE, Dunn AM, Brady MA, Starr NB, Blosser CG. *Pediatric Primary Care.* 5th ed. Philadelphia, PA: Saunders, 2013.

Dixon SD, Stein MT. *Encounters with Children: Pediatric Behavior and Development.* St. Louis, MO: Mosby, 2006.

Hagan JF, Shaw JS, Duncan P, eds. *Bright Futures: Guidelines for Health Supervision of Infants, Children, and Adolescents.* 3rd ed. Elk Grove Village, IL: American Academy of Pediatrics; 2008.

Holt K, Woolridge N, Story M, Sofka D, eds. *Bright Futures in Practice: Nutrition.* 3rd ed. Arlington, VA: National Center for Education in Maternal and Child Health; 2011.

Three-Year Visit (Preschool)

Frances K. Porcher

Nightmares, F51.5	Sleep terrors [night terrors], F51.4

I. GENERAL IMPRESSION

A. Three-year-old is active, increasingly independent, and easily understood by most people; is very self-determined and unpredictable; and is a master at attempting to negotiate.

II. NUTRITION

A. Requires approximately 100 kcal/kg (1000–1100 calories/day).

B. Fluoride supplement is necessary if water supply contains < 0.3 ppm fluoridation (see Appendix B).

C. Requires 2 servings of protein, 2 servings of fruit, 3 servings of vegetables, 7 servings of grains, and 16–24 oz of milk (skim, 1%, or 2%) each day.

D. Limit juice to 4–6 oz/day; offer water.

E. Child's serving is about ⅔ of a standard adult serving.

F. Uses a fork or spoon fairly well.

G. Needs structured mealtime environment, with family if possible.

H. Has 20 primary teeth, and second molars may have erupted.

III. ELIMINATION

A. Toilet trained for daytime, occasional accidents.

B. Regular pattern for bowel movements.

IV. SLEEP

A. Requires 10–12 hours of sleep a night.

B. One nap or quiet time/day.

C. Is common to arouse several times a night, may need brief comforting/reassurance.

D. May have night terrors or nightmares:
   1. Night terrors:
      a. Occur early after going to bed.
      b. Has partial arousal from very deep sleep; screams, thrashes about during the terror; returns to sleep without fully awakening and has no memory of incident in morning.
   2. Nightmares:
      a. Occur usually during the second half of night.
      b. Has scary dream followed by complete awakening; crying and fearful after awakening; may have trouble falling back to sleep; remembers and may talk about it in the morning.

V. GROWTH AND DEVELOPMENT

A. Graceful, agile, good posture.

B. Gains 4–6 lbs and 2–4 in./year.

C. Gross motor: Alternates feet when going up stairs; may ride tricycle; dresses self, including shoes but may need help with buttons and tying shoes; climbs, jumps, and hops.

D. Fine motor: Holds crayon with fingers; copies circle and cross; draws a person with two body parts; can snip with scissors.

E. Language: Has approximately 900–1500 words; uses longer sentences; can put 2–3 sentences together; uses plurals, pronouns, and some prepositions ("under," "on," "in," "out"); understands concepts of big/little, up/down; can tell name, gender, age; can recognize some colors; can name a friend; listens to adult conversations and may repeat what is heard; bilingual preschooler should be equally competent in both languages.

VI. SOCIAL DEVELOPMENT

A. Needs exposure to other children to play with in order to learn socialization; can separate easily from parents if wants to; can take turns; wants to help with simple chores (sweeping, wiping); wants to make own choices; starts to identify and name feelings (happy, sad); developing table and social manners (please, thank you); becoming aware of gender differences.

B. Discipline should involve distraction, warnings, and time out if necessary.

C. May regress when a new sibling arrives.

VII. IMMUNIZATIONS

A. See Appendix A: No scheduled immunizations at this visit; may need catch-up.

VIII. SAFETY

A. Needs constant vigilance, supervision, patience.

B. Safety-proof living and play environments and reinforce safety issues (stairs, streets).

C. Secure doors/windows.

D. Teach and reinforce water safety.

E. Teach and reinforce gun safety (locked, unloaded, ammunition stored apart from guns).

F. Remove/lock up toxic substances and all medicines.

G. Use car seat; continue to keep in backseat of vehicle.

H. Wear helmet when riding any toy with wheels (tricycle, scooter).

I. Use sunscreen (SPF 15 or higher) and wear sunglasses.

J. Teach and reinforce concepts of "good touch/bad touch/secret touch."

IX. ANTICIPATORY GUIDANCE

A. Promote active play indoors (imagination, safe toys) and outdoors (balls, jump ropes, toys with wheels).

B. Limit TV/computer viewing to 1–2 hours/day or less.

C. Read books together.

D. Encourage development of child's imagination (pretend play, tell stories).

E. Offer opportunities to make choices (clothes, books, activities); link with consequences.

F. Offer praise.

G. Promote toilet training if not already accomplished.

H. Promote dental health (brushing, flossing, dental visits).

I. Use consistent discipline as a way to learn rules, not just as punishment; use limit-setting.

J. Share mealtime with family if possible.

K. Avoid food struggles; offer food family eats, avoid making separate meals for child, avoid snacking if doesn't eat meal.

L. Offer nutritional snacks and avoid fast food/processed food.

BIBLIOGRAPHY

Burns CE, Dunn AM, Brady MA, Starr NB, Blosser CG. *Pediatric Primary Care*. 5th ed. Philadelphia, PA: Saunders, 2013.

Dixon SD, Stein MT. *Encounters with Children: Pediatric Behavior and Development*. 4th ed. St. Louis, MO: Mosby, 2006.

Hagan JF, Shaw JS, Duncan P, eds. *Bright Futures: Guidelines for Health Supervision of Infants, Children, and Adolescents*. 3rd ed. Elk Grove Village, IL: American Academy of Pediatrics; 2008.

Story M, Holt K, Sofka D, eds. *Bright Futures in Practice: Nutrition*. 2nd ed. Arlington, VA: National Center for Education in Maternal and Child Health; 2002.

Six-Year Visit (School Readiness)

Jane A. Fox

Attention-deficit hyperactivity disorder, combined type, F90.2	Mental disorder, not otherwise specified, F99
Attention-deficit hyperactivity disorder, predominantly hyperactive type, F90.1	Nightmares, F51.5
	Nonorganic encopresis, F98.1
Attention-deficit hyperactivity disorder, predominantly inattentive type, F90.0	Sleep terrors [night terrors], F51.4
	Sleepwalking [somnambulism], F51.3
Attention-deficit hyperactivity disorder, unspecified type, F90.9	Social phobia, unspecified, F40.10
Disturbance of activity and attention, F90.0	Other specified urinary incontinence, N39.498

I. GENERAL IMPRESSION

A. Six-year-old will be attending school perhaps for first time and is quite excited about it. The 6-year-old is becoming much more independent.

II. NUTRITION

A. Caloric and nutrient needs.
  1. 90 kcal/kg/day (1200 to 1400 cal/day) divided into 3 meals with 2 nutritious snacks.
  2. Limit junk food, nonnutritious foods.
  3. Refer to MyPlate (choosemyplate.gov/kids) for serving size, food group recommendations (see Appendix E).
  4. Encourage family meals as often as possible.

B. Oral hygiene.
   1. Semiannual dental visits.
   2. Regular tooth brushing twice/day.
   3. Fluoride supplement in diet or drinking water (see Appendix B).
   4. Discourage thumb sucking.

III. ELIMINATION

A. Most 6-year-olds are toilet trained but may have occasional accidents.
B. Frequency of bowel movements varies. Obtain parental input for what is normal for child; 1–3 times/day to 1 time every 2–3 days is acceptable.
C. Normal urine volume should be similar to adult: 650–1500 mL/day.
D. Urination frequency approximately 5–6 times/day.
E. Approximately 5–7% have problematic enuresis; 16% of 6-year-olds have nocturnal enuresis.
F. Occasional incontinence due to miscues/deep sleep not uncommon.

IV. SLEEP

A. 8–12 hours/night.
B. Encourage consistent bedtime routine.
C. Occasional nightmares are normal.
D. Night terrors/sleepwalking may emerge.

V. GROWTH AND DEVELOPMENT

A. Average weight gain/year: 2–3 kg (4–7 lbs.) for both boys and girls.
B. Average linear growth/year: 5–6 cm (2 in.) for both boys and girls.
C. AAP recommends use of BMI to screen for overweight and obesity in children beginning at 2 years of age. Plot on CDC-BMI for age growth charts available for both girls and boys.
D. Well-established vocabulary.
E. Can follow 3-step directions.
F. Moves from magical thinking to concrete operations.
G. Starts to grasp the concept of time.
H. Begins to understand feelings of others but still focused on self.
I. Grows more independent but feels less secure.

   J. Craves affection from parents/caregivers/teachers.

   K. Mastered skills.

      1. Personal.

         a. Independent in dressing, hygiene; feeds self, monitoring only as needed.

         b. Can recite address, phone number.

      2. Fine motor.

         a. Can draw/copy shapes.

         b. Can draw a man with 6 parts.

         c. Can print some letters, numbers.

      3. Language.

         a. Can articulate needs, but semantics may be incorrect.

         b. Recognizes most letters of alphabet.

         c. Can define at least 7 words.

         d. Can identify some opposites.

         e. Can learn now from language and logic.

      4. Gross motor.

         a. Can balance on each foot for 6 seconds.

         b. Can heel–toe walk forward and backward.

         c. Rides tricycle without problems.

VI. SOCIAL DEVELOPMENT

   A. The child is beginning to move from family relationships as primary focus to peer relationships as primary focus.

   B. Continues to use play to develop skills, competencies, and learn about his world.

   C. Social cooperation, morality, critical thinking, and self-concept are developing.

   D. Demonstrates cooperative play.

   E. Team/group activities encouraged (arts programs, organized clubs/sports, etc.); regular exercise encouraged.

   F. Making friends is primary social goal; developing "best friends."

   G. Developing conflict resolution skills.

VII. IMMUNIZATIONS

   A. Recommended.

      1. DTaP #5 if not done previously.

      2. IPV #4 if not done previously.

      3. MMR #2 if not done previously.

4. PPD #1 if not done previously.
5. Varicella #2 if not previously done.
6. Influenza annually.
B. Catch-up.
1. Hepatitis B series.
2. Varicella.
3. MMR.
4. DTaP.
5. Hepatitis A.
C. High-risk children.
1. Influenza (yearly).
2. Hepatitis A series.
3. Pneumococcal pneumonia vaccine.
4. PPD (yearly).
5. Meningococcal.
D. See Appendix A.

VIII. SAFETY

A. Motor vehicle.
1. Consistent use of appropriate safety restraints in motor vehicles.
2. Knows appropriate pedestrian safety rules.
3. Riding a motorcycle is discouraged; however, consistently uses helmet when passenger on motorcycle.
B. Sports/recreation.
1. Consistent use of appropriate protective equipment for all activities (biking, rollerblading, sports, boating, etc.).
2. Always wear a helmet when riding bike or rollerblading.
3. Discuss adequate hydration.
4. Ensure appropriate safety instruction provided for all activities.
5. Obtain swim lessons.
6. Use sunscreen of SPF 15 or higher and reapply as directed on container.
7. Discourage use of mini-bikes and ATVs.
C. Household.
1. Never leave child without appropriate supervision.
2. Teach appliance safety and monitor use.
3. Teach hazardous materials/medication safety. Keep out of reach and monitor use.
4. Teach fire safety. Develop family plan.

5. Teach gun safety. Keep guns out of reach, locked, unloaded. Store ammunition and guns separately.
6. Teach animal/pet responsibility and safety.

D. Social.
1. Teach phone number, address.
2. Teach use of 911.
3. Teach stranger safety.
4. Teach about "good touch/bad touch."

IX. ANTICIPATORY GUIDANCE

A. Preventive care.
1. Annual physical.
2. Semiannual dental visits.
3. Immunizations on schedule.

B. Home.
1. Establish family rules and remain consistent in enforcement.
2. Avoid corporal punishment for breaking rules.
3. Limit TV viewing to 1 hour/day.
4. Enforce good personal hygiene.
5. Avoid punishment for urinary or bowel incontinence.
6. Encourage family meals.
7. Encourage continued reading to and with child.
8. If parents work, ensure appropriate, safe supervision is provided before and after school.
9. Encourage responsibility for age-appropriate chores.
10. Develop fire safety plan for home.
11. Encourage physical activity: 1 hour or more each day.

C. Family/community.
1. Encourage and praise school activity, accomplishments.
2. Encourage socialization with peer groups in organized and unorganized activities.
3. Encourage consistent exercise; ensure proper supervision for all activities.
4. Discourage "hurried child syndrome"; no more than 1–2 activities/week.
5. Reinforce school/bus rules; encourage parents to become actively involved in school/community parent groups.
6. Encourage parents to teach/model moral behavior, good citizenship ("Do unto others as you would have them do unto you.").

D. Safety.
1. Ensure proper motor vehicle restraints consistently used.
2. Encourage swim lessons.
3. Reinforce proper bicycle use, rules, and use of helmet.
4. Reinforce use of proper safety equipment for all activities, including sunscreen SPF 15 or higher applied 30 minutes before going outdoors.
5. Reinforce proper pedestrian rules.
6. Reinforce proper gun safety and storing of ammunition separately.
7. Reinforce "good touch/bad touch" concepts.
8. Teach "just say no" concepts.
9. Discuss how to ask for help when needed.
10. Reinforce how to use telephone to call 911 in an emergency.
11. Ensure child knows address and phone number.
12. Reinforce age-appropriate child-proofing in residence and use of smoke detectors.
13. Reinforce fire safety; ensure family has plan for evacuation.
14. Don't leave child without proper supervision.
15. Discourage mini-bike and ATV use.

X. SCHOOL READINESS

A. Physical readiness.
1. Has met developmental milestones in cognitive, gross, and fine motor areas.
2. Cognitive, visual, hearing deficits addressed.
B. Emotional readiness.
1. Able to separate easily from parent.
2. Dresses without supervision.
3. Toilet trained.
4. Washes hands.
5. Follows instructions.
C. Screening and assessment tools.
1. Physical exam, including full neurologic evaluation.
2. Vision and hearing screening.
3. Developmental testing: Draw a man and Denver II recommended for ease of administration. Denver II is more comprehensive for children under age 4 years. At age 4, language domains are not as complete.
D. Anticipatory guidance.
1. Encourage and reinforce positive parental attitudes regarding school.
2. Prepare parent and child for separation, change in routine.

3. Have parent obtain list of school/classroom rules and review.
4. Have parent tour school and meet teacher prior to first day of school.
5. Prepare parent for child's potential fear/anxiety.
6. Prepare family to advocate for child in positive, supportive manner.

E. Potential concerns.
   1. School phobia.
   2. Lack of expected intellectual ability/progress.
   3. ADD/ADHD.
   4. Emotional immaturity.
   5. Behavioral problems related to classroom.
   6. Bullying.

BIBLIOGRAPHY

American Academy of Pediatrics. *Bright Futures: Guidelines for Health Supervision of Infants, Children, and Adolescents.* 4th ed. Elk Grove Village, IL: American Academy of Pediatrics; 2015.

Centers for Disease Control and Prevention. About child & teen BMI. http://www.cdc.gov/healthyweight /assessing/bmi/childrens_bmi/about_childrens_bmi.html. Accessed June 15, 2015.

Dixon SD, Stein MT. *Encounters with Children: Pediatric Behavior and Development.* 4th ed. St. Louis, MO: Mosby; 2006.

Seven- to Ten-Year Visit (School Age)

Elizabeth Godfrey Terry

Appendicitis, unspecified, K37

Asthma, J45

Attention-deficit hyperactivity disorder, combined type, F90.2

Attention-deficit hyperactivity disorder, predominantly hyperactive type, F90.1

Attention-deficit hyperactivity disorder, predominantly inattentive type, F90.0

Attention-deficit hyperactivity disorder, unspecified type, F90.9

Cardiac murmur, unspecified, R01.1

Chickenpox [Varicella], B01

Cystic fibrosis, E84

Dermatophytosis, unspecified, B35.9

Disturbances in tooth eruption, K00.6

Encounter for examination for adolescent development state, Z00.3

Heart disease, unspecified, I51.9

Hypertrophy of breast, N62

Impetigo, unspecified, L01.00

Irregular menstruation, unspecified, N92.6

Measles without complication, B05.9

Mental and behavioral disorders due to psychoactive substance use, F10–F19

Mumps without complication, B26.9

Myopia, bilateral, H52.13

Nightmares, F51.5

Nonorganic encopresis, F98.1

Nonorganic enuresis, F98.0

Osteochondropathy, unspecified of unspecified site, M93.90

Other childhood emotional disorders, F93.8

Other developmental disorders of scholastic skills, F81.89

Other juvenile osteochondrosis of hip and pelvis, unspecified leg, M91.80

Other voice and resonance disorders, R49.8

Rubella without complication, B06.9

Scabies, B86

Scoliosis, M41

Separation anxiety disorder of childhood, F93.0

Sickle-cell disorders, D57

Sleep apnea, unspecified, G47.30

Sleep disorders, G47

Sleep terrors [night terrors], F51.4

Sleepwalking [somnambulism], F51.3

Social phobia, unspecified, F40.10

I. OVERALL IMPRESSION

A. Early school agers are in routine of being in school, learning; now gaining skills to get along with many different personalities.

II. NUTRITION

A. Caloric and nutrient needs.
   1. Three full meals and 1–2 snacks a day.
   2. Needs vary depending upon amount of activity and development. Female, 1200–1600 calories (4–8 years, 1200 calories; 9–13 years, 1600 calories); male, 1400–1800 calories (4–8 years, 1400 calories; 9–13 years, 1800 calories). Calorie estimates based on a sedentary lifestyle. Increased physical activity will require additional calories: By 0 to 200 kcal/day if moderately physically active and by 200 to 400 kcal/day if very physically active.
   3. Refer to MyPlate for serving size, food group recommendations (see Appendix E).
   4. Whole grains preferred over refined-grain products; at least half the grains should be whole grains.
   5. Sweetened beverages and naturally sweet beverages, such as fruit juice, should be limited to 8 to 12 oz/day.
   6. Ages 4–8 years need 1000 mg of calcium and 600 IU of vitamin D/day. Ages 9–18 years need 1300 mg of calcium and 600 IU of vitamin D/day.
   7. Introduce and offer fish regularly, especially oily fish such as salmon, broiled or baked, and sardines. Avoid fish high in mercury content. Remove skin from poultry prior to serving. Offer more meat alternatives, such as legumes (beans) or tofu.
   8. Serve fresh, frozen, or canned vegetables and fruits at every meal.
B. Willing to try variety of foods from major food groups.
C. Appetite varies according to growth, activity.
D. May have big appetite during growth spurt and then cut back.
E. Good internal cues regarding appetite. Parents choose types of food and beverages served, and child chooses how much to eat.
F. Beginning steps toward obesity may start if child is not allowed to listen to internal cues.
G. Around 17.7% of children ages 6–11 are obese. Excess caloric intake and physical inactivity strongly associated with obesity.
H. Consider daily children's multivitamin if child is not consuming enough to get essential nutrients.

III. ELIMINATION

A. Enuresis occurs in 10% of 7-year-olds and 5% of 10-year-olds.
1. Children with this condition should receive complete exam to rule out underlying conditions such as urinary tract infections.
2. Children with sleep apnea at greater risk for enuresis.
B. Encopresis affects 1.5% of young school children.

IV. SLEEP

A. Need 9–11 hours/night.
B. Encourage and emphasize need for regular and consistent sleep schedule and bedtime routine.
C. Make bedrooms conducive to sleep—keep TV and computers out of bedroom.
D. Occasional nightmares or sleep disturbances such as night terrors, sleep walking.
E. May have fear of dark or of being alone (separation anxiety).
F. Emotional disturbances such as stress, anxiety, leading to insomnia.
G. Difficult bedtime behavior may develop.
H. Snoring, daytime sleepiness may be symptoms of sleep apnea.

V. GROWTH AND DEVELOPMENT

A. Musculoskeletal.
1. Document height, weight, and BMI once a year. BMI between 85th and 95th percentile for age and sex is considered at risk for overweight. Close supervision by healthcare provider may be considered. BMI values at or above the 95th percentile of the growth charts are categorized as obese.
2. Development not as rapid.
3. As body size increases, body fat stays relatively stable, giving slimmer appearance than preschool years.
4. Average height increase: A little over 2 in./year.
5. The closer to puberty, the greater the chances for increased growth.
6. Tends to be an increased growth rate between 6 and 8 years of age that may be accompanied by appearance of small amount of pubic hair.
7. If unusually short/tall for age, may need to consider possibility of growth disorder.

8. Appetite tends to vary due to growth fluctuations, but child should not be losing weight.

9. Orthopedic problems of this age group:

   a. Fractures, sprains, strains.

   b. Epiphyseal separations, dislocations.

   c. Scoliosis.

   d. Avascular necrosing lesions of epiphysis.
   - Legg-Calve-Perthes disease.
   - Osgood-Schlatter disease.

10. Motor skills improve in strength, balance, coordination.

B. Skin.

   1. Hair may become a little darker, skin becomes more adultlike.

   2. Look for changes in nevi or birthmarks and any signs of abuse or self-inflicted injuries. Note tattoos or piercings.

   3. Scabies, impetigo, ringworm, and head lice can be issues at this age.

C. Teeth.

   1. Should be able to brush teeth by themselves, still require some assistance or supervision.

   2. Brush with pea-sized amount of fluoride toothpaste after each meal or at least twice a day; floss once a day.

   3. Water supply should contain adequate fluoride; if not, consider fluoride supplement (see Appendix B).

   4. Eruption of permanent teeth occurs in order in which primary teeth are lost.

   5. Dental visits twice a year or according to a schedule recommended by dentist for exams, cleanings.

   6. Sealants as recommended.

   7. Problems with dental decay can peak during these years as well as periodontal diseases, often due to poor hygiene.

D. Eyes: Visual acuity of 20/20, although at about age 8 may begin to have myopia with no overt signs except school difficulty.

   1. Evaluate annually at primary healthcare visits or whenever a problem is suspected, such as visual acuity and ocular alignment. Screening examinations should be done at routine school checks or after the appearance of symptoms by those trained in vision assessment of school-age children. Screening emphasis should be directed to high-risk children, such as those with positive family history. Myopia is the most common refractive error in this age group and can be corrected with eyeglasses. Any child suspected of having an alignment problem or other eye health issues should have an ophthalmological examination by an eye doctor.

2. Children with presumed or diagnosed learning disabilities should undergo a comprehensive pediatric medical eye examination to identify and treat any undiagnosed vision impairment. Referrals should be made for appropriate medical, psychological, and educational evaluation and treatment of the learning disability.

E. Ears: Problems decrease due to further development of eustachian tubes and nasopharynx, although ear infections can still be frequent in younger school ages.

    1. Hearing tests are recommended at ages 8 and 10. Consider hearing screening if history of frequent ear infections or concerns about speech development.

F. Throat: Tonsillar tissue continues to enlarge, reaching its peak from 8 to 12 years when it levels off, begins to recess.

G. Immune system: Continues to mature; allergic conditions more common.

H. Hematopoietic system: Abnormal hemoglobin/hematocrit levels should not be attributed to dietary intake. Etiology should be established for any hemoglobin below 11.5 g.

I. Heart.

    1. Murmurs are often heard in these years.

    2. Any doubt of etiology requires referral to pediatric cardiologist.

    3. Circulation: Monitor blood pressure annually.

        a. Average pulse rate:
- Age 8: 78.
- Age 10: 74.

        b. Average blood pressure:
- Age 8: 105/60.
- Age 10: 111/66.

        c. Cholesterol screening: Recommended for all children at least once between the ages of 9 and 11 to reduce risk of cardiovascular disease.

J. Respiration rate.

    1. Age 8: 22 breaths/minute.

    2. Age 10: 20 breaths/minute.

K. Gastrointestinal system.

    1. Liver function is mature but still growing in size.

    2. Appendix: Open lumen and increased size increases risk of blockage, inflammatory reaction (appendicitis).

L. Genitourinary system.

    1. Urinary tract infections can be common, especially in girls; often asymptomatic at this age.

M. Nervous system: Essentially mature by age 10.

    1. Begins puberty.

a. Girls.
- Breast budding can begin as early as age 8; others not until 13, with the average being around age 10.
- Puberty before age 8: Girl should be evaluated for precocious puberty (twice as frequent in females as in males).
- Peak growth period (height, weight, muscle mass, etc.) occurs 1 year after puberty has begun.
- Menstruation usually begins 18 months to 2 years after onset of puberty, on average just before age 13.

b. Boys.
- Peak growth period occurs about 2 years after onset of puberty.
- Begin puberty about 1 year later than girls.
- First sign of puberty in boys is enlargement of testes, thinning and reddening of scrotum. This occurs on average at age 11 but may occur anytime between 9 and 14 years of age.
- Puberty before 9: Boy should be evaluated for precocious puberty.

2. Secondary sex characteristics.
a. Girls.
- Breast enlargement: 8–13 years.
- Axillary hair: 11–13 years.
- Pubic hair: 10–12 years.
- Menarche: 10–16 years.

b. Boys.
- Genitalia enlargement: 9–14 years.
- Axillary hair: 12–14 years.
- Facial hair: 11–14 years.
- Pubic hair: 12–15 years.

N. Language.
1. Although better able to express emotions and ideas, may talk in abstract terms without fully comprehending meaning of such speech.
2. Learning to communicate clearly with friends.

VI. SOCIAL DEVELOPMENT

A. Needs to master balance of feelings in dealing with successes, failures.
1. Self-concept (body self, social self, cognitive self) affects child's ability to be successful.
B. Successful accomplishments are of high priority for child in order to build positive self-image. Should feel successful with most day-to-day skills, activities, and chores.

C. Making friends is one of most important mid-childhood tasks.
1. Average number of friends: About five.
2. Sibling friendships may replace outside friends or need for them.
3. Selects friends of similar temperament, interests.
4. Often focus on "best friend" relationship, which can be more satisfying than large group.
D. Increasingly seeks peers for companionship.
E. Cliques may begin to form.
F. Parents and teachers are important significant others and will influence behavior, self-concept.
1. Encourage parents to share unscheduled spontaneous time with their child; time to be together, listen, and talk.
G. School issues.
1. School phobia.
2. Learning disorders.
3. Attention deficit hyperactivity disorder.
4. Bullying.
5. After-school care and activities.
6. Dealing with fears, disappointments, and stress.
7. Parent–teacher communication.

VII. IMMUNIZATIONS

A. Influenza vaccine.
1. Annual seasonal influenza immunization is recommended for all children 6 months of age and older.
2. Especially recommended for children with high-risk conditions such as asthma, diabetes, or neurological disorders.
3. For most healthy, nonpregnant persons ages 2 through 49 years, either live, attenuated influenza vaccine (LAIV) or inactivated influenza vaccine (IIV) may be used. However, LAIV should not be given to some people (see Appendix A).
4. Children 9 years of age and older need only 1 dose.
5. Children < 9 years receiving influenza vaccine for the first time require 2 doses (separated by at least 4 weeks). Some children in this age group who have been vaccinated previously will also need 2 doses (see Appendix A).
B. Varicella vaccine.
1. Children ages 7 through 18 years without evidence of immunity should receive 2 doses if not previously vaccinated or the second dose if only 1 dose has been administered.

2. For children ages 7 through 12 years, minimum interval between doses is 3 months, but accepted as valid if the second dose was given at least 28 days after the first dose.

C. Measles, mumps, rubella (MMR).

1. Children not previously vaccinated should receive 2 doses or the second dose for those who have received only 1 dose, with at least 28 days between doses.

D. Hepatitis A vaccine.

1. May be given if immunity against hepatitis A virus is desired, especially in populations at increased risk for infection. For any person aged 2 years and older who has not already received the HepA vaccine series, 2 doses of HepA vaccine separated by 6 to 18 months may be given.

E. Hepatitis B vaccine.

1. The 3-dose series should be given to those not previously vaccinated.

F. Pneumococcal vaccine.

1. To be given to children with certain underlying medical conditions, including a cochlear implant.

G. Meningococcal conjugate vaccines.

1. Routine vaccination against meningococcal disease is not recommended for children aged 2 months through 10 years except for those with high-risk conditions or at increased risk for disease, such as those with persistent complement component deficiency or anatomic or functional asplenia.

H. Human papillomavirus vaccine (HPV).

1. Routine vaccination of females and males begins at age 11 or 12 years but may start at age 9 years.

I. See Appendix A.

VIII. SAFETY/ANTICIPATORY GUIDANCE

A. Nutrition.

1. Offer nutrient-dense foods that include a wide variety of fruits, vegetables, whole grains, and nonfat or low-fat dairy foods.

2. Stress importance of parents being good role models. Child who sees parent enjoying a wide variety of nutritious foods is more likely to want them.

3. Encourage a healthy breakfast daily.

4. Encourage reading food labels when shopping, especially noting calories from fat, type of fat, sodium, cholesterol, vitamins, minerals, and serving size. Child can help read the labels.

5. Encourage family meals at home. Children who eat meals with family at home have a better quality diet.

6. Offer healthy ways of eating when eating out is necessary and remind parents to be mindful of portion sizes.

7. Encourage parents to closely supervise but involve child in family food preparation. Children are more likely to eat foods that they help prepare.

8. Encourage family use of USDA's Food Guide for Kids.

9. Child may need multivitamin if not eating enough to get essential nutrients, if an erratic eater, or if on a highly selective diet. Most healthy children eating well-balanced diets do not require supplementation.

10. Some children may still be picky eaters at this age so may have to slightly adjust portions or food groups in order ensure adequate intake; may eat more at snack times than at regular meals.

11. Offer water to drink instead of sugary drinks.

12. Healthy snacks 1–2 times a day can include:

    a. Fresh, canned, frozen vegetables or fruits. Keep cut-up veggies such as celery sticks, cucumber slices, or broccoli in the refrigerator. Offer hummus or low-fat dressings for dips. Try frozen grapes or bananas for fun treat.

    b. Cold skim or 1% milk, or calcium-fortified soy milk with whole-grain sugar-free cereal, peanut butter sandwich, or whole-grain crackers with hummus.

    c. Fruit smoothie made with fresh fruit, skim milk (or calcium-fortified milk alternative), ice, and a dash of vanilla or cinnamon.

    d. Nonfat or low-fat yogurt or cheese or cheese sticks.

    e. Air-popped or unbuttered popcorn.

    f. Baked tortillas or pretzels with salsa.

    g. Low-fat frozen yogurt, fruit juice bars (without added sugar).

    h. Use snack-size portions or bags to control serving size.

13. Encourage healthy eating behaviors, including no meals or snacking in front of TV. Parents should model these behaviors.

B. Sleep.

1. Stay consistent in routine activities such as daily mealtimes, playtimes, bedtime, wake-up time.

2. Avoid caffeine/other stimulants; limit food, drink before bedtime.

3. An hour or so before bedtime, begin a relaxing routine such as warm bath then a story in quiet bedroom.

4. Bed should only be used for sleeping, not for watching TV or homework. TVs and computers should be kept out of bedrooms.

5. Children who are overtired/have interrupted sleep may be more likely to have sleep disturbances such as night terrors.

C. Growth and development.
1. Musculoskeletal.
    a. Need an hour or more of moderate to vigorous age-appropriate daily physical activities such as team/individual sports, family activities, free play, walking, bicycling, chores, walking up and down stairs. Parents should model, prioritize, and promote regular physical activity, especially outdoor activity.
    b. Limit total amount of screen time (TV, computer) to < 1 to 2 hours a day.
    c. As they approach puberty, children tend to put on a little more weight, which is normal.
    d. Increases in BMI percentiles should be discussed with parents but in nonjudgmental, blame-free manner.
    e. Because fractures are common in this age group, children should wear appropriate protective sports gear and consume adequate calcium to decrease risk of fractures.
2. Skin.
    a. 30 minutes before going outside, on both sunny and cloudy days, thickly apply 1 oz of broad-spectrum UVA-UVB sunscreen with SPF 15+ to child's entire body, especially ears, nose, face, neck, shoulders, hands, and feet.
    b. When spending extended time outdoors, use a water-resistant, broad-spectrum sunscreen with an SPF of 30 or higher.
    c. Reapply sunscreen every 2 hours and after swimming or sweating heavily, regardless of whether sunscreen is waterproof.
    d. Use cool, comfortable clothing, especially clothes with a tight weave, to cover the body and protect from the sun.
    e. Wear a wide-brimmed hat to shield head, face, ears, and neck.
    f. Encourage sun avoidance between 10 a.m. and 4 p.m. when UV rays are the strongest. Seek shelter, shade, or umbrellas when out during those times. Remind that UV rays reflect and bounce back from sand, water, concrete, and snow, so even in shade, sun protection is needed.
3. Teeth.
    a. Dental visits twice a year (or according to schedule recommended by dentist) for exams, cleaning.
    b. Brush teeth at least twice a day with pea-sized amount of fluoride toothpaste; floss once a day.
    c. Still may need to help with or supervise brushing.
    d. Verify water source for adequate fluoride.

e. Care of baby teeth as important as permanent teeth. Early loss of baby teeth due to cavities or accidents can lead to spacing issues with premature rupture of permanent teeth, resulting in orthodontic issues.

f. Discuss importance of wearing mouth guards, helmets while playing sports.

4. Eyes.
   a. Wear sunglasses with 100% UVA-UVB protection whenever outside or in car.
   b. All youth in organized sports should be encouraged to wear appropriate eye protection, especially when engaged in high-risk sports and activities such as basketball, baseball/softball, lacrosse, hockey, and paintball, when using a BB gun, or when around yard debris. Mandatory protective eyewear for athletes who are functionally one-eyed and for athletes whose ophthalmologists recommend eye protection after eye surgery or trauma.
   c. Warn about dangers of fireworks to eyes; enjoy fireworks displays put on by professionals.

5. Puberty.
   a. Encourage honest, age-appropriate discussions about sex with child using accurate terminology and listening carefully to child's questions so parent only gives as much information as child requires.
   b. Concerns of girls about puberty:
      - Menstruation.
      - Breast development.
   c. Concerns of boys about puberty:
      - Voice change.
      - Wet dreams.
      - Involuntary erections.
      - Breast enlargement.
      - One testicle lower than other.

6. Cognitive and social development.
   a. Very sensitive to views of others.
   b. Appreciate having rules.
   c. Begin to have strong internal gauge of right and wrong.
   d. Friendship and teamwork are important parts of this stage of development.
   e. Eager for more independence but frustrated by what they cannot accomplish since they are still in the process of mastering skills.

Important to have sense of achievement, accomplishment to build strong self-esteem.

   f. Encourage an appropriately challenging academic schedule and a balance of extracurricular activities. This is determined by child's unique needs, skills, and temperament.

   g. Encourage exploration of activities and interests in a balanced way without the pressure of having to excel in everything.

   h. Encourage parents to promote child activities that are fun, increase self-confidence, and involve friends.

D. Safety.

  1. Auto.

    a. Children should be properly secured at all times while traveling in car.

    b. Children should be in a forward-facing car seat with a harness and tether until they reach the top height or weight limit allowed by the car seat's manufacturer. Children should ride in booster seats until the vehicle safety belts fit correctly, usually when they are around 4 ft 9 in. tall. This may not be until they are 8 to 12 years of age. Can move to safety belt when child can place his/her back firmly against vehicle seat back cushion with knees bent over vehicle seat cushion and be able to keep his or her feet flat on the floor. Lap belt must fit low and tight across upper thighs. Belt should rest over shoulder and across chest and not across the neck or face.

    c. Shoulder belt should never be placed under arm or behind child's back.

    d. Children should ride in the back seat at least until age 13.

    e. Keep all doors locked while in motion.

    f. Never leave young children alone in car.

    g. Children should not ride in truck beds or any other area of vehicle that does not have seat and seat belt.

    h. Children lack judgment, coordination, reflexes to drive other motorized vehicles such as mopeds, snowmobiles, mini-bikes, ATVs.

  2. Bicycle safety. Children who ride bikes should:

    a. Wear helmets at all times. Helmets should meet safety standards of the Consumer Product Safety Commission (www.cpsc.gov). Helmets should fit properly; parents may want to bring them in to check for proper fit. Parents should wear helmets as well to serve as a good role model.

    b. Know basic road rules such as obey all traffic signs/lights, stop and look both ways at intersecting points such as driveways/streets, ride in single file or on bike paths, ride in same direction as traffic.

    c. Not wear loose-fitting clothing, strings, ties that could get caught in bike chain or parts.

    d. Wear shoes with laces tied.

    e. Not wear earphones while riding.

3. Skateboard safety: Children should always wear helmet and never ride near traffic.

4. Water safety.

    a. Never allow child to swim alone or play unsupervised in or by water, even for a moment.

    b. Child should learn to swim and take lessons from qualified instructor.

    c. Backyard swimming pools should be enclosed with high, locked fence on all sides. Fences should be at least 4 ft high on all sides.

    d. Diving should not be allowed until underwater depth has been determined and checked for hazards.

    e. No swimming near boats, fishermen, unsupervised open water.

    f. Children should always wear a life jacket when in a boat.

    g. Parents should know how to perform CPR.

5. Fire and burn accidents.

    a. Install smoke detectors on all floors, particularly in or near sleeping areas.

    b. Keep fire extinguishers in kitchen, other areas where fire could start.

    c. Have family fire plan in place; practice regular fire drills.

    d. Discourage playing with matches, etc.

    e. To avoid scalding burns from water, heaters should never be set $> 120°F$ ($48.9°C$).

6. Home alone: Most children are not old enough until age 11 or 12. Child should be learning safety, security, emergency guidelines (calling parent, neighbor, 911) in preparation for emergencies or for when the time comes that the child is old enough to be left alone for short times, such as after school.

7. Gun safety: Guns, ammunition need to be stored and locked separately. Child needs to know to stay away from and alert parent should he encounter a gun at a friend's house or elsewhere.

8. Bullying: Children of this age can sometimes be the target of bullies. Child needs to know strategies for dealing with bullying. Strong friendships should be encouraged to avoid being bullied.

9. Sexual abuse.

    a. Most sexual abuse occurs between the ages of 8 and 12.

    b. In 80% of these cases, abuser is known to child.

    c. Reinforce "good touch/bad touch" concepts and awareness of possible scenarios that may occur. Promote abuse-prevention programs at school and encourage parents to listen carefully to child who might have a concern, particularly of a sexual nature.

10. Substance abuse.
    a. Begins with experimentation and casual use, often under peer pressure.
    b. Problem drinking often begins in grade school.
    c. Prevention of substance abuse needs to begin before adolescence.
    d. Secondhand smoke is a serious health hazard for children. Increases risk of developing asthma, bronchitis, middle-ear disease, pneumonia, wheezing and coughing spells, behavioral/cognitive problems.
    e. Children whose parents smoke are more than twice as likely to smoke themselves than are children of nonsmokers.

11. Media.
    a. In addition to < 1 to 2 hours of screen time per day and keeping TVs and computers out of bedrooms, remind parents about the importance of careful selection, watching together, and discussing programs their children watch.
    b. Encourage parents to be knowledgeable about online and social media.
    c. Keep computers in a central area of the house where computer activities can be monitored. Parents may want to consider purchasing online programs that allow them to monitor computer activity.
    d. Encourage parents to talk often with their children about online and social media safety and responsibility.
    e. Encourage parents to set a good example by limiting their own viewing time and engaging in other healthy activities.

BIBLIOGRAPHY

American Academy of Pediatric Dentistry. Guideline on periodicity of examination, preventive dental services, anticipatory guidance/counseling, and oral treatment for infants, children, and adolescents. *Reference Manual: Clinical Guidelines*. 2013;36(6):118-125.

American Academy of Pediatrics. Physicians recommend all children, ages 9-11, be screened for cholesterol. https://www.aap.org/en-us/about-the-aap/aap-press-room/pages/Physicians-Recommend-all -Children,-Ages-9-11,-Be-Screened-for-Cholesterol.aspx. Published November 14, 2011. Accessed June 5, 2015.

American Academy of Pediatrics. Policy statement: children, adolescents, and the media. *Pediatrics*. 2013;132(5):958-961.

American Academy of Pediatrics Committee on Infectious Diseases. Recommended childhood and adolescent immunization schedule, United States, 2015. *Pediatrics*. 2015;135(2):396-397.

American Academy of Pediatrics Committee on Nutrition. Prevention of pediatric overweight and obesity. *Pediatrics*. 2003;112(2):424-430.

American Academy of Pediatrics Committee on Sports Medicine and Fitness. Protective eyewear for young athletes. *Pediatrics*. 2004;113(3):619-622.

Bennett HJ. *Waking Up Dry: A Guide to Helping Children Overcome Bedwetting*. Elk Grove Village, IL: American Academy of Pediatrics; 2005.

Brooks LJ, Topol HI. Enuresis in children with sleep apnea. *J Pediatr*. 2003;142(5):515-518.

Centers for Disease Control and Prevention. Adolescent and school health: childhood obesity facts. http://www.cdc.gov/healthyyouth/obesity/facts.htm. Published April 24, 2015. Accessed April 30, 2015.

Centers for Disease Control and Prevention. Childhood obesity facts. http://www.cdc.gov/obesity/data/childhood.html. Updated June 19, 2015. Accessed August 30, 2015.

Centers for Disease Control and Prevention. Advisory Committee on Immunization Practices (ACIP). http://www.cdc.gov/vaccines/acip/. Accessed April 30, 2015.

Council on Communications and Media. From the American Academy of Pediatrics: policy statement—media violence. *Pediatrics*. 2009;124(5):1495-1503.

Daniels SR, Greer FR, and the Committee on Nutrition. Lipid screening and cardiovascular health in childhood. *Pediatrics*. 2008;122(1):198-208.

de Ferranti S, Washington RL. NHLBI guidelines on cholesterol in kids: what's new and how does this change practice? *AAP News*. 2012;33(2):1.

Dietz WH, Stern LM, eds. *American Academy of Pediatrics Guide to Your Child's Nutrition*. New York, NY: Villard; 1999.

eyeSmart. Eye screening for children. American Academy of Ophthalmology. http://www.geteyesmart.org/eyesmart/living/babies-children-teenagers-eye-health/children-eye-screening.cfm. Revised August 14, 2014. Accessed April 30, 2015.

Freeland-Graves JH, Nitzke S, Academy of Nutrition and Dietetics. Position of the academy of nutrition and dietetics: total diet approach to healthy eating. *J Acad Nutr Diet*. 2013;113(2):307-317.

Fryar CD, Carroll MD, Ogden CL. Prevalence of obesity among children and adolescents: United States, 1963–1965 through 2011–2012. Centers for Disease Control and Prevention. http://www.cdc.gov/nchs/data/hestat/obesity_child_11_12/obesity_child_11_12.htm. Updated September 19, 2014. Accessed May 2, 2015.

Gidding SS, Dennison BA, Birch LL, et al. Dietary recommendations for children and adolescents: a guide for practitioners. *Pediatrics*. 2006;117(2):544-559.

Ginsburg KR; American Academy of Pediatrics Committee on Communications; American Academy of Pediatrics Committee on Psychosocial Aspects of Child and Family Health. The importance of play in promoting healthy child development and maintaining strong parent-child bonds. *Pediatrics*. 2007;119(1):182-191.

Hagan JF, Shaw JS, Duncan P, eds. *Bright Futures: Guidelines for Health Supervision of Infants, Children, and Adolescents*. 3rd ed. Elk Grove Village, IL: American Academy of Pediatrics; 2008.

National Highway Transportation Safety Association. Parents central. http://www.safercar.gov/parents/index.htm

National Sleep Foundation [homepage]. http://www.sleepfoundation.org

Ogata BN, Hayes D. Position of the Academy of Nutrition and Dietetics: nutrition guidance for healthy children ages 2 to 11 years. *J Acad Nutr Diet*. 2014;114(8):1257-1276.

SHAPE America [homepage]. http://www.shapeamerica.org

Simon GR, Baker C, Barden GA, et al. 2014 recommendations for pediatric preventive health care. *Pediatrics*. 2014;133(3):568-570.

Skin Cancer Foundation. How to keep children sun-safe. http://www.skincancer.org/prevention/sun-protection/children/summer-tips

Eleven- to Thirteen-Year Visit (Preadolescent)

Mary J. Alvarado

Acne vulgaris, L70.0	Nontoxic goiter, unspecified, E04.9
Atherosclerotic heart disease, I25.1	
Human immunodeficiency virus [HIV] disease, B20–B24	Peripheral vascular disease, unspecified, I73.9
Iodine-deficiency related (endemic) goiter, unspecified, E01.2	Physical abuse, T76.12XA
	Psychological abuse, T74.32XA
Major depressive disorder, single episode, unspecified, F32.9	Scoliosis, M41
	Sexual abuse, T74.22XA

I. GENERAL IMPRESSION

    A. Preadolescence is time of rapid change and emotional vulnerability.

    B. Preteens need support, understanding, and caring from adults to effectively deal with the psychological changes of this period.

II. NUTRITION

    A. Nutritional requirements.

        1. Increased energy and protein requirement due to rapid growth.

        2. Require 2200–3000 calories/day.

        3. To meet increased need, increase milk and dairy products to 4 servings/day, bread group servings to 9 servings/day.

        4. One-fourth of daily calories is typically consumed in snacks; encourage fruit, cheese, milk beverages, raw vegetables, nuts.

     5. Diet should consist of 10–15% protein, 25–30% fat, 50–60% carbohydrates.

     6. Needs 8–15 mg of iron/day; iron is most commonly deficient nutrient.

     7. A well-balanced diet does not require supplementation; irregular eating patterns and/or high-calorie/low-nutrient snacking may lead to deficiencies requiring multivitamin.

B. Nutritional assessment.

     1. Calculate and plot body mass index (BMI) (see Appendix D).

     2. Evaluate 24-hour recall.

     3. Examine intake, eating patterns; ask about special diets or supplements.

     4. Assess for eating disorders.

     5. Monitor athletes' increased need for calories; advise on appropriate dietary changes.

     6. Provide guidance about nutrition annually.

     7. Refer to nutritionist if indicated.

III. ELIMINATION

A. Expect consistent pattern of elimination.

B. Changes may occur with irregular eating patterns, illness, diets, stress, eating disorders.

C. Check understanding of normal elimination and methods employed to deal with problems.

IV. SLEEP

A. Question about amount of sleep; aim for at least 8 hours/night.

B. Monitor for any difficulties, ability to cope.

C. Advise on sleep hygiene if necessary.

V. GROWTH AND DEVELOPMENT

A. Physical.

     1. Early adolescence is marked by rapid physical change. Tempo of adolescent development is variable and may be influenced by gender, health, socioeconomic status, genetics. Predictable sequence of events occurs over 2–6 years from onset, which on average is age 9–11 for girls and

age 10–12 for boys. The preadolescent may prefer to be examined with parent out of the room.

2. Perform complete physical exam with attention to the following:
   a. Document height, weight, and BMI annually (see Appendix D).
   b. Assess and document Tanner stage of pubertal development annually.
   c. Monitor blood pressure annually.
   d. Screen cholesterol once in this age group if following risk factors exist:
      - Parent with serum cholesterol > 240.
      - Family history unknown.
      - Parent/grandparent with stroke, peripheral vascular disease, coronary artery disease, sudden cardiac death younger than 55 years.
   e. Palpate thyroid gland; goiter may present in this age group.
   f. Examine spine for development/progression of scoliosis during rapid growth.
   g. Assess for presence/severity of acne.
   h. Ask about sexual activity; screen sexually active teens for sexually transmitted infections (STIs), evaluate risk for acquiring HIV.

B. Emotional.
   1. Rapid physical changes of early adolescence lead to increased self-consciousness and focus on external characteristics.
   2. Adolescent feels everyone is looking at him/her and questions if he/she is normal.
   3. Reassure about normal findings in the physical exam.
   4. Explain that each individual progresses through physical changes of puberty in same sequence but at his/her own pace.
   5. Ask about friends, family, school. Is there a best friend? A supportive adult? Monitor self-esteem.
   6. Ask about moods. Emotional lability is normal. Assess for excessive stress or depression.
   7. Ask about physical, emotional, or sexual abuse.
   8. Discuss safe use of Internet and online social networks. Remind to use caution when sharing personal information, photos, and videos by Internet and phone.

C. Intellectual.
   1. Adolescent begins to transition from concrete to abstract thinking; timing is variable. Some develop higher level thinking in early adolescence, some later or not at all. Abstract thinking gives adolescent better ability to reason and see other points of view. Individual may be able to think abstractly about algebra but not about decision making regarding risky

behaviors. Most young teens have limited ability to consider long-range health risks. Evaluate each preteen through conversation to tailor anticipatory guidance.

2. How is school performance? Ask about academic, athletic, personal goals. May still have impractical/unrealistic ideas.

3. What are responsibilities at home? Early adolescents should be encouraged to take on new responsibilities with supervision.

4. Ask about extracurricular activities. Encourage involvement in groups that interest him/her. Increasing communication skills helps with problem solving. Group discussions help adolescents learn to express themselves.

5. Advise to keep TV viewing, computer time, video games to < 2 hours/day. These activities interfere with opportunities to engage in communication with peers, family.

VI. SOCIAL DEVELOPMENT

A. Early adolescents begin to develop greater independence from parents, family. Remind parents that this is normal and healthy.

B. Establishment of reliable relationships with peers, other adults is important developmental task.

C. New peer group, which is usually same sex, provides opportunity to test, evaluate values/behaviors. It allows for sense of belonging and self-worth, and affords opportunity to build social competence.

D. Recognize that hairstyles, clothing, music preferences, piercings are expressions of individuality; often mirror others in peer group.

E. Preoccupation with own appearance is typical. Help parents anticipate greater privacy need.

F. Encourage variety of school/community activities to allow wider exposure to peers/interests.

G. Testing authority may occur. Encourage families to clearly establish and enforce guidelines for appropriate behavior. Identify consistent caring adult with whom adolescent is comfortable communicating.

H. Question about friends, peer groups, adult role models. Social isolation is not normal.

I. As with other areas of development, individuals progress at variable rates and often oscillate between dependence/independence.

J. Parents have an important role in minimizing negative peer influences; know who your child's friends are.

VII. IMMUNIZATIONS

A. Immunizations should be given according to recommended childhood immunization schedule (see Appendix A):
   1. Hepatitis B: Complete or initiate series.
   2. MMR: Give second dose now if not already administered.
   3. Tetanus toxoid (Tdap): Recommended at age 11–12 if at least 5 years since last dose. Subsequent doses every 10 years throughout adulthood.
   4. Varicella: Give if not previously immunized or unreliable history of disease. If 13 years or older, give 2 doses 4 weeks apart.
   5. Meningococcal: MCV.
   6. HPV: Recommend initiating series for males and females.
   7. Influenza: Recommend annually at start of flu season.

VIII. SAFETY

A. Unintentional injury is main cause of death and disability in this age group.
   1. Counsel about accident prevention: Seat belts, helmets, proper sports equipment, water-safety instruction, CPR.
   2. Instruct that firearms should be locked up, ammunition kept separate.
   3. Educate about dangers of drug use, both ingested and inhaled. Provide strategies to resist negative peer pressure.
   4. Discuss date rape prevention.
   5. Assess for depression, adolescents at high risk for suicide: Those with chronic illness or extreme stress (i.e., overachievers), athletes, those who feel unwanted.
   6. Assess for physical, emotional, sexual abuse.

IX. ANTICIPATORY GUIDANCE

A. Promotion of health.
   1. Review pubertal development of same and opposite sex.
   2. Explain menstruation and its management to females.
   3. Advise to get 8 hours of sleep every night.
   4. Encourage moderate to vigorous exercise for 30–60 minutes at least 3 times a week.
   5. Instruct to eat 3 nutritious meals/day. Snack on healthy foods such as fruits, vegetables, nuts, low-fat dairy. Choose foods rich in calcium, iron.

    6. Encourage maintaining healthy weight through exercise, appropriate eating habits.

    7. Remind to schedule dental exam every 6 months. Brush teeth twice a day. Floss daily.

    8. Educate about acne management.

    9. Provide safety instruction, avoidance of substance abuse and gang involvement.

B. Social development.

    1. Encourage participation in school activities.

    2. Advise to take on new responsibilities in home, school, community.

    3. Clarify parental limits, consequences of unacceptable behavior.

    4. Educate about safe use of the Internet and how to avoid exploitation.

C. Mental health.

    1. Encourage teens to consider their strengths and talents.

    2. Recommend talking with trusted adult/health professional if teen feels sad or helpless often.

    3. Advise against alcohol, drug use. Discuss strategies to resist negative peer pressure.

    4. Evaluate for potential abuse, counsel on avoiding date rape, gang involvement, abusive relationships.

D. Sexuality.

    1. Counsel on sexual abstinence. Encourage to identify supportive adult to provide accurate information. Invite adolescent to call the office for advice/information as needed. Explain confidentiality policy.

    2. If sexually active, discuss contraceptive methods, STI prevention. Counsel on abstinence.

    3. Educate about protection against STIs and pregnancy as indicated.

    4. Some early teens struggle with issue of sexual preference. Reassuring them that they will gradually form their own identity can be helpful. Some experimentation with the same sex is common but does not always predict future sexual orientation.

BIBLIOGRAPHY

American Academy of Pediatrics. *Bright Futures: Guidelines for Health Supervision of Infants, Children, and Adolescents.* 4th ed. Elk Grove Village, IL: American Academy of Pediatrics; 2015.

Elster AB, Kuznets NJ. *AMA Guidelines for Adolescent Preventive Services (GAPS): Recommendations and Rationale.* Baltimore, MD: Williams & Wilkins; 1994.

Fisher J, Wildey L. Developmental management of adolescents. In: Burns CE, Dunn AM, Brady MA, Starr NB, Blosser CG. *Pediatric Primary Care: A Handbook For Nurse Practitioners.* 5th ed. Philadelphia: W.B. Saunders; 2013.

Fox J, ed. *Primary Health Care of Infants, Children, and Adolescents.* 2nd ed. St. Louis, MO: Mosby; 2002.

Gutgesell ME, Payne N. Issues of adolescent psychological development in the 21st century. *Pediatr Rev.* 2004;25(3):79-85.

Knapp S, Swager LWM, Nield LS. Game over: helping a teenager quit a video game addiction. *Consultant for Pediatricians.* 2014;13(6):266-268.

Neinstein LS, ed. *Adolescent Health Care: A Practical Guide.* 5th ed. Philadelphia, PA: Lippincott Williams & Wilkins; 2008.

Fourteen- to Eighteen-Year Visit (Adolescent)

Mary Lou C. Rosenblatt and Beth Richardson

Abdominal and pelvic pain, R10

Acanthosis nigricans, L83

Anemia, unspecified, D64.9

Anxiety disorder, generalized, F41.1

Catatonic schizophrenia, F20.2

Constipation, K59.0

Diabetes mellitus, E10–E14

Diabetes mellitus, family history of, Z98.3

Disorders of the sleep-wake schedule, G47.2

Disorder of thyroid, unspecified, E07.9

Dysmenorrhea, unspecified, N94.6

Eating disorders, F50

Essential (primary) hypertension, I10

Hallucinations, unspecified, R44.3

Hyperlipidemia, unspecified, E78.5

Hypertrophy of tonsils, J35.1

Insomnia, unspecified, G47.00

Iron deficiency anemia, unspecified, D50.9

Major depressive disorder, single episode, unspecified, F32.9

Mental and behavioral disorders due to psychoactive substance use, F10–F19

Morbid (severe) obesity due to excess calories, E66.01

Narcolepsy and cataplexy, G47.4

Nutritional deficiency, unspecified, E63.9

Obesity, E66

Sleep apnea, unspecified, G47.30

Sleep disorders, G47

Visible peristalsis, R19.2

I. GENERAL IMPRESSION

A. This well visit is an opportunity to provide health care for individual who is faced with many developmental challenges on road to adulthood.

B. Introduce yourself and your role to teen and parent. Explain that you need information from both parent and teen and will spend some time just with teen to check on his/her concerns.

C. Be knowledgeable of your state's confidentiality and consent statutes and explain how that will be handled in practice. Assure both teen and parent that your first goal is well-being of teen.

D. Listening skills are especially important with teens. Show interest in their concerns and address them. "Hear" pauses, hesitation, and body language, and validate your understanding of meaning of nonverbal communication with teen.

E. Be nonjudgmental and gather information before giving advice.

F. Have supply of well-written and informative handouts on variety of issues.

G. Involve parents by finding out what advice they give on sensitive subjects, such as substance abuse and sex. Interaction between parent and teen will give feedback on what is discussed in home and how open they are with each other. Encourage both parent and teen to talk about these subjects together.

H. Ask about responsibilities teen has at home. Many parents advance privileges based on teen's ability to take care of his/her chores. This can also support fair negotiations that take place in family.

I. Use tool such as HEADSSS (Home and environment, Education and employment, Activities, Drugs, Sexuality, Suicide and depression, Safety) assessment to take snapshot of teen's life and identify problem areas to focus on during acute visits.

   1. HEADSSS assessment: Ask open-ended questions about home, education, activities, drug use and depression, sexuality, suicide, and safety.

J. Have resources available if issues such as drug abuse, school problems, physical/sexual abuse, depression, sexual activity, pregnancy are present.

K. If an undesired behavior that is identified through screening can be dealt with during primary care office visit, state desired behavior, offer health information detailing risks of undesired behavior, benefit of change, and alternatives. If teen can commit to change, set goal and timeframe, offer support and resources, and set up follow-up time.

II. NUTRITION

A. History.
   1. Ask for 24-hour diet recall.
   2. Are any foods/food groups avoided and why?
   3. Is milk consumed? Skim, 2%, whole?
   4. Is meat eaten? What types?
   5. What fruits, vegetables does teen eat? How much juice is consumed?
   6. Trying to gain or lose weight? How?
   7. Are meals skipped? Is breakfast eaten?

8. Are meals eaten on run or sitting down with family?
9. What types of "junk" foods are consumed? How much?
10. How often does teen eat at fast food restaurants? What foods?
11. Does teen watch TV and snack?
12. How much soda is consumed? Regular or diet?
13. What types of exercise is teen involved in?
14. Does teen spend time thinking about how to be thin?
15. Has teen tried dieting, diet pills, laxatives, vomiting to control weight?
16. Does teen ever eat in secret?
17. Is teen dieting to fit into weight class for sports?
18. Are any nutritional supplements taken?

B. Teaching.
1. Use MyPlate (see Appendix E) to encourage healthy eating practices and to review daily requirements of protein, calcium, vitamins, fiber.
2. Recognize that teen is likely making more choices on own, can start to read labels, becomes conscious of nutritional value.
3. Skipping breakfast may make it harder to concentrate in school and may lead to more hunger after school, possibly poor nutritional choices.
4. Skipping meals may lead to more hunger, poor food choices.
5. Encourage teen to talk with parent about planning meals, snacks.
6. Encourage trying new foods.
7. When limiting soda, drink more water, avoid excessive calories from juice products.
8. Discuss sources of calcium.
9. 5–8% of teen girls have iron-deficiency anemia.
10. Teens risk dental decay with high-sugar diets, poor dental hygiene.
11. 13–15% of children and adolescents are estimated to be overweight.
12. Teach behavioral techniques for weight management, such as goal setting, self-monitoring, positive reinforcement, problem solving, social support.
13. Incidence of eating disorders has increased and is estimated to affect 7% of male adolescents and 13% of female adolescents. Eating disorders can be associated with depression, substance abuse, low self-esteem.
14. Discourage rapid weight gain/loss to fit into weight class for sports.
15. Discourage major weight/dietary restrictions during growth spurt.

C. Physical exam.
1. Chart height, weight, body mass index (BMI); review growth curves with teen.
2. BMI at or above 95th percentile is considered overweight/obese. For obese teens, BMI is objective measure that is useful in motivating them to recognize their risks of developing heart disease, diabetes.

D. Labs.
   1. Screen hematocrit at beginning or ending puberty visit or both to check for anemia due to rapid growth, poor nutrition, menstrual losses.
   2. Glucose if there is family history of diabetes, symptoms of diabetes, or obesity and acanthosis nigricans.
   3. Cholesterol for adolescents with heart disease, hypertension, diabetes, or if there is family history of heart disease or hyperlipidemia.
E. Treatment plan.
   1. Encourage healthy eating practices.
   2. Encourage good exercise habits.
   3. For teens just starting to exercise, start slow, for example, walking for 20 minutes 3 times/week so they can build up their exercise tolerance.
   4. For teens with special diets, such as vegetarian diets, be prepared to assess dietary content, give advice/referral resource to offer nutritional guidance, support.
   5. For obese teens, offer support and encouragement. When motivated, they may be ready for weight-loss program. Suggest starting by keeping daily food diary to look for problem areas in diet. Behavioral techniques, mentioned earlier, may be enough for some teens to get started with healthier eating practices. In supportive environment, family involvement may help to cut down excess intake. Some teens benefit from professional weight-loss programs. Refer morbidly obese patients to medical weight-loss program.
   6. When eating disorders are suspected, careful assessment and monitoring are needed. Denial is common and should not offer reassurance. Patients require nutritional, medical management as well as mental health assessment and referral. Referral to eating disorder program will offer comprehensive approach to assessment and management.

III. ELIMINATION

A. Teens are normally independent in their elimination practices.
B. Constipation.
   1. Infrequent and/or difficult passage of feces.
   2. Common cause of abdominal pain.
C. History.
   1. What are bowel habits?
   2. When was last bowel movement? Hard and dry? Any abdominal pain?
   3. How long has constipation been a problem?
   4. Is fiber present in teen's diet?

5. What is fluid intake?
6. Does teen avoid public or school restrooms?
7. Does schedule allow time to use bathroom?
8. Have laxatives or stool softeners been tried? How often?
9. Ask about other signs of thyroid disease, such as menstrual disorder, dry skin, brittle hair, lethargy, and weight gain.

D. Teaching.
1. Describe gastrocolic reflex (peristalsis of colon induced by entrance of food into empty stomach).
2. Describe bowel function and need for fluid and fiber to keep stool moist and moving through GI tract.

E. Physical exam for suspected constipation.
1. Firm loops of bowel may be palpable on thin patients.
2. Rectum is typically filled with hard stool.
3. Passage of hard stool may cause anorectal pain or bleeding.

F. Labs.
1. Abdominal film may be needed in case of abdominal pain, after ruling out other systems as sources of pain.
2. Make sure female patients are not pregnant before sending for X-ray.

G. Treatment plan for constipation.
1. Encourage drinking plenty of water.
2. Help teen plan on how to add fiber to diet.
3. Encourage good toilet habits, such as right after meals.
4. Consider use of stool softener.
5. In addition to the above, sitz baths may help anal fissure heal.
6. Follow up in 1–2 weeks.

IV. SLEEP

A. Teenagers need 9–10 hours of sleep per night. Most teens do not get it.
B. Sleep history.
1. Does teen feel rested or tired?
2. What are concerns about sleep? Frequency? Duration?
3. What are usual bedtimes and wake-up times?
4. Are naps taken? If so, do they interfere with sleep later that night?
5. Has family complained about teen's snoring?
6. Does teen fall asleep in class? Other times?
7. What are school hours?
8. What are after-school activities?

      9. Does teen have job? How many hours?

   10. How many hours are spent on homework?

   11. Does teen care for child or have other household responsibilities?

   12. Is there family history of sleep disorders?

   13. Is teen depressed, sad, moody?

   14. Are stimulants (coffee, tea, soda, OTC medications, illicit drugs) used to stay awake longer?

   15. Does teen have TV, radio/stereo, computer, phone in bedroom? Are these in use when trying to go to sleep and delaying bedtime?

C. Teaching.

    1. Insomnias are most frequent sleep disorder during adolescence.

    2. Insomnias involve problems falling asleep, staying asleep, waking too early.

    3. Delayed sleep phase syndrome is inability to fall asleep at appropriate time, but if left to fall asleep naturally would fall asleep late, get up late. These teens will be sleepy if awakened to attend school.

    4. Teens may be motivated to stay up late, sleep late. If teen can awaken by his/her own motivation but not for school, this may be form of school refusal.

    5. Insomnia may occur due to stress, anxiety, poor sleep habits.

    6. Excessive daytime sleepiness can be caused by chronic sleep deprivation, usually due to busy schedule.

    7. Sleep apnea may be associated with obesity; symptoms include snoring, apneic periods during sleep, nighttime waking, and daytime sleeping.

    8. Narcolepsy is uncommon disorder that has an onset of 10–25 years of age. Components include sleep attacks, catalepsy, sleep paralysis, and/or hallucinations. There is evidence of genetic component.

D. Physical.

    1. Does teen appear alert?

    2. Does teen appear sad or depressed?

    3. Note blood pressure and pulse.

    4. Is teen obese?

    5. Is teen comfortable and able to breathe through both nostrils?

    6. Are tonsils enlarged?

E. Lab.

    1. To rule out sleep apnea, consider sleep study if teen/family reports snoring, frequent wake ups, apneic periods, daytime sleep.

F. Treatment plan.

    1. Have teen track sleep patterns for 1–2 weeks.

    2. Any question of depression needs assessment.

3. Have teen/parent look at schedule and commitments. Are there ways to decrease workload for overloaded teen?
4. Cut down on caffeine products, including OTC stimulants.
5. Cut out nap time.
6. Use bedroom for sleep only and put TV, computer, etc., elsewhere.
7. Teach relaxation techniques.
8. Identify stressors and write them down. If stressors are complex, consider counseling.
9. Stick to regular schedule of bedtime and waking up.
10. Encourage weight loss for obese teens.
11. Refer teens with nasal breathing problems/enlarged tonsils to ENT specialist.
12. Refer teens with difficult sleep problems, including those who do not do well with above plan, to sleep clinic.

V. GROWTH AND DEVELOPMENT

A. While some teens are able to state concerns, others may hope you will mention possible concerns for them, such as height, weight, pubertal development. Comfortable way to start such conversation may be "Some teens worry about being shorter (or taller, heavier, thinner) than their friends. I wonder if you have any concerns about this . . . "
B. Use growth charts to help see progress over time, relate their parameters to their blood relatives or point out what future growth is likely.
C. Tanner or sexual maturity rating (SMR) also may be reassuring.
D. For development outside of expected range, evaluate for medical cause.
E. Height.
   1. 33–60% of adult bone growth occurs during adolescence.
   2. 20–25% of final adult height occurs in puberty.
F. Weight: 50% of ideal adult body weight is gained during adolescence.
G. SMR: By middle adolescence most teens are in latter classes of Tanner or SMR scales. Spermarche occurs at about SMR 2.5. Menarche usually occurs at SMR 3 or 4. Using SMR can help teens to see where they are in puberty and what can be expected without having to compare themselves to friends.
   1. Menstrual history.
      a. Age at menarche?
      b. Frequency, duration, quantity of menstrual periods?
      c. Last menstrual period (LMP)?
      d. Dysmenorrhea and treatments used?

H. Psychosocial developmental tasks.
1. Increased independence from parents, inviting conflicts over control.
2. Peer group involvement intensifies. Conformity with peer values. Less time for family. Teams, clubs, gangs may become important.
3. Interest in dating, sexual experimentation. Preoccupation with romantic fantasy. Sexual orientation more evident to peers.
4. Identity and individuality grow. Increased acceptance of body image, more established ego and sexual identity. Increased intellectual abilities, emotional feelings. Vocational ideas more realistic.
5. Sense of omnipotence and immortality that may lead to high-risk behaviors.
6. Improved ability with abstract thought.

VI. SOCIAL DEVELOPMENT

A. Family.
1. Who are family members living with teen?
2. What is level of communication between members?
3. What are supports? Conflicts?
4. What are house rules? Who makes them?
5. What are teen's responsibilities?
6. Is there a curfew?
7. Does teen drive family car? What supervision is given?
B. School.
1. What is teen's school performance? Any recent changes?
2. What does teen like or dislike about school?
3. How does teen relate to classmates? To teachers?
4. Are there learning problems? Has teen been evaluated by school?
5. Are there behavior problems? How have those been addressed?
6. What is educational/vocational plan?
7. Has teen dropped out of school?
8. Is teen planning to get a GED?
9. If chronic illness, is there teaching plan in place for missed days?
C. Peers.
1. Who are teen's friends?
2. Is there a best friend?
3. Is there a trusted adult to talk to?
4. Does teen prefer to be with friends or alone?
5. What are interests and activities of peer group?
6. Does parent know teen's friends?

D. Interests.
  1. What are teen's activities? Hobbies?
  2. Does teen have a job? How many hours? Safety hazards on job?
  3. Does teen like to read?
  4. Does teen enjoy sports? Exercise?
E. Dating.
  1. What are house rules about dating?
  2. What advice have parents given about dating?
  3. Is teen thinking about dating?
  4. Does teen have romantic feelings about anyone?
      a. Is this person male or female?
      b. If these feelings are for same-sex person, does teen feel support from parents? Friends? Community?
F. Sexual history.
  1. Is teen thinking about sexual relationship or has he or she had sexual relations?
  2. Able to talk with parent about being sexually active?
  3. Aware of risks of sexual activity (emotional, sexually transmitted infections [STIs], pregnancy)?
  4. Vulnerable to these risks?
  5. Reason for being sexually active? Does teen feel pressured?
  6. Specific sexual behaviors (vaginal/anal intercourse or oral-genital sex)?
  7. Teen's age at first intercourse?
  8. Number of lifetime partners?
  9. How old is current partner? Is there more than one partner now?
  10. Are condoms used? Hormonal contraception? Spermicides?
  11. Does teen know how to use male/female condom?
  12. Does teen know about emergency contraception (EC)? Does teen who only uses condoms have prescription for EC?
  13. Any history of or current symptoms of STIs?
  14. Any history of pregnancy? Pregnancy scares? LMP?
  15. History of pregnancy termination? If so, how is teen coping?
  16. For teen parents, what are stresses? Support?
  17. Does teen feel safe in current relationship?
  18. In dating situations, has teen been hit or pushed? What did she/he do?
G. Substance use.
  1. Does teen know risks of substance use?
  2. Do any friends smoke cigarettes, drink alcohol, use inhalants, marijuana, other drugs?

3. Does teen smoke cigarettes, drink alcohol, use inhalants, marijuana, other drugs?
4. If teen does use substances, use screen such as CAGE (Cut down, Annoyed, Guilty, Eye-opener) to obtain more information (have resource available to teen who needs substance abuse treatment):

   C: Do you think you should cut down your use of _____?

   A: Do you get angry or annoyed when people tell you that you should cut down your use of _____?

   G: Do you feel guilty about your use of _____?

   E: Do you use this substance as eye-opener to get going in morning?
5. Does teen drink alcohol or use other drugs when driving?
6. Does teen attend parties where alcohol is served?
7. What plans are there to get home safely? Does teen have to deal with parents for this type of situation?

H. Antisocial behavior.
1. Does teen skip school?
2. Has teen had trouble with the law?
3. Does teen belong to or associate with a gang?

VII. IMMUNIZATIONS

A. May not have completed recommended vaccinations.
B. Immunization status can be reviewed at each visit.
1. Tdap: Booster usually given between 11 and 12 years but before 16 years, then every 10 years.
2. MMR: 2 doses needed before school entry.
3. Hepatitis B: Recommended for all adolescents, especially those at risk (sexually active, injection drug abusers, work-related exposure to blood/body fluids). Routine vaccination of infants began in 1991; may be in need of immunization. Two-dose regimen for 11- to 15-year-olds; 3-dose regimen for others.
4. Varicella: Needed if there is no history of varicella disease. If history is unclear, vaccine is well tolerated, more cost effective than serologic testing in most cases. Two doses given more than 4 weeks apart needed if 13 years of age or older.
5. Influenza: Recommended for teens with chronic illness (i.e., asthma, sickle cell disease, HIV, etc.) or those living with persons with impaired immunity. Can be given to others who want immunity. Cannot be given to individuals with egg allergy.

6. Hepatitis A: Vaccination recommended for those living in high-risk areas; 2 doses needed, at least 6 months apart.
7. *Neisseria meningitidis*: Vaccination recommended in many states for college freshmen living in dormitories.
8. HPV: Vaccination recommended before sexual intercourse begins to help prevent HPV infection, genital warts for all teens.

C. See Appendix A.

VIII. SAFETY

A. Self-protection.
   1. Does teen have any self-defense skills?
   2. Is teen aware of surroundings when in public?
   3. Does teen travel with friends?
   4. Has teen been victim of any attack in past? Any fear of someone threatening harm currently? Are parents/authorities aware?
   5. Does teen feel safe in school?
   6. Can teen walk away from conflict if she/he feels fear/anger?
   7. Does teen get into fights regularly?
   8. Is teen exposed to violence in home, community, media?
   9. Does teen have access to gun? What are rules for gun safety?
   10. Does teen carry a weapon? Why?
B. Injury prevention.
   1. Does teen wear seat belts?
   2. Does teen wear a helmet?
   3. Does teen plan to take driver's education classes?
   4. Does teen drive at night or with friends?
   5. Does teen use alcohol/other drugs?
   6. Does teen routinely take risks?
   7. Has teen had injuries in past?
   8. Does teen use power tools/lawn equipment?
C. Suicide prevention.
   1. Does teen or family worry about teen being depressed?
   2. Has teen lost pleasure in usual interests?
   3. Weight loss or gain?
   4. Sleep problem: Too much or too little?
   5. Increased/decreased activity level?
   6. Daily fatigue?
   7. Feelings of worthlessness, excessive/inappropriate guilt?

8. Decreased concentration or ability to make decisions?

9. Asking teen about mood can be done at every visit and is especially important if teen visits frequently or if physical complaints do not seem to make sense.

10. Recurrent thoughts of death or suicide? (If teen is suicidal, have resources, such as ability to escort to emergency department for psychiatric evaluation, immediately available.)

IX. ANTICIPATORY GUIDANCE

A. Many opportunities to give advice exist during history and physical exam.

B. Giving information in nonjudgmental way allows teen to make up his/her own mind about how to improve his/her health.

C. Puberty: Acknowledge where individual is regarding pubertal development and how development is likely to proceed.

D. Health care.
   1. Have yearly physical exam.
   2. See dentist twice/year, practice good dental hygiene.
   3. Keep up with routine vision care.
   4. Discuss use of sunscreen and skin cancer prevention.

E. Injury prevention.
   1. Wear seat belt when traveling in car.
   2. Wear helmet when riding bike, skates, scooter, motor bike/cycle.
   3. Wear appropriate protection when engaging in sports.
   4. Drowning prevention includes learning how to swim, not swimming alone, never abusing substances while doing water activities, entering unknown depths feet first.
   5. When operating equipment such as power tools, lawn mowers, and tractors, know safety rules and use appropriate safety equipment.
   6. Leading causes of death and injury of young drivers are inexperience, risk taking (speeding, dares), distraction (driving with friends, talking on cell phones), driving at night. Parents who recognize these risks can outline safety plan (curfew, supervision, no driving with peers until parent feels teen is ready, contracting for no substance abuse) for young driver going through "rite of passage."
   7. Ask parents to remove guns from home. If not an option, guns/ammunition need to be stored separately, in locked boxes. Especially important for parents of depressed teens to realize risk guns pose to their teen.
   8. Learn CPR.

F. Self-exam.
   1. Teach females self-administered breast exam. Use breast model to show how lumps may feel. Reassure teen that most lumps in her age group are not cancer.
   2. Teach males self-administered testes exam. Reinforce that concerns are okay to talk about. Teach warning signs for testicular tumors, torsion, and epididymitis.
G. Nutrition.
   1. Eat breakfast.
   2. Eat a low-fat diet.
   3. Watch junk food, soda consumption.
   4. Use MyPlate (see Appendix E) to evaluate diet.
   5. Encourage maintenance of healthy weight.
H. Exercise.
   1. Do aerobic exercise 3 times/week.
   2. Look for ways to increase exercise opportunities in daily life.
I. Peer pressure and self-esteem.
   1. Pick good friends who are interested in positive activities.
   2. Look at best qualities and feel good about them.
   3. Participate in activities because of desire to, not because everyone else is doing so.
   4. Figure out personally important goals, make sure friends do not derail.
J. Body modification: Tattoos and piercings.
   1. Reasons for getting a tattoo range from expressing independence to being part of a group. Some teens may be self-described "risk takers" who may also engage in drug use and sexual activity.
   2. Parental consent may be required in some locales.
   3. Advise teens that tattoos should be considered permanent because removal is expensive, time consuming, and may leave a scar.
   4. Tattoos and piercings may become infected. Advise teens to research sterile practices of the tattoo/piercing establishment. Postcare hygiene needs to be strictly followed.
   5. Teens should not get a tattoo or piercing if they are upset or intoxicated.
   6. Alternatives such as temporary tattoos or magnetic piercing look-a-likes may satisfy a passing need.
K. Stress reduction.
   1. Encourage setting aside time to rest and gather thoughts.
   2. Get plenty of sleep at night.
   3. Eat varied, nutritious diet.

4. Encourage physical activity.
5. Teach deep breathing and counting to 10 if feeling stressed or angry.
6. Keep lines of communication open with parent/guardian.
7. Get help from adult in teen's life if teen has much stress.
8. Try to keep open communication with family.
9. Have resources available for depressed teens.
10. Arrange emergency evaluation for suicidal intent/severe depression.

L. Substance abuse.
1. Do not smoke cigarettes or marijuana.
2. Do not drink alcohol or use inhalants or other drugs.
3. Do not drive if intoxicated. Have teen make plan with parents about what to do if out and driver providing ride becomes intoxicated.
4. Point out risks of substance use, including health consequences, accidents, school performance, impact on family/friends, legal implications, gateway to other drug use.
5. Make sure athletes are aware of risks of performance-enhancing drugs.

M. Sex.
1. Consider benefits of abstinence, such as ability to focus on personal and academic goals, less complicated breakups, STI prevention.
2. Consider risks of sexual activity, such as emotional stress, pregnancy, STIs.
3. Discuss how to deal with issues important to individual teen: Sex drive, peer pressure, older partners, partners who refuse to use protection, desire to have baby.
4. If teen decides sexual activity is right for him/her, advise use of condoms and make sure teen knows how to leave room at top of male condom for ejaculate and that female condoms can cover part of external genitalia.
5. Be frank about risks of STIs, especially HIV and other viral infections.
6. Educate about all types of appropriate birth control.
7. Make sure teens are aware of emergency contraception and how to obtain it.
8. For sexually active teens, screen for STIs.
9. For sexually active females, perform yearly Pap smear.
10. Encourage teen to talk with adult in his/her life about sex if able.
11. If teen identifies as minority sexual identity (gay, lesbian, bisexual, transgendered), make sure teen has resources, support.
12. If teen is pregnant, outline options and encourage parental involvement.

BIBLIOGRAPHY

Dixon SD, Stein MT. *Encounters with Children: Pediatric Behavior and Development.* 4th ed. St. Louis, MO: Mosby; 2006.

Goldenring JM, Cohen E. Getting into adolescent heads. *Contemp Pediatr.* 1998;5(7):75-90.

Jellinek M, Patel BP, Froehle MC, eds. *Bright Futures in Practice: Mental Health—Volume I. Practice Guide.* Arlington, VA: National Center for Education in Maternal and Child Health; 2002.

Joffe A, Blythe MJ, eds. *Handbook of Adolescent Medicine.* Philadelphia, PA: Hanley and Belfus; 2009.

Kleigman RM, Stanton BF, St. Geme JW, Schor NF, eds. *Nelson Textbook of Pediatrics.* 20th ed. Philadelphia, PA: Elsevier; 2016.

Neinstein LS. *Nelson's Adolescent and Young Adult Health Care: A Practical Guide.* 6th ed. Philadelphia, PA: Lippincott Williams & Wilkins; 2015.

Rosen D, The Committee on Adolescence. Clinical report: identification and management of eating disorders in children and adolescents. *Pediatrics.* 2003;111(1):204-211.

Shore W, Leanza F, Chaisson N, eds. *Adolescent Medicine, An Issue of Primary Care: Clinics in Office Practice.* Philadelphia, PA: Elsevier; 2014.

Common Childhood Disorders

Dermatological Problems

Linda Gilman, Megan Reynolds, Samantha Casselman, and Judith O'Haver

Acne, unspecified, L70.9

Allergic contact dermatitis, L23

Allergic urticaria, L50.0

Atopic dermatitis, L20

Contact dermatitis, unspecified, L25

Idiopathic urticaria, L50.1

Impetigo, unspecified, L01.00

Irritant contact dermatitis, L24

Pediculosis due to *Pediculus humanus capitis*, B85.0

Pityriasis versicolor, B36.0

Tinea barbae and tinea capitis, B35.0

Urticaria, unspecified, L50.9

I. APPROACH TO PATIENT WITH A RASH: HPI

A. Consider location, duration, distribution, secondary changes, associated symptoms (i.e., pruritus, scale), color.

B. Consider history such as age of the patient, other medical conditions, medications, recent illness or travel, other family members with similar symptoms.

C. Obtain a history of treatment of the rash/lesion, as it may change its morphology.

D. Description of actual lesion:

1. Macule: Flat lesion less than 1 cm.

2. Patch: Flat lesion larger than 1 cm.

3. Papule: Solid elevated lesion less than 1 cm.

4. Plaque: Solid elevated lesion greater than 1 cm.

5. Nodule: A palpable well-circumscribed lesion less than 1 cm.

6. Tumor: Solid palpable lesion greater than 1 cm.

7. Wheals: Caused by edema, so variation in size is often associated with pruritus. Characteristic is the individual lesions may disappear in 24 hours.

8. Vesicle: Lesion filled with fluid less than 1 cm.
9. Bulla: Lesion filled with fluid greater than 1 cm.
10. Pustule: A fairly well-circumscribed lesion of upper layers of skin filled with pus.

E. Secondary findings, including crusts, erosions, scars, excoriations, and scale often accompany many dermatological conditions. Determination of the appearance of the primary lesion, associated symptoms, and characteristics, along with secondary findings, are helpful in determination of the cause of the dermatitis.

II. ACNE

A. Etiology.
1. Interaction of the following:
   a. An alteration in the shedding process of the keratinocytes that line the pilosebaceous unit.
   b. An increase in sebum production.
   c. Proliferation of *Propionibacterium acnes* (*P. acnes*).
   d. The release of inflammatory mediators (Kim & Mancini, 2013). Open and closed comedones occur when there is an occlusion caused by the abnormal cornification and desquamation of the pilsebaceous duct and trapping of sebum (Tom & Friedlander, 2008). The presence of *P. acnes* on the skin causes the upregulation of many cytokines (Mancini et al, 2011).

B. Occurrence.
1. Affects 85% of adolescents aged 12–24 (Bhate & Williams, 2013).
2. Neonatal acne, which occurs in infants starting from birth to 4 weeks of age, affects up to 20% of newborns (Mancini et al, 2011).
3. Infantile acne, which occurs from roughly 4 weeks of age to 1 year of age, affects boys more often than girls (Mancini et al, 2011).
4. Midchildhood acne (age 1–7) is never considered normal, due to the fact that the adrenal secretion effectively ends after the first year of life until about the age of 7 (Mancini et al, 2011). Preadolescent acne affects children between the ages of 7 and 11 and adolescent acne begins about the age of 11 (Eichenfield et al, 2013).

C. Clinical manifestations.
1. Lesions often precede puberty.
2. Types of lesions direct treatment.

3. Comedones (both open and closed) are made when there is an increase in the activity and production of the sebaceous gland with abnormal follicular differentiation with increased keratinization, microbial hypercolonization of follicular canal, and increased inflammation, which occurs primarily through the activation of the adaptive immune system (Gollnick & Zouboulis, 2014). Inflammatory acne generally consists of erythematous papules, nodules, or cystlike nodular lesions, which are caused when follicles are colonized by *P. acnes*, with the inflammation occurring via the production of inflammatory mediators (Kim & Mancini, 2013). Mixed acne comprises both the inflammatory and comedonal components.

D. Physical findings.
  1. Acne appears in locations with increased sebum production, including the face, back, and shoulders. Comedonal acne can be found mostly in the "T-zone" across the forehead, on the nose, and on the chin. Inflammatory acne and mixed variations of acne can be found on the face, back, neck, and shoulders.
  2. Acne is categorized clinically as mild, moderate, or severe. There are no current agreed-upon standards of classifying acne. Acne can also contribute to anxiety, low self-esteem, embarrassment, social withdrawal, and depression (Tom & Friedlander, 2008).

E. Diagnostic tests.
  1. Generally, acne is a clinical diagnosis.
  2. Suspicion of possible adrenal or gonadal involvement for midchildhood acne should include Tanner staging and the following laboratory tests: Serum-free and serum-total testosterone, DHEA-S, FSH, LH, 17α-hydroxyprogesterone, prolactin, and an ACTH (Tom & Friedlander, 2008). A bone age assessment is the most useful tool for screening androgenicity (Tom & Friedlander, 2008).
  3. Isotretinoin therapy requires enrollment into the iPledge system, monthly pregnancy tests for childbearing females, complete blood count (CBC), triglycerides, and liver function tests (www.ipledgeprogram .com). Providers need to be registered in the system to order this therapy.

F. Differential diagnosis.
  1. Perioral dermatitis.
  2. Tinea faceii.
  3. Keratosis pilaris.
  4. Papular sarcoid.

G. Treatment.
1. Depends on lesion type, severity, and patient tolerance.
2. Acne patients should follow up with a provider 3 months after treatment has been initiated.
3. Refer to the treatments in **Table 21-1**.
4. **Table 21-2**, **Table 21-3**, and **Table 21-4** go into more detail about the different medications that can be used for acne treatment and their concentrations, doses, and side effects.

Table 21-1 Common Acne Treatments

Generic name	Brand name	Dosage Forms Available
Adapalene	Differin	Cream, gel, topical solution
Azelaic acid	Azelex	Cream
Azithromycin	Zithromax	Injection, oral liquid, tablet
Benzoyl peroxide	Brevoxyl, Zoderm	Cream, Lotion, soap
Clindamycin-benzoyl peroxide	BenzaClin	Gel
Tetracycline	Sumycin	Capsule, suspension, tablet
Tretinoin	Retin-A	Capsule, cream, gel, topical solution

Table 21-2 Fixed-Dose Combination Prescription Acne Therapies

Active Ingredients	Product	Age Indication
BP and clindamycin	BenzaClin gel (Dermik)	≥ 12 years of age
	Duac gel (Stiefel labs)	≥ 12 years of age
	Acanya gel (Medicis Pharma)	≥ 12 years of age
BP and adapalene	Epiduo gel (Gladerma)	≥ 9 years of age
Clindamycin and tretinoin	Ziana gel (Medicis Pharma)	≥ 12 years of age
	Veltin gel (Stiefel Labs)	≥ 12 years of age
BP and erythromycin	Benzamycin gel (Dermik)	≥ 12 years of age

Source: Kim W, Mancini AJ. Acne in childhood: an update. *Pediatr Ann.* 2013;42(10):418-427. Reproduced with permission of SLACK Incorporated.

Table 21-3 Topical Anti-infective Agents

Drug: Generic (Brand)	Dose	Formulations	Side Effects/Adverse Effects	Special Considerations
Azelaic acid (Azelex, Finacea)	Apply 2 times/day	Cream: 20% Gel: 15%	Itching, stinging, burning; may cause hypopigmentation	
Bacitracin (Baciguent)	Apply 1–3 times/day	Ointment	Contact dermatitis	Use with caution for persons with myasthenia gravis.
Benzoyl peroxide	Facial wash: apply 1–2 times/day	Gel: 2.5%, 5%, 10% 5% mixed with glycolic acid Solution: 5% mixed with erythromycin	Local irritation, photosensitivity, dryness	Do not use simultaneously with retinoids. Bleaching agent; avoid contact with hair and clothing.
Clindamycin (Cleocin-T)	Apply 2 times/day	Gel, lotion, solution: 10%	Dry skin, redness, peeling itching, oiliness Rarely with topical application: gastrointestinal upset, diarrhea, colitis, shortness of breath	Contraindicated for persons with history of ulcerative colitis or antibiotic-associated colitis.
Erythromycin (Erycette, A/T/S 2%, Benzamycin)	Apply 1–2 times/day	Gel, ointment: 2% Solution: 1.5%, 2%	Stinging, burning, dryness, peeling, redness	
Mupirocin (Bactroban)	Apply 3 times/day	Ointment: 2%	Burning, itching, headache, nausea, rash	
Neomycin (Myciguent)	Apply 1–3 times/day	Ointment	Skin irritation, burning, rash, ototoxicity	Use with caution for persons with impaired renal function.
Polymyxin B/neomycin (Neosporin cream)	10,000 units/g; 3.5 mg/g, respectively; apply 1–3 times/day	Cream	Skin irritation, rash, allergic response	Contraindicated for persons with myasthenia gravis.
Polymyxin B/Bacitracin/neomycin (Neosporin ointment)	400 units/g; 3.5 mg/g and 5000 units/g, respectively; apply 1–3 times/day	Ointment		

Table 21-4 Oral Anti-infective Agents Used to Treat Acne

Drug: Generic (Brand)	Dose Range	Indication	Side Effects/Adverse Effects	Special Considerations
Azithromycin (Zithromax)	500 mg as 1 dose then 250 mg daily for 5 days	MRSA	Diarrhea, nausea, severe allergic response including anaphylaxis or Stevens-Johnson syndrome	Use caution for persons with pneumonia, impaired liver or kidney function, or prolonged QT interval.
Erythromycin	250–750 mg 2 times/day	Acne	Gastrointestinal upset, decreased liver function, anaphylaxis, cardiac dysrhythmia	Diarrhea associated with use may indicate *Clostridium difficile* infection. Simultaneous use of clindamycin is contraindicated.
Clindamycin hydrochloride (Cleocin)	150–450 mg every 6 hours	MRSA	Rash, diarrhea, nausea, jaundice, pseudomembranous colitis	Simultaneous use of erythromycin is contraindicated. Use with caution for persons with history of colitis or atopy.
Cefaclor (Ceclor, Ceclor CD)	250–500 mg every 8 hours ER-375 mg every 12 hours	Skin or subcutaneous infections	Nausea, diarrhea, rash, arthralgia	Use with caution for persons with penicillin sensitivity or history of colitis.
Cefadroxil monohydrate (Duricef)	1 g/day	Skin or subcutaneous infections	Diarrhea, nausea, rash	Use with caution for persons with penicillin sensitivity or history of colitis.

Drug	Dosage	Use	Adverse Effects	Precautions
Cephalexin (Keflex)	250 mg every 6 hours or 500 mg every 12 hours	Skin or subcutaneous infections	Nausea, diarrhea, increased liver enzymes	Use with caution for persons with penicillin sensitivity or history of colitis.
Ciprofloxacin (Cipro)	400–750 mg orally, every 8–12 hours	Adverse skin infections	Rash, diarrhea, nausea, dizziness, headache, tendinitis, peripheral neuropathy	Use with caution for persons with alkaline urine, seizure disorder, renal impairment, or exposure to excessive sunlight.
Levofloxacin (Levaquin)	500–750 mg daily	Adverse skin infections	Nausea, diarrhea, constipation, headache, hypoglycemia, prolonged QT interval, liver failure, anemias, tendon rupture, acute renal failure	Use with caution for persons with CNS disorders, steroid use, diabetes, or impaired renal function.
Amoxicillin/ clavulanate (Augmentin)	250 mg every 8 hours or 500 mg every 12 hours	*Staphylococcus aureus*, *Escherichia coli*, *Klebsiella* spp.	Nausea, diarrhea, vaginitis, headache, transient elevation of liver functions, transient anemia	Use with caution for persons with liver dysfunction. Contraindicated if prior liver symptoms occurred with Augmentin.
Dicloxacillin sodium (Dynapen)	250–500 mg every 6 hours	*Staphylococcus*	Nausea, gastrointestinal upset (take 1 hour before or 2 hours after eating)	
Trimethoprim– sulfamethoxazole (Bactrim)	1 DS 2 times/day	MRSA	Gastrointestinal distress, urticaria, rash, aplastic anemia, agranulocytosis, hepatic disease	Contraindicated during pregnancy in third trimester. Contraindicated for persons with folate deficiency. Use with caution for persons with G6PD deficiency or asthma.

(continues)

Table 21-4 Oral Anti-infective Agents Used to Treat Acne (*continued*)

Drug: Generic (Brand)	Dose Range	Indication	Side Effects/Adverse Effects	Special Considerations
Doxycycline (Vibramycin, Atridox)	100 mg 2 times/day	Acne vulgaris	Photosensitivity, lightheadedness, vertigo, gastrointestinal upset, diarrhea, vaginitis, pseudotumor cerebri, hepatotoxicity, CNS symptoms	In pregnancy, fetal tooth damage and bone damage are possible. Use with caution in persons with renal or liver impairment or SLE.
	50–100 mg 2 times/day	Acne rosacea		
	100 mg 2 times/day for 7 days	MRSA		
Minocycline (Minocin, Solodyn)	100 mg 2 times/day	Acne vulgaris Acne rosacea MRSA		
Tetracycline	250–500 mg 2 times/day	Acne vulgaris Acne rosacea		

Abbreviations: CNS, central nervous system; G6PD, glucose-6-phosphate dehydrogenase; MRSA, methicillin-resistant *Staphylococcus aureus*; SLE, systemic lupus erythematosus.

H. Follow-up.
1. Acne patients should follow up with a provider 3 months after treatment begins to assess for care-plan effectiveness.
2. Clinicians should order lab work as indicated by therapy.
3. Clinicians should assess for compliance as well as overall acne improvement at every visit.

I. Complications.
1. Scarring.
2. Self-esteem issues.

J. Education.
1. Application and administration of medications with potential side effects.
2. Improvement occurs over months; therefore, adherence to regimen imperative.
3. Avoid harsh products to skin as may exacerbate dryness.
4. Topical emollients as needed.
5. Photoprotection, as many of the acne products may make skin more photosensitive.

III. ATOPIC DERMATITIS/ECZEMA

A. Etiology.
1. Atopic dermatitis (AD), commonly known as eczema, is a chronic skin condition characterized by pruritic, inflammatory patches that wax and wane throughout childhood.
2. It is hypothesized that a deficiency in the fillagrin gene causes the skin barrier to weaken (Eichenfield et al, 2014).

B. Occurrence.
1. AD has been reported to affect up to 25% of children worldwide (Eichenfield et al, 2014). It is one of the most widely treated dermatologic conditions of childhood requiring regular follow-up for medication and symptom management.
2. AD typically presents as early as infancy and is commonly associated with a strong family history of atopic conditions.
3. Approximately 70–80% of children will outgrow AD (Eichenfield et al, 2014).

C. Physical examination.
1. Erythema.
2. Edema.
3. Xerosis.

4. Erosions/excoriations.
5. Oozing and crusting.
6. Hypo-/hyperpigmentation.
7. Lichenification (thickening of the skin).
8. Distribution of affected areas will vary with age (Eichenfeld et al, 2014).
    a. Infants and children typically present with eczematous plaques on the face, neck, and extremities.
    b. Flexural involvement is common in the antecubital and popliteal fossa among all age groups, and involvement commonly spares the groin and axilla.
    c. The hands, ankles, and feet are also common locations for AD in school-age children and adolescents.
9. See **Box 21-1** for differential diagnosis.

D. Diagnosis/testing.
   1. Presence of clinical features.
   2. Thorough medical and family history.
   3. Formal testing is often not necessary.
   4. Lab evaluation: Commonly elevated serum IgE.

E. Symptoms.
   1. Pruritus.
   2. Inflammation with associated papulation, excoriation, exudation, and bleeding.
   3. Aside from physical findings, quality of life (QoL) may be negatively impacted in the patient and family.

F. Complications.
   1. Secondary infection.
      a. Staphylococcus or group A beta-hemolytic streptococci.

Box 21-1 Differential Diagnosis

- Psoriasis
- Tinea
- Contact dermatitis
- Scabies
- Seborrheic dermatitis
- Ichthyoses
- Cutaneous T-cell lymphoma

Source: Reprinted from Eichenfield L, Tom WL, Chamlin SL, et al. Guidelines of care for the management of atopic dermatitis part 1: diagnosis and assessment of atopic dermatitis. *J Am Acad Dermatol.* 2014;70(2);338-351, with permission from Elsevier.

2. Increased risk for viral infections.
   a. Molloscum contagiosum, verucca vulgaris, and herpes simplex.
3. Scarring and hyper/hypopigmentation.
4. Side effects of topical steroids.
   a. Skin thinning, stretch marks, telangiectasia, adrenal suppression.

G. Treatment.
   1. Ointments/creams: Topical steroids remain the gold standard for treatment of AD. Additionally, calcineurin inhibitors (e.g., Tacrolimus) may be utilized for thinner areas of skin (face, axilla, or groin) or for maintenance therapy to provide reprieve from topical steroid use. Ointments preferred over creams due to increased association of stinging/burning with creams. See **Table 21-5**.
   2. Emollients: Equally important, emollient use with petroleum jelly or fragrance free, thick creams should be utilized as often as is necessary to provide relief. Application of moisturizers provides a barrier to the skin and topical medications.

Table 21-5 Topical Treatment Dependent on Location of Atopic Dermatitis

Location of AD	Topical Treatment
Face, axilla, or groin	Hydrocortisone 2.5%
	Protopic™ (0.03% < 12 years old; 0.1% > 12 years old)
	Elidel™ 1%
Body	Triamcinolone 0.1% (maintenance therapy)
	Fluocinonide 0.05% (moderate to severe, short term)
	Clobetasol 0.05% (severe, short term)
Scalp	Dermasmooth FS scalp oil
	Betamethasone valerate lotion
	Clobetasol/fluocinonide foam
Hands/feet	Triamcinolone 0.1%
	Fluocinonide 0.05%
	Clobetasol 0.05%

Source: Reprinted from Schachner LA, Hansen RC, eds. *Pediatric Dermatology.* 4th ed. London: Mosby Elsevier; 2011, with permission from Elsevier.

3. Bathing: Soaking in lukewarm water 5–10 minutes a day should be recommended for patients with AD. Cleansers are preferred over soaps, and all products should be fragrance free and designed for sensitive skin.

4. Quality of life: Factors that negatively impact QoL for patients with AD should be addressed. Poor sleep is often a complaint due to itching throughout the night. Commonly recommended medications include antihistamines for sedation and may consider nonsedating formulations for suspicion for seasonal or environmental allergies.

H. Patient education considerations.

1. Nurse-led programs to support AD teaching in the clinic have been found to improve AD severity, with significant improvements in disease severity and QoL (Grillo, Gassner, Marshman, Dunn, & Hudson, 2006).

2. Proper assessment of the patient's and family's needs for patient education should be evaluated by the provider to promote family-centered care and patient satisfaction.

3. A combination of tools to promote patient education can include one-on-one counseling, educational videos, pamphlets, and web-based learning.

4. Promotion of patient and family knowledge of the condition and management at home should improve disease severity and decrease the need for unnecessary clinic visits and secondary infections.

IV. IMPETIGO

A. Etiology.

1. A superficial bacterial skin infection. It is more common in exposed areas with disruptions in the skin due to minor trauma.

2. In North America, is generally caused by Staphylococcus aureus or group A β-hemolytic streptococcus.

3. Lesions are characterized by honey-colored, crusted lesions or bullae surrounded by a narrow margin of erythema.

B. Occurrence.

1. Common in ages 2–7 years.

2. Incubation 1–10 days.

3. Predisposing factors such as poor hygiene and antecedent lesions such as insect bite, scabies, or pruritus from eczema or contact dermatitis.

C. Clinical manifestations.

1. Two major forms.

a. Nonbullous form: Underlying erythematous base with clear vesicles that rupture, enlarge, and spread, resulting in honey-colored crusts with erosion of the epidermis.

     b. Bullous form: Rapidly forming fragile bullae filled with clear fluid progressing to cloudy fluid before rupture. The recent erupted bullae leave an erythematous shiny base. They heal centrally, leaving crusted annular formation. This form may leave a scalded skin appearance.

     c. May be associated with regional adenopathy.

D. Physical findings.

   1. Moist crusted lesions generally on exposed areas such as face and hands.

   2. There are areas of erythematous swollen skin with blisters and honey crusts.

E. Diagnostic tests.

   1. Gram stain and bacterial culture for identification of causative organism.

   2. Diagnosis usually made by clinical presentation.

F. Differential diagnosis.

   1. Herpes simplex.

   2. Varicella zoster.

   3. Contact dermatitis.

   4. Atopic dermatitis.

   5. Fungal infections.

   6. Folliculitis.

   7. Ecthyma.

G. Treatment.

   1. Topical antibiotics if superficial nonbullous or localized to one or more lesions.

   2. Remove crusts by soaking with warm compresses.

   3. Topical antibiotic ointment such as Mupirocin 2% to lesions 3 times a day till clearing occurs. Re-evaluate if no improvement in 3–5 days or associated with systemic symptoms.

   4. If systemic treatment is needed due to multiple lesions that are widely separated with a deeper skin involvement such as face, buttocks, and knees, administer one of the following:

     a. Cephalexin.

     b. Augmentin: Dose based on amoxicillin component of the antibiotic.

     c. Failure to respond may suggest infection with methicillin-resistant Staph aureus, necessitating change of antibiotics to clindamycin or trimethoprim-sulfamethoxazole. Suggest obtaining confirmatory culture of lesions.

H. Patient education.

   1. Continue medication for 10 days; do not stop if lesions have cleared.

   2. Stress handwashing technique: Use separate towels and wash linens in hot water.

   3. Advise to keep nails short and filed to minimize spread of bacteria.

    4. May return to school after antibiotic therapy for 48 hours or if lesions are covered.

    5. Stress impetigo is spread by direct and indirect contact.

I. Follow-up.

    1. If not responding to treatment in 4–5 days or developing systemic symptoms.

    2. Acute glomerulonephritis is a major concern, and it can be a sequel of infection with Streptococcus pyogenes. Parents to call immediately if child has dark-colored urine or if edema is noted.

V. CONTACT DERMATITIS

A. Etiology.

    1. Contact dermatitis is an eczematous eruption resulting from either direct irritation to the skin from an irritating substance or delayed hypersensitive reaction to an allergen, resulting in nonspecific intracellular edema and inflammation.

B. Occurrence.

    1. Irritant contact dermatitis may occur at any age, though it is more common in young infants due to skin sensitivity and exposure to primary irritants such as diaper products, urine, and feces.

    2. Allergic contact dermatitis, such as associated with nickel exposure from metals in jewelry and snaps, topical products, and plants: Reaction is caused by delayed hypersensitivity reaction to contact with the allergen (T-cell mediated—Type IV immune response).

C. Clinical manifestations of allergic contact dermatitis.

    1. Localized rash with discrete borders and shapes.

    2. Usually is pruritic.

    3. Skin lesions are usually in the distribution of the contacting allergen and may appear as erythematous papular lesions, blisters, vesicles, or just erythematous linear rash.

    4. Lesions appear a day or two after exposure to allergen and may last for weeks without further exposure.

D. Clinical manifestations of irritant contact dermatitis.

    1. Rash appears almost immediately after contact.

    2. Rash more diffuse and located in the area of irritation.

    3. Rash is inflammatory and is time-dependent to skin response to irritant.

    4. Rash does not require prior sensitization to occur.

E. Physical findings.
   1. Localized erythematous rash with discrete border and shapes.
   2. Rash matches the contact site of the irritant.
   3. The irritant rash is characterized by burning, not itching.
   4. Skin folds are usually spared.
F. Diagnostic tests.
   1. Patch testing is gold standard for diagnosis.
G. Differential diagnosis.
   1. Infection (impetigo, candida, herpes).
   2. Langerhans cell histiocytosis.
   3. Atopic dermatitis/nummular eczema.
   4. Nutritional deficiencies.
   5. Psoriasis.
   6. Seborrheic dermatitis.
H. Treatment.
   1. Identify and eliminate future exposure to irritant or allergen.
   2. Cool compresses to irritant contact dermatitis area for comfort.
   3. Barrier ointments, thickly applied, such as petroleum jelly or zinc oxide to reduce friction and protect skin from irritant.
   4. Low potency topical corticosteroids with allergic dermatitis to the groin or diaper area or moderate to high potency for limited use for 2–3 weeks as needed if affected areas are not face, groin, or folds.
   5. In severe cases of allergic dermatitis, systemic corticosteroids may be used with a tapering course to avoid rebound of the dermatitis.
   6. May use antihistamines for severe cases of itching. Generally the sedation associated with these products makes them effective for nighttime use.
   7. Suggest cotton clothing and avoidance of perfumed products and cleansers.
I. Complications.
   1. Secondary bacterial infection.
J. Education.
   1. Identify offending substance and avoid. Limited exposure may exacerbate symptoms.
   2. Protect skin by wearing protective clothing or skin barrier creams.
   3. Prevention is the only approach to reducing incidence of contact dermatitis.
   4. Wash clothing in hot soapy water after exposure to remove allergen.
   5. Use antihistamines for sedation if sleep is an issue.
   6. Use topical steroids as directed. If symptoms escalate, may need to be reevaluated for consideration of further testing or systemic steroids.

VI. URTICARIA

A. Etiology.
1. Urticaria is a common allergic skin reaction characterized by well-circumscribed localized or generalized erythematous raised skin lesions (hives, wheals, or welts) of various sizes accompanied by intense pruritus. Factors included in the reaction are immune globulin E (IgE) response and complement activation. The immunological response is the release of histamine and leukotrienes, resulting in urticaria. A chronic type of urticaria exists and may occur frequently and last longer than 6 weeks. Histamine is the primary mediator to a variety of antigens.
B. Occurrence.
1. Common in pediatric population.
2. Approximately 25% of children will experience urticaria in childhood.
3. Chronic form more common in those children with a history of allergies, asthma, or atopic disease.
4. The cause is variable, and triggering agent may be difficult to ascertain. Common triggers are infection, medications, foods, insect bites, or systemic disease, or can be idiopathic.
C. Clinical manifestations.
1. Lesions are itchy, edematous, discrete, and/or confluent.
2. Lesions may be erythematous macules, papules, plaques, or wheals. May be annular or incomplete rings.
3. Lesions may be surrounded by a pale color.
4. Lesions may extend into tissue, resulting in angioedema, where there is an abundant number of mast cells; however, lesions usually involve the dermis.
5. By definition, individual lesions are transient and resolve within 24 hours; however, new lesions may appear.
D. Physical exam.
1. Erythematous wheals, plaques that change shape over time, usually pruritic.
2. Blanching of lesions when applying pressure.
3. Lesions appear to be migratory.
E. Diagnostic tests.
1. If suspect IgE-mediated urticarial, then future skin testing may be considered.
2. If suspect underlying infectious disease such as hepatitis or EBV, then consider titers.
F. Differential diagnosis.
1. Drug reaction.
2. Viral exanthema.

      3. Erythema multiforme.

      4. Urticarial vasculitis.

G. Treatment.

      1. Avoid triggers such as heat, alcohol, aspirin, tight-fitting itchy clothing.

      2. Colloidal oatmeal baths for comfort.

      3. Cool compresses for comfort.

      4. Antihistamines given every day to prevent the release of histamine from the mast cells.

      5. Acute urticaria usually is time limited, but chronic urticaria may take years to resolve.

H. Complications.

      1. Referral to pediatric allergist if patient does not respond to treatment.

I. Education.

      1. Keep a daily diary, most common causes of urticaria: Food or drug allergies, insect bites, exposure to plants such as poison ivy or poison oak.

      2. Give antihistamines daily to stabilize the response of mast cells.

      3. If associated with respiratory compromise, consider education on emergency treatment and dispense Epi-Pen with instructions appropriate for size of child.

VII. TINEA VERSICOLOR

A. Etiology.

      1. Tinea versicolor is a common superficial fungal skin infection caused by *Malassezia furfur*, which is found on healthy skin, especially if lipophilic, and thrives in hot, humid environments.

      2. Infection localizes to the stratum corneum and is characterized by hypopigmented or hyperpigmented macules and patches on the chest and back.

B. Occurrence.

      1. Tinea versicolor most often affects adolescents and young adults age 15–24.

      2. Seen worldwide, however more common in the tropics and summer months among 10- to 19-year-olds.

      3. Occasionally affects infants.

C. Clinical manifestations.

      1. Patient presents with hypopigmented patches of various sizes that generally do not itch.

D. Physical findings.
1. Characteristic macule covered with fine scale that coalesces to form confluent patches.
2. Localized on neck, upper chest, back, and upper arms.
3. Lesions are tan or reddish brown; color varies depending on darkness or lightness of skin.
E. Diagnostic tests.
1. Diagnosis may be made through potassium hydroxide (KOH) scraping with direct microscope examination.
2. The hyphae are short and have a "spaghetti and meatball" appearance.
F. Differential diagnosis.
1. Seborrheic dermatitis.
2. Pityriasis alba.
3. Postinflammatory hypopigmentation.
4. Vitiligo.
5. Pityriasis rosea.
G. Treatment.
1. Apply selenium sulfide 2.5% (Selsun lotion) daily for 7–10 days. Bathe, dry with coarse bath towel, apply Selsun to lesions, lather with small amount of water, and leave on for 10 minutes. Rinse thoroughly and dry with rough towel. May use monthly after initial treatment to prevent recurrence.
2. Systemic treatments are reserved for patients who do not respond to topical therapy.
3. Repigmentation occurs over months.
H. Follow-up.
1. Recheck in 2–4 weeks.
2. If lesions do not improve, consider oral treatment.
3. Referral to dermatology if no improvement.
I. Complications.
1. None.
J. Education.
1. Recurrence is common.
2. Pigment changes are gradual over a period of 4–6 months.

VIII. TINEA CAPITIS

A. Etiology.
1. Tinea capitis is a common dermatophyte infection of the scalp.
2. When present, must be treated systemically as topical agents are not effective.

3. The infection is often transmitted after a break in the skin.
4. Tinea capitis is caused by a common dermatophyte/fungi capable of infecting or colonizing hair follicles.
5. *Trichophyton tonsurans* is the main cause of 90% of tinea capitis infections. However, *Microsporum canis* and *Epidermophyton* may also be isolated.

B. Occurrence.
   1. Tinea capitis is spread by person-to-person contact, fomites, and, in some cases, from contact with infected animals. The peak incidence is school age, 3–7 years of age, and it occurs more in males than females.
   2. It is more common in African-American children.

C. Clinical manifestations.
   1. Two major forms:
      a. Noninflammatory form: Areas of alopecia with characteristic black dots caused by breaking of hairs shaft at base of hair follicle.
         • Lesions are round with patchy hair loss, and the lesions are usually pruritic.
         • Lesions may have erythematous plaques with follicular papules and crusting.
      b. Inflammatory form known as a kerion: Contains swollen hairless lesions with suppurative folliculitis. The area is boggy with tender plaques and pustules and is associated with local lymphadenopathy.

D. Physical findings.
   1. Oval patch of hair loss with erythema.
   2. Area of hair loss has black dots and broken hairs surrounding the oval patch of hair loss.
   3. Scaling itchy crusts involve the surrounding lesions.
   4. Kerions present with scaling pustules or a boggy, indurated, purulent, pruritic, raised plaque with localized lymphadenopathy.

E. Diagnostic tests.
   1. Gold standard is scrapings from the lesion and a KOH preparation.
   2. Fungal culture.
   3. Wood's lamp and fluorescencing the lesion; if Microsporum is the offending species, a green fluorescence will be noted.
   4. The most common offending species Trichophyton does not flourescence.

F. Differential diagnosis.
   1. Seborrheic dermatitis.
   2. Atopic dermatitis.
   3. Psoriasis.
   4. Alopecia areata.

5. Impetigo.
6. Bacterial folliculitis.
7. Trichotillomania.
8. Traction alopecia.

G. Treatment.
1. First line of treatment is with Griseofulvin. Dosing depends on preparation of the medication (microsize or ultramicrosize). It is given for 6–8 weeks.
2. Griseofulvin is to be taken with high-fat foods such as whole milk, ice cream, or bacon.
3. Adjunctive therapy, selenium sulfide shampoo 2.5% to suppress viable spores and decrease the spread of infection.
4. Terbinafine is generally more effective for treatment of *T. tonsurans*.
5. If kerion is present, treat as tinea capitis; may need oral steroids if extensive inflammation present to prevent scarring. This should be used in conjunction with the antifungal medication.
6. If kerion is present, may need to treat for secondary bacterial infection.

H. Follow-up.
1. Four weeks to evaluate progress.
2. Laboratory monitoring is generally not indicated in asymptomatic and otherwise healthy children.

I. Complications.
1. Permanent hair loss and scarring of infected area of skin.
2. Antifungal oral medications have many drug interactions.

J. Education.
1. Children should be discouraged from sharing clothing, especially hats and scarfs.
2. Watch pets for any suspicious lesions.
3. At onset of therapy, wash all hats and hair utensils.
4. Stress importance of completing therapy.
5. Family members should use selenium sulfide or ketoconazole shampoo for several weeks following diagnosis on one member in family.

IX. HEAD LICE (*PEDICULOSIS HUMANUS CAPITIS*)

A. Etiology.
1. Head lice (*Pediculus humanus capitis*) are ectoparasites that grasp the hair shaft and lay their eggs (nits). The eggs need warmth to hatch, therefore, most nits are found close to the scalp. They hatch within 6–9 days. Once hatched, the lice rely on human hosts for survival.

B. Occurrence.
   1. Estimates vary; however, reports suggest 6–12 million are infected annually.
   2. Infection is more common in school-age children as they are more likely to have head-to-head contact.
   3. Contact may be also from fomites such as combs and brushes (Canyon, Speare, & Muller, 2002).
C. Clinical manifestations.
   1. Pruritus is common; however, initially the patient is often asymptomatic.
   2. Nits are adherent to the hair shaft and often noted post auricular and nape of neck. Usually these are white to tan brown and are 0.5–0.8 mm in size.
   3. Live lice may be noted throughout scalp.
   4. Secondary infection may be present with associated lymphadenopathy.
D. Physical findings.
   1. Adherent nits to shaft of hair.
   2. Presence of live louse.
   3. Secondary excoriations or infections to scalp.
   4. Lymphadenopathy may be present.
E. Diagnostic tests.
   1. Clinical examination.
   2. Microscopic exam of nits or lice is possible to confirm diagnosis but usually not needed.
F. Differential diagnosis.
   1. Pseudonits (hair casts).
   2. Hair products that leave residue in hair.
   3. Seborrheic dermatitis.
G. Treatment.
   1. Pediculicides: There are many topical products available both over the counter and by prescription, with varying safety profiles and efficacy. Resistant patterns vary regionally, which may affect treatment choice; however, important to determine if actual resistance versus reinfestation. Some products require a second application to increase efficacy. There are also herbal remedies that have been tried with various reported success. Occlusive treatments generally have poor success as the lice have the ability to appear dead initially and then resurrect in a few hours and continue the life cycle.
   2. Examine close contacts for infestation and treat if necessary.
   3. Clothing, bedding, and head-gear should be washed in hot water and dried on high heat.

4. Nits should be removed if possible to prevent hatching and for cosmetic reasons; however, "no nit" policies in schools are not warranted.

5. Topical corticosteroids may be indicated for pruritus or associated dermatitis related to infestation.

6. Secondary infections should be treated with antibiotics.

7. Severe pruritus or sleep disturbance may warrant systemic antihistamine therapy.

H. Follow-up.

1. Usually not warranted unless resistant infection.

I. Complications.

1. Secondary infection.

2. Pruritus.

J. Education.

1. Directions for administration of pediculicide of choice.

2. Directions for examination of close contacts.

3. Cleaning and housekeeping directions to prevent spread and reinfestation. The CDC has a fact sheet that is helpful for family teaching.

4. Directions for use of topical corticosteroids and use of antihistamines if warranted.

5. Directions for nit removal.

6. Reassurance that this does not indicate poor hygiene and is a common occurrence for children.

BIBLIOGRAPHY

Acne.org. Accutane (isotretinoin): everything you need to know about accutane, including user reviews. http://www.acne.org/accutane.html. Accessed June 15, 2015.

Amer A. Can you spot the cause of this girl's scalp lesion? *Consultant for Pediatrics.* 2004;13(8):345, 346-349.

Balkrishnan R, Kulkarni AS, Cayce K, Feldman SR. Predictors of healthcare outcomes and costs related to medication use in patients with acne in the United States. *Cutis.* 2006;77(4):251-255.

Bhate K, Williams HC. Epidemiology of acne vulgaris. *Br J Dermatol.* 2013;168(3):474-485.

Canyon DV, Speare R, Muller R. Spatial and kinetic factors for the transfer of head lice (*Pediculus capitis*) between hairs. *J Invest Dermatol.* 2002;119(3):629-631.

Centers for Disease Control. Parasites—lice—head lice. http://www.cdc.gov/parasites/lice/head. Updated September 24, 2013. Accessed June 15, 2015.

Eichenfield LF, Krakowski AC, Piggott C, et al. Evidence-based recommendations for the diagnosis and treatment of pediatric acne. *Pediatrics.* 2013;131(Suppl 3):S163-S186.

Eichenfield L, Tom WL, Chamlin SL, et al. Guidelines of care for the management of atopic dermatis part 1: diagnosis and assessment of atopic dermatitis. *J Am Acad Dermatol.* 2014;70(2):338-351.

Ely J, Rosenfeld S, Stone M. Diagnosis and management of Tinea infections. *Am Fam Physician.* 2014;90(10):702-711.

Gollnick HP, Zouboulis CC. Not all acne is acne vulgaris. *Dtsch Arztebl Int.* 2014;111(17):301-312.

Grillo M, Gassner L, Marshman G, Dunn S, Hudson P. Pediatric atopic eczema: the impact of an educational intervention. *Pediatr Dermatol.* 2006;23(5):428-36.

Hamm H, Johr R, Mayer J. Principles of diagnosis in pediatric dermatology. In: Schachner LA, Hansen RC, eds. *Pediatric Dermatology.* 3rd ed. Edinburgh: Mosby; 2003:59-86.

Hartman-Adams H, Bonvard C, Juckett G. Impetigo: diagnosis and treatment. *Am Fam Physician.* 2014;15;90(4):229-235.

Herro E, Jacob SE. An update on pediatric allergic contact dermatitis patch testing for common allergens. *Consultant for Pediatricians.* 2014;13(8):305-355.

iPledge [homepage]. http://www.ipledgeprogram.com. Accessed June 15, 2015.

Johansen NG. What's causing this boy's hair loss? *Consultant for Pediatrics.* 2014;13(1):8-9.

Kim W, Mancini AJ. Acne in childhood: an update. *Pediatr Ann.* 2013;42(10):418-427.

Krowchuk DP, Mancini AJ. Head lice. In: Krowchuk DP, Mancini AJ, eds. *Pediatric Dermatology: A Quick Reference Guide.* Elk Grove Village, IL: American Academy of Pediatrics; 2007:221-224.

Kwan JM, Jacobs SE. Contact dermatitis in the atopic child. *Pediatr Ann.* 2012;41(10):422-23, 426-428.

Lewis LS. Impetigo treatment & management. Medscape. http://emedicine.medscape.com/article/965254 -treatment. Updated September 10, 2014. Accessed June 18, 2015.

Mancini AJ, Baldwin HE, Eichenfield LF, Friedlander SF, Yan AC. Acne life cycle: the spectrum of pediatric disease. *Semin Cutan Med Surg.* 2011;30(3 Suppl):S2-S5.

McEvoy B, Nydegger R, Williams G. Factors related to patient compliance in the treatment of acne vulgaris. *Int J Dermatol.* 2003;42(4):274-280.

Meinking TL, Taplin D, Kalter DC, Eberle MW. Comparative efficacy of treatment for *Pediculosis capitis* infestations. *Arch Dermatol.* 1986;122(3):267-271.

Park C, Kim G, Patel I, Chang J, Tan X. Improving adherence to acne treatment: the emerging role of application software. *Clin Cosmet Investig Dermatol.* 2014;7:65-72.

Schachner LA, Hansen RC, eds. *Pediatric Dermatology.* 4th ed. London: Mosby Elsevier; 2011.

Taketomo CK, Hodding JH, Kraus DM. *Pediatric & Neonatal Dosage Handbook.* 20th ed. Hudson, OH: Lexi-Comp, Inc.; 2014.

Tom WL, Friedlander SF. Acne through the ages: case-based observations through childhood and adolescence. *Clin Pediatr (Phila).* 2008;47(7):639-651.

Wang V. Boy is itching for relief. *Contemp Pediatr.* 2013;30(4):21-22.

Eye Disorders

Frances K. Porcher

I. ALLERGIC CONJUNCTIVITIS

Acute upper respiratory infection, unspecified, J06.9	Epiphora, H04.2
Allergic rhinitis due to pollen, J30.1	Other chronic allergic conjunctivitis, H10.45
Allergic rhinitis, unspecified, J30.4	Other seasonal allergic rhinitis, J30.2
Asthma, J45	

A. Definition.
  1. Inflammation or infection of bulbar and/or palpebral conjunctiva.
B. Etiology.
  1. Allergens such as pollen, molds, animal dander, smoke, dust.
C. Occurrence.
  1. Common in all age groups.
  2. Often seasonal.
  3. May have had recent upper respiratory infection.
D. Clinical manifestations.
  1. Watery, red eyes.
  2. Itching or burning bilaterally.
  3. Excessive tearing.
E. Physical findings.
  1. Diffuse conjunctival hyperemia.
  2. Boggy conjunctiva.
  3. Stringy, mucoid discharge.
  4. May see concurrent asthma, atopic dermatitis, or allergic rhinitis.
F. Diagnostic tests.
  1. None.
  2. Culture if conjunctivitis is persistent or does not respond to treatment.

G. Differential diagnosis.

Acquired stenosis of unspecified nasolacrimal duct, H04.559	Injury of conjunctiva and corneal abrasion without foreign body, unspecified eye, initial encounter, S05.00XA
Conjunctivitis, unspecified, H10.9	Viral conjunctivitis, unspecified, B30.9

1. Bacterial or viral conjunctivitis.
2. Nasolacrimal duct obstruction.
3. Corneal abrasion.

H. Treatment.
1. Eliminate offending agent.
2. Systemic oral antihistamine (Loratadine [Claritin], Cetirizine [Zyrtec]).
3. Topical ophthalmic mast-cell stabilizer (Cromolyn, Alomide).
4. Topical ophthalmic antihistamine/mast-cell stabilizer combination (Patanol, Bepreve).
5. Artificial tears.
6. Cool, wet compresses.

I. Follow-up.
1. Routine follow-up not necessary.
2. Return if fails to improve in 2–3 days or worsens.

J. Complications.

Adverse effect of drug or medicament, unspecified, T88.7

Other specified bacterial agents as the cause of diseases classified elsewhere, B96.89

1. Allergic reaction to medication.
2. Secondary bacterial infection.

K. Education.
1. Avoid rubbing eyes.
2. Use meticulous handwashing.
3. Avoid wearing eye makeup until resolved.
4. Avoid use of contact lenses until resolved.
5. Will last about 10–14 days.

II. BACTERIAL CONJUNCTIVITIS

Acute serous otitis media, H65.0

Conjunctival hyperemia, unspecified eye, H11.439

Conjunctivitis, unspecified, H10.9

A. Etiology.
  1. *Haemophilus influenzae (H. influenzae).*
  2. *Streptococcus pneumoniae.*
  3. *Moraxella catarrhalis.*
  4. *Staphylococcus aureus* (less common).
B. Occurrence.
  1. Common in school-age children.
  2. Accounts for 80% of pediatric acute conjunctivitis.
C. Clinical manifestations.
  1. Red eyes.
  2. Purulent discharge, with matted eyelids on awakening.
  3. May complain of gritty sensation in eye.
  4. Usually starts unilaterally, becoming bilateral.
D. Physical findings.
  1. Diffuse and marked conjunctival hyperemia.
  2. Purulent or mucopurulent discharge.
  3. May see concurrent otitis media (especially with *H. influenzae*).
E. Diagnostic tests.
  1. Culture in infants younger than 1 month of age, multiple cases in a daycare/school; unless conjunctivitis is persistent or does not respond to treatment.
F. Differential diagnosis.

Acquired stenosis of unspecified nasolacrimal duct, H04.559	Herpesviral keratitis, B00.52
Blepharitis, H01.0	Injury of conjunctiva and corneal abrasion without foreign body, unspecified eye, initial encounter, S05.00XA
Chlamydial conjunctivitis, A74.0	
Corneal ulcer, H16.0	
Gonococcal infection of eye, A54.3	Viral conjunctivitis, unspecified, B30.9

  1. Viral conjunctivitis.
  2. Chlamydial conjunctivitis (refer to ophthalmologist).
  3. Neisseria gonorrhoeae conjunctivitis (refer to ophthalmologist).
  4. Nasolacrimal duct obstruction.
  5. Blepharitis.
  6. Corneal abrasion or ulcer (refer to ophthalmologist).
  7. Herpes simplex (refer to ophthalmologist).
G. Treatment.
  1. Medications:
    a. Erythromycin ophthalmic ointment.
    b. Trimethoprim-polymixin B ophthalmic ointment or drops (Polytrim) (> 2 months of age).

     c. Moxifloxacin (VIGAMOX) or Moxeza (> 4 months of age).

     d. Levofloxacin (Quixin) (> 1 year of age).

  2. Treat conjunctivitis-otitis syndrome (usually caused by *H. influenzae*) for otitis only; concurrent use of topical antibiotic not necessary.

  3. Cool, wet compresses.

  4. Discontinue use of contact lenses immediately, see ophthalmologist if symptoms do not improve in 12–24 hours.

  5. To ophthalmologist if reduction of visual acuity or presence of photophobia (concern for keratitis, iritis).

H. Follow-up.

  1. No routine follow-up necessary.

  2. Recheck if fails to improve in 2–3 days or worsens.

I. Complications.

Sepsis, unspecified organism, A41

Visual impairment including blindness (binocular or monocular), H54

---

  1. Systemic infection.

  2. Blindness.

J. Education.

  1. Continue treatment for at least 7 days or for at least 3 days after symptoms have resolved.

  2. Very contagious; meticulous handwashing and no sharing of linens.

  3. No school or daycare until antibiotic treatment for 24 hours.

  4. Instillation of ophthalmic ointment will blur vision.

III. CHLAMYDIAL CONJUNCTIVITIS

Chlamydial pneumonia, J16.0

Conjunctival hyperemia, unspecified eye, H11.439

Cough, R05

Other specified disorders of nose and nasal sinuses, J34.8

Tachypnea, not elsewhere classified, R06.82

Viral conjunctivitis, unspecified, B30.9

Viral pneumonia, not otherwise classified, J12

A. Etiology.

  1. Chlamydia trachomatis.

B. Occurrence.

  1. Neonatal occurrence, acquired from infected cervix during birth.

  2. Adult occurrence, acquired through sexual contact.

C. Clinical manifestations.
   1. Purulent discharge.
   2. May occur in one or both eyes.
   3. Neonatal infection appears from day 2 to week 8.
D. Physical findings.
   1. Mucopurulent discharge.
   2. Hyperemic conjunctiva.
   3. May see *Chlamydophila pneumoniae* in infants.
E. Diagnostic tests.
   1. Giemsa-stained epithelial cells from conjunctival scraping.
   2. Conjunctival culture from swab (requires special tissue culture techniques).
   3. Immunofluorescent staining of conjunctival scraping.
   4. Chlamydial antigen test.
F. Differential diagnosis.

Congenital glaucoma, Q15.0	Gonococcal infection of eye, A54.3
Conjunctivitis, unspecified, H10.9	Viral conjunctivitis, unspecified, B30.9

   1. *Neisseria gonorrhoeae* conjunctivitis (refer to ophthalmologist).
   2. Bacterial conjunctivitis.
   3. Viral conjunctivitis.
   4. Congenital glaucoma (refer to ophthalmologist).
G. Treatment.
   1. Refer all neonates for evaluation and treatment (systemic oral erythromycin).
   2. Refer mother and mother's sexual partner for evaluation and treatment.
   3. Report to appropriate authority (sexually transmitted infection).
H. Follow-up.
   1. Return in 3 days to monitor eye infection.
   2. Return sooner if infant has signs of pneumonia or parental concerns.
I. Complications.
   1. Other sexually transmitted infections.
J. Education.
   1. Review good handwashing with family.
   2. Mother and partner need treatment because disease is usually transmitted vaginally during birth.
   3. Eye infection can be associated with pneumonia that started during first 6 weeks with cough, rhinorrhea, tachypnea.
   4. Infant may need second round of erythromycin; efficacy is 80%.

IV. VIRAL CONJUNCTIVITIS

Acute pharyngitis, J02	Conjunctival hyperemia, unspecified
Acute upper respiratory infection,	eye, H11.439
unspecified, J06.9	Viral conjunctivitis, unspecified, B30.9

A. Etiology.
 1. Adenovirus 3, 4, 7 (most common).
 2. Herpes simplex.
 3. Varicella zoster.
 4. Coxsackie.
B. Occurrence.
 1. Common in all age groups.
 2. Very contagious; 8-day incubation period.
C. Clinical manifestations.
 1. Pinkish-red eyes.
 2. Watery or serous discharge, with crusty eyelids on awakening.
 3. May complain of gritty sensation in eye.
 4. May complain of sore throat, upper respiratory infection, flulike symptoms.
 5. One or both eyes involved.
 6. Vesicles on skin around eye (herpes).
D. Physical findings.
 1. Diffuse conjunctival hyperemia with follicles.
 2. Watery or serous discharge.
 3. Discomfort, not acute pain.
 4. Preauricular and submandibular adenopathy.
 5. May see concurrent pharyngitis and/or upper respiratory infection.
 6. Vesicular lesions on skin around eyes (herpes).
 7. Normal vision.
E. Diagnostic tests.
 1. None.
 2. Culture if conjunctivitis is persistent or does not respond to treatment.
F. Differential diagnosis.

Acquired stenosis of unspecified nasolacrimal duct, H04.559	Injury of conjunctiva and corneal abrasion without foreign body,
Blepharitis, H01.0	unspecified eye, initial encounter,
Conjunctivitis, unspecified, H10.9	S05.00XA
Corneal ulcer, H16.0	Other chronic allergic conjunctivitis, H10.45

    1. Bacterial conjunctivitis.

    2. Allergic conjunctivitis.

    3. Nasolacrimal duct obstruction.

    4. Blepharitis.

    5. Corneal abrasion or ulcer (refer to ophthalmologist).

G. Treatment.

    1. Antibiotics not indicated.

    2. Cool, wet compresses.

    3. Artificial tears.

    4. Refer if suspect conjunctivitis due to herpes.

H. Follow-up.

    1. No routine follow-up necessary.

    2. Recheck if fails to improve in 10–14 days; sooner if worsens.

I. Complications.

Other specified bacterial agents as the cause of diseases classified elsewhere, B96.89

    1. Secondary bacterial infection.

J. Education.

    1. Very contagious; meticulous handwashing and no sharing of linens.

    2. Avoid touching eyes.

    3. Will last about 12–14 days.

    4. No school or daycare until discharge is resolved.

V. CONGENITAL NASOLACRIMAL DUCT OBSTRUCTION (DACRYOSTENOSIS)

A. Definition.

Acquired stenosis of unspecified nasolacrimal duct, H04.559

    1. Defect of lacrimal drainage system resulting in blockage.

B. Etiology.

    1. Imperforate membrane at distal end of nasolacrimal duct.

C. Occurrence.

    1. Occurs in up to 6% of all newborn infants.

    2. Both eyes involved, 33%; one eye involved, 66%.

D. Clinical manifestations.

    1. Persistent, excessively watery eyes.

    2. Mucopurulent discharge.

    3. Matted eyes on awakening.

E. Physical findings.
   1. Watery eyes, often overflowing onto cheek.
   2. Sclera clear.
   3. Reflux of mucopurulent discharge from punctum easily obtained with gentle pressure over nasolacrimal sac.
   4. May see concurrent erythema or irritation of skin around eyes.
F. Diagnostic tests.
   1. Gentle pressure over nasolacrimal sac produces mucopurulent discharge from punctum.
G. Differential diagnosis.

Blepharitis, H01.0	Dacryocystitis of unspecified lacrimal passage, unspecified H04.309
Conjunctivitis, unspecified, H10.9	Viral conjunctivitis, unspecified, B30.9

   1. Viral conjunctivitis.
   2. Bacterial conjunctivitis.
   3. Blepharitis.
   4. Dacryocystitis.
H. Treatment.
   1. Massage lacrimal sac several times a day.
   2. If secondarily infected, treat with anti-infective (see *Bacterial Conjunctivitis* on page 210).
   3. Refer to ophthalmologist if not resolved by 12 months of age.
I. Follow-up.
   1. Recheck at all well-baby exams and as needed.
J. Complications.

Cellulitis of unspecified orbit, H05.019
Conjunctivitis, unspecified, H10.9
Dacryocystitis of unspecified lacrimal passage, unspecified H04.309

   1. Bacterial conjunctivitis.
   2. Dacryocystitis.
   3. Periorbital or orbital cellulites.
K. Education.
   1. Wash hands before touching infant's eyes.
   2. Teach massage technique: Place index finger over lacrimal sac, exert gentle downward pressure, and slide finger downward toward mouth.

VI. BLEPHARITIS

A. Definition.

Blepharitis, H01.0

Conjunctivitis, unspecified, H10.9

Inflammation of eyelid, unspecified, H01.9

B. Etiology.
 1. Seborrhea.
 2. Staphylococcal.
 3. Pediculosis pubis or pediculosis capitis.
C. Occurrence.
 1. Can occur in all age groups.
D. Clinical manifestations.
 1. Red eyelid margin.
 2. Itching or burning of eyelid margin.
 3. Crusting or scaling of eyelid margin.
 4. Commonly bilateral and chronic or recurrent.
E. Physical findings.
 1. Seborrhea.
 a. Easy-to-remove yellow, greasy scales along base of eyelashes.
 b. May see concurrent and similar scales on eyebrows, scalp, external ears.
 2. Staphylococcal.
 a. Fibrinous, difficult-to-remove scales along base of eyelashes.
 b. Inflammation or ulceration of lid margins.
 c. Loss of eyelashes.
 d. May see concurrent conjunctivitis.
 3. Pediculosis.
 a. Lice along lid margins.
 b. May see concurrent pubic or head lice.
F. Diagnostic tests.
 1. Culture of lid margin indicated only if fails to respond to treatment.
G. Differential diagnosis.

Acquired stenosis of unspecified nasolacrimal duct, H04.559	Other chronic allergic conjunctivitis, H10.45
Conjunctivitis, unspecified, H10.9	Seborrheic dermatitis, unspecified, L21.9
Contact dermatitis, unspecified, unspecified cause, L25.9	
Other atopic dermatitis, L20.8	Viral conjunctivitis, unspecified, B30.9

    1. Conjunctivitis (allergic, bacterial, or viral).

    2. Nasolacrimal duct obstruction.

    3. Atopic or contact dermatitis.

    4. Seborrheic dermatitis.

H. Treatment.

    1. Clean eyelid margins twice a day with diluted baby shampoo.

    2. Seborrhea blepharitis: Treat eyebrows, scalp, ears with selenium sulfide shampoo.

    3. Staphylococcal blepharitis: Apply topical anti-infective ointment (erythromycin ophthalmic ointment or bacitracin/polymyxin B ophthalmic ointment).

    4. Pediculosis blepharitis: Remove parasite by smothering with ophthalmic petrolatum along lid margins.

I. Follow-up.

    1. No routine follow-up necessary.

    2. Recheck if fails to improve; sooner if worsens.

J. Complications.

Conjunctivitis, unspecified, H10.9

Hordeolum externum unspecified eye, unspecified eyelid, H00.019

Hordeolum internum unspecified eye, unspecified eyelid, H00.029

---

    1. Loss of eyelashes.

    2. Conjunctivitis.

    3. Hordeolum or chalazion.

K. Education.

    1. Frequent handwashing.

    2. Discourage rubbing of eyes.

VII. HORDEOLUM

Hordeolum externum unspecified eye, unspecified eyelid, H00.019

Hordeolum internum unspecified eye, unspecified eyelid, H00.029

A. Definition.

    1. Infection of meibomian glands (internal hordeolum) or glands of Zeis or Moll (external hordeolum or stye) of eyelid.

B. Etiology.

    1. Usually Staphylococcal aureus.

C. Occurrence.

    1. Can occur at any age.

D. Clinical manifestations.
   1. Internal: Painful and tender eyelid, red eye, usually without pustule.
   2. External: Painful and tender eyelid, red eye, usually with pustule.
E. Physical findings.
   1. Internal: Large, erythematous, tender mound of one eyelid with associated mild conjunctival hyperemia.
   2. External: Smaller, more superficial eyelid pustule with associated mild conjunctival hyperemia.
F. Diagnostic tests.
   1. None indicated.
G. Differential diagnosis.

Abscess of eyelid unspecified eye, unspecified eyelid, H00.039

Chalazion unspecified eye, unspecified eyelid, H00.19

---

   1. Eyelid abscess.
   2. Chalazion.
H. Treatment.
   1. Frequent, warm compresses.
   2. May use topical antiinfective ointment (erythromycin ophthalmic ointment or bacitracin/polymyxin B ophthalmic ointment).
   3. Refer if mass fails to disappear after several weeks (may need surgical incision and drainage).
I. Follow-up.
   1. No routine follow-up necessary.
   2. Recheck if fails to resolve or worsens.
J. Complications.

Cellulitis of unspecified orbit, H05.019

---

   1. Orbital or eyelid cellulitis.
K. Education.
   1. Frequent handwashing.
   2. Avoid rubbing eyes.

VIII. CHALAZION

A. Definition.

Chalazion unspecified eye, unspecified eyelid, H00.19

Hordeolum externum unspecified eye, unspecified eyelid, H00.019

B. Etiology.
   1. Granulomatous inflammation.
C. Occurrence.
   1. Can occur at any age.
D. Clinical manifestations.
   1. Hard painless mass in upper or lower eyelid.
   2. Not red or pustular.
   3. Chronic appearance.
E. Physical findings.
   1. Firm, nontender nodule in upper or lower eyelid.
   2. Not erythematous or pustular.
   3. No eye discharge.
F. Diagnostic tests.
   1. None indicated.
G. Differential diagnosis.

Abscess of eyelid unspecified eye, unspecified eyelid, H00.039	Hordeolum internum unspecified eye, unspecified eyelid, H00.029
Acute and unspecified inflammation of lacrimal passages, H04.3	Hordeolum externum unspecified eye, unspecified eyelid, H00.019
Cellulitis of unspecified orbit, H05.019	

   1. Hordeolum (internal or external).
   2. Orbital cellulitis.
   3. Dacryocystitis (inflammation of the lacrimal sac).
   4. Eyelid abscess.
H. Treatment.
   1. Most spontaneously subside without treatment.
   2. Surgical removal if size distorts vision.
I. Follow-up.
   1. No routine follow-up necessary.
   2. Recheck if fails to improve or worsens.
J. Complications.

Other subjective visual disturbances, H53.19

   1. Distorted vision secondary to size of lesion.
K. Education.
   1. Frequent handwashing.
   2. Avoid rubbing eyes.

IX. CHEMICAL BURN

A. Definition.

Burn of unspecified eye and adnexa, part unspecified, initial encounter, T26.40XA	Other specified disorders of eye and adnexa, H57.8
Corneal scar and opacity, unspecified, H17.9	Visual discomfort, unspecified, H53.149
Ocular pain, bilateral, H57.13	

   1. Instillation of alkali or acid solution or substance to eye. True emergency needs immediate referral to ophthalmologist.
B. Etiology.
   1. Installation of alkali or acid solution or substance into eye.
C. Occurrence.
   1. Boys > girls.
   2. 11- to 15-year olds have highest rate of injury.
D. Clinical manifestations.
   1. Eye pain.
   2. Unable to open eye(s).
E. Physical findings.
   1. Eyelid burn.
   2. Opacity of corneal tissue, pale surrounding tissue.
   3. Photophobia.
   4. Tearing, swollen corneas.
F. Diagnostic tests.
   1. None.
G. Differential diagnosis.

Contusion of eyelid and periocular area, S00.1
Foreign body on external eye, T15

   1. Foreign body.
   2. Type of chemical burn.
   3. Eyelid injury.
H. Treatment.
   1. Emergency treatment is immediate irrigation with copious amounts of water or saline.
   2. Emergency referral to ophthalmologist.
I. Follow-up.
   1. Per ophthalmologist.

J. Complications.

Visual loss, unspecified H54.7

   1. Loss of vision.

K. Education.
   1. Prevention is most important.
   2. Need to know name of chemical in eye; acid burns affect cornea and anterior chamber of eye.
   3. Alkali burns can continue for days.

X. CORNEAL ABRASION (SUPERFICIAL)

A. Definition.

Epiphora, H04.2	Visual loss, unspecified, H54.7
Ocular pain, bilateral, H57.13	
Injury of conjunctiva and corneal abrasion without foreign body, unspecified eye, initial encounter, S05.00XA	Visual discomfort, unspecified, H53.149

   1. Scratched, abraded, or denuded cornea.

B. Etiology.
   1. Usually due to accidental contact with object (fingernail, branches, bushes, paper, contact lens overwear).

C. Occurrence.
   1. Can occur at any age.

D. Clinical manifestations.
   1. Pain.
   2. Excessive tearing.
   3. Photophobia.
   4. Decreased vision.

E. Physical findings.
   1. May see uneven light reflection or cloudiness of cornea.
   2. May see foreign body.
   3. After staining with fluorescein and using cobalt-blue light or Wood's lamp, will see area of green staining (persists with blinking).
   4. Decreased visual acuity.

F. Diagnostic tests.
   1. Fluorescein staining and cobalt-blue light or Wood's lamp.

G. Differential diagnosis.

Foreign body on external eye, T15

    1. Foreign body.

H. Treatment.

    1. Instill topical ophthalmic anti-infective ointment (erythromycin ophthalmic ointment or bacitracin/polymyxin B ophthalmic ointment).

    2. Patching not recommended.

I. Follow-up.

    1. Recheck in 24–48 hours, or sooner if worsens.

J. Complications.

Visual loss, unspecified, H54.7

    1. Infection.

    2. Impaired vision.

K. Education.

    1. Frequent handwashing.

    2. Avoid use of contact lenses for at least 1 week following healing of abrasion.

XI. FOREIGN BODY (CONJUNCTIVAL, CORNEAL)

A. Definition.

Epiphora, H04.2	Visual discomfort, unspecified, H53.149
Foreign body on external eye, T15	Visual disturbance, unspecified, H53.9

B. Etiology.

    1. Usually object is airborne.

C. Occurrence.

    1. Can occur at any age.

D. Clinical manifestations.

    1. Excessive tearing.

    2. Photophobia.

    3. Sensation that something is in eye.

E. Physical findings.

    1. Excessive tearing.

    2. Use bright light or magnification to visualize corneal and conjunctival surfaces for foreign body.

    3. May need to evert upper eyelid to find foreign body.

F. Diagnostic tests.
    1. None.
G. Differential diagnosis.

Perforated corneal ulcer, unspecified eye, H16.079

---

    1. Infection.
    2. Perforation of ocular globe.
H. Treatment.
    1. Test visual acuity.
    2. Remove foreign body if possible with moistened, cotton-tipped applicator.
    3. After removal of foreign body, inspect for corneal abrasion using fluorescein.
    4. Topical ophthalmological antibiotic to prevent superinfection (Erythromycin ointment preferable).
    5. Patching not routinely recommended.
    6. Oral nonsteroidal anti-inflammatory drug (ibuprofen) as needed for pain.
    7. Refer to ophthalmologist if large abrasion or unable to find foreign body.
I. Follow-up.
    1. Recheck in 24 hours or sooner if worsens.
J. Complications.
    1. Infection.
    2. Damage to cornea.
K. Education.
    1. Avoid rubbing eyes.
    2. Teach prevention of eye injuries (protective eyewear).

XII. HEMORRHAGE (SUBCONJUNCTIVAL)

A. Definition.

Conjunctival hemorrhage, bilateral, H11.33

Injury of blood vessel(s) of unspecified body region, T14.5

B. Etiology.
    1. Sudden increase in intrathoracic pressure (coughing, sneezing).
    2. Direct ocular trauma.
C. Occurrence.
    1. Can occur at any age.

D. Clinical manifestations.
 1. Ruptured blood vessel in eye.
E. Physical findings.
 1. Blotchy, bulbar erythema of conjunctiva.
F. Diagnostic tests.
 1. None.
G. Differential diagnosis.
 1. Ocular trauma.
H. Treatment.
 1. None; will spontaneously resolve in 5–7 days.
 2. Refer to ophthalmologist if due to trauma.
I. Follow-up.
 1. No routine follow-up necessary.
 2. Recheck if fails to disappear in 5–7 days, or worsens.
J. Complications.
 1. Usually none.
K. Education.
 1. Teach measures to avoid increasing intrathoracic pressure.

XIII. HYPHEMA

A. Definition.

Hyphema, bilateral, H21.03
Ocular pain, bilateral, H57. 13
Visual loss, unspecified H54.7

 1. Blood in anterior chamber of eye.
B. Etiology
 1. Usually due to blunt or perforating trauma to eye.
C. Occurrence.
 1. Variable.
D. Clinical manifestations.
 1. Bright or dark red area near iris.
 2. Painful.
E. Physical findings.
 1. Bright or dark red fluid level between cornea and iris.
F. Diagnostic tests.
 1. X-rays, CT scan for other injuries.

G. Differential diagnosis.

Foreign body in conjunctival sac, T15.1

---

1. Type of foreign body.

H. Treatment.
    1. Immediate referral to ophthalmologist.
I. Follow-up.
    1. Per ophthalmologist.
J. Complications.

Visual loss, unspecified, H54.7

---

1. More extensive ocular injury.
2. Rebleeding, which may result in vision impairment.

K. Education.
    1. Children sometimes take weeks for vision to return to normal.
    2. Prevention is best.
    3. Encourage parents to continue follow-up as recommended by ophthalmologist.

XIV. OCULAR TRAUMA

A. Definition.

Diplopia, H53.2	Other visual disturbances, H53.8
Ocular pain, bilateral, H57.13	Visual loss, unspecified H54.7
Other specified disorders of eye and adnexa, H57.8	

---

1. Indirect or direct serious injury to eye.

B. Etiology.
    1. Fireworks, sticks, stones, BB shots.
    2. Sports related.
C. Occurrence.
    1. One-third of all causes of acquired blindness.
    2. Males > females 4:1.
D. Clinical manifestations.
    1. Double, blurred, or decreased vision.
    2. Eye pain or pain in surrounding area.
    3. Tearing.
E. Physical findings.
    1. Unable to open eye.

      2. Tearing.

      3. Corneal redness.

F. Diagnostic tests.

      1. X-rays if orbital fracture or nasal fracture is suspected.

G. Differential diagnosis.

Fracture of facial bones, unspecified, initial encounter for closed fracture, S02.92XA

Ocular laceration without prolapse or loss of intraocular tissue, unspecified eye, initial encounter, S05.30XA

Perforated corneal ulcer, unspecified eye, H16.079

---

      1. Laceration to ocular globe or orbit.

      2. Perforation to ocular globe or orbit.

      3. Orbital wall fracture.

H. Treatment.

      1. Referral to ophthalmologist.

I. Follow-up.

      1. Per ophthalmologist.

J. Complications.

Visual impairment including blindness (binocular or monocular), H54

---

      1. Extensive ocular injury.

      2. Blindness.

      3. Infection.

K. Education.

      1. Prevention: Use of goggles or glasses when spraying.

      2. Do not instill any medication.

      3. Immediate referral to ophthalmologist.

XV. PRESEPTAL CELLULITIS (PERIORBITAL CELLULITIS)

A. Definition.

Cellulitis of unspecified orbit, H05.019	Generalized edema, R60.1
Chronic sinusitis, unspecified, J32.9	Other specified disorders of eye and adnexa, H57.8
Erythematous condition, unspecified, L53.9	
Fever of other and unknown origin, R50	Periapical abscess without sinus, K04.7

---

      1. Inflammation and infection of eyelids and periorbital tissue.

B. Etiology.
 1. Staphylococcal aureus (including community-acquired methicillin-resistant *Staphylococcus aureus* [MRSA]).
 2. *Streptococcus pneumoniae.*
 3. *Streptococcus pyogenes.*
 4. *Haemophilus influenzae* type B.
C. Occurrence.
 1. Common in young children secondary to trauma, infected wound, insect bite, severe sinusitis, dental abscess.
D. Clinical manifestations.
 1. Red, painful swelling around eye.
 2. May or may not have fever.
 3. History of local trauma to area, insect bite, sinusitis, dental abscess.
E. Physical findings.
 1. Erythematous, edematous, tender, warm area around eye.
 2. Regional adenopathy.
F. Diagnostic tests.
 1. Complete blood count (will indicate leukocytosis in severe cases).
 2. Blood culture.
 3. Head computed tomography scan (helps delineate extent of disease).
G. Differential diagnosis.

Conjunctivitis, unspecified, H10.9	Malignant neoplasm of unspecified retina, C69.20
Contact dermatitis, unspecified, unspecified cause, L25.9	Nasal cavity, C30.0
Malignant neoplasm of connective and soft tissue, unspecified, C49.9	

 1. Severe contact dermatitis.
 2. Severe conjunctivitis.
 3. Ophthalmic malignancy or tumor (retinoblastoma, rhabdomyosarcoma, neuroblastoma).
H. Treatment.
 1. Uncomplicated and older than 2 months of age: Ceftriaxone then oral antibiotics, oral antiinfective (amoxicillin-clavulanate, cephalexin, or erythromycin).
 2. If concerned for MRSA, use either monotherapy with oral clindamycin or combination therapy with oral trimethoprim-sulfamethoxazole and either amoxicillin, amoxicillin-clavulanate, cefpodoxime, or cefdinir.

    3. Complicated/extensive or younger than 2 months of age: Requires hospitalization and intravenous antibiotics.

I. Follow-up.

    1. Daily follow-up is necessary to monitor for rapid improvement.

J. Complications.

Hordeolum and other deep inflammation of eyelid, H00.0

Visual loss, unspecified, H54.7

---

    1. Spread of infection with possible abscess formation.

    2. Loss of vision.

K. Education.

    1. Frequent handwashing.

    2. Teach prevention (avoid trauma, use insect repellent, cleanse wounds).

BIBLIOGRAPHY

Burns CE, Dunn AM, Brady MA, Starr NB, Blosser CG. *Pediatric Primary Care*. 5th ed. Philadelphia, PA: Saunders; 2013.

Centers for Disease Control and Prevention. Pink eye: usually mild and easy to treat. http://www.cdc.gov/Features/Conjunctivitis. Updated May 15, 2015. Accessed May 26, 2015.

Gerstenblith AT, Rabinowitz MP, eds. *The Wills Eye Manual: Office and Emergency Room Diagnosis and Treatment of Eye Disease*. 6th ed. Baltimore, MD: Lippincott Williams & Wilkins; 2012.

Hunter A. Problems related to the head, eyes, ears, nose, throat or mouth. In: Barnes K, ed. *Paediatrics—A Clinical Guide for Nurse Practitioners*. Philadelphia, PA: Butterworth-Heinemann; 2003:88-115.

Kliegman RM, Stanton BF, St. Geme JW III, Schor NF, Behrman RE. *Nelson Textbook of Pediatrics*. 19th ed. Philadelphia, PA: Saunders; 2011.

Nelson LB, Olitsky SE, eds. *Harley's Pediatric Ophthalmology*. 6th ed. Philadelphia, PA: Lippincott Williams & Wilkins; 2014.

Trobe JD. *The Physician's Guide to Eye Care*. 4th ed. San Francisco, CA: American Academy of Ophthalmology; 2012.

Ear Disorders

Jane A. Fox

I. FOREIGN BODY

Hearing loss, unspecified, unspecified ear, H91.90

Foreign body, ear, T16

Otalgia, H92.0

Otitis externa, H60

Otorrhoea, H92.1

A. Etiology.
1. Usually results from young children or their companions placing stones, erasers, vegetables (beans, peas, string beans), paper, jellybeans, toy parts, or small alkaline batteries in their ear(s).
2. Insects may become lodged in ear.
3. Chronic irritation or inflammation (e.g., otitis externa may result from putting objects in ear).
B. Occurrence.
1. Most common between 2 and 4 years of age.
C. Clinical manifestations.
1. Presenting complaints may include:
a. Pain or itching.
b. Decreased hearing.
c. Buzzing if insect is in ear canal.
d. Feeling of fullness in ear or pressure.
e. Discharge from ear.
D. Physical findings.
1. Foreign object or insect visualized on otoscopic exam.
2. Check all body orifices if foreign body found in one.
3. Carefully check ear after removal of foreign object for additional ones.
E. Diagnostic tests.
1. Usually none.

F. Differential diagnosis.

Acute serous otitis media, H65.0	Impacted cerumen, bilateral, H61.23
Contact dermatitis, unspecified, unspecified cause, L25.9	Otitis externa, H60
	Psoriasis, L40

1. Foreign body: Object or insect is visualized on otoscopic exam.
2. Otitis media (OM).
3. Otitis externa.
4. Trauma.
5. Impacted cerumen.
6. Dermatologic disorders (psoriasis or eczema).

G. Treatment.
  1. Remove foreign body. If bleeding occurs, object must be removed.
  2. Have child lie down, restrain head if needed.
  3. ***Do not irrigate*** if foreign body is vegetable or wood and/or suspect perforation of tympanic membrane (TM).
  4. Insect in ear: Kill insect by filling ear canal with mineral oil or alcohol before removal. Ticks: Dislodge ticks by filling canal with 70% alcohol and then remove.
  5. Removal of objects.
     a. Best: Remove objects using an otoscope with an opening head for visualization.
     b. Objects that are soft and unwedged.
        • Remove by irrigation with tepid water (body temperature) and water pick on low setting or an 18-gauge butterfly catheter with needle cut off. Pulsating water should help dislodge object.
        • Insert pliable tubing into ear canal behind foreign body.
  6. If object does not completely occlude canal, can use ear loop, curette, forceps for removal.
  7. Refer to otolaryngologist if:
     a. Object is an alkaline battery.
     b. Object cannot be easily removed.
     c. Ear canal is swollen or bleeding.
     d. Object is tightly wedged in canal.
     e. Child is unable to cooperate.

H. Follow-up.
  1. Generally none, well-child care.

I. Complications.

Perforation of tympanic membrane, H72

  1. Perforation of TM.

J. Education.
   1. Advise parents not to attempt to remove foreign body.
   2. Tell parents some bleeding may occur after removal.
   3. Cleaning ear canal is not necessary.

II. HEARING LOSS: CONDUCTIVE, SENSORINEURAL

Acute serous otitis media, H65.0

Allergic rhinitis, unspecified, J30.4

Cholesteatoma of middle ear, H71

Conductive hearing loss, bilateral, H90.0

Conductive hearing loss, unilateral with unrestricted hearing on the contralateral side, H90.1

Conductive hearing loss, unspecified, H90.2

Congenital malformation of ear, unspecified, Q17.9

Congenital malformation of face and neck, unspecified, Q18.9

Foreign body in ear, T16

Hearing loss, unspecified, unspecified ear, H91.90

Impacted cerumen, bilateral, H61.23

Injury of face, unspecified, initial encounter, S09.93XA

Other congenital malformations of middle ear, Q16.4

Other congenital malformations of skull and face bones, Q75

Other developmental disorders of speech and language, F80.8

Other developmental disorders of speech and language, unspecified, F80.9

Otitis externa, H60

Perforation of tympanic membrane, H72

Sensorineural hearing loss, bilateral, H90.3

Sensorineural hearing loss, unilateral with unrestricted hearing on the contralateral side, H90.4

Sensorineural hearing loss, unspecified, H90.5

Specific developmental disorders of speech and language, F80

Specific speech articulation disorder, F80.0

A. Etiology.
   1. Genetic or hereditary factors, environmental or acquired diseases, malformations.
   2. Trauma.
   3. Congenital perinatal infections.
   4. Medications (ototoxicity).
   5. About 33% of cases of hearing impairment: Cause unknown.

B. Occurrence.
  1. About 15% of school-age children have significant conductive hearing losses.
  2. OM and its sequelae most common cause of conductive hearing losses during childhood.
  3. Acquired conductive hearing losses most common types of hearing loss in childhood.
C. Clinical manifestations.
  1. *Conductive hearing loss* (middle ear hearing loss).
     a. Decreased hearing.
     b. May have history of middle ear effusions.
     c. OM and its sequelae.
     d. Foreign body and/or impacted cerumen.
     e. May report delayed language and speech development or parental concern about child's ability to hear.
     f. Allergies.
     g. Head or ear trauma.
     h. Middle ear anomalies.
     i. Cholesteatoma can cause hearing loss.
  2. Sensorineural hearing loss (perceptive or nerve deafness): May report distortion of sound and problems in discrimination of sounds. Hearing loss often involves high-range frequencies, speech difficulties.
D. Physical findings.
  1. Conductive hearing loss (middle ear hearing loss).
     a. Possible:
        • Otitis externa.
        • OM.
        • Foreign body.
        • Impacted cerumen.
        • Growths or tumors, cholesteatomas.
        • TM perforation.
     b. Rinne test on affected side; bone conduction (BC), air conduction (AC).
     c. Weber test sounds lateralized to involved side.
     d. Average hearing loss 27–31 dB (mild), may be intermittent, may occur in one or both ears.
  2. Sensorineural hearing loss (perceptive or nerve deafness).
     a. Possible dysmorphic facial features suggesting presence of syndrome.
     b. Head and/or neck anomalies.

      c. Anomalies of pinnae and external ear canals.

      d. Weber test sounds louder in unaffected ear.

      e. Rinne test: In normal ear or ear with sensorineural hearing loss, AC, BC.

  3. Audiometric testing: Soft sounds not well perceived, loud sounds perceived almost normally. In older children, if normal in high and low frequencies but poor in middle frequencies, suspect congenital hearing loss.

  4. Acquisition of language skills affected.

E. Diagnostic tests.

  1. Evoked otoacoustic emissions (EOAE) testing (can be performed on children of all ages): Newer type of newborn screening, 10 minutes.

  2. Automated auditory brainstem response (AABR): For newborn screening, 10 minutes.

  3. Brainstem auditory evoked response (BAER): Newborn screening, 90 minutes; often used in children of all ages who are unable to cooperate for audiometry testing.

  4. Behavioral observation audiometry.

  5. Pure tone audiometry for children 5 years of age.

  6. Tympanometry identifies a middle ear effusion.

  7. Impedance audiometry.

  8. Language screening: Early Language Milestone Scale.

F. Differential diagnosis.

Conductive hearing loss, bilateral, H90.0	Sensorineural hearing loss, bilateral, H90.3
Conductive hearing loss, unilateral with unrestricted hearing on the contralateral side, H90.1	Sensorineural hearing loss, unilateral with unrestricted hearing on the contralateral side, H90.4
Conductive hearing loss, unspecified, H90.2	
Mixed conductive and sensorineural hearing loss, unspecified, H90.8	Sensorineural hearing loss, unspecified, H90.5

  1. Careful history and thorough physical examination, including screening and laboratory data, essential in identifying those at risk and in early detection of hearing losses.

  2. Hearing disorders classified into three categories:

      a. Conductive hearing loss.

      b. Sensorineural hearing loss.

      c. Mixed conductive sensorineural loss.

G. Treatment.
  1. Refer for audiologic testing.
  2. Surgery for conductive hearing loss (usually bilateral myringotomy with tubes).
  3. Refer to multidisciplinary team, hearing center, or ear, nose, and throat (ENT) specialist if hearing impairment detected.
  4. For sensorineural loss:
      a. Amplification (hearing aids; bilateral is best) benefits most children.
      b. Cochlear implants with sensorineural loss have been FDA approved for use in eligible children beginning at 12 months of age. Best results if done by 18 months of age followed by intense therapy. These children are better able to speak, hear, and comprehend sound than their peers who received implants when they were older.
H. Follow-up.
  1. Determined by type and cause of hearing loss.
  2. Well-child care.
I. Complications.

Specific developmental disorders of speech and language, F80

---

  1. Speech and language disorders.
J. Education.
  1. Early detection imperative to minimize negative consequences for language, other development.
  2. Disease process, type of loss, causes. Conductive loss usually reversible, sensorineural loss often irreversible.
  3. To decrease incidence of communication disorder in child with middle ear disease:
      a. When speaking to child, turn off sources of background noise (e.g., dishwasher, television, radio, stereo, computer games, etc.).
      b. Make sure child is looking directly at speaker and that speaker has child's attention.
      c. Speak louder than normal.
      d. Child should sit in front of classroom (may need referral for full evaluation of hearing needs).
  4. Effects on child.
      a. Speech and language development.
      b. Social development.
      c. Learning process.

5. Needs of child.
   a. Emotional.
   b. Social.
   c. Educational.
6. Parents' role.
   a. Care and function of hearing aids, if indicated.
   b. Medic alert bracelet.
7. Parent support groups.
8. Support groups for the child.
9. Prevention: Limit exposure to loud noise.

III. OTITIS EXTERNA

Contact dermatitis, unspecified, unspecified cause, L25.9	Psoriasis, L40
Otitis externa, H60	Seborrheic dermatitis, unspecified, L21.9
Perforation of the tympanic membrane, H72	

A. Etiology.
   1. Bacteria: *Pseudomonas aeruginosa* (most common); *Streptococcus* species, *Staphylococcus epidermidis, Proteus* species, *Mycoplasma* species. Acute bacterial infection discharge is scant white mucus but may be thick. Chronic bacterial infection is bloody discharge, especially in place of granulation tissue.
   2. Fungi: *Aspergillus* species, *Candida* organisms. Typical fluffy and white to off-white discharge. But may be black, gray, bluish-green, or yellow.
   3. Excess cerumen or loss of protective cerumen from exposure to excess moisture.
   4. Trauma to the ear canal caused by overzealous cleaning with a cotton-tipped applicator or a foreign body.
   5. Allergic reaction to chemical or physical agents; contact dermatitis.
   6. Excessive wetness from swimming, bathing, or high humidity.
   7. Excessive dryness; child or family history of eczema, psoriasis, seborrhea.
   8. Purulent OM with perforation of the TM and drainage may masquerade as otitis externa, usually painless with no swelling of the canal.
B. Occurrence.
   1. Most common in hot, muggy weather, summer months.
   2. Persons who are swimmers or divers are more susceptible.

    3. Higher incidence in those with smaller ear canals.

    4. Males and females equally affected.

    5. Affects all ages.

C. Clinical manifestations.

    1. Ear pain and itching (common in fungal infections) in the ear, especially when chewing or pressure on tragus.

    2. Feeling of fullness or obstruction of ear.

    3. Frequently, a history of exposure to water.

    4. Purulent discharge and hearing loss (conductive) possible.

D. Physical findings.

    1. Pain on movement of pinna or tragus.

    2. Periauricular adenitis may occur, but not necessary for diagnosis.

    3. External canal: Gross edema and erythema of canal, accumulation of moist debris in canal. Patient may resist insertion of ear speculum.

    4. TM often difficult to visualize and may be mildly inflamed but is mobile on insufflation.

E. Diagnostic tests.

    1. No tests specific to diagnosing otitis externa.

    2. Gram stain and culture of discharge may be helpful, particularly when fungal cause is suspected.

F. Differential diagnosis.

Contact dermatitis, unspecified, unspecified cause, L25.9	Malignant neoplasm of middle ear, C30.1
	Mastoiditis, unspecified, H70.9
Foreign body in ear, unspecified ear, initial encounter, T16.9XXA	Nonspecific lymphadenitis, unspecified, I88.9
Foreign body in left ear, initial encounter, T16.2XXA	Other infective otitis externa, H60.3
	Perforation of tympanic membrane, H72
Foreign body in right ear, initial encounter, T16.1XXA	Supparative and unspeficied otitis media, H66
Furuncle, unspecified, L02.92	

    1. Cyst, furuncle, or abscess.

    2. Foreign body.

    3. OM with perforation.

    4. Dental infection.

    5. Mastoiditis.

    6. Postauricular lymphadenopathy.

    7. Eczema or other dermatologic condition.

    8. Malignant otitis externa.

G. Treatment.
   1. Clean debris from canal: Insert small gauze wick or absorbent sponge into external canal to carry antibiotic corticosteroid solution into canal if needed (severe swelling).
   2. Topical treatment is always needed to treat otitis externa.
      a. Otic antibiotic and steroid combinations highly effective (e.g., 2% acetic acid otic solution [VoSol] with hydrocortisone VoSol HC otic).
      b. Ciprofloxacin hydrochloride/hydrocortisone otic suspension (Cipro HC Otic Suspension) has broad spectrum for covering resistant organisms or combination eardrops of antibiotics, hydrocortisone, propylene glycol.
         • Not recommended for children younger than 1 year of age.
         • Advise parents to warm bottle in hands for 1–2 minutes before use and then place 3 drops in affected ear(s) 2 times a day for 7 days.
      c. Ofloxacin solution 0.3% otic drops (Floxin) every 12 hours.
         • Highly effective if *Pseudomonas aeruginosa* and *Staphylococcus aureus (S. aureus)* are causes in patients 1 year of age and older.
         • Age 1–12 years: 5 drops in affected ear(s) 2 times daily for 10 days.
         • Older than 12 years of age: 10 drops in affected ear(s) twice daily for 10 days.
         • Analgesics for pain (acetaminophen or acetaminophen with codeine). See **Table 23-1**.
   3. Oral antibiotics only if signs of invasive infection.
      a. Cellulitis of auricle.
      b. Fever.
      c. Tender postauricular lymph nodes.
   4. Keep ear dry.
   5. Do not use cotton swabs.
H. Follow-up.
   1. Mild cases: None.
   2. Immediate recheck: Pain worsens, does not improve in 48–72 hours, or sensitivity to eardrops.
   3. Return visit in 2–3 days if marked cellulitis or TM was not visualized.
   4. Return visit if symptoms recur.
   5. Telephone if severe pain.
   6. Recheck in 10 days and continue treatment, if not completely resolved.
I. Complications.

Acquired stenosis of external ear canal, H61.3	Other infective otitis externa, H60.3
Furuncle, unspecified, L02.92	Transient ischemic deafness,
Malignant otitis externa, H60.2	unspecified ear, H93.019

Table 23-1 Treatments for Otalgia in AOM

Treatment Modality	Comments
Acetaminophen, ibuprofen	Effective analgesia for mild to moderate pain. Readily available. Mainstay of pain management for AOM.
Home remedies (no controlled studies that directly address effectiveness)	May have limited effectiveness.
Distraction	
External application of heat or cold	
Oil drops in external auditory canal	
Topical agents	
Benzocaine, procaine, lidocaine	Additional, but brief, benefit over acetaminophen in patients older than 5 y.
Naturopathic agents	Comparable to amethocaine/phenazone drops in patients older than 6 y.
Homeopathic agents	No controlled studies that directly address pain.
Narcotic analgesia with codeine or analogs	Effective for moderate or severe pain. Requires prescription; risk of respiratory depression, altered mental status, gastrointestinal tract upset, and constipation.
Tympanostomy/myringotomy	Requires skill and entails potential risk.

Source: Lieberthal AS, Carroll AE, Chonmaitree T, et al. The diagnosis and management of acute otitis media. *Pediatrics.* 2013;131(3):e964-e999. Reproduced with permission by the AAP.

1. Cellulitis of surrounding tissue.
2. Irritated furunculosis.
3. Malignant otitis externa (uncommon) seen in chronically ill or immuno-suppressed children.
4. Stenosis of auditory canal.
5. Transient conductive hearing loss.

J. Education.
   1. Explain cause and treatment plan.
      a. Keep ear(s) dry: No swimming during acute phase, can use cotton coated with petroleum jelly or lamb's wool when showering or shampooing to occlude canal; remove immediately when finished.

    b. Side effects of eardrops: Local stinging or burning sensation and rash where drops have come in contact with skin.

    c. Avoid earplugs and use of cotton swabs.

    d. Acute pain should subside within 48 hours.

2. Keep foreign objects out of ears.

3. Prevention of recurrence (common): Instill 2–3 drops of isopropyl alcohol in ear canals after swimming or showering or during hot, humid weather; shake excess water out of ears but not too often.

IV. ACUTE OTITIS MEDIA (AOM)

Acute pharyngitis, unspecified, J02.9	Perforation of tympanic membrane, H72
Acute serous otitis media, H65.0	
Acute upper respiratory infection, unspecified, J06.9	Otitis media, unspecified, H66.9
Chronic serous otitis media, H65.2	Respiratory syncytial virus as the cause of diseases classified elsewhere, B97.4
Fever of other and unknown origin, R50	
Influenza due to unidentified influenza virus with other respiratory manifestations, J11.1	

A. Etiology.

1. *Streptococcus pneumoniae (S. pneumoniae)* (most common causative organism).

2. Nontypeable *Haemophilus influenzae (H. influenzae)* causes about 27% of the bacterial otitis.

3. *Moraxella catarrhalis (M. catarrhalis).*

4. *Streptococcus pyogenes* (group A beta-hemolytic streptococci) account for less than 5% of AOM cases.

5. *S. aureus* and *Pseudomonas aeruginosa:* Common in chronic serous OM, especially if perforation of TM present.

    a. Group A beta-hemolytic streptococci, *Escherichia coli, S. aureus:* More common in neonates.

6. Viruses, particularly respiratory syncytial virus, influenza virus (types A and B), and adenovirus, increase the risk, possibly by impairing Eustachian tube function. Infants have increased susceptibility to OM, possibly due to short horizontal position of Eustachian tube.

7. Viruses may be involved in about 40% of cases of AOM.

8. Bacterial resistance is increasing problem: Certain strains of *H. influenzae* and most strains of *M. catarrhalis* are resistant to amoxicillin

because of beta-lactamase production. Another concern is drug-resistant *S. pneumoniae* (DRSP).

9. The groups most at risk for DRSP are:
   a. Children younger than 24 months of age.
   b. Those who have recently received beta-lactam drugs, were recently treated with antibiotics, and/or had a recent ear infection.
   c. Children exposed to large numbers of other children (e.g., daycare attendance in children 2 months to younger than 5 years of age, or household crowding in children older than 2 years of age).
   d. Those with immune deficiencies (e.g., sickle cell disease, HIV, malignancy). The proportion of penicillin-resistant *S. pneumoniae* strains may be 40–50%, and half of these may be highly resistant.

B. Occurrence.
   1. After upper respiratory infection (URI), OM most common disease of childhood; peak prevalence from 6 to 36 months of age. Incidence declines at about 6 years of age.
   2. Incidence has dramatically increased since 1985; greatest in children younger than 2 years of age.
   3. By 3 years of age, most have had at least 1 acute infection; 33% have had 3.
   4. Those with first episode early in life have increased risk for developing chronic ear disease.
   5. More common in boys than in girls.
   6. Caucasians, Native Alaskans, Native Americans have higher incidence than African Americans.
   7. More frequent in low-income and large families and those children in group daycare settings.
   8. Those immunocompromised, including those with AIDS, have higher incidence.
   9. Smoking in household increases incidence.
   10. Bottle-fed infants have higher incidence than breastfed infants.
   11. Incidence, prevalence of otorrhea: Tympanostomy tubes in place longer.

C. Clinical manifestations.
   1. Diagnosis of AOM requires (diagnosis certainty imperative):
      a. History of acute onset of signs and symptoms (less than 48 hours) and fever; pulling, tugging, rubbing at affected ear.
      b. Presence of middle ear effusion.
      c. Signs and symptoms of middle ear inflammation.
      d. Distinct erythema of TM or distinct otalgia (discomfort clearly related to the ear[s] that causes sleep disturbances and/or interferes with normal activity).
   2. Most common younger than 2 years of age.

3. Neonate may present with irritability or feeding difficulty. This may be the indication of a septic focus.

4. Occasionally asymptomatic.

5. Fever in 50% of cases.

6. Other associated symptoms: Irritability, disturbed sleep, restlessness, rhinorrhea or URI, cough, malaise, sore throat, stiff neck, refusal of bottle, change in eating habits, vomiting, diarrhea.

7. May report recent URI, previous ear infections, allergies, taking bottle to bed, infant supine when feeding from bottle, attending daycare, other siblings sick.

8. Hearing loss.

9. New onset of otorrhea not due to acute otitis externa.

D. Physical findings.

1. Fever is common (50% of cases).

2. Signs of URI or allergies.

3. Possible red, enlarged tonsils (pharyngitis).

4. Cervical nodes often enlarged.

5. Otoscopic findings (stringent otoscopic diagnostic criteria endorsed for management decisions): Middle ear effusion must be present as evidenced by any of the following: Bulging TM, decreased or absent mobility of the TM as noted with pneumatic otoscopy, air fluid level behind the TM, otorrhea, acoustic reflectometry.

E. Diagnostic tests.

1. Pneumatic otoscopy to assess mobility of TM.

2. Tympanometry: To supplement but not replace pneumatic otoscopy, for children older than 6 months of age.

3. Acoustic reflectometry.

4. Tympanocentesis with culture and sensitivity testing is diagnostic of organism.

F. Differential diagnosis.

Acute tonsillitis, J03	Mastoiditis, unspecified, H70.9
Chronic sinusitis, unspecified, J32.9	Nonspecific lymphadenitis, unspecified, I88.9
Foreign body in left ear, initial encounter, T16.2XXA	Nonsuppurative otitis media, unspecified, H65.9
Foreign body in right ear, initial encounter, T16.1XXA	Other specified disorders of Eustachian tube, unspecified ear, H69.80
Furuncle, unspecified, L02.92	Otitis externa, H60
Immunodeficiency, unspecified, D84.9	Periapical abscess without sinus, K04.7
Impacted teeth, K01.1	Temporomandibular joint disorders, K07.6

1. Otitis externa, otitis media with effusion (OME), sinusitis.
2. Mastoiditis, furuncle.
3. Foreign body, trauma.
4. Eustachian tube dysfunction (ETD).
5. Lymphadenitis.
6. Dental abscess, tonsillitis, impacted teeth.
7. Temporomandibular joint (TMJ) dysfunction.
8. Immune deficiency.

G. Treatment (**Table 23-1** and **Table 23-2**).

1. Pain management, especially during the first 24 hours, is a priority regardless of whether antimicrobial agents are prescribed. Acetaminophen and ibuprofen are the mainstays. Adequate dosage is important. Warm compresses and eardrops with benzocaine and antipyrine (Auralgan) may help. Immediate treatment for pain is very important.

2. May also consider prescribing aqueous lidocaine ear drops up to 3 times in 24 hours. Some studies indicate reduction in pain, but others concluded limited evidence that ear drops are effective.

Table 23-2 Recommendations for Initial Management for Uncomplicated AOM[a]

Age	Otorrhea With AOM[a]	Unilateral or Bilateral AOM[a] With Severe Symptoms[b]	Bilateral AOM[a] Without Otorrhea	Unilateral AOM[a] Without Otorrhea
6 mo to 2 y	Antibiotic therapy	Antibiotic therapy	Antibiotic therapy	Antibiotic therapy or additional observation
≥ 2 y	Antibiotic therapy	Antibiotic therapy	Antibiotic therapy or additional observation	Antibiotic therapy or additional observation[c]

[a] Applies only to children with well-documented AOM with high certainty of diagnosis.
[b] A toxic-appearing child, persistent otalgia more than 48 h, temperature ≥102.2°F (39°C) in the past 48 h, or if there is uncertain access to follow-up after the visit.
[c] This plan of initial management provides an opportunity for shared decision-making with the child's family for those categories appropriate for additional observation. If observation is offered, a mechanism must be in place to ensure follow–up and begin antibiotics if the child worsens or fails to improve within 48 to 72 h of AOM onset.
Source: Lieberthal AS, Carroll AE, Chonmaitree T, et al. The diagnosis and management of acute otitis media. *Pediatrics.* 2013;131(3):e964-e999. Reproduced with permission by the AAP.

3. Observation involves deferring treatment for 48–72 hours in otherwise healthy children 6 months to 2 years of age with nonsevere illness at presentation *and* uncertain diagnosis and in children ages 2 years and older who present without severe symptoms *or* an uncertain diagnosis. There should also be a reliable parent or caregiver able to obtain medication if needed and adequate facilities for follow-up and reevaluation.

4. Prescribe antibiotics with caution. More than 80% of cases resolve spontaneously. Antibiotic therapy is recommended for AOM (bilateral or unilateral) in:

   a. All children 6 months and older with severe signs or symptoms (i.e., moderate or severe otaglia, otaglia for at least 48 hours, or temperature 102.2°F (39°C) or higher.

   b. Children with bilateral AOM who are younger than 24 months of age without severe signs or symptoms (i.e., mild otaglia for less than 48 hours, temperature less than 102.2°F (39°C).

5. Duration of antibiotic therapy: Children with severe symptoms or under 2 years of age: 10-day course of treatment; children age 2 to 5 years of age with mild or moderate AOM: 7-day course of oral antibiotics; children 6 years and older with mild to moderate symptoms: 5–7 days of antibiotics is adequate.

6. Prescribe antibiotic therapy or offer observation with close follow-up based on joint decision making with the parents or caregivers for:

   a. Unilateral AOM in children 6 months to 23 months of age without severe signs or symptoms.

   b. Bilateral or unilateral AOM in children 24 months or older without severe signs or symptoms (i.e., mild otaglia for less than 48 hours, temperature less than 102.2°F (39°C).

   c. If observation is used, must have mechanism in place to ensure follow-up and begin antibiotic therapy if child worsens or fails to improve within 48–72 hours of onset of symptoms.

7. For children age 2 years and older who appear well, discuss treatment options with parents which include:

   a. Wait and see prescription (WASP) or safety-net antibiotic prescription (SNAP). These are a prescription for an appropriate antibiotic written to be filled within 5 days of the office visit. Parents are instructed not to fill the prescription unless symptoms worsen at any time or symptoms do not improve during the waiting period of 48–72 hours. Instruct parents that child's condition may quickly progress to a more severe case and to call and make a return visit if this occurs.

   b. Five-day course of high-dose amoxicillin (if no history of allergy).

8. Prescribe amoxicillin (drug of choice) if causative organism unknown (most cases), if the child has not received amoxicillin in the past 30 days, if the child does not have concurrent purulent conjunctivitis, or if the child is not allergic to penicillin. Because of cost and adverse effects, amoxicillin is the initial antibiotic of choice.

9. High-dose amoxicillin is recommended as the first-line treatment in most patients.

10. If child attends daycare, has received amoxicillin in the past 30 days, has concurrent purulent conjunctivitis, or has a history of AOM unresponsive to amoxicillin (suspect beta-lacatamase-positive *H. influenzae* or *M. catarrahalis*), prescribe an antibiotic with additional beta-lactamase coverage. Initiate therapy with high-dose amoxicillin-clavulanate (90 mg/kg/day of amoxicillin, with 6.4 mg/kg/day of clavulanate, a ratio of 14:1, given in two divided doses; this is less likely to cause diarrhea).

11. If allergic to penicillin, treatment with a cephalosporin is recommended. Recent data suggests cross-reactivity among penicillin and cephalosporins is lower than reported. The American College of Allergy, Asthma and Immunology and Joint Council of Asthma, Allergy and Immunology recommend a cephalosporin in cases without severe and/or recent penicillin allergy reaction history when skin test is not available.

12. Macrolides (erythromycin and azithromycin) have limited efficacy against *H. influenzae* and *S. pneumoniae*.

13. Palatability of oral suspensions has been studied and may lead to active rejection such as spitting out the suspension. Cefuroxime, cefpodoxime, and clindamycin may benefit from adding taste-favoring products such as chocolate or strawberry to mask the bitter taste and unpleasant aftertaste.

14. If child is vomiting or is unable to tolerate oral medication, prescribe ceftriaxone (50 mg/kg, IM in 1 or 2 sites in the anterior thigh, or IV). This has demonstrated to be effective for the initial or repeat antibiotic treatment of AOM.

15. Clinical improvement should be noted within 48–72 hours after antibiotics have been initiated. If patient has persistent symptoms of AOM and unimproved otologic findings (persistent fever, ear pain, irritability, TM findings of redness, bulging, or otorrhea) after initial treatment, consider changing the antibiotic (see **Table 23-3**). If initially treated with amoxicillin, prescribe amoxicillin-clavulanate. If initially prescribed amoxicillin-clavulanate or oral third-generation cephalosporin IM ceftriaxone (50 mg/kg), a 3-day course has been shown to be more effective than a 1-day regimen.

Table 23-3 Recommended Antibiotics for (Initial or Delayed) Treatment and for Patients Who Have Failed Initial Antibiotic Treatment

Initial Immediate or Delayed Antibiotic Treatment		Antibiotic Treatment After 48–72 h of Failure of Initial Antibiotic Treatment	
Recommended First-line Treatment	*Alternative Treatment (if Penicillin Allergy)*	*Recommended First-line Treatment*	*Alternative Treatment*
Amoxicillin (80–90 mg/kg per day in 2 divided doses)	Cefdinir (14 mg/kg per day in 1 or 2 doses)	Amoxicillin-clavulanate[a] (90 mg/kg per day of amoxicillin, with 6.4 mg/kg per day of clavulanate in 2 divided doses)	Ceftriaxone, 3 d Clindamycin (30–40 mg/kg per day in 3 divided doses), with or without third-generation cephalosporin
or	Cefuroxime (30 mg/kg per day in 2 divided doses)	or	Failure of second antibiotic
Amoxicillin-clavulanate[a] (90 mg/kg per day of amoxicillin, with 6.4 mg/kg per day of clavulanate [amoxicillin to clavulanate ratio, 14:1] in 2 divided doses)	Cefpodoxime (10 mg/kg per day in 2 divided doses)	Ceftriaxone (50 mg IM or IV for 3 d)	Clindamycin (30–40 mg/kg per day in 3 divided doses) plus third-generation cephalosporin
			Tympanocentesis[b]
	Ceftriaxone (50 mg IM or IV per day for 1 or 3 d)		Consult specialist[b]

Abbreviations: IM, intramuscular; IV, intravenous.

[a] May be considered in patients who have received amoxicillin in the previous 30 d or who have the otitis-conjunctivitis syndrome.

[b] Perform tympanocentesis/drainage if skilled in the procedure, or seek a consultation from an otolaryngologist for tympanocentesis/drainage. If the tympanocentesis reveals multidrug-resistant bacteria, seek an infectious disease specialist consultation.

[c] Cefdinir, cefuroxime, cefpodoxime, and ceftriaxone are highly unlikely to be associated with cross-reactivity with penicillin allergy on the basis of their distinct chemical structures.

Source: Lieberthal AS, Carroll AE, Chonmaitree T, et al. The diagnosis and management of acute otitis media. *Pediatrics.* 2013;131(3):e964-e999. Reproduced with permission by the AAP.

16. Although trimethoprim-sulfamethoxazole and erythromycin-sulfisoxazole have been used successfully in the past to treat AOM, pneumococcal surveillance studies have shown that resistance to these two combination agents is substantial. If amoxicillin is not initially effective, these two agents are not appropriate therapy.

17. Children with frequent AOM: Evaluate for anemia. If iron deficiency is diagnosed (hemoglobin 10 g/dL), begin iron supplementation to achieve at least a hemoglobin level of 11 g/dL.

18. Recurrent AOM: American Academy of Pediatrics and the CDC suggest placement of tympanostomy tubes rather than antibiotic prophylaxis. Tympanostomy tubes (performed by an ENT surgeon) are options in children with chronic middle ear fluid (3 months or 4 persistent episodes) who fail to respond to antimicrobial therapy; children with recurrent AOM; those with suppurative complications; and those with ETD.

19. Tympanocentesis (performed by an ENT specialist) and culture of exudate: If diagnosis is uncertain, child is seriously ill or toxic, response to antibiotic therapy is unsatisfactory, suppurative complications develop, OM in newborn or in immunologically deficient patients, or AOM develops despite receiving antibiotic therapy.

20. If tympanocentesis is not available, obtain nasopharyngeal specimen. Most middle ear pathogens derive from pathogens colonizing the nasopharynx. Not all nasopharnyx pathogens enter the middle ear and cause AOM. Therefore, if the nasopharyngeal culture is negative for specific bacteria, those bacteria are likely not the AOM pathogen.

21. Recommend pneumococcal conjugate vaccine to all children according to schedule of the Advisory Committee on Immunization Practices, AAP, and AAFP.

22. Recommend annual influenza vaccine for all children 6 months of age and older.

23. Encourage exclusive breastfeeding for at least 6 months of life and to continue for at least the first year and beyond as long as mutually desired by mother and baby.

24. Encourage avoidance of exposure to tobacco smoke.

25. Lifestyle changes: Avoid supine bottle-feeding (bottle propping) and reduce or eliminate pacifier use in the second 6 months of life. Reducing the incidence of URIs during infancy and early childhood by altering childhood daycare attendance patterns may significantly decrease the incidence of AOM.

26. If tympanocentesis is not available, obtain nasopharyngeal specmen. Most middle ear pathogens derive from pathogens colonizing the nasopharnx. Not all nasopharnyx pathogens enter the middle ear and cause AOM. Therefore, if the nasopharyngeal culture is negative for specific bacteria, those bacteria are likely not the AOM pathogen.

27. Refer for audiologic testing if fail hearing screen.

28. Consult/refer to physician: Infant younger than 2 months of age, signs of meningitis.
29. ENT referral: Hearing loss or delayed speech, 3 infections in 6 months or 4 in 12 months.

H. Follow-up.
1. Younger than 3 months of age: Revisit 1 to 2 days (higher incidence of treatment failure).
2. Children 3 months of age and older: Revisit in 48–72 hours if no improvement or condition worsens (need to change antibiotics).
3. Return visit if caregiver reports child's symptoms have worsened or failed to respond to the initial antibiotic therapy within 48–72 hours to determine if change in therapy is indicated.
4. Return visit 4–8 weeks to evaluate for OME and reinforce teaching.
5. Persistent AOM: Prescribe second-line antibiotic (e.g., amoxicillin-clavulanate, cefuroxime, or ceftriaxone IM); recheck every 2–4 weeks until resolved.
6. Return visit if signs or symptoms of ear infection, trouble hearing, fever with/without ear pain.

I. Complications.

Acute serous otitis media, H65.0	Mastoiditis, unspecified, H70.9
Benign intracranial hypertension, G93.2	Meninigitis, unspecified, G03.9
Birth injury to facial nerve, P11.3	Nonsuppurative otitis media, unspecified, H65.9
Cholesteatoma of middle ear, H71	Other developmental disorders of speech and language, F80.89
Hearing loss, unspecified, unspecified ear, H91.90	Partial loss of ear ossicles, unspecified ear, H74.329
Intracranial and intraspinal phlebitis and thrombophlebitis, G08	Perforation of tympanic membrane, H72
Labyrinthitis, H83.0	Tympanosclerosis, unspecified ear, H74.09

1. Perforation of TM.
2. Hearing loss, language delay.
3. Persistent AOM, persistent OME.
4. Mastoiditis, cholesteatoma.
5. Meningitis.
6. Facial nerve paralysis.
7. Labyrinthitis.

8. Tympanosclerosis.
9. Ossicle necrosis.
10. Pseudotumor cerebri.
11. Cerebral thrombophlebitis.

J. Education.
1. Causes of ear infections.
2. Risk factors/modification: Passive smoke, bottle propping, allergies, sinusitis, use of pacifier after age 6 months, breastfeeding (may protect), immunizations.
3. Treatment plan: If antibiotics prescribed, call if symptoms worsen or do not improve in 48 hours; give exactly as prescribed.
4. Pain relief measures.
5. Importance of follow-up.

V. OTITIS MEDIA WITH EFFUSION

Acute serous otitis media, H65.0	Hypertrophy of tonsils, J35.1
Allergic rhinitis, unspecified, J30.4	Irritability and anger, R45.4
Chronic otitis externa, unspecified, unspecified ear, H60.60	Other specified disorders of Eustachian tube, unspecified ear, H69.80
Enlarged lymph nodes, unspecified, R59.9	Perforation of tympanic membrane, H72
	Sleep disorders, G47
Hearing loss, unspecified, unspecified ear, H91.90	Specific developmental disorders of speech and language, F80

A. Etiology.
1. Multifactorial: ETD, infection, allergies.
2. Bacteria are same as for AOM, except frequency of *H. influenzae* is greater in OME.
3. If TM perforated in chronic OME: *S. aureus* and *P. aeruginosa* most likely causative organisms.

B. Occurrence.
1. See AOM section on page 241.
2. Usually follows episode of AOM.
3. Children who are diagnosed with AOM during the first year of life are much more likely to develop chronic OME.
4. Sixty-six percent of children with AOM have middle ear effusion or high-negative middle ear pressure 2 weeks after diagnosis; 33% have middle ear effusion 1 month after diagnosis, regardless of antibiotic therapy.
5. OME most common cause of hearing loss in children.

C. Clinical manifestations.
1. May be asymptomatic.
2. Complaint of hearing loss (older children).
3. Possible language delay.
4. Feeling of fullness in affected ear, clogged/crackling sensation in ear, "talking in tunnel."
5. Irritability.
6. Sleep disturbances.
7. Poor school performance.
8. Allergies.
9. Frequent episodes of OM.
D. Physical findings.
1. Possible indicators of allergies.
2. Possible enlarged tonsils.
3. Possible cervical lymphadenopathy.
4. External canal may have discharge.
5. TM: Often retracted or convex, opaque; diffuse light reflex; may be translucent with air-fluid level or air bubbles present or amber with blue-gray fluid noted, no visible landmarks.
6. Pneumatic otoscopy: Decreased or irregular mobility to both negative and positive pressure.
7. Weber test: Lateralization to involved ear.
8. Rinne test: BC, AC (abnormal).
9. Hearing impairment.
10. Tympanometry: Fluid present.
E. Diagnostic tests.
1. Pneumatic otoscopy should be used as the primary diagnostic method for OME. Tympanometry can be used to confirm the diagnosis.
2. Tympanometry: Tympanogram is flat with an effusion.
3. Audiometry.
4. Acoustic reflectometry.
5. Otoacoustic emissions.
6. Tympanocentesis.
F. Differential diagnosis.

Acute serous otitis media, H65.0	Hearing loss, unspecified, unspecified ear, H91.90
Congenital malformation, unspecified, Q89.9	Malignant neoplasm of nasopharynx, unspecified, C11.9

1. All possible causes of hearing loss.
2. Anatomic abnormalities.

      3. AOM.

      4. Nasopharyngeal carcinoma (if unilateral OME).

G. Treatment.

      1. Most cases of OME resolve spontaneously within 3 months.

      2. Document at each visit: Laterality, duration of effusion, and presence and severity of associated symptoms.

      3. Distinguish the child who is at risk for speech, language, or learning problems from other children with OME and more quickly evaluate hearing, speech, and language and need for intervention in children at risk.

      4. Refer for hearing evaluation when OME persists for 3 months or longer; at any time there is a language delay or learning problems; or if a significant hearing loss is suspected in a child with OME.

      5. Not recommended for treatment of OME in an otherwise healthy child 2 months through 12 years: Antibiotics, nasal steroids, antihistamines, and decongestants are not indicated for OME and should not be prescribed.

      6. Myringotomy and tympanostomy tubes: *Consider* for children 6 months to 12 years of age who have had bilateral effusion for a total of 3 months or longer with documented hearing deficiency (defined as a 20-dB hearing threshold level or worse in the better hearing ear) or for children with recurrent AOM who have evidence of middle ear effusion (MEE) at the time of assessment for tubes.

H. Follow-up.

      1. Return visit in 1 month, sooner if acute symptoms develop.

I. Complications.

Acute serous otitis media, H65.0

Hearing loss, unspecified, unspecified ear, H91.90

Specific developmental disorders of speech and language, F80

---

      1. Hearing loss, speech delay.

      2. Recurrent AOM.

J. Education.

      1. Diagnosis; OME usually resolves spontaneously without treatment in 3 months.

      2. Treatment plan.

      3. Signs of hearing loss.

      4. Modify risk factors.

      5. Relationship between speech and language development and hearing.

      6. Importance of follow-up.

VI. EUSTACHIAN TUBE DYSFUNCTION (ETD)

A. Etiology.
   1. Eustachian tube is narrower and oriented horizontally in children, which predisposes them to ventilation and drainage problems.
   2. URI.
   3. Pressure changes that occur, such as with plane travel, may lead to acute ETD.
   4. OM, serous effusions, cholesteatoma may cause chronic ETD from negative middle ear pressure.
   5. Gastroesophageal reflux (GERD).
   6. Enlarged adenoids.
   7. Allergies.
   8. Down syndrome (associated with small Eustachian tubes).
   9. Smoking.
B. Occurrence.
   1. Most common in children younger than 5 years.
   2. Usually decreases with age but may persist to adulthood.
C. Clinical manifestations.
   1. Presenting complaints may include:
      a. Fullness, clogged feeling in ear.
      b. Ear discomfort (may be relieved by "popping ears").
      c. Hearing loss.
      d. Symptoms can be unilateral or bilateral.
      e. Allergic symptoms.
      f. Dizziness or lightheadedness.
D. Physical findings.
   1. Retracted TM, effusion, decreased movement on pneumoscopy.
   2. Nasal obstruction.
   3. Tuning fork test lateralizes to the affected ear if conductive hearing loss present.
E. Diagnostic tests.
   1. Usually none.
   2. Tympanography will confirm diagnosis.
   3. Audiometry may be needed to determine hearing loss.
F. Differential diagnosis.
   1. OM.
   2. OME.
   3. Otitis externa.
   4. Sinus infection.

   5. Perforation of the TM.

   6. Bullous myringitis.

   7. Patulous Eustachian tube (Eustachian tube remains open for a prolonged period of time).

 G. Treatment.

   1. Decongestants.

     a. Pseudoephedrine (Sudafed, Actifed) OR:

     b. Topical nasal sprays (avoid use longer than 3 days): Phenylephrine (Neo-Synephrine topical), oxymetazoline (Afrin).

   2. Nasal steroids (especially helpful to those with allergic rhinitis, most approved for children 6 years and older).

     a. Beclomethasone (Beconase).

     b. Budesonide (Rhinocort).

     c. Fluticasone (Flonase) approved for those 4 years of age and older.

     d. Fluticasone furoate (Veramyst) approved for those 2 years of age and older.

     e. Mometasone (Nasonex) approved for those 2 years of age and older.

   3. Second generation H1 antihistamines (may be beneficial for those with allergic rhinitis).

     a. Loratadine (Claritin).

     b. Desloratadine (Clarinex).

     c. Fexofenadine (Allegra).

     d. Cetirizine (Zyrtec).

   4. Antibiotics: Not usually indicated unless AOM present.

     a. Amoxicillin for 10 days is most effective.

   5. Tympanic perforation or ventilation tubes present.

     a. Topical antibiotic drops with topical steroid if discharge present.

     b. Neomycin-polymyxin-hydrocortisone (Cortisporin) otic drops.

     c. Ciprofloxacin-hydrocortisone (Cipro HC).

   6. Pain management.

     a. Anti-inflammatories such as acetaminophen or ibuprofen, others.

   7. GERD: Omeprazole (Prilosec).

   8. Patulous (abnormally open) Eustachian tube: Premarin nose drops or nasal spray.

 H. Follow-up.

   1. Check tubes every 3 months, if present.

   2. If OME present, check for resolution in 3 months.

   3. Return visit if symptoms worsen or change.

I. Complications.
1. TM perforation.
2. Hearing loss.
3. Cholesteatoma.
4. Meningitis.
5. Brain abscess.
6. Labyrinthitis.
7. Subdural empyema.
8. Subperiosteal abscess.
9. Facial paralysis.
10. Death.
J. Education.
1. Diagnosis: Importance of treating cause.
2. Treatment plan.
3. Modification of risk factors.
4. Importance of follow-up.
5. Relationship between speech, language and hearing.

BIBLIOGRAPHY

American Academy of Family Physicians; American Academy of Otolaryngology-Head and Neck Surgery; American Academy of Pediatrics Subcommittee on Otitis Media With Effusion. Otitis media with effusion. *Pediatrics.* 2004;113(5):1412-1429.

American Academy of Pediatrics Subcommittee on Management of Acute Otitis Media. Diagnosis and management of acute otitis media. *Pediatrics.* 2004;113(5):1451-1465.

Block SL. Improving the diagnosis of acute otitis media: "seeing is believing." *Pediatr Ann.* 2013;42(12):485-490.

Lieberthal AS, Carroll AE, Chonmaitree T, et al. The diagnosis and management of acute otitis media. *Pediatrics.* 2013;131(3):e964-e999.

Stool SE, Berg AO, Berman S, et al. Managing otitis media with effusion in young children. In: *Quick Reference Guide for Clinicians.* Rockville, MD: Agency for Health Care Policy and Research; 1994.

Vernacchio L, Vezina R, Mitchell AA. Management of acute otitis media by primary care physicians: trends since the release of the 2004 American Academy of Pediatrics/American Academy of Family Physicians clinical practice guideline. *Pediatrics.* 2007;120(2):281-287.

Sinus, Mouth, Throat, and Neck Disorders

Susan G. Rains

I. ALLERGIC RHINITIS

Allergic rhinitis, unspecified, J30.4	Other seasonal allergic rhinitis, J30.2
Cough, R05	Other specified disorders of nose and
Dyspnea, unspecified, R06.00	nasal sinuses, J34.8
Halitosis, R19.6	Sneezing, R06.7
Other chronic allergic conjunctivitis, H10.45	Wheezing, R06.2

A. Etiology.
1. Atopic predilection.
   a. Very common atopic disease of childhood second only to asthma.
   b. Often same mediators that produce asthma.
   c. Genetic factors: Increased IgE production in response to allergens.
2. Environmental factors.
   a. Common allergens.
      - Seasonal (rare in children younger than 3 years of age).
        o Nonflowering, wind-pollinated plants.
        o Tree pollens: Early spring.
        o Grasses: Late spring and early summer.
        o Weeds: Fall.
      - Acute: Sudden-onset hypersensitivity reaction caused by environmental exposure to an allergen. Symptoms generally occur within 30 minutes, and once exposure to the offending allergen ceases, they generally resolve within 24 hours.
      - Perennial: Animal dander, dust (mites), molds (spores), mildew, feathers, cockroaches.

B. Occurrence.
   1. Affects about 40% of children and 30% of adolescents.
   2. If one parent affected, child has 30% chance of developing allergies; both parents, 70% chance.
   3. The incidence in males is slightly higher.
   4. The incidence in children < 2 years of age is rare as it requires repeated exposure to offending, inhaled allergens. A child in this age group with persistent nasal symptoms may more likely be a case of adenoidal hypertrophy or chronic sinusitis.

C. Clinical manifestations.
   1. Stuffy nose, sneezing, itching, runny nose, noisy breathing/snoring, cough, halitosis, frequent clearing of throat, plugged ears, wheezing.
   2. Possibly associated signs of allergic conjunctivitis: Itchy, injected conjunctiva, puffy lids, tearing or clear mucous drainage in eye.
   3. Has significant decrement on measurements of vigilance and a broad range of cognitive functioning.

D. Physical findings.
   1. Nasal mucosa is usually pale, edematous, boggy.
   2. Thin, watery rhinorrhea.
   3. Allergic salute may cause external, transverse crease near end of nose.
   4. Nasal obstruction may cause mouth breathing.
   5. Allergic shiners (dark circles under eyes), due to venous pooling.
   6. Nose and eyes may be pruritic.
   7. Cobblestoning of the conjunctiva.
   8. Cobblestoning of the post-pharyngeal wall.

E. Diagnostic tests.
   1. Nasal smear for presence of eosinophils: 10% is positive (intranasal steroids may decrease percentage).
   2. Skin testing.

F. Differential diagnosis.

Acute atopic conjunctivitis, bilateral, H10.13	Cystic fibrosis, E84
Acute upper respiratory infection, unspecified, J06.9	Deviated nasal septum, J34.2
	Foreign body in nostril, T17.1
	Headache, R51
Allergic rhinitis due to food, J30.5	Nasal polyp, unspecified, J33.9
Allergic rhinitis, unspecified, J30.4	Other specified disorders of nose and nasal sinuses, J34.8
Choanal atresia, Q30.0	
Chronic sinusitis, unspecified, J32.9	Sebaceous cyst, L72.3

1. Infection.
    a. Viral upper respiratory infection (URI): Red and swollen turbinates, thicker, more purulent rhinorrhea; duration 10–14 days, clustered fall–spring.
    b. Sinusitis: Possibly symptoms of URI, also headache, facial pressure; duration longer than viral URI but more limited than solely allergic rhinitis.
2. Nasal foreign body: Unilateral purulent nasal discharge, foul odor.
3. Nasal polyp, dermatoid cyst, nasal glioma.
4. Cystic fibrosis (patients often have nasal polyps and chronic sinusitis).
5. Choanal atresia, deviated septum.
6. Vasomotor rhinitis: Sudden appearance and disappearance of symptoms in response to irritants.
7. Rhinitis medicamentosus: Abuse of nasal spray/drops.
8. Drug- or food-induced rhinitis.

G. Classification.
1. Mild, moderate, severe.
2. Intermittent or persistent.

H. Treatment.
1. Avoidance.
    a. Minimize exposure to dust mites, especially in child's bedroom: Remove wall-to-wall carpets, curtains, bed ruffles, stuffed animals; wash cotton bedding in hot water frequently, use nonallergenic bedding covers.
    b. Minimize exposure to animal dander.
    c. Minimize exposure to pollens: Close windows, use air conditioning, filters on air systems, keep humidity low in home, remove house plants.
    d. Avoid activities such as leaf raking, lawn mowing, furniture dusting.
    e. Avoid talcs, perfumes, cigarettes, wood smoke.
2. Pharmacotherapy.
    a. Antihistamines.
        • First generation: Avoid, especially in young children as they can cause paradoxical agitation and may be dangerous in infants.
        • Second generation: Loratadine (Claritin, generic and brand preparations now available over the counter [OTC]), age 2–5 years: 5 mg PO daily; > 6 years: 10 mg. Cetirizine (Zyrtec, generic and brand preparations now available OTC; now approved for children ≥ 6 months of age), age 6–12 months: 2.5 mg once daily; age 12 months–2 years: 2.5 mg, may increase to max of 2.5 mg q 12 hours; age 2–5 years: 2.5–5 mg PO daily;

> 6 years: 10 mg. Fexofenadine (Allegra), age 2–11 years: 30 mg bid; age ≥ 12 years: 60 mg tab bid or 180 mg daily. Desloratidine (Clarinex), age 6–11 months: 1 mg/day; 12 months–5 years: 1.25 mg/day; 6–11 years: 2.5 mg/day; age ≥ 12 years: 5 mg/day. Levoceterizine (Xyzal), 2–5 years: 1.25 mg q HS; 6–11 years: 2.5 mg HS; age ≥ 12 years: 5 mg HS.

b. Intranasal steroids, e.g., fluticasone propionate (Flonase); mometasone furoate (Nasonex); triamcinolone acetonide (Nasocort AQ); are all FDA approved in the U.S. for children 2 years and above.
   - 2–12 years of age: 1 spray each nostril once per day.
   - Older than 12 years of age: 2 sprays/nostril.

c. Mast cell stabilizers: Topical Cromolyn (NasalCrom): 1 spray tid–qid, 2–4 weeks for effect (available OTC).

d. Nasal antihistamine: Patanase (Olopatadine), ages 6–11 years: 1 spray/nostril bid; > 12 years: 2 sprays/nostril bid. Astelin (Azelastine nasal), age 2–5 years: 1 spray of 0.1 % sol. bid; 6–12 years: 1 spray of 0.1% OR 0.15% sol. Q nostril bid; age > 12 years: 2 sprays of 0.15% sol. bid.

e. Nasal decongestants (not recommended due to rebound effect secondary to abuse).
   - Oral often combined with antihistamines.
   - Topical not recommended due to rebound and abuse potential.

f. Ipratropium bromide: Useful in the treatment of rhinorrhea; age > 5 years: 2 sprays (0.06%) in each nostril qid.

g. Antileukotriene agents: Only Montelukast (Singulair) is approved in the U.S. for treatment of allergic rhinitis: Perennial: age 6–23 months: 4 mg PO daily, and starting at this age group for seasonal; age 2–5 years: 4 mg PO daily; age 6–14 years: 5 mg daily; age ≥ 15 years: 10 mg daily.

3. Immunotherapy (hyposensitization): "Allergy shots," especially recommended for children who suffer perennially and do not respond to medications.

4. Adjunct therapies:
   a. Nasal irrigation with sterile, warm saline has been shown to decrease the symptoms, primarily the rhinorrhea of allergic rhinitis.
   b. Warnings concerning alternative and complementary therapies:
      - Ingestion of St. John's wort will lead to a decrease in levels of loratadine and fexofenadine.
      - Patients with weed pollen allergies may have severe reactions when taking Echinacea purpura.

I. Follow-up.
   1. 2–4 weeks after initial treatment, sooner if needed, then 3–6 months.
J. Complications.

Acute serous otitis media, H65.0	Hearing loss, unspecified, unspecified ear, H91.90
Anosmia, R43.0	Malocclusion, unspecified, K07.4
Chronic sinusitis, unspecified, J32.9	Other voice and resonance disorders, R49.8

   1. Chronic sinusitis.
   2. Recurrent otitis media.
   3. Hoarseness.
   4. Loss of smell or hearing.
   5. High-arched palate, dental malocclusion from chronic mouth breathing.
K. Education.
   1. Chronicity of problem.
   2. Avoidance of allergens (recent evidence that exposure to cats, dogs in first year of life decreases development of allergies later in childhood).
   3. Medication administration and side effects.

II. APHTHOUS STOMATITIS

Deficiency of other specified B group vitamins, E53.8	Intestinal malabsorption, unspecified, K90.9
Diseases of lips, K13.0	Iron deficiency anemia, unspecified, D50.9
Enlarged lymph nodes, unspecified, R59.9	Lesions of oral mucosa, unspecified, K13.70
Fever of other and unknown origin, R50	Recurrent oral aphthae, K12.0

A. Etiology.
   1. Commonly known as canker sores, aphthous stomatitis is recurrence of painful, discrete, shallow ulcers on unattached mucous membranes of mouth.
   2. Considered to be immune-mediated destruction of epithelium, cause is multifactorial, including infection, autoimmune disease, allergies, nutritional deficiencies, and trauma.
   3. Associated risk factors.
      a. Genetic: Positive family history.
      b. Deficiencies of iron, vitamin B12, folic acid.

      c. Chronic illness such as IBD, celiac disease, immune suppression, lupus, juvenile rheumatoid arthritis (JRA).

      d. Nonsteroidal anti-inflammatory drug (NSAID) or angiotension-convering enzyme (ACE) inhibitor usage.

      e. Childhood: Higher incidence (peak 10–19 years).

B. Occurrence.

  1. Incidence: Up to 20% of population.

  2. Precipitating factors.

      a. Stress/trauma: Emotional, physical, hormonal.

      b. Foods: Chocolate, nuts, tomatoes.

      c. Malabsorption syndromes.

C. Clinical manifestations.

  1. Aphthous minor: 80% of cases: 1–5 mm lesions; heal in 5–12 days; no scarring.

  2. Considered severe (15% of cases) by some experts if lesions are large (> 1 cm) and by others solely if there are multiple lesions; persist up to 4 weeks; may scar.

  3. Patient complains of single or multiple painful sores in mouth.

  4. Tingling or burning may precede appearance of lesions.

D. Physical findings.

  1. Painful yellow, gray, ulcerative lesions with erythematous halo on mucosa.

  2. 1–5 ulcerative oval or circular ulcers with an erythematous periphery and pale white/gray or yellow center.

  3. Size: 2–10 mm.

  4. Absence of systemic symptoms (i.e., fever, lymphadenopathy).

E. Diagnostic tests.

  1. None.

F. Differential diagnosis.

Enlarged lymph nodes, unspecified, R59.9	Fever of other and unknown origin, R50
Enteroviral vesicular pharyngitis, B08.5	Herpesviral infection, unspecified, B00.9

  1. Infections:

      a. Herpes simplex (rare).

        • Small, irregular vesicles that rupture and leave ulcers.

        • Red at periphery with gray center.

        • Patient often febrile with significant lymphadenopathy.

- Recurrent herpes infections remain localized to lips, rarely cross mucocutaneous junction.
- Primary infections sometimes involve oral mucosa.
  b. Coxsackie—hand, foot, and mouth disease.
- Sometimes ulcers in the mouth (and will have papules on hands and feet, perhaps buttocks).
 2. Traumatic (injury).
 3. Herpangina: Ulcerative pharyngitis (not stomatitis); fever, lymphadenopathy.
 4. Angular cheilitis: Erythematous, painful fissures at corners of the mouth. May be caused by lipsucking, sensitivity to agent with which in contact. Treatment is topical with an antibiotic, antiyeast, or low-dose steroid ointment.
 5. Autoimmune disease: IBD, lupus, Reiter's syndrome.
G. Treatment.
 1. Supportive.
    a. Oral analgesics such as acetaminophen or ibuprofen.
    b. Topical anesthetics: Especially prior to eating/drinking.
    - Viscous Xylocaine dabbed on lesions with cotton swab.
    - Mouthwashes.
      o Diphenhydramine elixir: Antacid suspension (aluminum and magnesium hydroxide combination): Mix 1:1 (parent can do this). Do not allow more than 1/2 teaspoon total of preparation every 3–4 hours for young children as they will probably swallow the medication rather than "swish and spit."
      o Pharmacist may add lidocaine 1% for older child to swish and spit.
    - 0.1% triamcinolone (Kenalog) in Orabase: Dab on lesions qid.
    c. Avoid acidic, salty foods and drinks.
    d. Good oral hygiene.
    - Rinse mouth frequently with clear water.
    - Offer water to young children frequently, especially after eating or drinking other fluids.
H. Follow-up.
 1. None if healed.
 2. If slow to heal or accompanied by systemic symptoms or dermatologic lesions, must be evaluated.
 I. Complications.
 1. Generally none. Young child may refuse to drink.
 2. Referral if persists 3 weeks or no urine output for 12 hours.
 J. Education.
 1. Avoidance of triggers/precipitating factors.

III. CAT-SCRATCH DISEASE (CSD)

Cat-scratch disease, A28.1

Conjunctivitis, unspecified, H10.9

Disorder of the skin and subcutaneous tissue, unspecified, L98.9

Enlarged lymph nodes, unspecified, R59.9

Fever of other and unknown origin, R50

Granuloma of unspecified orbit, H05.119

Other benign neoplasm of skin of unspecified part of face, D23.30

A. Etiology.
   1. Bacteria *Bartonella henselae* infects humans via cat saliva entering the body through a scratch or bite. Fleas from the cat may also be a vector for the microorganism.
   2. Reports vary, but in some studies, up to 99% of patients have had contact with a kitten or cat within the previous 6 months; 50% have history of a scratch.
B. Occurrence.
   1. More common in children (younger than 18 years), especially boys.
   2. 20,000 cases/year in United States, primarily July–January.
C. Clinical manifestations.
   1. Typical cat-scratch disease.
      a. Primary skin lesion (papule) appears 3–10 days following inoculation.
      b. Regional (primarily unilateral) lymphadenopathy develops in about 2 weeks and sometimes persists for months. 85% have a single node.
      c. Fever, which may be prolonged (up to 2 weeks) in two-thirds of patients; also malaise, headache, and anorexia.
      d. 10% of nodes may suppurate spontaneously.
      e. May have hepatosplenic disease.
   2. Less common clinical manifestations:
      a. Parinaud oculoglandular syndrome.
      b. Neuroretinitis-posterior segment ocular disease.
      c. Encephalopathy.
      d. Radiculopathy.
      e. Facial nerve palsy.
      f. Guillain-Barré syndrome.
      g. Cerebral arteritis.
      h. Transverse myelitis.

       i. Glomerulonephritis.

       j. Thrombocytopenia purpura.

       k. Osteomyelitis.

       l. Arthritis/arthralgia.

       m. Endocarditis.

D. Physical findings (in typical CSD).

    1. Nonpruritic vesicle or papule(s) over site of inoculation.

    2. Lymphadenopathy of area that drains site of inoculation. Most commonly axillary and epitrochlear nodes, then head, neck, and groin in descending order of frequency.

    3. Skin over affected nodes is warm, taut, tender, indurated.

E. Diagnostic criteria:

    1. History of cat or flea contact regardless of presence of inoculation site.

    2. Clinical presentation of tender, regional unilateral lymphadenopathy.

    3. Difficult to culture, though can be done. Serology probably most useful though many patients will have positive serology due to past exposure to *B. henselae.*

      • IgG titers of < 1:64 suggest no disease; those between 1:64 and 1:256 are unequivocal and should be repeated in 10–14 days. Titers > 1:256 suggest acute disease. IgM more sensitive for acute disease but produced briefly.

      • Immunoglobulin testing will pick up various strains of bartonella; may be necessary to do PCR testing to differentiate. (Klotz)

    4. Negative cultures for other causes of adenopathy.

    5. Sterile node aspirate.

F. Differential diagnosis.

Asymptomatic HIV infection status, Z21	Methicillin susceptible *Staphylococcus aureus* infection as the cause of diseases classified elsewhere, B95.61
Cytomegaloviral disease, unspecified, B25.9	Mycobacterial infection, unspecified, A31.9
Enlarged lymph nodes, unspecified, R59.9	Streptococcus, group A, as the cause of diseases classified elsewhere, B95.0
Infectious mononucleosis, unspecified without complication, B27.90	Streptococcus, group B, as the cause of diseases classified elsewhere, B95.1
Localized swelling, mass and lump, neck, R22.1	Toxoplasmosis, unspecified, B58.9

1. Other causes of lymphadenopathy.
   a. Common viral and bacterial infections such as group A beta-hemolytic streptococci (GABHS), staphylococci (especially methicillin resistant *Staphylococcus aureus* [MRSA]) cytomegalovirus (CMV), Epstein-Barr virus (EBV; infectious mono), HIV.
2. Subacute and chronic lymphadenopathy more likely associated with mycobacterium and toxoplasmosis.
3. Neck masses from other sources.

G. Treatment.
   1. Symptomatic.
      a. Antipyretics and analgesics.
      b. Moist wraps/compresses.
      c. Aspiration of painful nodes (avoid I&D).
      d. Antimicrobial treatment for severely ill patients or those with other chronic condition. Not suggested for regional CSD.
      e. For patients with significant lymphadenopathy, prolonged, severe disease or complications: Azithromycin (Zithromax): 500 mg day 1, 250 mg days 2–5; younger children 10 mg/kg day 1, 5 mg/kg days 2–5.
      f. Other antibiotics with anecdotal evidence of efficacy: Ciprofloxacin, rifampin, trimethoprim-sulfamethoxazole, gentamicin.

H. Follow-up.
   1. Every week until resolution of symptoms, dependent on severity of symptoms.

I. Complications.

Enlarged lymph nodes, unspecified, R59.9	Osteomyelitis of vertebra, site unspecified, M46.20
Erythema nodosum, L52	Other specified diseases of liver, K76.89
Focal chorioretinal inflammation, juxtapapillary, unspecified eye, H30.019	Viral meningitis, unspecified, A87.9
Myelitis, unspecified, G04.91	Viral pneumonia, not otherwise classified, J12

1. Parinaud oculoglandular syndrome: Inoculation of conjunctiva results in ipsilateral preauricular or submandibular lymphadenopathy.
2. Less commonly: Encephalitis, aseptic meningitis, neuroretinitis, thrombocytopenia purpura, erythema nodosum, pneumonia, hepatosplenomegaly, osteomyelitis, endocarditis.

J. Education.
1. Avoid scratches by decreasing rough play with kittens or cats.
2. Immediately cleanse wounds from cats.

IV. CERVICAL LYMPHADENITIS

Abnormal weight loss, R63.4	Mycobacterial infection, unspecified, A31.9
Acute lymphadenitis, unspecified, L04.9	
Acute pharyngitis, J02	Nonspecific lymphadenitis, unspecified, I88.9
Acute upper respiratory infection, unspecified, J06.9	Other fatigue, R53.83
Cat-scratch disease, A28.1	Other specified diseases of liver, K76.89
Cough, R05	
Disorder of circulatory system, unspecified, I99.9	Other specified types of non-Hodgkin lymphoma, unspecified site, C85.80
Enlarged lymph nodes, unspecified, R59.9	Pain in joint, M25.5
Fever of other and unknown origin, R50	Protein-calorie malnutrition, unspecified, E46
Generalized hyperhidrosis, R61	
Infectious mononucleosis, unspecified without complication, B27.90	Streptococcus, group A, as the cause of diseases classified elsewhere, B95.0
Infectious mononucleosis, unspecified without complication, B27.90	Streptococcus, group B, as the cause of diseases classified elsewhere, B95.1
Methicillin susceptible *Staphylococcus aureus* infection as the cause of diseases classified elsewhere, B95.61	
Mucocutaneous lymph node syndrome [Kawasaki], M30.3	Toxoplasmosis, unspecified, B58.9
	Rubella without complication, B06.9

A. Etiology.
1. Enlargement of lymph glands of neck generally due to:
    a. Infection, which causes proliferation and invasion of inflammatory cells.
        • Viruses:
            o Upper respiratory: Respiratory syncytial virus (RSV), adenoviruses, enteroviruses, influenza, parainfluenza, rhinoviruses—which usually resolve more quickly than other etiologies.
            o EBV.

- o CMV: Rare.
- o Rubella, rubeola, roseola: Rare.
- o Varicella zoster: Rare.
- o Herpes simplex virus (HSV).
- o Coxsackie.
- o HIV: Rare.
- Bacteria:
  - o *Staphylococcus aureus* and GABHS: 40–80% of cases.
  - o Anaerobes: Rare.
  - o Corynebacterium diphtheriae.
  - o *Bartonella henselae* (cat-scratch disease).
  - o Gram-negative rods (rare): *Haemophilus influenzae*, pseudomonas, salmonellae, shigellae, *Francisella tularensis* (tularemia).
- Mycobacterium.
  - o Mycobacterium tuberculosis.
  - o Nontuberculous mycobacteria (NTM).
- Spirochetes.
- Rickettsiae.
- Fungi, including *Histoplasma capsulatum* (histoplasmosis): Rare.
- Protozoa, including *Toxoplasma gondii* (toxoplasmosis): Rare.

   b. Other causes.
- Neoplasms that cause infiltration of neoplastic cells: Rare.
- Histiocytosis.
- Collagen vascular diseases: JRA, lupus.
- Sarcoidosis.
- Kawasaki disease.
- Postvaccination: DTaP, polio, typhoid.
- Drugs-phenytoin, INH.

B. Occurrence.
   1. About 40% of all children have palpable cervical lymph nodes.
   2. Most cases of cervical lymphadenitis resulting from common bacterial and viral infections occur in toddler and preschool age groups.
   3. Etiologic and age-related occurrence.
      a. Neonate.
- Acute unilateral cervical lymphadenitis: *S. aureus*.
- "Cellulitis-adenitis" syndrome: Late-onset group B streptococcus.
      b. Younger than 5 years of age.
- Acute pyogenic cervical lymphadenitis: *S. aureus* and GABHS.
- Nontuberculous mycobacteria (NTM) lymph node infection.
- Kawasaki disease (also usually unilateral).

     c. School-age and adolescents: More likely chronic cervical lymphadenitis than acute pyogenic disease.

C. Clinical manifestations.

  1. Acute bilateral cervical lymphadenitis generally caused by URI or strep pharyngitis. Sometimes associated with EBV (infectious mononucleosis), though should have posterior cervical nodes.

  2. Acute unilateral cervical lymphadenitis variably associated with fever and suppuration, most often caused by staph and group A streptococcus, and sometimes anaerobes.

  3. Subacute and chronic lymphadenitis, though often unilateral, is found in CSD, toxoplasmosis, and mycobacterial infections. Nodes become fluctuant and are generally nontender.

  4. Painless, possibly matted nodes and especially those in the supraclavicular area are more likely malignant.

  5. Associated symptoms.

     a. With URI: Fever, sore throat, cough.

     b. Lymphoma, tuberculosis (TB): Fever, night sweats, weight loss.

     c. Collagen vascular disease or serum sickness: Fever, fatigue, arthralgias.

D. Physical findings.

  1. General.

     a. Signs of malnutrition, including poor growth: Suggestive of chronic disease.

     b. Generalized adenopathy and hepatosplenomegaly: Suggestive of malignancy or other noninfectious illnesses and some infectious diseases such as EBV, HIV, TB, histoplasmosis.

  2. Enlargement of the lymph nodes: > 1 cm.

     a. Node-bearing areas: Occipital, cervicofacial, axillary, epitrochlear, inguinal, popliteal.

     b. Nodes may be warm, mobile, fixed, fluctuant, solid, smooth.

  3. Presentation, distribution, associated diseases.

     a. Acute posterior cervical lymphadenopathy: Rubella, infectious mononucleosis.

     b. Supraclavicular or posterior cervical lymphadenopathy: Risk for malignancy.

     c. Cervical lymphadenopathy, associated generalized lymphadenopathy: Viral infection.

     d. Generalized lymphadenopathy: Associated with leukemia, lymphoma, collagen vascular disease.

     e. Nodes bilateral and soft (not fixed): Viral infection.

    f. Tender nodes, possibly fluctuant, not fixed: More likely bacterial.

    g. Redness and warmth: Acute pyogenic process.

    h. With fluctuance: Abscess formation.

    i. Matted or fluctuant nodes, skin overlying red but not warm: TB.

    j. Nodes hard and fixed, without signs of acute inflammation: Associated malignancy.

  4. Associated physical signs.

    a. Markedly red pharynx, possibly exudates, soft palate petechiae: GABHS.

    b. Swelling, redness, tenderness of gums: Periodontal disease.

    c. Edema of the soft tissues of the neck: Diphtheria.

    d. Sinus tract formation: TB.

    e. Gingivostomatitis: HSV.

    f. Herpangina: Coxsackievirus.

    g. Rash: Infectious mono, scarlet fever.

    h. Pallor, petechiae, bruises, sternal tenderness.

    i. Hepatosplenomegaly: Leukemia.

E. Diagnostic tests.

  1. Appropriate for suspicion of specific entity.

  2. Throat culture.

  3. PPD.

  4. CBC.

  5. Erythrocyte sedimentation rate (ESR) or (CRP) C-reactive protein.

  6. Blood cultures.

  7. Liver enzymes.

  8. Serology for specific microorganisms.

  9. Chest X-ray.

  10. Ultrasound of nodes.

  11. Echocardiogram, electrocardiogram.

  12. Fine-needle aspiration for Gram stain and culture.

  13. Biopsy: If malignancy suspected.

F. Differential diagnosis.

Localized swelling, mass and lump, neck, R22.1

---

  1. Neck masses.

    a. Congenital lesions are generally painless and most likely identified in infancy.

      • Thyroglossal duct cyst: Midline between thyroid bone and suprasternal notch, moves upward.

- Branchial cleft cyst: Smooth, fluctuant, proximal, anterior border of sternocleidomastoid muscle, though possibly in 3 separate areas of that muscle: preauricular down to supraclavicular.
- Sternocleidomastoid tumor: Mass in belly of the muscle caused by perinatal injury; associated torticollis.
- Cervical ribs: Bony anomaly.
- Cystic hygroma: Fluid filled, easily transilluminated.
- Hemangioma.
- Laryngocele: Cystic mass extending through the thyroid membrane.
- Dermoid cyst: Midline cyst, also contains solid components.
- Parotitis: Swelling crosses angle of jaw; mumps.

2. To summarize: It is reasonable to safely observe nodes that are bilateral, < 3 cm in size, nonerythematous nor exquisitely tender. Treat empirically if: No accompanying systemic symptoms, node > 2–3 cm, unilateral, or erythematous and tender.

G. Treatment.
   1. Acute unilateral cervical lymphadenitis.
      a. Oral:
         - Methicillin susceptible *Staphylococcus aureus* (MSSA), group A streptococcus, or oral anaerobes (periodontal disease).
         - Patient nontoxic, no abscesses or cellulitis: Amoxicillin-clavulanate (based on amoxicillin component): 40 mg/kg/day divided bid for 10 days (max 1.75 g/day).
         - MSSA and group A strep.
            o Cephalexin 25–100mg/day, divided tid or qid (max 4g/day).
            o Cefadroxil 30 mg/kg/day divided bid (max 2g/day).
         - MSSA, community-acquired MRSA (CA-MRSA), group A strep, oral anaerobes.
            o Clindamycin 30 mg/kg/day divided qid or tid (max 1.8 g/day).
         - MSSA, CA-MRSA, or *Bartonella henselae.*
            o Trimethoprim-sulfamethoxazole (> 2 months) 10 mg/kg/day divided bid (max 320 mg/day) (dosed according to trimethoprim component).
         - Patients should respond to empiric therapy within 48–72 hours. If they do not, or they worsen, they should be promptly reevaluated.
      b. Patient toxic or immunocompromised.
         - IV cefazolin, nafcillin, clindamycin, ampicillin-sulbactam, linezolid, oxacillin, piperacillin-tazobactam, vancomycin.

- Oral analgesia, warm compresses.
- Incision and drainage for suppurative, fluctuant nodes.
c. Consider referral for biopsy if significant lymphadenopathy (> 2 cm in diameter) persists for 2 weeks, no decrease in size after 4–6 weeks, or node(s) are supraclavicular, lack inflammation, are firm or rubbery, develop ulceration, fail to respond to antibiotic treatment, or there are systemic symptoms (e.g., fever, weight loss, hepatosplenomegaly).
d. Cervical lymphadenitis abscess: Refer for fine-needle aspiration or excision (I&D).
H. Follow-up.
1. Call if node enlarges, becomes markedly tender, erythematous, indurated.
2. Call if child appears toxic, has difficulty breathing or swallowing.
3. If being treated for bacterial infection, call if not better in 48 hours (fever down, tenderness decreased, size of node stable).
4. Recheck at end of treatment.
5. Recheck if node(s) persist longer than several weeks.
I. Complications.
1. Bacterial: Suppuration, bacteremia.
2. Undiagnosed infectious process or malignancy.
J. Education.
1. Address family's fears: Primarily those of malignancy.
2. Compliance with medications.
3. Observation: When to call, return to clinic.
4. Hydration.

V. EPISTAXIS

Allergic rhinitis, unspecified, J30.4	Epistaxis, R04.0
Acute upper respiratory infection, unspecified, J06.9	Essential (primary) hypertension, I10
Disorder of the skin and subcutaneous tissue, unspecified, L98.9	Hepatomegaly, not elsewhere classified, R16.0
Enlarged lymph nodes, unspecified, R59.9	Rash and other nonspecific skin eruption, R21
	Volume depletion, E86

A. Etiology.
   1. Bleeding from the nose can be anteriorly from nares (commonly Kiesselbach plexus) or posteriorly into nasopharynx. The nasal mucosa has rich yet relatively unprotected blood supply. The mucosa is thin, especially in children.
   2. Causative factors.
      a. Inflammation.
         - Infectious processes.
         - Allergies.
      b. Neoplasms, polyps.
      c. Trauma.
         - External injury.
         - Nose picking.
         - Foreign bodies.
         - Chemical or caustic agents (including drugs).
   3. Rarely.
      a. Systemic illnesses.
         - Hematologic diseases.
         - Hypertension.
B. Occurrence.
   1. Very common in children.
   2. Highest incidence 2–10 years of age.
   3. Often familial history.
C. Clinical manifestations.
   1. Complaints of persistent, recurrent nosebleeds.
   2. May have history of:
      a. Recent or current URI.
      b. Allergies (especially nasal).
      c. Tarry stools.
      d. Medication or drug use.
      e. Persistent bleeding or bruising.
      f. Family history of epistaxis or bleeding disorders.
      g. Trauma: Nose picking or foreign body insertion.
D. Physical findings.
   1. Vital signs may reflect hypovolemia or underlying cause such as hypertension.
   2. Inspection of nose (pushing the tip of the nose up facilitates inspection of the anterior structures), nasopharynx, and oropharynx may reveal:
      a. Bleeding most commonly from medial anterior nares, especially Kiesselbach's plexus.

      b. Dry, crusted mucosa.

      c. Excoriation of mucosa, site of bleeding.

   3. General exam may find lymphadenopathy, hepatomegaly, petechial rashes, or pale skin, mucosa, nail beds.

E. Diagnostic tests.

   1. Vital signs, including blood pressure.

   2. Hematocrit or CBC with platelets.

   3. If severe and persistent, laboratory evaluation for bleeding disorder begins with:

      a. CBC with platelets.

      b. Prothrombin time (PT) and activated partial thromboplastin time (aPTT).

F. Differential diagnosis.

Disease of blood and blood-forming organs, unspecified, D75.9	Foreign body in nostril, T17.1
Disorder of kidney and ureter, unspecified, N28.9	Nasal polyp, unspecified, J33.9
Essential (primary) hypertension, I10	Other specified symptoms and signs involving the circulatory and respiratory systems, R09.89

   1. Bleeding disorder: If severe and recurrent, child younger than 2 years, positive family history.

   2. Polyps, vascular abnormalities.

   3. Foreign body.

   4. Hypertension, renal disease.

G. Treatment.

   1. Elevate head and lean forward.

   2. Pinch nares together for at least 10 minutes (may check after 5 minutes).

   3. Ice to nasal dorsum may be added but has not been shown to hasten resolution.

   4. Packing (preferably absorbable), topical vasoconstrictive medications such as oxymetazoline (Afrin), phenylephrine (Neo-Synephrine), or epinephrine (1:1000) may be needed. They can be applied with a cotton pledget to the nasal mucosa.

   5. Referral to ENT if unmanageable or prolonged or abnormalities of nose.

   6. If on nasal steroids, discontinue.

H. Follow-up.

   1. Hct, 6–12 hours after bleed if concern for anemia.

   2. Return if unmanageable and/or persistent.

I. Complications.
　1. Possibly mild anemia.
　2. Rare: Airway obstruction, aspiration, vomiting.
J. Education.
　1. Prevention.
　　a. Humidification of air in home, especially bedroom.
　　b. Nasal saline sprays, drops.
　　c. Petroleum jelly applied sparingly to anterior nares.
　　d. Protective athletic gear.
　　e. Discouragement of nose-picking behaviors and vigorous blowing.
　2. Reassurance: Amount of blood always looks greater than it is.

VI. FOREIGN BODY, NASAL

Cough, R05	Foreign body in nostril, T17.1
Dysphagia, unspecified, R13.10	Other abnormalities of breathing, R06.89
Foreign body in nasal sinus, 17.0	Vomiting, unspecified, R11.10

A. Etiology.
　1. Small objects are often inserted into nose by children, causing full or partial obstruction of nares.
B. Occurrence.
　1. Frequent, especially in young children age 3–6 years.
C. Clinical manifestations.
　1. Child may have been observed.
　2. Initially, local symptoms of obstruction: Swelling, sneezing, mild discomfort.
　3. Subsequently, persistent, purulent, unilateral discharge; may be bloody or foul smelling.
　4. Epistaxis.
D. Physical findings.
　1. Dependent on length of time obstruction has been present: See previously listed symptoms. Obstruction is almost always unilateral.
　2. Examiner may be able to visualize object with nasal speculum or otoscope.
　3. Common objects include beads, buttons, toy parts, pebbles, candle wax, food, paper, cloth, button batteries (which are quite concerning, as they can quickly cause significant tissue damage).
　4. Tend to locate in floor of nasal passage or in the upper nasal fossa.

E. Diagnostic tests.
1. Nasal X-rays can be helpful in identification of radiopaque foreign bodies.
F. Differential diagnosis.

Chronic adenoiditis, J35.02

Chronic sinusitis, unspecified, J32.9

Nasal polyp, unspecified, J33.9

---

1. Infection.
   a. Rhinosinusitis.
   b. Adenoiditis.
2. Polyps.
3. Nasal tumors.
G. Treatment.
1. Purulent discharge may need to be suctioned in order to visualize object.
2. An older child may be told to occlude one side of nares and blow vigorously.
3. Using an Ambu bag to the mouth while occluding the nonobstructed side of the nose has been used as a method to expel the object.
4. Removal requires:
   a. Good lighting.
   b. Topical anesthesia (generally lidocaine).
   c. Vasoconstrictor drugs (0.5% epinephrine, oxymetazoline, phenylephrine) may be needed to reduce mucosa edema.
   d. Straight or alligator forceps, cerumen spoon (curved, wire ones best).
   e. Narrow tip suction.
   f. Passing a thin, lubricated, 5–6 Fr balloon-tipped catheter past the foreign body, inflating balloon and pulling forward.
   g. Batteries should be removed within 1 hour of insertion as they are quite damaging.
   h. Saline nose drops after removal to soothe mucosa. Possibly antibacterial ointment applied sparingly.
      • Saline will sting if foreign body is a battery. Use sterile water for irrigation.
H. Follow-up.
1. None, if successful removal and signs of infection clear within 1–2 days.
2. Referral to ENT if unable or unlikely to remove easily.
3. Consider behavioral/emotional assessment if it is recurrent problem or developmentally inappropriate behavior.

I. Complications.
  1. Chronic infection if undetected and/or not removed.
  2. Trauma to nares from removal procedure.
J. Education.
  1. Close observation of children by caregivers.
  2. Limit access by small children to small objects.
  3. **Note:** If child swallows foreign body, especially coin, radiographic survey must be done to ensure object is in stomach. Child must be observed closely for hoarseness, dysphagia, drooling, gagging, vomiting, coughing, choking, and airway compromise, including inspiratory stridor.

VII. INFECTIOUS MONONUCLEOSIS

Abdominal and pelvic pain, R10	Other fatigue, R53.83
Acquired hemolytic anemia, unspecified, D59.9	Other specified disorders of white blood cells, D72.89
Acute pharyngitis, J02	Rash and other nonspecific skin eruption, R21
Acute tonsillitis, J03	
Enlarged lymph nodes, unspecified, R59.9	Splenomegaly, not elsewhere classified, R16.1
Fever of other and unknown origin, R50	Spontaneous ecchymoses, R23.3
Infectious mononucleosis, unspecified without complication, B27.90	Streptococcus, group A, as the cause of diseases classified elsewhere, B95.0
Inflammatory liver disease, unspecified, K75.9	Streptococcus, group B, as the cause of diseases classified elsewhere, B95.1
Myalgia, M79.1	Thrombocytopenia, unspecified, D69.6
Myocarditis, unspecified, I51.4	

A. Etiology.
  1. EBV (which is a herpesvirus).
  2. Clinical symptoms result from proliferation of b-lymphocytes in the epithelial cells of the pharynx, parotid duct, lymph nodes, spleen.
  3. Spread primarily in saliva.
  4. Latent, lifelong infection occurs and may be reactivated during immunosuppression.

B. Occurrence.
1. Humans.
   a. Endemic worldwide in younger children, especially third-world countries.
   b. One-third of cases in adolescents in more affluent populations of developed countries, more prevalent in Caucasians.
   c. Almost all adults in United States are seropositive for EBV.
C. Clinical manifestations.
1. Primary EBV infection.
   a. Incubation is 30–50 days.
   b. Primary EBV infection in adolescents presents in > 50% of cases with:
      • Fatigue, malaise, myalgia.
      • Generalized lymphadenopathy.
      • Pharyngitis.
      • Possibly fever or prodrome of malaise and fever.
   c. Younger children may experience mild febrile episode, rash, abdominal pain.
D. Physical findings.
1. Tonsillitis, pharyngitis: Possibly exudative.
2. Palatal petechiae (transient).
3. Lymphadenopathy.
   a. Anterior and posterior cervical nodes, also axillary or inguinal nodes.
   b. Large, mildly (if at all) tender.
   c. Epitrochlear and posterior cervical nodes highly indicative.
4. Almost always splenomegaly, possibly hepatomegaly.
   a. Spleen is generally palpable 2–3 cm below the costal margin.
   b. Persists for 2–4 weeks past resolution of other symptoms.
5. Rash is common but variable as it may be erythematous, petechial, urticarial scarlatiniform or present more like erythema-multiforme.
   a. If treated with ampicillin drug or derivative, approximately 80% of young adults with this disease will develop a rash.
6. Sometimes eyelid edema.
E. Diagnostic tests.
1. "Monospot" (mononucleosis rapid slide agglutination test for heterophile antibodies disease process) 25% false negative in the first week of the disease. In children younger than 12 years of age, monospot detects 25–50% of cases.
2. Commercial diagnostic kits that detect the heterophil antibody and are often used in outpatient settings are about 98% sensitive.

3. CBC with differential.
   a. Lymphocytosis with up to 20,000 white blood cells.
   b. Up to 40% atypical lymphocytes.
   Note: 50% lymphocytes with 10–20% atypical lymphocytes is diagnostic.
   c. Mild thrombocytopenia 50% of cases.
   d. Positive monocytes on differential.
4. Liver enzymes.
   a. Mild hepatitis common.
   b. Usually asymptomatic.
5. EBV serology: Indicated in acutely ill patient.
   a. If monospot negative and strong suspicion.
   b. VCA-IgM test if monospot negative and urgent diagnosis needed, such as in a competitive athlete.
6. Throat culture.
   a. Rule out other causes.
   b. 5–25% cases have concurrent GABHS infection.

F. Differential diagnosis.

Acute pharyngitis, J02	Leukemia, unspecified not having
Acute tonsillitis, J03	achieved remission, C95.90
Adenovirus infection, unspecified site, B34.0	Rubella without complication, B06.9
Asymptomatic HIV infection status, Z21	Streptococcus, group A, as the cause of diseases classified elsewhere, B95.0
Cytomegaloviral disease, unspecified, B25.9	Streptococcus, group B, as the cause of diseases classified elsewhere, B95.1
Herpesviral infection, unspecified, B00.9	Toxoplasmosis, unspecified, B58.9

1. Other causes of infectious mononucleosis-like syndrome (in descending order of incidence):
   a. CMV.
   b. Toxoplasmosis gondii.
   c. HIV-mucocutaneous lesions, diarrhea, nausea and vomiting, weight loss.
   d. Human herpesvirus.
   e. Rubella.

    2. Pharyngitis/tonsillitis.

        a. GABHS: Absence of hepatosplenomegaly; fatigue less prominent.

        b. Other bacterial causes.

        c. Viruses other than EBV.

    3. Leukemias.

    4. Infectious mononucleosis should be suspected in any febrile patient with sore throat plus palatal petechiae, splenomegaly, posterior cervical, and possibly axillary, epitrochlear, or inguinal adenopathy.

    5. Due to its rarity, if abdominal pain is severe and in the LUQ, it should be taken quite seriously.

G. Treatment.

    1. Supportive.

        a. Analgesics and antipyretics.

        b. Hydration support if needed.

        c. Corticosteroids may be indicated (though there is significant disagreement as to their efficacy) if:

- Impending airway obstruction or dehydration secondary to severe tonsillopharyngitis.
- Massive splenomegaly.
- Myocarditis.
- Hemolytic anemia.
- Hemophagocytic syndrome.

H. Follow-up.

    1. Fatigue may persist months after recovery. Patient should be allowed to resume school and activities as energy level permits.

    2. Splenomegaly.

        a. Risk of rupture is estimated at 0.1% (50% are spontaneous).

        b. Recheck at weekly intervals.

        c. Avoid contact sports at least 3–4 weeks until fully recovered and spleen no longer palpable.

        d. Consider selective ultrasonography, such as when an athlete would like to return to competitive sports in < 4 weeks.

I. Complications.

Dermatitis due to substances taken internally, L27	Other specified respiratory disorders, J98.8
Infarction of spleen, D73.5	Volume depletion, E86

    1. Additional complications are rare but include:

        a. Dehydration.

        b. Antibiotic-induced rash (most commonly when ampicillin or amoxicillin antibiotic used for concurrent bacterial infection).

     c. Thrombocytopenia.
     d. Airway obstruction.
     e. Acute interstitial nephritis.
     f. Hemolytic anemia.
     g. Myocarditis.
     h. Neurologic abnormalities.
     i. Cranial nerve palsies.
     j. Encephalitis.
     k. Retrobulbar neuritis.

J. Education.
    1. Close personal contact is required for transmission.
    2. Recovery often biphasic, with worsening of symptoms after period of improvement.
    3. Full recovery may take months.
    4. Patient should not donate blood.

VIII. PHARYNGITIS

Acute pharyngitis, J02	Other viral agents as the cause of diseases classified elsewhere, B97.89
Adenovirus infection, unspecified site, B34.0	Peritonsillar abscess, J36
Diphtheria, unspecified, A36.9	Rheumatic fever without heart involvement, I00
Enterovirus as the cause of diseases classified to other chapters, B97.11	Streptococcus, group A, as the cause of diseases classified elsewhere, B95.0
Infectious mononucleosis, unspecified without complication, B27.90	Streptococcus, group B, as the cause of diseases classified elsewhere, B95.1

A. Etiology.
    1. Inflammation of mucous membranes and underlying structures of pharynx and tonsils, usually caused by infection.
    2. Causative agents.
       a. Respiratory viruses, including rhinovirus, adenovirus, coxsackievirus, EBV.
       b. GABHS.
       c. Group C beta-hemolytic strep (not a cause of rheumatic fever), *Neisseria gonorrhoeae* rarely.
       d. Mycoplasma pneumoniae: Possibly 10% occurrence in adolescents.
       e. Corynebacterium diphtheriae.

  f. *Arcanobacterium haemolyticum:* Cause of pharyngitis primarily in adolescents. Rash similar to that of scarlet fever without desquamation. Unresponsive to penicillin (PCN), erythromycin is drug of choice.

  g. *Fusobacterium necrophorum:* Cause of acute pharyngitis in adolescents and cause of Lemierre syndrome.

B. Occurrence.

  1. Peak incidence late fall through early spring.

  2. Younger children more commonly present in winter months and with viral pharyngitis.

  3. GABHS has proclivity for 5- to 15-year age group, also peaking in winter.

C. Clinical manifestations.

  1. Viral pharyngitis.

    a. Gradual onset.

    b. Cough, coryza, diarrhea more common.

  2. Coxsackievirus (see *Physical Findings*).

  3. Streptococcal.

    a. Rapid onset.

    b. See *Physical Findings*.

    c. Incubation 2–4 days.

D. Physical findings.

  1. Viral pharyngitis.

    a. Sore throat, dysphagia.

    b. Low-grade fever.

    c. Possibly diarrhea.

  2. Coxsackievirus.

    a. Fever, headache.

    b. GI complaints.

    c. Possibly papular rash of hand, foot, and mouth disease.

    d. Possibly ulcerative lesions in mucosa of mouth.

  3. Streptococcal GABHS.

    a. Moderate to high fever, headache.

    b. Red pharynx: Beefy red, swollen uvula and tonsils.

    c. Yellow, blood: Tinged exudates.

    d. Petechiae on soft palate, strawberry (coated) tongue.

    e. Tender cervical lymphadenopathy.

    f. Multiple GI complaints.

    g. Accompanying scarlatiniform rash: Red, sandpaper-like, clustered in body's "hot spots" (axillae, neck, inguinal, anticubital, popliteal areas).

E. Diagnostic tests.
   1. Throat swab for rapid antigen detection test for GABHS. Negative should also have follow-up throat culture (can also identify carrier state).
   2. Heterophile antibody test for EBV.
   3. CBC.
F. Differential diagnosis.

Allergic rhinitis, unspecified, J30.4	Other streptococcus as the cause of diseases classified elsewhere, B95.4
Infectious mononucleosis, unspecified without complication, B27.90	

   1. Viral vs. bacterial entity.
      a. Infectious mononucleosis.
      b. Group C or G streptococcus.
      c. Other bacteria: *Fusobacterium necrophorum*.
      d. May be important pathogen in cause of pharyngitis in adolescents and young adults.
   2. Allergic rhinitis.
G. Treatment.
   1. Nonpharmacologic.
      a. Encourage fluids: May prefer hot or cold for pain relief.
   2. Pharmacologic.
      a. Topical and oral analgesics and antipyretics.
      b. Antimicrobials: In general, 10 days of treatment is recommended duration of therapy to achieve maximal eradication of GAS in the pharynx. Penicillin V recommended:
      • Children < 27 kg: 250 mg bid or tid for 10 days.
      • Children > 27 kg: 500 mg bid or tid for 10 days.
      • IM benzathine penicillin G: If compliance, vomiting issues.
         o Children < 27 kg: 600,000 units (Bicillin C-R 900/300).
         o Children > 27 kg: 1.2 million units.(Bicillin L-A).
      • Amoxicillin: Substituted for taste issues (may benefit 40% of children with adenotonsillar disease, who yield beta-lactamase-producing bacteria, and is effective for otitis media, which is often associated with pharyngitis).
         o 50 mg/kg/day PO (max 1 gm/day) for 10 days divided bid or tid.

- PCN-allergic options:
  - ○ Clindamycin < 70 kg: 7 mg/kg/dose tid for 10 days; > 70 kg: 600 mg tid x 10 days (max 300 mg tid x 10 days).
  - ○ Clarithromycin: Child: 15 mg/kg/day (max: 250 mg/dose), divided q12h for 10 days.
  - ○ Azithromycin: 12 mg/kg/day for 5 days (max 500 mg/day).
- First-generation cephalosporin such as cephalexin: Also appropriate if retreatment necessary.
- **Note:** As many as 5% of PCN-allergic people are also allergic to cephalosporins. People with type 1 allergy to PCN should not be treated with a cephalosporin.
- Due to increased treatment failure with PCN, some clinicians are using a first-generation cephalosporin in all nonallergic patients.
  - ○ Cephalexin (25–40 mg/kg/day in 2 divided doses for 10 days).
- Other cephalosporins also have indication for GAS treatment: Cefprozil, Cefpodoxime, cefdinir, cefadroxil, cefaclor, cefuroxime, loracarbef, cefixime, ceftibuten. Ceftriaxone must be administered for 3 consecutive days for effective treatment.
- If illness recurs shortly after treatment:
  - ○ May be retreated with same drug.
  - ○ IM penicillin if compliance an issue.
  - ○ Narrow-spectrum cephalosporin (cephalexin).
  - ○ Amoxicillin-clavulanate potassium.

H. Follow-up.
   1. Routine reculturing is not necessary.
   2. Encourage patients to call if:
       a. Unable to complete course of medication or retain medication.
       b. Siblings complain of sore throat within 2–5 days: Amoxicillin-clavulanate 90 mg/6.4 mg per kg/day. If allergic: 6 months to 12 years of age, cefdinir 7 mg/kg bid or 14 mg/kg daily; 13 years, 300 mg bid 10 days.
       c. No improvement in patient in 48 hours, reevaluate for other causes, complications.
       d. Signs and symptoms of renal complications.
       e. Drug reaction.
   3. Possible assessment of carrier state, which is common, and patients are low risk to transmit and develop invasive disease. Most common scenario is a carrier who is experiencing repeated intercurrent episodes of viral

pharyngitis. (In true GAS, pharyngitis response to antimicrobial therapy is rapid.) Treatment of carriers is indicated only in very specific cases such as those involving rheumatic fever or glomerulonephritis outbreaks or recurrent, symptomatic GAS pharyngitis in a family after appropriate therapy. Ten-day course of either:
  a. Clindamycin.
  b. Amoxicillin/clavulanate.
  c. ENT referral for possible tonsillectomy.
    • Multiple bouts of GAS (6 episodes in 1 year or 3–4 in 2 consecutive years) despite adequate treatment.
    • Significant upper airway obstruction.
    • Peritonsillar abscess.

I. Complications.

Acute lymphadenitis, unspecified, L04.9	Mastoiditis, unspecified, H70.9
Acute nephritic syndrome with diffuse mesangial proliferative glomerulonephritis, N00.3	Peritonsillar abscess, J36
Acute rheumatic heart disease, unspecified, I01.9	Streptococcal pharyngitis, 02.0

  1. Streptococcal pharyngitis.
    a. Suppurative.
      • Peritonsillar abscess.
      • Cervical lymphadenitis.
      • Mastoiditis.
    b. Acute rheumatic fever.
    c. Poststrep glomerulonephritis.
      • Children under 7 years most at risk.
      • Role of antibiotics for prevention uncertain.
    d. Pediatric autoimmune neuropsychiatric disorder associated with group A streptococci (PANDAS).
      • Symptoms include sudden onset of OCD and ADHD behaviors, tics, or rapid worsening of existing behaviors and evidence of recent or active streptococcal infection.

J. Education.
  1. Transmission is person to person via respiratory tract secretions.
  2. Medication compliance is essential.
  3. May return to school/daycare 24 hours after beginning antibiotic therapy.

IX. RHINOSINUSITIS

Acute upper respiratory infection, unspecified, J06.9	Glossodynia, K14.6
	Halitosis, R19.6
Allergic rhinitis, unspecified, J30.4	Headache, R51
Ataxia, unspecified, R27.0	Otalgia, H92.0
Chronic frontal sinusitis, J32.1	Other and unspecified speech disturbances, R47.8
Chronic rhinitis, J31.0	
Chronic sinusitis, unspecified, J32.9	Other combined immunodeficiencies, D81.89
Cough, R05	Other fatigue, R53.83
Cystic fibrosis, E84	Other specified disorders of nose and nasal sinuses, J34.8
Dyspnea, unspecified, R06.00	
Exophthalmic conditions, H05.2	Toxic effect of smoke, accidental (unintentional), initial encounter, T59.811A
Gastroesophageal reflux disease without esophagitis, K21.9	

A. Etiology.
   1. Each case of viral rhinitis is also rhinosinusitis because mucous membranes of nasal passages, sinus cavities are identical.
   2. Sinusitis is inflammation of mucous membranes lining, paranasal sinuses, commonly used to describe bacterial rhinosinusitis.
   3. Factors that increase risk of sinusitis are:
      a. Smoke exposure.
      b. Cold and dry inspired air.
      c. Preceding or concurrent URI.
      d. Allergic rhinitis.
      e. Swimming.
      f. Gastroesophageal reflux.
      g. Cystic fibrosis.
      h. Immunodeficiency.
      i. Ciliary dyskinesia.
      j. Factors associated with nasal obstruction.
      k. Daycare attendance.
   4. Stagnation of secretions occurs within sinus cavities, becoming culture medium for bacteria.
   5. Common pathogens.
      a. Streptococcus pneumoniae.
      b. *Haemophilus influenzae.*
      c. Moraxella catarrhalis.

B. Occurrence.
1. Complication of 5–10% of viral upper respiratory illnesses in children.
2. In young children, occurs primarily in maxillary sinuses, ethmoids secondly.
3. Frontal sinusitis is rare prior to age 10 years.
C. Clinical manifestations.
1. Acute bacterial sinusitis.
   a. A child or adolescent has a URI and presents with:
      • Persistent illness that includes any quality or color of nasal discharge or daytime cough or both lasting > 10 days without improving.
      • Worsening course (worsening or new onset of nasal discharge, daytime cough, or after initially improving development of fever).
      • Severe onset: Fever of 102.2°F (39°C) or higher with purulent nasal discharge for 3 consecutive days or longer.
D. Physical findings.
1. Nasal discharge of any quality.
2. Erythema and edema of the turbinates are nonspecific findings.
3. Percussion of the sinuses is not useful.
4. Transillumination in children is very difficult and unreliable.
   a. History of symptoms is much more important than physical exam as bad breath, fatigue, headache, and decreased appetite are not specific indicators of sinusitis.
   b. Assessment of nasal discharge is important, primarily in a temporal context (i.e., purulent nasal discharge is significant initially and with fever, and if it persists for at least 3 days).
   c. Most physical findings without history of symptoms cannot be distinguished from those of a viral URI.
E. Diagnostic tests.
1. X-rays: Findings on plain radiographs correlate poorly with disease and should not be used.
2. CT scan with contrast or MRI of paranasal sinuses when suspicion of orbital or central nervous system complications.
F. Differential diagnosis.

Acute upper respiratory infection, unspecified, J06.9	Deviated nasal septum, J34.2
Allergic rhinitis, unspecified, J30.4	Foreign body in nostril, T17.1
Choanal atresia, Q30.0	Hypertrophy of adenoids, J35.2

      1. Viral URI.
      2. Allergic rhinitis.
      3. Drug induced (rhinitis medicamentosa).
      4. Tumors: Polyps, neoplasms, adenoidal hypertrophy.
      5. Foreign body.
      6. Septal deviation, choanal atresia.

G. Treatment.

    1. Indication:

      a. Antibiotic therapy initiated for acute bacterial rhinosinusitis (ABRS) with severe onset or worsening course.

      b. Option of 3-day observation of children with persistent illness (nasal discharge of any quality, daytime cough that may be worse at night or both, persisting for > 10 days without improvement).

    2. ABRS in children.

      a. Children aged 2 years or older with uncomplicated ABRS that is mild to moderate, who do not attend daycare, and who have not been treated with an antimicrobial agent in the last 4 weeks and in communities with a high (or unknown) prevalence of nonsusceptible *S. pneumoniae*:

        • Amoxicillin 80–90 mg/kg/day, divided BID, max 2 gm/dose.

      b. Children with moderate to severe illness or who are under 2 years of age, attending child care, or have been recently treated with an antimicrobial agent in the past 4 weeks:

        • Amoxicillin-clavulanate 80–90 mg/kg/day of amoxicillin component in 2 divided doses, max 2 gm/dose.

      c. Allergy to PCN:

        • Cefdinir, cefuroxime, cefpodoxime.

        • Ceftriaxone 50 mg/kg x 1 IM dose may be used for vomiting patients, observing for response and following with PO course of therapy.

        • Serious allergic reaction to second- and third-generation cephalosporins with history of nonsevere PCN allergy is now thought to be negligible.

        • Microbial resistance precludes current use of sulfamethoxazole-trimethoprim or azithromycin for the treatment of ABRS.

      d. Length of treatment:

        • At least 10 days.

        • Some recommendations for therapy to be continued for 7 days after resolution of symptoms.

e. If no response or worsening of symptoms within 72 hours of beginning treatment, change antibiotic or initiate antibiotic if initially observing for 3 days.

3. Normal saline nasal irrigation or lavage assists drainage and ventilation.
4. Topical nasal steroids: May decrease swelling of turbinates and aid ostia to drain.
5. Mucolytics: May help mucous clearance.
6. Antihistamines: Nonsedating helpful if allergic component.
7. Decongestants: Controversial benefit.
8. Humidified air.
9. Encourage fluids.
10. Ensure yearly influenza vaccination.
11. Administration of pneumococcal vaccine on appropriate schedule and update as newer vaccines with additional strains are developed.
12. Treat reflux if present.

H. Follow-up.
1. Patient to call if no response to medications in 72 hours, sooner if worsens.
2. Recheck in 2 weeks.
3. Referral to ENT or allergist if indicated or refractory.

I. Complications.

Asthma with (acute) exacerbation, unspecified, J45.901	Intracranial and intraspinal phlebitis and thrombophlebitis, G08
Cellulitis of unspecified orbit, H05.019	
Extradural and subdural abscess, unspecified, G06.2	Optic neuritis, unspecified, H46.9
Intracranial abscess and granuloma, G06.0	Osteomyelitis of vertebra, site unspecified, M46.20

1. Periorbital and intraorbital inflammation and infection.
2. Intracranial complications such as cavernous sinus thrombosis, subdural empyema, brain abscess (most common in previously healthy male adolescents subsequent to frontal sinusitis).
3. Exacerbation of asthma.
4. Optic neuritis.
5. Osteomyelitis of maxilla or frontal bone.

J. Education.
1. Prevention: Avoid allergens and treat allergies when appropriate.
2. Encourage humidified air at home unless it exacerbates mildew, mold allergies.

3. Emphasize that most rhinitis and sinusitis are viral in etiology, and antibiotics are not indicated.
4. Encourage compliance with prescribed antimicrobial agents.
5. Advise patient against diving (including scuba).

BIBLIOGRAPHY

American Academy of Pediatrics, Subcommittee on Management of Sinusitis and Committee on Quality Improvement. Clinical practice guideline: management of sinusitis. *Pediatrics*. 2001;108(3):798-808.

Centers for Disease Control and Prevention. Infant deaths associated with cough and cold medications—two states, 2005. *MMWR Morb Mortal Wkly Rep*. 2007;56(1):1-4.

Centers for Disease Control and Prevention. Epstein-Barr virus and infectious mononucleosis. http://www.cdc.gov/epstein-barr/index.html. Updated January 7, 2014. Accessed April 14, 2015.

Centor RM. Expand the pharyngitis paradigm for adolescents and young adults. *Ann Intern Med*. 2009;151(11):812-815.

Chervinsky P, Philip G, Malice MP, et al. Montelukast for treating fall allergic rhinitis: effect of pollen exposure in 3 studies. *Ann Allergy Asthma Immunol*. 2004;92(3):367-373.

Choby BA. Diagnosis and treatment of streptococcal pharyngitis. *Am Fam Physician*. 2009;79(5):383-390.

Chow AW, Benninger MS, Brook I, et al. IDSA clinical practice guideline for acute bacterial rhinosinusitis in children and adults. *Clin Infect Dis*. 2012;54(8):e72-e112.

Cutler DL, Banfield C, Affrime MB. Safety of mometasone furoate nasal spray in children with allergic rhinitis as young as 2 years of age: a randomized controlled trial. *Pediatr Asthma Allergy Immunol*. 2006;19(3):146-153.

Dulin MF, Kennard TP, Leach L, Williams R. Management of cervical lymphadenitis in children. *Am Fam Physician*. 2008;78(9):1097-1098.

Feder HM Jr. Periodic fever, aphthous stomatitis, pharyngitis, adenitis: a clinical review of a new syndrome. *Curr Opin Pediatr*. 2000;12(3):253-236.

Florin TA, Zaoutis TE, Zaoutis LB. Beyond cat scratch disease: widening spectrum of Bartonella henslae infection. *Pediatrics*. 2008;121(5):e1413-e1425.

Heim SW, Maughan KL. Foreign bodies in the ear, nose, and throat. *Am Fam Physician*. 2007;76(8):1185-1189.

Klotz SA, Ianas V, Elliott SP. Cat scratch disease. *Am Fam Physician*. 2011;83(2):152-155.

Kucik CJ, Clenney T. Management of epistaxis. *Am Fam Physician*. 2005;71(2):305-311.

Leung AK, Robson WL. Childhood cervical lymphadenopathy. *J Pediatr Health Care*. 2004;18(2):3-7.

McBride DR. Management of aphthous ulcers. *Am Fam Physician*. 2000;62(1):149-154, 160.

Milgrom H, Biondi R, Georgitis JW, et al. Comparison of ipratropium bromide 0.03% with beclamethasone dipropriate in the treatment of perennial rhinitis in children. *Ann Allergy Asthma Immunol*. 1999;83(2):105-111.

Mullins RJ, Heddle R. Adverse reactions associated with echinacea: the Australian experience. *Ann Allergy Asthma Immunol*. 2002;88(1):42-51.

Pickering LK, Kimberlin DW, Long SS. *Red Book: 2012 Report of the Committee on Infectious Diseases*. 29th ed. Elk Grove Village, IL: American Academy of Pediatrics; 2012.

Shulman ST, Bisno AL, Clegg HW, et al. Clinical practice guideline for the diagnosis and management of group A streptococcal pharyngitis: 2012 update by the Infectious Diseases Society of America. *Clin Infect Dis*. 2012;55(10):1279-1282.

Wald ER, Applegate KE, Bordley C, et al. Clinical practice guideline for the diagnosis and management of acute bacterial sinusitis in children aged 1 to 18 years. *Pediatrics*. 2013;132(1):e262-e280.

Welch M. *Guide to your child's allergies and asthma*. Elk Grove Village, IL: American Academy of Pediatrics; 2010.

Respiratory Disorders

Nancy Valentine

I. CROUP

Acquired deformity of chest and rib, M95.4

Acute laryngotracheitis, J04.2

Acute obstructive laryngitis [croup], J05.0

Acute pharyngitis, J02

Bronchitis, not specified as acute or chronic, J40

Bronchopneumonia, unspecified organism, J18.0

Cough, R05

Cyanosis, R23.0

Dyspnea, unspecified, R06.00

Edema of larynx, J38.4

Erythematous condition, unspecified, L53.9

Fever of other and unknown origin, R50

Generalized anxiety disorder, F41.1

Irritability and anger, R45.4

Laryngeal spasm, J38.5

Other diseases of pharynx, J39.2

Other fatigue, R53.83

Other specified disorders of nose and nasal sinuses, J34.8

Other specified respiratory disorders, J98.8

Other voice and resonance disorders, R49.8

Somnolence, R40.0

Stridor, R06.1

Stupor, R40.1

Tachycardia, unspecified, R00.0

Tachypnea, not elsewhere classified, R06.82

Wheezing, R06.2

A. Etiology.
   1. Acute upper airway obstruction in children, most often caused by viral infection.
      a. Most common form of viral croup is laryngotracheitis resulting from inflammation and edema of larynx, subglottic area.
         • The most common viral etiology is due to parainfluenza, enterovirus, and rhinovirus; influenza A and B, RSV, and measles are less common etiologies.

    b. Spasmodic croup is similar to viral croup but is not associated with fever and symptoms; lasts only hours, not days.
- Onset typically occurs during night in a child who has been well.
- May represent allergic reaction to viral antigen.

    c. Laryngotracheobronchitis (LTB) and laryngotracheobronchopneumonia (LTBP) involve upper airway; also affect lower airway, specifically bronchi.
- Same viral agents are common to LTB and LTBP.
- Bacterial superinfection occurs more commonly in this croup variant; includes *Staphylococcus aureus, Streptococcus pyogenes, Streptococcus pneumoniae, Haemophilus influenzae, Corynebacterium diphtheria.*
  - Agents are infrequent causes but tend to cause more severe illness.

B. Occurrence.
1. Viral croup occurs at 6 months to 5 years of age, with peak in second year of life.
2. Affects boys more than girls.
3. Occurs in late fall, early winter; correlates with the activity of viral agents causing the syndrome.
4. Symptoms typically last 3–7 days.

C. Clinical manifestations.
1. Gradual onset with rhinorrhea, sore throat, mild fever.
2. Disease has wide spectrum, from very mild illness to severe illness.
3. Harsh, "seal-like" barking cough.
4. Hoarseness.
5. Inspiratory stridor.
6. Increasing obstruction.
    a. Tachycardia, tachypnea—usually not > 50 breaths/min.
    b. Suprasternal, supraclavicular, substernal, and intercostal retractions.
    c. Paradoxical abdominal and chest wall movement.
    d. Progressive restlessness and anxiety correlates with hypoxemia.

D. Physical findings.
1. Normal or mildly elevated temperature.
2. Mild erythema and edema of nasal mucosa.
3. Inspiratory stridor.
4. Hoarseness.
5. Harsh, barky cough.

6. Nontoxic appearing.
7. On auscultation, normal breath sounds except transmission of stridor.
8. With increased obstruction: Wheezing, prolonged expiration, decreased breath sounds.

E. Diagnostic tests.
  1. Diagnosis made on basis of history and clinical presentation.
  2. Imaging is not usually necessary in the ambulatory setting; posteroanterior neck X-ray.
     a. Classic "steeple sign": Narrowed air column consistent with narrowing of subglottic space seen in an anteroposterior (AP) film.
     b. Lateral view is useful in ruling out epiglottitis, retropharyngeal abscess, or radiopaque foreign body.
  3. A complete blood count (CBC) is usually nonspecific but may suggest viral lymphocytosis.
  4. Clinical croup score can classify severity of illness and aid in decision making regarding hospitalization.

F. Differential diagnosis.

Acute epiglottitis without obstruction, J05.10	Peritonsillar abscess, J36
Diphtheria, unspecified, A36.9	Retropharyngeal and parapharyngeal abscess, J39.0
Foreign body in larynx, T17.3	

  1. Epiglottitis: Toxic appearing, drooling, high fever, acute onset, age range typically 3–7 years.
  2. Laryngeal foreign body: History, age (usually 6 months to 2 years), abrupt onset, lack of preceding respiratory symptoms.
  3. Retropharyngeal or peritonsillar abscess: Severe throat pain, refusal to swallow or speak, fever to 105°F (40.6°C).
  4. Bacterial tracheitis: Affects children of any age, acute onset with respiratory stridor, high fever, and copious and purulent secretions. This is a rare but life-threatening upper airway disease.
  5. Diphtheria: Characteristic thin, gray membrane (pseudomembrane) that extends from tonsil to associated soft/hard palate. Caused by toxin produced from the bacteria.

G. Treatment.
  1. Most children have mild airway obstruction that resolves without specific treatment.

    2. Supportive care at home includes making the child comfortable, avoiding fatigue and anxiety; encourage fluids and antipyretics for fever.

    3. Cool mist vaporizer may be used.

    4. Nebulized epinephrine has been beneficial for children with more severe croup in the emergency department or hospital setting.

    5. Corticosteroids.

       a. Systemic or nebulized corticosteroids are mainstay of both outpatient and inpatient treatment.

       b. Decrease edema of laryngeal mucosa.

       c. Single dose 0.6 mg/kg dexamethasone given orally or IM or 2 mg dose of nebulized budesonide.

       d. Clinical improvement in 6–12 hours.

       e. Efficacy did not vary according to route of administration.

       f. Facilitates clinical improvement, decreases hospitalizations, and fewer follow-up visits.

    6. Nebulized racemic epinephrine may be used for patients in moderate to severe distress.

    7. Criteria for hospitalization:

       a. Signs of moderate to severe airway obstruction.

       b. Increased work of breathing and respiratory distress.

       c. Hypoxemia.

       d. Restlessness, anxiety, or fatigue.

       e. Change in level of consciousness.

       f. Dehydration.

H. Follow-up.

    1. Call healthcare provider immediately if signs of respiratory distress increase.

    2. Increased respiratory rate.

    3. Stridor at rest.

    4. Increased retractions.

    5. Change in level of consciousness, restlessness, or anxiety.

    6. Cyanosis.

I. Complications.

    1. Acute deterioration in respiratory status requires hospitalization/intubation.

J. Education.

    1. Croup usually lasts 3–7 days; typically worse at night.

    2. Give guidelines about oral intake (fluids) and urine output.

3. Use of bathroom mist, cool night air, cool-mist vaporizer to relieve symptoms.
4. Signs of increasing respiratory distress and hypoxemia.
5. Good handwashing; containment of coughs/sneezes prevents spread of illness.
6. Maintain calm, reassuring manner. Avoid situations that provoke stress or crying, which can worsen respiratory distress.
7. Children may have repeated episodes of croup.
8. Antibiotics are not indicated for viral croup.
9. Avoid secondhand smoke exposure.

II. BRONCHIOLITIS

Acute bronchiolitis due to other specified organisms, J21.8	Other specified disorders of nose and nasal sinuses, J34.8
Acute upper respiratory infection, unspecified, J06.9	Primary sleep apnea of newborn, P28.3
Anorexia, R63.0	Pulmonary collapse, J98.1
Cough, R05	Respiratory syncytial virus as the cause of diseases classified elsewhere, B97.4
Dyspnea, unspecified, R06.00	Tachypnea, not elsewhere classified, R06.82
Feeding difficulties, R63.3	
Fever of other and unknown origin, R50	Vomiting, unspecified, R11.10
Other fatigue, R53.83	Wheezing, R06.2

A. Etiology.
1. Bronchiolitis is a common viral illness characterized by edema, inflammation, increased mucus production, and necrosis of the epithelial cells lining the small airways.
   a. Respiratory syncytial virus (RSV), bronchiolitis is most common cause of acute lower respiratory infection (LRI) in first 2 years of life.
   b. Bronchiolitis is also caused by parainfluenza 1 and 3, adenovirus, rhinoviruses, influenza, and human metapneumovirus.
2. Transmission.
   a. Highly contagious.
      • Virus shed in 3–8 days and up to 30 days with underlying disease.

- Virus spreads by large droplet aerosols generated by coughing, sneezing.
- Transmitted by direct contact with nasopharyngeal secretions from infected person.
  - Virus survives on skin approximately 20 minutes.
  - Virus survives on gowns/tissues approximately 30–60 minutes.
  - Virus survives on hard, nonporous surfaces approximately 6 hours.
- High-risk factors for more severe disease: Prematurity, chronic lung disease, congenital heart disease, immunosuppression.
  b. Reinfection occurs throughout life.

B. Occurrence.
1. Seasonal prevalence.
   a. Yearly epidemics in early winter/spring.
   b. In temperate climates, typically start in November and persist through April.
   c. Strains A and B circulated concurrently during outbreaks; strain A more dominant.
   d. By age 2, 90% of children have been infected with RSV.
   e. Bronchiolitis is the most common cause of hospitalization of infants in the first year of life.
   f. Adolescents, adults with RSV have symptoms of upper respiratory tract infection and cough.

C. Clinical manifestations.
1. Initial presentation.
   a. Mild upper respiratory infection (URI) with rhinorrhea and nasal congestion.
   b. Low-grade fever for 2–3 days.
   c. Poor appetite.
   d. Hoarse cough progresses to deep, wet cough.
   - Often paroxysmal.
   - Often associated with post-tussive vomiting.
   - Associated with wheezing.
2. Clinical progression.
   a. LRT involvement evident by:
   - Tachypnea: 60–80 breaths/minute.
   - Increased respiratory effort: Grunting, nasal flaring, and retractions.
   - Coughing, wheezing.

      b. Neonatal presentation:
- Lethargy, irritability.
- Poor feeding.
- URI symptoms.
- Apnea: Occurrence is inversely proportional to age.

D. Physical findings.
1. Increased work of breathing.
    a. Nasal congestion with thick purulent secretions.
    b. Respirations rapid, shallow with accessory muscle use, retractions.
    c. Nasal flaring, grunting, head bobbing.
    d. Paroxysmal cough, wheezing, crackles.
    e. Prolonged expiratory phase, chest hyperexpansion and hyperresonance.
    f. Liver and spleen may be palpable secondary to chest hyperexpansion.
    g. Hypoxemia correlates with severity of tachypnea.
    h. Paradoxical abdominal and chest wall movement.

E. Diagnostic tests.
1. Diagnosis often made on basis of clinical presentation, physical findings, epidemiology.
    a. Definitive diagnosis may not be necessary in infants with mild disease.
    b. If diagnosed clinically on the basis of history and physical exam, X-ray and lab studies should not be done routinely.
2. Chest X-ray (CXR).
    a. Hyperinflation may be only abnormality: Flattened diaphragms, increased lucency.
    b. Peribronchial thickening and increased interstitial markings.
    c. Subsegmental consolidation in upper and middle lobes: Patchy atelectasis or consolidation due to atelectasis.
3. Oximetry: To determine oxygenation status.
4. Laboratory tests.
    a. Reverse transcriptase-polymerase chain reaction (RT-PCR) assays are often more sensitive than virus isolation or antigen detection methods.
- Specimen obtained by nasal swab.
- Serologic tests are not used for routine diagnosis.

F. Differential diagnosis.

Acute upper respiratory infection, unspecified, J06.9	Foreign body in other parts of respiratory tract causing other injury, unspecified, initial encounter, T17.808A
Allergic rhinitis, unspecified, J30.4	
Asthma, J45	
Bacterial pneumonia, unspecified J15.9	Heart failure, unspecified, I50.9
	Immunodeficiency, unspecified, D84.9
Chlamydial infection, unspecified, A74.9	
Congenital malformation of heart, unspecified, Q24.9	Pneumonia due to mycoplasma pneumonia, J15.7
	Sleep apnea, unspecified, G47.30
Cough, R05	Tachypnea, not elsewhere classified, R06.82
Dyspnea, unspecified, R06.00	
Enlarged lymph nodes, unspecified, R59.9	Viral pneumonia, not otherwise classified, J12
Fever of other and unknown origin, R50	Whooping cough, unspecified species without pneumonia, A37.90

1. Apnea is often a presenting sign in young infants.
2. Pneumonia: Viral URI symptoms and coryza with low-grade fever; bacterial pneumonia; abrupt onset with high fever; *Mycobacterium pneumoniae* (insidious onset and nontoxic appearance).
3. Asthma: Pattern of symptoms, absence of fever, inspiratory wheezing, prolonged expiratory phase.
4. Foreign body aspiration: Typically in toddler; may be detected on X-ray or by bronchoscopy.
5. Aspiration: Swallowing study to determine silent or free aspiration.
6. Chlamydial infection: Manifests from 3 to 19 weeks of age, afebrile, repetitive, staccato cough with tachypnea; wheezing is rare; cervical lymphadenopathy.
7. Immunodeficiency: Systemic illness following vaccination with live virus; severe, life-threatening illness with viral infection.
8. Congenital heart disease: Accompanied by heart murmur, signs of congestive heart failure (CHF), poor feeding, poor growth.
9. GER.

G. Treatment.
   1. Treatment is supportive, maintaining adequate hydration, oxygenation; monitor closely for increasing respiratory distress.
      a. Management of nasal congestion and rhinitis.
      b. Use of antipyretics.
      c. Guidelines for feeding and urine output.
      d. Recognition of signs of increasing respiratory distress.
      e. Patients have a worsening of clinical symptoms, with peak at day 3–4 of illness.
      f. Bronchodilators are not routinely recommended.
      g. Consider a monitored trial of bronchodilator if infant has history of previous wheezing and continue only if a clinical response is documented.
   2. Criteria for hospitalization.
      a. Age (younger more likely).
      b. Tachypnea/hypoxemia.
      c. Hydration management.
H. Follow-up.
   1. Most infants improve within 4–6 days.
      a. Guidelines for parents to call healthcare provider: Increased respiratory distress, poor fluid intake, or low urine output.
      b. Close outpatient follow-up by telephone or visit may be indicated.
I. Complications.

Other disorders of lung, J98.4	Respiratory syncytial virus as the cause of diseases classified elsewhere, B97.4
Pneumothorax, J93	Wheezing, R06.2

   1. Acute complications.
      a. Respiratory failure, apnea: Rarely secondary bacterial infection.
      b. Spontaneous pneumothorax due to air trapping, airway narrowing.
      c. Worsening of chronic lung disease.
      d. Mortality 1–5%, with higher rates in high-risk groups.
   2. Long-term complications.
      a. Recurrent episodes of wheezing.
      b. Infants have airway hyperreactivity and impaired pulmonary function for up to 10 years after RSV infection.
J. Education.
   1. Hand hygiene.
   2. Avoid secondhand smoke exposure.

3. Encourage breastfeeding for the first 6 months of life.
4. Post-illness.
   a. Reinfection common; having RSV offers no immunity to subsequent infections.
   b. May have period of prolonged wheezing after infection.
   c. Recurrent wheezing is common, especially with URIs.
   d. Cough and other signs resolve gradually over 1–2 weeks.
K. Prevention.
   1. Palivizumab (Synagis) is a monocloncal antibody that is recommended by the AAP for high-risk infants during the RSV season.
      a. High-risk infants include premature infants < 29 weeks gestation and children with certain underlying medical conditions.

III. INFLUENZA

Abdominal and pelvic pain, R10	Myalgia, M79.1
Acute obstructive laryngitis [croup], J05.0	Nausea, R11.0
Acute pharyngitis, J02	Other abnormalities of breathing, R06.89
Acute upper respiratory infection, unspecified, J06.9	Other fatigue, R53.83
Anhedonia, R45.84	Other general symptoms and signs, R68.89
Conjunctivitis, unspecified, H10.9	Pulmonary collapse, J98.1
Cough, R05	Shortness of breath, R06.02
Cyanosis, R23.0	Somnolence, R40.0
Dyspnea, unspecified, R06.00	Stupor, R40.1
Fever of other and unknown origin, R50	Tachycardia, unspecified, R00.0
Generalized anxiety disorder, F41.1	Tachypnea, not elsewhere classified, R06.82
Headache, R51	
Hyperventilation, R06.4	Viral pneumonia, not otherwise classified, J12
Influenza due to unidentified influenza virus with other respiratory manifestations, J11.1	Vomiting, unspecified, R11.10
Irritability and anger, R45.4	Wheezing, R06.2

A. Etiology.
  1. Influenza is a highly contagious respiratory illness caused by influenza viruses.
     a. Influenza viruses are orthomyxoviruses.
     b. Type A and B are primary pathogens, responsible for community outbreaks.
     c. Influenza A viruses are subcategorized based on surface (H) and neuraminidase (N).
        - Subtypes include H1N1, H1N2, and H3N2.
  2. Influenza is spread by large-particle respiratory droplet.
     a. Close contact with person with influenza.
     b. Direct contact with articles contaminated with nasopharyngeal secretions.
     c. Virus is shed 1 day prior to developing symptoms.
        - Children may shed virus several days prior to developing symptoms and can remain infectious more than 10 days.
        - Immunocompromised persons may shed virus for weeks to months.
     d. Incubation period is 1–4 days, with average of 2 days after exposure.
B. Occurrence.
  1. Peak of flu season can occur from December through March.
  2. About 1% of children require hospitalization annually.
  3. Influenza can cause URI, croup, bronchiolitis, pneumonia.
C. Clinical manifestations.
  1. Abrupt onset of fever with rigors, chills.
  2. Pharyngitis.
  3. Cough.
  4. Diffuse myalgia.
  5. Extreme fatigue, headache, and generalized malaise.
  6. Gastrointestinal symptoms: Abdominal pain, nausea, vomiting.
  7. Conjunctivitis.
  8. With severe disease: Irritability, change in mental status.
  9. Symptoms progressively worsen over 12–24 hours.
  10. May present with nonspecific signs of febrile illness, limited respiratory symptoms.
  11. Symptoms typically resolve in 3–7 days.
D. Physical findings.
  1. High fever.
  2. Tachycardia, tachypnea.

   3. Nonproductive cough.
   4. If lower respiratory tract infected, physical findings consistent with pneumonia or bronchiolitis.
E. Diagnostic tests.
   1. Identification of virus or viral antigen in nasopharyngeal secretions.
      a. Specimens should be obtained within 72 hours of illness because of decrease in viral shedding after that time.
      b. Specimen obtained by swab, nasal aspirate, or wash.
      c. Viral culture.
      d. Rapid diagnostic tests via fluorescent antibody staining, enzyme-linked immunoassay, or optical immunoassay.
         • Rapid tests are more sensitive on pediatric specimens than adult specimens.
         • Some tests detect both influenza A and B; some detect only one strain.
      e. RT-PCR.
   2. Diagnosis of specific flu-related complications.
   3. CXR normal or areas of atelectasis.
F. Differential diagnosis.

Acute bronchiolitis due to other specified organisms, J21.8

Bronchitis, not specified as acute or chronic, J40

Viral pneumonia, not otherwise classified, J12

---

   1. Other lower respiratory illness (e.g., bronchiolitis, LTB, pneumonia).
G. Treatment.
   1. Encourage fluids.
   2. Antipyretics for fever (never use salicylates in children or adolescents).
   3. Monitor for complications of influenza.
   4. Antiviral therapy.
      a. Recommendations for selection of antiviral drugs are made annually: www.cdc.gov.
      b. Must be administered within 48 hours of onset of illness.
      c. Oral oseltamivir (Tamiflu) is the drug of choice for management of influenza for children over 2 weeks of age. Adverse effects: Nausea and vomiting in the first 2 days of treatment. Taking Tamiflu with food can reduce these side effects.
      d. Inhaled Zanamivir is an acceptable alternative for children but is more difficult to administer and has more side effects. Side effects include: Diarrhea, nausea, cough, stuffy nose, and headache.

Zanamivir may cause bronchospasm and is not recommended for anyone with underlying lung disease, such as asthma.

e. Confusion and abnormal behavior have been reported with both antiviral drugs and may be more common in children.

H. Follow-up.

1. Call healthcare provider immediately if signs of respiratory distress increase.
   a. Increased respiratory rate, shortness of breath.
   b. Increased retractions.
   c. Change in level of consciousness, restlessness, or anxiety.
   d. Cyanosis.
2. Close telephone follow-up for those at high risk for flu-related complications.

I. Complications.

Asthma, J45	Viral pneumonia, unspecified, J12.9
Bacterial pneumonia, unspecified, J15.9	
Diabetes mellitus, E10-E14	Volume depletion, E86

1. Viral and bacterial pneumonia.
2. Severe illness requiring hospitalization.
3. Dehydration.
4. Worsening of chronic illness, including CHF, asthma, or diabetes.
5. Death.

J. Education.

1. Certain people are at greater risk for complications, including young children, pregnant women, the elderly, and those with certain medical conditions, such as asthma and heart conditions.
2. Prevention.
   a. Yearly influenza vaccine is recommended for all people 6 months and older.
   b. Intranasal vaccine is an option for healthy children with no contraindications for the intranasal vaccine.
      • Trivalent and quadrivalent inactivated vaccines are administered IM for children > 6 months of age.
      • Children 6 months to 8 years of age require 2 doses of vaccine in the first year they received the vaccine, administered 1 month apart to produce sufficient antibody response.

   c. Influenza vaccine can be given to children with egg allergy with the following cautions: Appropriate resuscitation equipment should be available, and the child should be monitored for 30 minutes after the immunization.

   d. Good handwashing, avoidance of ill contacts during influenza outbreaks.

  3. Post-illness.

   a. Treat with antiviral agents within 48 hours after onset of symptoms to reduce duration of illness.

   b. Recognize signs of severe illness requiring medical intervention, including shortness of breath, dyspnea, cyanosis, change in level of consciousness.

   c. Encourage fluids to maintain adequate hydration and urine output.

   d. Acetaminophen for treatment of myalgia, headache, fever.

   e. Recurrent wheezing is common, especially with URIs.

   f. Avoid secondhand smoke exposure.

IV. BRONCHITIS

Acute bronchitis, J20	Mycoplasma infection, unspecified
Acute pharyngitis, J02	site, A49.3
Acute upper respiratory infection, unspecified, J06.9	Mycosis, unspecified, B49
	Other disorders of lung, J98.4
Bronchitis, not specified as acute or chronic, J40	Other specified bacterial agents as the cause of diseases classified elsewhere, B96.89
Chest pain, unspecified, R07.4	
Chronic bronchitis, unspecified, J42	Respiratory syncytial virus as the cause of diseases classified elsewhere, B97.4
Chronic rhinitis, J31.0	
Cough, R05	
Fever of other and unknown origin, R50	Vomiting, unspecified, R11.10
	Wheezing, R06.2

  A. Etiology.

   1. Acute bronchitis is produced by inflammation of the bronchioles, bronchi, and trachea.

2. Most commonly occurs after viral infection.
   a. Rhinovirus, RSV, influenza, parainfluenza, adenovirus, coxsackievirus, paramyxoviruses can be etiologic agent.
3. Most commonly occurs in children < 2 years of age with another peak seen in children ages 9–15.
4. May occur with bacterial, mycoplasmal, or fungal infection.
5. May occur as result of inflammation caused by frequent viral infection, secondhand smoke exposure, and air pollution.
6. Chronic bronchitis is poorly defined in children due to symptom overlap with asthma and reactive airway disease states.

B. Occurrence.
1. Peak months in young children are related to high RSV activity.
2. Peak incidence is in winter months.
3. Chronic/recurrent bronchitis: Cough lasting > 1 month or 4 episodes within 1 year.

C. Clinical manifestations.
1. Mild URI symptoms, including rhinitis and pharyngitis.
2. Dry hacking cough begins 3–4 days after onset of rhinitis.
3. Cough often becomes productive after a few days.
4. Older patients may complain of chest pain, worse with coughing.
5. As cough progressively worsens, the child has more signs of generalized illness.
6. Younger children may have post-tussive vomiting.
7. Normal temperature or mild elevation.

D. Physical findings.
1. Physical findings vary with phase of illness.
2. Initially clear or mucopurulent nasal secretions.
3. Auscultation initially may be normal.
4. Cough is dry, hacking in nature.
5. Normal or slightly elevated temperature.
6. Over next week, cough becomes productive as condition progresses to include lower respiratory symptoms.
   a. Coarse crackles with variable wheezing may be present.
   b. Moderate to severe productive cough, chest pain.
   c. Post-tussive vomiting, thick yellow mucopurulent sputum.
7. Elevated temperature is likely during this time.

E. Diagnostic tests.
1. Diagnosis is often diagnosis of exclusion (see *Differential Diagnosis*).
2. Assessment of general health status, including height, weight, signs of chronic pulmonary disease.
3. Elevated neutrophil count or C-reactive protein is suggestive of bacterial etiology.
4. CXR is usually normal but may show peribronchial thickening.
5. Pulmonary function testing may demonstrate airway hyperactivity characteristic of asthma.
F. Differential diagnosis.

Asthma, J45	Foreign body in other parts of
Bronchiectasis, J47	respiratory tract causing
Bronchopulmonary dysplasia	other injury, unspecified,
originating in the perinatal period,	initial encounter, T17.808A
P27.1	Gastroesophageal reflux
Chronic rhinitis, J31.0	disease without esophagitis,
Chronic sinusitis, unspecified, J32.9	K21.9
Food in other parts of respiratory	Irritability and anger, R45.4
tract causing other injury, initial	Other disorders of lung, J98.4
encounter, T17.828A	Wheezing, R06.2

1. Asthma: Pattern of symptoms, absence of fever, expiratory wheezing, prolonged expiratory phase.
2. Bronchiectasis: Recurrent pulmonary infections, anorexia, irritability, poor growth, digital clubbing, rule out other chronic pulmonary disorders.
3. Bronchopulmonary dysplasia: History of prematurity, treatment with oxygen therapy, and/or mechanical ventilation during neonatal period.
4. Immunodeficiency: Systemic illness following vaccination with live virus; severe life-threatening illness with viral infection.
5. GER: Barium swallow demonstrates reflux of barium into esophagus; esophageal pH monitoring.
6. Sinusitis: Purulent rhinitis lasting 2 weeks, facial/dental pain, headache, pressure over affected area.
7. Foreign body aspiration: Typically in toddler, unilateral physical findings, X-ray, or by bronchoscopy.

G. Treatment.
1. Treatment is supportive.
2. Cough suppressants should be avoided in children with productive cough.
3. Rest as needed.
4. Avoidance of environmental irritants.
5. Empiric trial of bronchodilator therapy and oral steroids.
6. Acetaminophen for chest pain, fever.
7. Antibiotic therapy may be considered if bacterial infection is strongly suspected (prolonged symptoms, patient's age, high fever).
8. Humidification of air promotes comfort.
9. Chest physiotherapy may be indicated if productive cough, coarse crackles on exam.

H. Follow-up.
1. If cough for 2 weeks or worsens, fever, or signs of respiratory distress: Contact healthcare provider.

I. Complications.

Acute serous otitis media, H65.0

Chronic sinusitis, unspecified, J32.9

Viral pneumonia, not otherwise classified, J12

---

1. In healthy children, bronchitis is not a serious illness.
2. In chronically ill children, may develop concurrent otitis, sinusitis, pneumonia.

J. Education.
1. Avoid large daycare settings for young children to minimize frequency of viral infection.
2. Avoid secondhand smoke exposure.
3. Bronchitis is usually caused by viral infection; antibiotics are not effective.
4. Acute bronchitis is a benign, self-limited illness usually lasting 2 weeks.
5. Should consult with healthcare providers before administering cough suppressants.
6. If child has signs of respiratory distress, contact healthcare provider.
7. If cough does not resolve within 2 weeks or worsens or fever recurs, contact healthcare provider.

V. PERTUSSIS

Acute upper respiratory infection, unspecified, J06.9	Other specified disorders of white blood cells, D72.89
Conjunctival hemorrhage, bilateral, H11.33	Primary sleep apnea of newborn, P28.3
Cough, R05	Pulmonary collapse, J98.1
Cyanosis, R23.0	Sneezing, R06.7
Epiphora, unspecified, unspecified lacrimal gland, H04.209	Spontaneous ecchymoses, R23.3
Fever of other and unknown origin, R50	Syncope and collapse, R55
Other abnormalities of breathing, R06.89	Viral pneumonia, not otherwise classified, J12
Other fatigue, R53.83	Vomiting, unspecified, R11.10
Other specified disorders of nose and nasal sinuses, J34.8	Whooping cough, unspecified species without pneumonia, A37.90

A. Etiology.
1. Pertussis: Highly contagious, vaccine-preventable bacterial infection caused by *Bordetella pertussis,* less commonly by *B. parapertussis* (Gram-negative coccobacillus).
2. Transmission: Airborne, occurs by contact with respiratory droplets of infected person or by indirect contact with contaminated surfaces.
3. Disease is endemic in United States, with all 50 states reporting cases annually.
4. Most cases in United States occur between June and October.
B. Occurrence.
1. Pertussis causes disease in every age group.
   a. Significantly impacts nonimmunized or partially immunized young children; can cause severe disease. Highest mortality in infants younger than 6 months of age.
2. Incubation period is 7–10 days, with a range of 5–21 days.
3. Persons with pertussis are considered infectious from 7 days after exposure to 3 weeks after person enters paroxysmal stage.
   a. Pertussis is most contagious from catarrhal stage until 2 weeks after onset of cough without appropriate therapy.

C. Clinical manifestations.
1. Pertussis is lengthy disease lasting 6–10 weeks, divided into 3 stages.
   a. Catarrhal stage lasts 1–2 weeks, may not be recognized in infants younger than 3 months.
      • Characterized by URI symptoms such as rhinorrhea, sneezing, mild cough, low-grade fever.
   b. The paroxysmal stage lasts 2–4 weeks or longer.
      • Characterized by paroxysmal cough/bouts of rapid cough, sudden coughing.
      • Have color change, bulging eyes, tearing, tongue protrusion.
      • May be triggered by feeding, crying, excitement, activity.
      • May have multiple episodes each hour during peak but appear well between episodes.
      • May have characteristic whoop during forceful inspiration.
      • Post-tussive vomiting, exhaustion are common following episode.
      • Infants < 6 months of age may have less typical presentation. The characteristic whoop may be absent, but apnea, choking, and gagging may occur.
   c. Convalescent stage lasts 1–2 weeks, but cough can persist for several months. During this stage, cough and post-tussive vomiting decrease.
D. Physical findings.
1. Cough.
   a. Catarrhal stage: Mild.
   b. Paroxysmal cough: Associated with cyanosis, lacrimation, exhaustion, post-tussive vomiting.
   c. Subconjunctival hemorrhages and petechiae on head and neck.
2. Breath sounds are normal, unless significant atelectasis or pneumonia.
E. Diagnostic tests.
1. Consider in cases of prolonged cough with history of post-tussive vomiting, whoop, paroxysmal cough.
2. Culture is "gold standard" for laboratory diagnosis but is used less often.
   a. Most likely to be positive during catarrhal stage to peak of paroxysmal stage.
   b. Use calcium alginate or Dacron swab of posterior nasopharynx for 15–30 seconds or by nasal wash and plate on specialized media, incubate for 7 days.
3. PCR is replacing culture as the diagnostic test of choice at many hospitals.
   a. PCR is a rapid, sensitive, and specific test for *B. pertussis* even late in the course of illness.
   b. Do not use calcium alginate swabs for PCR as it is inhibitory to PCR.

4. Serology.
   a. Enzyme immunoassay detects antibody to *B. pertussis* in acute and convalescent samples: Not helpful during acute illness and difficult to interpret in immunized persons.
5. CBC: Leukocytosis with lymphocytosis in catarrhal and early paroxysmal stages.
   a. Present in infants and young children but not in adolescents.
F. Differential diagnosis.

Acute bronchiolitis due to other specified organisms, J21.8	Chlamydial infection, unspecified, A74.9
Acute bronchiolitis due to respiratory syncytial virus, J21.0	Cytomegaloviral disease, unspecified, B25.9
Adenovirus infection, unspecified site, B34.0	Whooping cough due to *Bordetella parapertussis*, A37.1

1. Adenoviral infection: Presence of fever distinguishes from pertussis.
2. Mycoplasma infection: Causes prolonged cough, but fever, systemic symptoms, crackles on auscultation help differentiate from pertussis.
3. *B. parapertussis* infection: Less severe illness.
4. In infancy, consider chlamydia, cytomegalovirus (CMV).
G. Treatment.
   1. Most children beyond infancy can be managed at home.
   2. Macrolides are treatment of choice for infected persons and close contacts.
   3. Azithromycin, erythromycin, or clarithromycin are first-line agents for treatment and prophylaxis.
      a. Do not use erythromycin in infants < 1 month of age because of association with infantile hypertrophic pyloric stenosis (IFPS).
   4. Dosing.
      a. Less than 30 days of age:
         • Azithromycin 10 mg/kg/day as single daily dose for 5 days.
         • All infants < 30 days of age who receive macrolides should be monitored for IFPS during and for 1 month following completion of course.
      b. 1–5 months of age.
         • Azithromycin 10 mg/kg/day as single daily dose for 5 days.
         • Erythromycin 40–50 mg/kg/day in 4 divided doses for 14 days.
         • Clarithromycin 15 mg/kg/day in 2 divided doses for 7 days.

c. Infants 6 months of age or older and children.
- Azithromycin 10 mg/kg/day as single daily dose on day 1 (maximum dose 500 mg), then 5 mg/kg/day (maximum dose 250 mg) on days 2–5.
- Erythromycin 40–50 mg/kg/day in 4 divided doses for 14 days.
- Clarithromycin 15 mg/kg/day in 2 divided doses for 7 days.

d. Adults.
- Azithromycin 500 mg as single daily dose on day 1, then 250 mg on days 2–5.
- Erythromycin 2 g/day in 4 divided doses for 14 days.
- Clarithromycin 1 g/day in 2 divided doses for 7 days.

5. Alternatively use trimethoprim-sulfamethoxazole (TMP-SMX), 8–12 mg/kg/day divided every 12 hours for 14 days, if unable to take macrolides or culture resistant to macrolides.

6. Those with pertussis should be considered contagious until treatment with appropriate therapy for 5 days.

7. Treat all household and close contacts, including daycare and school, regardless of age, immunization status, symptoms. The recommended dosing and antibiotics are the same as treatment regimen.

8. In addition to chemoprophylaxis, for children younger than 7 years of age who are not immunized or partially immunized, follow schedule for accelerated vaccination.

9. Reportable disease to local and state health departments.

H. Follow-up.
1. Guidelines for parents to call healthcare provider for poor fluid intake, low urine output, change in level of consciousness, cyanosis, or respiratory distress.
2. Close outpatient follow-up by telephone to monitor and reassure family.

I. Complications.

Acute serous otitis media, H65.0	Other disorders of electrolyte and fluid balance, not elsewhere classified, E87.8
Bacterial pneumonia, unspecified, J15.9	
Conjunctival hemorrhage, bilateral, H11.33	Primary sleep apnea of newborn, P28.3
Convulsions, unspecified, R56.9	Spontaneous ecchymoses, R23.3
Encephalopathy, unspecified, G93.40	Viral pneumonia, unspecified, J12.9
Epistaxis, R04.0	

1. Infants younger than 6 months of age have highest rate of hospitalization, secondary pneumonia, and seizures.
2. Children with history of prematurity or underlying chronic heart, pulmonary, or neurologic disease are at high risk for severe disease.
3. Apnea.
4. Secondary infection causing viral or bacterial pneumonia or otitis media.
   a. Secondary bacterial pneumonia causes most pertussis-related deaths.
5. Neurologic complications include encephalopathy and seizures.
6. Sequelae of violent coughing, including conjunctival hemorrhage, central nervous system (CNS) hemorrhage, pneumothorax, epistaxis, petechiae.
7. Fluid and electrolyte imbalances.
8. Death: Infants < 1 year of age are at highest risk.

J. Education.
1. *B. pertussis* is preventable with appropriate immunizations.
2. Pertussis is very contagious and spread by direct or indirect contact with respiratory droplets.
3. Good handwashing and containment of coughs/sneezes prevent spread of illness.
4. Guidelines about adequate hydration and nutrition.
5. Children may continue to have cough for several months.
6. Provide adequate rest and avoid activity that triggers cough.
7. Need for antibiotic treatment of all household and close contacts.
8. Household and close contacts are considered contagious until completed 5 days of erythromycin therapy.
9. Need for accelerated immunization for contacts < 7 years of age partially immunized/not immunized.
10. Avoid secondhand smoke exposure.
11. Tdap booster is now recommended for all adults over the age of 19.

VI. ASTHMA

Acute bronchiolitis due to other specified organisms, J21.8

Acute upper respiratory infection, J06.9

Allergic rhinitis, unspecified, J30.4

Asthma, J45

Atopic dermatitis, L20

Chest pain, unspecified, R07.4

Conjunctivitis, unspecified, H10.9

Cough, R05

Chronic rhinitis, J31.0

Chronic sinusitis, unspecified, J32.9

Family history of asthma and other chronic lower respiratory diseases, Z82.5

Family history of diseases of the skin and subcutaneous tissue, Z84.0

Family history of other specified conditions, Z84.89

Localized swelling, mass and lump, head, R22.0

Nasal polyps, 471.9

Other fatigue, R53.83

Other seasonal allergic rhinitis, J30.2

Other specified respiratory disorders, J98.8

Otitis, 382.9

Pneumonia, unspecified organism, J18.9

Pruritus, unspecified, L29.9

Rhinorrhea, clear, J34.8

Shortness of breath, R06.02

Sleep disorder, unspecified, G47.9

Sneezing, R06.7

Wheezing, R06.2

A. Etiology.
1. Asthma is chronic inflammatory disorder of the airways due to airflow obstruction and inflammation. Many cells and cellular elements play a role in the changes in the airways.
   a. Mast cells, eosinophils, T-lymphocytes, neutrophils.
2. May have genetic predisposition (with critical interaction with environment).
3. The characteristics of asthma are:
   a. Symptoms of episodic airflow obstruction that is reversible.
   b. Airway inflammation.
   c. Increased airway responsiveness to variety of stimuli.
4. Hyperresponsiveness.
   a. Chronically inflamed airways are hyperresponsive.
   b. When exposed to "triggers," there is bronchoconstriction and airflow limitation.
   c. Inflammation contributes to airway edema and increased mucous production.
   d. Cough and wheeze are characteristic of asthma but are also common nonspecific symptoms associated with many other clinical entities.
5. Common triggers.
   a. Inhalant allergens: Animal allergens, house dust mites, cockroach allergens, molds, outdoor allergens.
   b. Irritants: Active/passive tobacco smoke exposure, indoor and outdoor air pollution, strong odors, chemical cleaning products.

    c. Viral illness.
- URI, sinusitis, rhinitis, otitis, LRI.
- Viral illness is primary trigger for asthma in young children.

    d. Weather: Rapid change in weather; hot, humid weather; or cold air.

    e. Exercise.

    f. Emotions or stress.

    g. Occupational exposures: Farm and barn exposures, formaldehydes, paint fumes, smoke, strong odors.

    h. Aspirin sensitivity (more common in adults): Includes other nonsteroidal anti-inflammatory drugs (NSAIDs).

    i. Sulfite sensitivity: In many processed foods, dried fruit, salad bars, beer, wine.

    j. Risk factors:
- Atopy: Family history or eczema.
- Gender: Preadolescent boys are at higher risk.
- Smoking: History of mother smoking perinatally.
- Respiratory viral disease.

    k. Aggravating factors: Smoking, gastroesophageal reflux (GER), sinusitis.

B. Occurrence.
1. Most common serious chronic illness among children.
2. Onset at any age from infancy to old age; 50–80% of children with asthma develop symptoms before 5 years of age.

C. Clinical manifestations.
1. Recurrent wheezing.
2. Dry, persistent cough, nocturnal cough.
3. Recurrent chest tightness or shortness of breath, chest pain.
4. Sputum production.
5. Exercise-induced cough, wheezing, shortness of breath, or chest tightness.
6. In younger children, difficulty keeping up with peers.
7. Atopic profile.
    a. Eczema.
    b. Seasonal or perennial allergy symptoms.
    c. Rhinitis, sneezing, itching and rubbing of nose, throat clearing.
    d. Conjunctivitis.
8. Fatigue secondary to sleep disturbance.
9. Poor school performance secondary to sleep disturbance.

D. Physical findings.
  1. Upper respiratory tract.
     a. Allergic shiners, "allergic salute" (characteristic crease at bridge of nose due to chronic rhinitis).
     b. Conjunctivitis.
     c. Boggy, pale nasal mucosa, mucosal swelling, clear rhinorrhea, nasal polyps, nasal flaring.
     d. Grunting.
  2. Chest exam.
     a. Normal chest examination does not rule out asthma.
     b. Bilateral wheezing, end-expiratory wheezing on forced expiration.
     c. Prolonged expiratory phase; rapid, shallow respirations.
     d. Hyperresonance to percussion.
     e. Hyperexpansion of chest, increased anterior–posterior diameter.
     f. Intercostal, suprasternal, and/or subcostal retractions.
     g. In infants, paradoxical breathing.
     h. In young children, pushing with abdominal musculature on expiration.
     i. Dry, tight-sounding cough.
E. Diagnostic tests.
  1. Detailed medical history.
     a. Family history of allergy, asthma, eczema, dermatitis.
     b. Identify symptoms consistent with asthma.
     c. Identify pattern of symptoms that occur or worsen in presence of specific triggers.
        • Consider diagnosis after 3 episodes of cough and/or wheezing, once alternative diagnoses are excluded.
  2. Focused physical examination with special attention on the upper respiratory tract, chest, and skin.
  3. Laboratory procedures.
     a. Spirometry.
        • Age limited; difficult to accurately test children younger than 5–7 years of age in most settings.
        • Pre- and postbronchodilator to validate reversibility.
          o May be normal.
          o Essential for diagnosis.
          o Test annually to establish baseline pulmonary function.
     b. Peak flow is monitoring tool, not diagnostic tool.
  4. CXR: Important in newly diagnosed asthmatic, rules out alternative diagnoses.

5. Special studies.
   a. Sinus X-rays or CT to evaluate sinusitis.
   b. pH probe or barium swallow to evaluate GER.
   c. Allergy testing.
      • Referral to board-certified allergist to administer skin tests and interpret.
      • RAST testing: Not as sensitive as skin testing, results not immediate.
      • Allergic bronchitis, wheezy bronchitis.
      • Recurrent bronchiolitis or pneumonia.
         ○ Even children with mild persistent asthma have significant airway inflammation.
         ○ Without adequate anti-inflammatory therapy, there may be airway remodeling or irreversible changes in asthma airway.
6. Asthma classification.
   a. Severity: Intrinsic to the disease process.
      • First step in initiating therapy for patient who has not been taking long-term controller medication.
   b. Control: Fluctuates over time.
   c. Impairment: Assessment component for severity and control; effect of asthma on quality of life and functional capacity.
   d. Risk: Assessment component for severity and control; refers to future impact on quality of life and functional capacity.
   e. Four categories: Intermittent, mild persistent, moderate persistent, and severe persistent. See **Figure 25-1** through **Figure 25-3** at the end of the asthma section.
      • Symptoms > 2 times per week, nighttime symptoms > 2 times a month.
      • Asymptomatic and normal peak flow between exacerbations.
      • Exacerbations brief; intensity may vary.
      • May have severe or lethal episodes.
   f. Mild persistent asthma.
      • Symptoms 2 times per week but less than daily. Nighttime symptoms 2 times a month.
      • Exacerbations may affect activity.
      • Nighttime symptoms 2 times per month.
   g. Moderate persistent asthma.
      • Daily symptoms, daily use of inhaled quick-relief bronchodilators.
      • Nighttime symptoms 1 time a week.
      • Exacerbations affect activity, occur 2 times per week; may last days.

h. Severe persistent.
- Continual symptoms; frequent exacerbations, nighttime symptoms.
- Limited physical activity.

F. Differential diagnosis.

Acute bronchiolitis due to other specified organisms, J21.8	Intestinal malabsorption, unspecified, K90.9
Bronchopulmonary dysplasia originating in the perinatal period, P27.1	Other diseases of vocal cords, J38.3
	Other disorders of lung, J98.4
Cystic fibrosis, E84	Pyothorax with fistula, J86.0
Foreign body in respiratory tract, part unspecified, T17.9	Slow fetal growth, unspecified, P05.9
Gastroesophageal reflux disease without esophagitis, K21.9	

1. Vocal cord dysfunction: Paradoxical adduction of vocal cords during inspiration (often in adolescent girls). Symptoms of distress, including inspiratory wheezing, and are out of proportion to clinical exam, including normal oxygen saturations. Diagnosis established by direct visualization of vocal cords using flexible rhinolaryngoscopy or flexible laryngoscopy.
2. Congenital pulmonary malformations: Radiologic testing, bronchoscopy to rule out abnormality.
   a. Tracheoesophageal fistula.
   b. Vascular ring, sling, or extrinsic mass.
3. Foreign body aspiration: Focal findings on auscultation; medical history key.
4. Bronchopulmonary dysplasia: History of prematurity, treatment with oxygen therapy, mechanical ventilation during neonatal period.
5. Viral bronchiolitis: Virus may be identified by antigen testing or culture; may be trigger for asthma. Asthma differentiated by pattern of symptoms over time.
6. GER: Reflux of barium into esophagus by barium swallow or esophageal pH monitoring. Can be aggravating factor in asthma control.
7. Cystic fibrosis: Genetic disease characterized by excessive production of thick, tenacious respiratory secretions, chronic pulmonary infection, malabsorption, subsequent poor growth.

G. Treatment.
   1. Goals of treatment.
      a. No coughing, shortness of breath/rapid breathing, wheezing, chest tightness.
      b. No nighttime awakenings because of asthma symptoms.
      c. Normal activities, including play, sports, exercise.
      d. No absences from school or activities or work (for parent or caregiver).
      e. Normal lung function.
   2. Key principles.
      a. Prevent airway inflammation by eliminating or avoiding triggers.
      b. Asthma can be controlled, not cured.
      c. Reverse and suppress inflammation.
   3. Nonpharmacologic therapy.
      a. Patient education.
      b. Objective measures of lung function using peak flow monitoring and follow-up spirometry.
      c. Control or avoid aggravating factors.
   4. Pharmacologic therapy.
      a. Simplify treatment plan whenever possible.
      b. Classification of severity guides choice and frequency of therapy.
      c. Persistent asthma is most effectively controlled with daily anti-inflammatory medications.
      d. National Asthma Education and Prevention guidelines support aggressive therapy to achieve rapid control of symptoms and then step down to lowest level of therapy to maintain control.
      e. Goals in treatment of acute episode are:
         • Rapid reversal of acute airway obstruction.
         • Identify causes of asthma episode.
         • Adjust chronic maintenance to prevent recurrence of asthma flare.
         • Inhaled beta 2-agonist is quick-relief medication for all levels of severity and treatment of choice for prevention of exercise-induced asthma.
         • Short "burst" of oral glucocorticoids is used to reduce inflammation during acute episode.
      f. For estimated comparative daily dosages for inhaled corticosteroids, see **Figure 25-4** at the end of the asthma section.
   5. Build child/family and healthcare provider partnership.
      a. Understand and address reasons for adherence problems in asthma.
      b. Explore patient/family misconceptions about asthma.
      c. Agree on goals and expectations of treatment.
      d. Jointly develop treatment plan.

H. Follow-up.
1. Before increasing medications, investigate reasons for poor asthma control.
    a. Improper inhaler technique.
    b. Adherence issues, knowledge deficit.
    c. Environmental exposures.
    d. Exacerbation of aggravating conditions (e.g., GER, sinusitis).
2. Many children have multiple caretakers.
    a. Each caretaker must have access to medications, appropriate devices, asthma action plan.
    b. Provide information to all caregivers, including daycare providers, teachers, coaches, school nurses.
    c. Ensure reliable, immediate access to medications in all settings, including school.
3. Regular use of quick-relief medicine indicates deterioration in control of asthma and need to assess maintenance therapy.
4. Regular follow-up visits are encouraged to achieve and maintain control with appropriate intensity of therapy.
5. Monitor child for side effects of medications.
6. Refer to asthma specialist for difficult-to-control asthma (See **Figure 25-1** through **Figure 25-3** and **Figure 25-5** through **Figure 25-10**).
    a. For children younger than 5 years of age: Consider referral at step 2; refer at steps 3 and 4.
    b. For children older than 5 years of age: Consider referral at step 3; refer at step 4.
7. Peak-flow monitoring to establish personal best: More specific than predicted value.
8. At each encounter, reassess concerns and correct misconceptions.
9. Monitor quality of life on regular basis.
10. Recognize and address barriers to asthma self-management.
11. Assess source of social support for child and family.
12. Assess child and family satisfaction with asthma care.
13. Yearly influenza vaccine for child and household contacts.
I. Complications.

Pneumothorax, J93

Viral pneumonia, not otherwise classified, J12

1. Pneumothorax, pneumonia.
2. Acute exacerbation requiring hospitalization, intubation, mechanical ventilation.
3. Death.

J. Education.

1. Asthma education should begin at diagnosis and continue at every encounter: Include child as developmentally appropriate and all caregivers.
2. Key components.
   a. Basic asthma facts to enable child and family to understand rationale for treatment decisions and asthma self-management.
   b. Roles of medications in treating acute symptoms and achieving/maintaining asthma control.
   c. Environmental avoidance and control measures.
   d. Teach relevant skills: How to use devices such as spacers, other medication-delivery devices, peak-flow meter; have child demonstrate relevant skills at each encounter.
   e. Provide asthma action plan: Daily maintenance therapy, including avoidance of triggers, plan for recognizing and treating worsening asthma, and when to seek medical attention.
3. Establish goals of therapy jointly and monitor child and family's perception of progress toward reaching goals.

Figure 25-1 Classifying asthma severity and initiating treatment in children 0–4 years of age.

Assessing severity and initiating therapy in children who are not currently taking long-term control medication

Components of Severity		Classification of Asthma Severity (0–4 years of age)			
		Intermittent	Persistent		
			Mild	Moderate	Severe
Impairment	Symptoms	≤ 2 days/week	> 2 days/week but not daily	Daily	Throughout the day
	Nighttime awakenings	0	1–2x/month	3–4x/month	> 1x/week
	Short-acting beta₂-agonist use for symptom control (not prevention ot EIB)	≤ 2 days/week	> 2 days/week but not daily	Daily	Several times per day
	Interference with normal activity	None	Minor limitation	Some limitation	Extremely limited
Risk	Exacerbations requiring oral systemic corticosteroids	0–1/year	≥ 2 exacerbations in 6 months requiring oral systemic corticosteroids, or ≥ 4 wheezing episodes/1 year lasting > 1 day AND risk factors for persistent asthma		
		Consider severity and interval since last exacerbation. ◄——— Frequency and severity may fluctuate over time. ———► Exacerbations of any severity may occur in patients in any severity category.			
Recommended Step for Initiating Therapy		Step 1	Step 2	Step 3 and consider short course of oral systemic corticosteriods	
		In 2–6 weeks, depending on severity, evaluate level of asthma control that is achieved. If no clear benefit is observed in 4–6 weeks, consider adjusting therapy or alternative diagnosis.			

Key: EIB, exercise-included bronchospasm.

Notes:

- The stepwise approach is meant to assist, not replace, the clinical decision making required to meet individual patient needs.

- Level of severity is determined by both impaiment and risk. Assess impairment domain by patient's/caregiver's recall of previous 2–4 weeks. Symptom assessment for longer periods should reflect a global assessment such as inquiring whether the patient's asthma is better or worse since the visit. Assign severity to most severe category in which any feature occurs.

- At present, there are inadequate data to correspond frequencies of exacerbations with different levels of asthma severity. For treatment purposes, patients who had ≥ 2 exacerbations requiring oral systemic corticosteroids in the past 6 months, or ≥ 4 wheezing episodes in the past year, and who have risk factors for persistent asthma may be considered the same as patients who have persistent asthma, even in the absence of impairment levels consistent with persistent asthma.

Source: National Institutes of Health, National Heart, Lung, and Blood Institute. *Expert Panel Report 3: Guidelines for the Diagnosis and Management of Asthma*. Bethesda, MD: National Heart, Lung, and Blood Institute; 2007.

Figure 25-2 Classifying asthma severity and initiating treatment in children 5–11 years of age.

Assessing severity and initiating therapy in children who are not currently taking long-term control medication

Components of Severity		Classification of Asthma Severity (5–11 years of age)			
		Intermittent	Persistent		
			Mild	Moderate	Severe
Impairment	Symptoms	≤ 2 days/week	> 2 days/week but not daily	Daily	Throughout the day
	Nighttime awakenings	≤ 2x/month	3–4x/month	> 1x/week but not nightly	Often 7x/week
	Short-acting beta₂-agonist use for symptom control (not prevention ot EIB)	≤ 2 days/week	> 2 days/week but not daily	Daily	Several times per day
	Lung function	• Normal FEV₁ between exacerbations • FEV₁ > 80% predicted • FEV₁/FVC > 85%	• FEV₁ = > 80% predicted • FEV₁/FVC > 80%	• FEV₁ = 60–80% predicted • FEV₁/FVC = 75–80%	• FEV₁ < 60% predicted • FEV₁/FVC < 75%
Risk	Exacerbations requiring oral systemic corticosteroids	0–1/year (see note)	≥ 2/year (see note) ⟶		
		Consider severity and interval since last exacerbation. Frequency and severity may fluctuate over time for patients in any category. Relative annual risk of exacerbations may be FEV₁.			
Recommended Step for Initiating Therapy		Step 1	Step 2	Step 3, medium dose ICS option	Step 3, medium dose ICS option, or step 4 and consider short course of oral systemic corticosteroids
		In 2–6 weeks, evaluate level of asthma control that is achieved and adjust therapy accordingly.			

Key: EIB, exercise-included bronchospasm; FEV₁, forced expiratory volume in 1 second; FVC, forced vital capacity; ICS, inhaled corticosteroids.

Notes:

- The stepwise approach is meant to assist, not replace, the clinical decision making required to meet individual patient needs.

- Level of severity is determined by both impairment and risk. Assess impairment domain by patient's/caregiver's recall of previous 2–4 weeks and spirometry. Assign severity to the most severe category in which any feature occurs.

- At present, there are inadequate data to correspond frequencies of exacerbations with different levels of asthma severity. In general, more frequent and intense exacerbations (i.e., requiring urgent, unscheduled care, hospitalization, or ICU admission) indicate greater underlying disease severity. For treatment purposes, patients who had ≥ 2 exacerbations requiring oral systemic corticosteroids in the past year may be considered the same as patients who have persistent asthma, even in the absence of impairment levels consistent with persistent asthma.

Source: National Institutes of Health, National Heart, Lung, and Blood Institute. *Expert Panel Report 3: Guidelines for the Diagnosis and Management of Asthma.* Bethesda, MD: National Heart, Lung, and Blood Institute; 2007.

Figure 25-3 Classifying asthma severity and initiating treatment in youths ≥ 12 years of age and adults.

Assessing severity and initiating treatment for patients who are not currently taking long-term control medications

Components of Severity		Classification of Asthma Severity ≥ 12 years of age			
		Intermittent	Persistent		
			Mild	Moderate	Severe
Impairment Normal FEV₁/FVC: 8-19 yr 85% 20-39yr 80% 40-59yr 75% 60-80yr 70%	Symptoms	≤ 2 days/week	> 2 days/week but not daily	Daily	Throughout the day
	Nighttime awakenings	≤ 2x/month	3-4x/month	> 1x/week but not nightly	often 7x/week
	Short-acting beta₂-agonist use for symptom control (not prevention ot EIB)	≤ 2 days/week	> 2 days/week but not daily, and not more than 1x on any day	Daily	Several times per day
	Interference with normal activity	None	Minor limitation	Some limitation	Extremely limited
	Lung function	• Normal FEV₁ between exacerbations • FEV₁ > 80% predicted • FEV₁/FVC normal	• FEV₁ = > 80% predicted • FEV₁/FVC > 80%	• FEV₁ > 60% but <80% predicted • FEV₁/FVC reduced 5%	• FEV₁ < 60% predicted • FEV₁/FVC reduced > 5%
Risk	Exacerbations requiring oral systemic corticosteroids	0-1/year (see note)	≥ 2/year (see note) ⟶ ◀── Consider severity and interval since last exacerbation. ──▶ Frequency and severity may fluctuate over time for patients in any severity category. Relative annual risk of exacerbations may be related to FEV₁.		

Recommended Step for Initiating Treatment	Step 1	Step 2	Step 3 and consider short course of oral systemic corticosteroids	Step 4 or 5
	In 2-6 weeks, evaluate level of asthma control that is achieved, and adjust therapy accordingly.			

Key: FEV₁, forced expiratory volume in 1 second; FVC, forced vital capacity; ICU, intensive care unit.

Notes:

■ The stepwise approach is meant to assist, not replace, the clinical decision making required to meet individual patient needs.

■ Level of severity is determined by assessment of both impairment and risk. Assess impairment domain by patient's/caregiver's recall of previous 2–4weeks and spirometry. Assign severity to the most severe category in which any feature occurs.

■ At present, there are inadequate data to correspond frequencies of exacerbations with different levels of asthma severity. In general, more frequent and intense exacerbations (i.e., requiring urgent, unscheduled care, hospitalization, or ICU admission) indicate greater underlying disease severity. For treatment purposes, patients who had ≥ 2 exacerbations requiring oral systemic corticosteroids in the past year may be considered the same as patients who have persistent asthma, even in the absence of impairment levels consistent with persistent asthma.

Source: National Institutes of Health, National Heart, Lung, and Blood Institute. *Expert Panel Report 3: Guidelines for the Diagnosis and Management of Asthma.* Bethesda, MD: National Heart, Lung, and Blood Institute; 2007.

Figure 25-4 Estimated comparative daily dosages for inhaled corticosteroids in children.

Drug	Low Daily Dose Child 0–4	Low Daily Dose Child 5–11	Median Daily Dose Child 0–4	Median Daily Dose Child 5–11	High Daily Dose Child 0–4	High Daily Dose Child 5–11
Beclomethasone HFA						
40 or 80 mcg/puff	NA	80–160 mcg	NA	> 160–320 mcg	NA	> 320 mcg
Budesonide DPI						
90, 180, or 200 mcg/inhalation	NA	180–400 mcg	NA	> 400–800 mcg	NA	> 800 mcg
Budesonide inhaled						
inhalation suspension for nebulization (child dose)	0.25–0.5 mg	0.5 mg	> 0.5–1.0 mg	1.0 mg	> 1.0 mg	2.0 mg
Flunisolide						
250 mcg/puff	NA	500–750 mcg	NA	1000–1250 mcg	NA	> 1250 mcg
Flunisolide HFA						
80 mcg/puff	NA	160 mcg	NA	320 mcg	NA	≥ 640 mcg
Fluticasone						
HFA/MDI: 44, 110, or 220 mcg/puff	176 mcg	88–176 mcg	> 176–352 mcg	> 176–352 mcg	> 352 mcg	> 352 mcg
DPI: 50, 100, or 250 mcg/inhalation	NA	100–200 mcg	NA	> 200–400 mcg	NA	> 400 mcg
Mometasone DPI						
200 mcg/inhalation	NA	NA	NA	NA	NA	NA
Triamcinolone acetonide						
75 mcg/puff	NA	300–600 mcg	NA	> 600–900 mcg	NA	> 900 mcg

Key: HFA, hydrofluoroalkane; NA, not approved and no data available for this age group.

Notes:

- The most important determinant of appropriate dosing is the clinician's judgment of the patient's response to therapy. The clinician must monitor the patient's response on several clinical parameters and adjust the dose accordingly. The stepwise approach to therapy emphasizes that once control of asthma is achieved, the dose of medication should be carefully titrated to the minimum dose required to maintain control, thus reducing the potential for adverse effect.

- Some doses may be outside package labeling, especially in the high-dose range. Budesonide nebulizer suspension is the only ICS with FDA approved labeling for children < 4 years of age.

- Metered-dose inhaler (MDI) dosages are expressed as the actuator dose (the amount of the drug leaving the actuator and delivered to the patient), which is the labeling dosage in the United States. This is different from the dosage expressed as the valve dose (the amount of the drug leaving the valve, not all of which is available to the patient), which is used in many European countries and in some scientific literature. Dry powder inhaler (DPI) doses are expressed as the amount of drug in the inhaler following activation.

- For children < 4 years of age: The safety and efficacy of ICS in children < 1 year has not been established. Children < 4 years of age generally require delivery of ICS (budesonide and fluticasone HFA) through a face mask that should fit snugly over nose and avoid nebulizing in the eyes. Wash face after each treatment to prevent local corticosteroid side effects. For budesonide, the dose may be administered 1–3 times daily. Budesonide suspension is compatible with albuterol, ipratropium, and levalbuterol nebulizer solutions in the same nebulizer. Use only jet nebulizers, as ultrasonic nebulizers are ineffective for suspensions.

- For fluticasone HFA, the dose should be divided 2 times daily: the low dose for children < 4 years is higher than for children 5–11 years of age due to lower dose delivered with face mask and data on efficacy in young children.

Source: National Institutes of Health, National Heart, Lung, and Blood Institute. *Expert Panel Report 3: Guidelines for the Diagnosis and Management of Asthma*. Bethesda, MD: National Heart, Lung, and Blood Institute; 2007.

Figure 25-5 Assessing asthma control and adjusting therapy in children 0–4 years of age.

Components of Control		Classification of Asthma Control (0–4 years of age)		
		Well Controlled	Not Well Controlled	Very poorly Controlled
Impairment	Symptoms	≤ 2 days/week	> 2 days/week	Throughout the day
	Nighttime awakenings	≤ 1x/month	> 1x/month	> 1x/week
	Interference with normal activity	None	Some limitation	Extremely limited
	Short-acting beta₂-agonist use for symptom control (not prevention ot EIB)	≤ 2 days/week	> 2 days/week	Several times per day
Risk	Exacerbations requiring oral systemic corticosteroids	0–1/year	2–3/year	> 3/year
	Treatment-related adverse effects	Medication side effects can vary in intensity from none to very troublesome and worrisome. The level of intensity does not correlate to specific of control but should be considered in the overall assessment of risk.		
Recommended Action for Treatment		• Maintain current treatment. • Regular follow-up every 1–6 months. • Consider step down if well controlled for at least 3 months.	• Step up (1 step) and • Reevaluate in 2–6 weeks. • If no clear benefit in 4–6 weeks, consider alternative diagnosis or adjusting therapy. • For side effects, consider alternative treatment options.	• Consider short course of oral systemic corticosteroids. • Step up (1–2 steps) and • Reevaluate in 2 weeks. • If no clear benefit in 4–6 weeks, consider alernative diagnosis or adjusting therapy. • For side effects, consider alternative treatment options.

Key: EIB, exercise-induced bronchospasm.

Notes:

■ The stepwise approach is meant to assist, not replace, the clinical decision making required to meet individual patient needs.

■ The level of control is based on the most severe impairment or risk category. Assess impairment domain by caregiver's recall of previous 2–4 weeks. Symptom assessment for longer periods should reflect a global assessment such as inquiring whether the patient's asthma is better or worse since the last visit.

■ At present, there are inadequate data to correspond frequencies of exacerbations with different levels of asthma control. In general, more frequent and intense exacerbations (i.e., requiring urgent, unscheduled care, hospitalization, or ICU admission) indicate poorer disease control. For treatment purposes, patients who had ≥ 2 exacerbations requiring oral systemic corticosteroids in the past year may be considered the same as patients who have not-well-controlled asthma, even in the absence of impairment levels consistent with not-well-contolled asthma.

■ Before step up in therepy:

— Review adherence to medications, inhaler technique, and environmental control.

— If alternative treatment option was used in a step, discontinue it and use preferred treatment for that step.

Source: National Institutes of Health, National Heart, Lung, and Blood Institute. *Expert Panel Report 3: Guidelines for the Diagnosis and Management of Asthma.* Bethesda, MD: National Heart, Lung, and Blood Institute; 2007.

Figure 25-6 Assessing asthma control and adjusting therapy in children 5–11 years of age.

Components of Control		Classification of Asthma Control (5–11 years of age)		
		Well Controlled	**Not Well Controlled**	**Very Poorly Controlled**
Impairment	Symptoms	≤ 2 days/week but not more than once on each day	> 2 days/week or multiple times on ≤ 2 days/week	Throughout the day
	Nighttime awakenings	≤ 1x/month	≥ 2x/month	≥ 2x/week
	Interference with normal activity	None	Some limitation	Extremely limited
	Short-acting beta$_2$-agonist use for symptom control (not prevention of EIB)	≤ 2 days/week	> 2 days/week	Several times per day
	Lung function • FEV$_1$ or peak flow • FEV$_1$/FVC	> 80% predicted/ personal best > 80%	60–80% predicted/ personal best 75–80%	< 60% predicted/ personal best < 75%
Risk	Exacerbations requiring oral systemic corticosteroids	0–1/year	≥ 2/year (see note)	
		Consider severity and interval since last exacerbation		
	Reduction in lung growth	Evaluation requires long-term follow-up.		
	Treatment-related adverse effects	Medication side effects can vary in intensity from none to very troublesome and worrisome. The level of intensity does not correlate to specific levels of control but should be considered in the overall assessment of risk.		
Recommended Action for Treatment		• Maintain current step. • Regular follow-up every 1–6 months. • Consider step down if well controlled for at least 3 months.	• Step up at least 1 step and • Reevaluate in 2–6 weeks. • For side effects consider alternative treatment options.	• Consider short course of oral systemic corticosteroids, • Step up (1–2 steps) and • Reevaluate in 2 weeks. • For side effects, consider alternative treatment options.

Key: EIB, exercise-induced bronchospasm; FEV$_1$, forced expiratory volume in 1 second; FVC, forced vital capacity.

Notes:

■ The stepwise approach is meant to assist, not replace, the clinical decision making required to meet individual patient needs.

■ The level of control is based on the most severe impairment or risk category. Assess impairment domain by patient's/caregiver's recall of previous 2–4 weeks and spirometry/or peak flow measures. Symptom assessment for longer periods should reflect a global assessment such as inquiring whether the patient's asthma is better or worse since the last visit.

■ At present, there are inadequate data to correspond frequencies of exacerbations with different levels of asthma control. In general, more frequent and intense exacerbations (i.e., requiring urgent, unscheduled care, hospitalization, or ICU admission) indicate poorer disease control. For treatment purposes, patients who had ≥ 2 exacerbations requiring oral systemic corticosteroids in the past year may be considered the same as patients who have persistent asthma, even in the absence of impairment levels consistent with persistent asthma.

■ Before step up in therepy:

— Review adherence to medications, inhaler technique, and environmental control, and comorbid conditions.

— If alternative treatment option was used in a step, discontinue it and use preferred treatment for that step.

Source: National Institutes of Health, National Heart, Lung, and Blood Institute. *Expert Panel Report 3: Guidelines for the Diagnosis and Management of Asthma.* Bethesda, MD: National Heart, Lung, and Blood Institute; 2007.

Figure 25-7 Assessing asthma control and adjusting therapy in youths ≥ 12 years of age and adults.

Components of Control		Classification of Asthma Control (≥ 12 years of age)		
		Well Controlled	Not Well Controlled	Very Poorly Controlled
Impairment	Symptoms	≤ 2 days/week	> 2 days/week	Throughout the day
	Nighttime awakenings	≤ 2x/month	1–3x/week	≥ 4x/week
	Interference with normal activity	None	Some limitation	Extremely limited
	Short-acting beta₂-agonist use for symptom control (not prevention of EIB)	≤ 2 days/week	> 2 days/week	Several times per day
	FEV_1 or peak flow	> 80% predicted/ personal best	60–80% predicted/ personal best	< 60% predicted/ personal best
	Validated questionnaires ATAQ ACQ ACT	0 ≤ 0.75ᵃ ≥ 20	1–2 ≥ 1.5 16–19	3–4 N/A ≤ 15
Risk	Exacerbations requiring oral systemic corticosteroids	0–1/year	≥ 2/year (see note)	
		Consider severity and interval since last exacerbation		
	Progressive loss of lung function	Evaluation requires long-term follow-up care.		
	Treatment-related adverse effects	Medication side effects can vary in intensity from none to very troublesome and worrisome. The level of intensity does not correlate to specific levels of control but should be considered in the overall assessment of risk.		
Recommended Action for Treatment		• Maintain current step. • Regular follow-ups every 1–6 months to maintain control. • Consider step down if well controlled for at least 3 months.	• Step up 1 step and • Reevaluate in 2–6 weeks. • For side effects, consider alternative treatment options.	• Consider short course of oral systemic corticosteroids. • Step up 1-2 steps and • Reevaluate in 2 weeks. • For side effects, consider alternative treatment options.

Key: EIB, exercise-induced bronchospasm; ICU, intensive care unit.
ᵃACQ values of 0.76–1.4 are inderminate regarding well-controlled asthma.

Notes:

- The stepwise approach is meant to assist, not replace, the clinical decision making required to meet individual patient needs.

- The level of control is based on the most severe impairment or risk category. Assess impairment domain by patient's recall of previous 2–4 weeks and by spirometry/or peak flow measures. Symptom assessment for longer periods should reflect a global assessment, such as inquiring whether the patient's asthma is better or worse since the last visit.

- At present, there are inadequate data to correspond frequencies of exacerbations with different levels of asthma control. In general, more frequent and intense exacerbations (i.e., requiring urgent, unscheduled care, hospitalization, or ICU admission) indicate poorer disease control. For treatment purposes, patients who had ≥ 2 exacerbations requiring oral systemic corticosteroids in the past year may be considered the same as patients who have not-well-controlled asthma, even in the absence of impairment levels consistent with not-well-controlled asthma.

- Validated questionnaires for the impairment domain (the questionnaires do not asses lung function or the risk domain):
  ATAQ = Asthma Therapy Assessment Questionnaire© (See sample in "Component 1: Measures of Asthma Assessment and Monitoring.")
  ACQ = Asthma Control Questionnaire© (user package may be obtained at www.qoltech.co.uk or juniper@qoltech.co.uk)
  ACT = Asthma Control Test™ (See sample in "Component 1: Measures of Asthma Assessment and Monitoring.")
  Minimal Important Difference: 1.0 for the ATAQ; 0.5 for the ACQ; not determined for the ACT.

- Before step up in therapy:
  — Review adherence to medications, inhaler technique, and environmental control, and comorbid conditions.
  — If an alternative treatment option was used in a step, discontinue and use the preferred treatment for that step.

Source: National Institutes of Health, National Heart, Lung, and Blood Institute. *Expert Panel Report 3: Guidelines for the Diagnosis and Management of Asthma.* Bethesda, MD: National Heart, Lung, and Blood Institute; 2007.

Figure 25-8 Stepwise approach for managing asthma in children 0–4 years of age.

Intermittent Asthma	Persistent Asthma : Daily Medication Consul with asthma specialist if step 3 care or higher is required. Consider consultation at step 2.

Step 1
Preferred:
SABA PRN

Step 2
Preferred:
Low-dose ICS
Alternative:
Cromolyn or montelukast

Step 3
Preferred:
Medium-dose ICS

Step 4
Preferred:
Medium-dose ICS + either LABA or montelukast

Step 5
Preferred:
High-dose ICS + either LABA or montelukast

Step 6
Preferred:
High-dose ICS + either LABA or montelukast
Oral systemic corticosteroids

Step up if needed
(first, check adherence, inhaler technique, and environmental control)

Assess control

Step down if possible
(and asthma is well controlled at least 3 months)

Patient Education and Environmental Control at Each Step

Quick-Relief Medication for All Patients

- SABA as needed for symptoms. Intensity of treatment depends on severity of syptoms.
- With viral respiratory infection: SABA q 4–6 hours up to 24 hours (longer with physician consult). Consider short course of oral systemic corticosteroids if exacerbation is severe or patient has history of previous severe exacerbations.
- Caution: Frequent use of SABA may indicate the need to step up treatment. See text for recommendations on initiating daily long-term control therapy.

Key: Alphabetical order is used when more than one treatment option is listed within either preferred or alternative therapy. ICS, inhaled corticosteroid; LABA, inhaled long-acting beta$_2$-agonist; SABA, inhaled short-acting beta$_2$-agonist.

Notes:

■ The stepwise approach is meant to assist, not replace, the clinical decision making required to meet individual patient needs.

■ If alternative treatment is used and response inadequate, discontinue it and use the preferred treatment before stepping up.

■ If clear benefit is not observed within 4–6 weeks and patient/family medication technique and adherence are satisfactory, consider adjusting therapy or alternative diagnosis.

■ Studies on children 0–4 years of age are limited. Step 2 preferred therapy is based on Evidence A. All other recommendations are based on expert opinion and extrapolation from studies in older children.

Source: National Institutes of Health, National Heart, Lung, and Blood Institute. *Expert Panel Report 3: Guidelines for the Diagnosis and Management of Asthma.* Bethesda, MD: National Heart, Lung, and Blood Institute; 2007.

Figure 25-9 Stepwise approach for managing asthma in children 5–11 years of age.

Intermittent Asthma	Persistent Asthma : Daily Medication Consul with asthma specialist if step 4 care or higher is required. Consider consultation at step 3.

Step 1
Preferred:
SABA PRN

Step 2
Preferred:
Low-dose ICS
Alternative:
Cromolyn,
LTRA,
Nedocromil, or
theophylline

Step 3
Preferred:
EITHER:
Low-dose ICS +
either LABA,
LTRA or
theophylline
OR
Medium-dose
ICS

Step 4
Preferred:
Medium-dose
ICS + LABA
Alternative:
Medium-dose
ICS + either
LTRA or
theophylline

Step 5
Preferred:
High-dose ICS +
LABA
Alternative:
High-dose ICS
+ either LTRA
or theophylline

Step 6
Preferred:
High-dose ICS
+ LABA + oral
systemic
corticosteroid
Alternative:
High-dose ICS
+ either LTRA
or theophylline
+ oral systemic
corticosteroid

Step up if needed
(first, check adherence, inhaler technique, environmental control, and comorbid conditions)
Assess control
Step down if possible
(and asthma is well controlled at least 3 months)

Each step: Patient education, environmental control, and management of comorbidities.

Steps 2–4: Consider subcutaneous allergen immunotherapy for patients who have allergic asthma (see notes).

Quick-Relief Medication for All Patients
- SABA as needed for symptoms. Intensity of treatment depends on severity of symptom: up to 3 treatments at 20-minute intervals as needed. Short course of oral systemic corticosteroids may be needed.
- Caution: Increasing use of SABA or use > 2 days a week for symptom relief (not prevention of EIB) generally indicates inadequate control and the need to step up treatment.

Key: Alphabetical order is used when more than one treatment option is listed within either preferred or alternative therapy. ICS, inhaled corticosteroid; LABA, inhaled long-acting beta$_2$-agonist; LTRA, leukotriene receptor antagonist; SABA, inhaled short-acting beta$_2$-agonist.

Notes:

- The stepwise approach is meant to assist, not replace, the clinical decision making required to meet individual patient needs.

- If alternative treatment is used and response inadequate, discontinue it and use the preferred treatment before stepping up.

- Step 1 and step 2 medications are based on Evidence A. Step 3 ICS + adjunctive therapy and ICS are based on Evidence B for efficacy of each treatment and extrapolation from comparator trials in older children and adults—comparator trials are not available for this age group; steps 4–6 are based on expert and extrapolation from studies in older children and adults.

- Immunotherapy for steps 2–4 is based on Evidence B for house-dust mites, animal danders, and pollens; evidence is weak or lacking for molds and cockroaches. Evidence is strongest for immunotherapy with single allergens. The role of allergy in asthma is greater in children than in adults. Clinicians who administer immunotherapy should be prepared and equipped to identify and treat anaphylaxis that may occur.

Source: National Institutes of Health, National Heart, Lung, and Blood Institute. *Expert Panel Report 3: Guidelines for the Diagnosis and Management of Asthma.* Bethesda, MD: National Heart, Lung, and Blood Institute; 2007.

Figure 25-10 Stepwise approach for managing asthma in youths ≥ 12 years of age and adults.

Intermittent Asthma	Persistent Asthma : Daily Medication Consul with asthma specialist if step 4 care or higher is required. Consider consultation at step 3.

Step 1
Preferred:
SABA PRN

Step 2
Preferred:
Low-dose ICS
Alternative:
Cromolyn, LTRA, nedocromil,or theophylline

Step 3
Preferred:
Low-dose ICS + LABA
OR
Medium-dose ICS
Alternative:
Low-dose ICS + either LTRA or theophylline, or zileuton

Step 4
Preferred:
Medium-dose ICS + LABA
Alternative:
Medium-dose ICS + either LTRA or theophylline, or zileuton

Step 5
Preferred:
High-dose ICS + LABA
AND
Consider omalizumab for patients who have allergies

Step 6
Preferred:
High-dose ICS + LABA + oral corticosteroid
AND
Consider omalizumab for patients who have allergies

Step up if needed
(first, check adherence, environmental control, and comordid conditions)

Assess control

Step down if possible
(and asthma is well controlled at least 3 months)

Each step: Patient education, environmental control, and management of comorbidities.
Steps 2–4: Consider subcutaneous allergen immunotherapy for patients who have allergic asthma (see notes).

Quick-Relief Medication for All Patients

- SABA as needed for symptoms. Intensity of treatment depends on severity of symptoms: up to 3 treatments at 20-minute Intervals as needed. Short course of oral systemic corticosteroids may be needed.
- Use of SABA > 2 days a week for symptom relief (not prevention of EIB) generallly indicates inadequate control and the need to step up treatment.

Key: Alphabetical order is used when more than one treatment option is listed within either preferred or alternative therapy. EIB, excercise-induced bronchospasm; ICS, inhaled corticosteroid; LABA, long-acting inhaled beta₂-agonist; LTRA, leukotriene receptor antagonist; SABA, inhaled short-acting beta₂-agonist.

Notes:

- The stepwise approach is meant to assist, not replace, the clinical decision making required to meet individual patient needs.

- If alternative treatment is used and response inadequate, discontinue it and use the preferred treatment before stepping up.

- Zileuton is a less desirable alternative due to limited studies as adjunctive therapy and the perferred treatment before function. Theophylline requires monitoring of serum concentration levels.

- In step 6, before oral systemic cortcosteroids are introduced, a trail of high-dose ICS + LABA + either LTRA, theophylline, or zileuton may be considered, although this approach has not been studied in clinical trials.

- Step 1, 2, and 3 perferred therapies are based on Evidence A; step 3 alternative therapy is based on Evidence A for LTRA, Evidence B for theophylline, and Evidence D for zileuton. Step 4 preferred therapy is based on Evidence B, and alternative therapy is based on Evidence B for LTRA and theophylline and Evidence D for zileuton. Step 5 perferred therapy is based on Evidence B. Step 6 perferred therapy is based on (EPR—2 1997) and Evidence B for omalizumab.

- Immunotherapy for steps 2–4 is based on Evidence B for house-dust mites, animal danders, and pollens; evidence is weak or lacking for molds and cockroaches. Evidence is strongest for immunotherapy with single allergens. The role of allergy in asthma is greater in children than in adults.

- Clinicians who administer immunotherapy or omalizumab should be prepared and equipped to identify and treat anaphylaxis that may occur.

Source: National Institutes of Health, National Heart, Lung, and Blood Institute. *Expert Panel Report 3: Guidelines for the Diagnosis and Management of Asthma.* Bethesda, MD: National Heart, Lung, and Blood Institute; 2007.

VII. PNEUMONIA

Abdominal distension (gaseous), R14.0

Acquired deformity of chest and rib, M95.4

Acute nasopharyngitis [common cold], J00

Acute pharyngitis, J02

Acute serous otitis media, H65.0

Acute upper respiratory infection, unspecified, J06.9

Anorexia, R63.0

Bacterial pneumonia, unspecified, J15.9

Bronchopneumonia, unspecified organism, J18.0

Chest pain on breathing, R07.1

Chronic rhinitis, J31.0

Conjunctivitis, unspecified, H10.9

Convulsions, unspecified, R56.9

Cough, R05

Cyanosis, R23.0

Diarrhea, unspecified, R19.7

Dyspnea, unspecified, R06.00

Enlarged lymph nodes, unspecified, R59.9

Fever of other and unknown origin, R50

Headache, R51

Irritability and anger, R45.4

Lobar pneumonia, unspecified organism, J18.1

Meningismus, R29.1

Nausea, R11.0

Otalgia, H92.0

Other cardiac sounds, R01.2

Other fatigue, R53.83

Other specified acquired deformities of musculoskeletal system, M95.8

Other specified disorders of white blood cells, D72.89

Other voice and resonance disorders, R49.8

Parainfluenza virus pneumonia, J12.2

Pleural effusion in other conditions classified elsewhere, J91.8

Pneumonia due to methicillin-susceptible Staphylococcus aureus, J15.211

Pneumonia due to mycoplasma pneumonia, J15.7

Pyothorax without fistula, J86.9

Respiratory syncytial virus as the cause of diseases classified elsewhere, B97.4

Sneezing, R06.7

Tachycardia, unspecified, R00.0

Tachypnea, not elsewhere classified, R06.82

Urticaria, unspecified, L50.9

Viral pneumonia, not otherwise classified, J12

Viral pneumonia, unspecified, J12.9

Volume depletion, E86

Vomiting, unspecified, R11.10

Wheezing, R06.2

A. Etiology.
1. Pneumonia is inflammation and infection of lung parenchyma due to infectious pathogens.
2. It represents wide spectrum of signs/symptoms and disease severity.
3. Pathogens vary depending on age of patient.
4. Classification.
   a. By pathogen (bacterial, including mycoplasma or viral).
   b. By anatomic location: Lobar, interstitial, bronchopneumonia.
5. Common viral pathogens.
   a. RSV; adenovirus; parainfluenza 1, 2, 3; influenza A and B; rhinovirus.
   b. Transmission: Highly contagious.
      • Transmitted by direct contact with nasopharyngeal secretions from infected person.
      • Pneumonia results from spread of infection along airways.
         o Causes direct injury to respiratory epithelium, resulting in airway obstruction, abnormal secretion, and necrotic debris in airway lumen and lymphocytic infiltrations of interstitium and lung parenchyma.
         o Small airways are obstructed, resulting in poor oxygenation and air trapping, which leads to ventilation and perfusion mismatch.
6. Common bacterial pathogens.
   a. *Streptococcus pneumoniae, Mycoplasma pneumoniae, Streptococcus* (group A) *pyogenes, Staphylococcus aureus.*
   b. Transmission: Contagious.
      • Bacterial pathogens may be aspirated or inhaled, rarely by hematogenous spread.
      • Transmitted via person-to-person contact by large droplet aerosolization during coughing/sneezing.
      • Viral infection damages host's normal airway defense mechanisms, facilitating secondary bacterial infection.
   c. *S. pneumoniae.*
      • Many have *S. pneumoniae* colonization in upper respiratory tract.
      • Gram-positive encapsulated diplococci produce local edema.
         o Organism is distributed into adjacent areas of lung, resulting in typical focal lobar consolidation.
         o More than 90 serotypes exist.

d. *S. aureus.*
- Gram-positive organism; beta-lactamase producer.
- Produces exoproducts, enzymes, toxins, which contribute to virulence of this organism.
- Causes confluent bronchopneumonia; often unilateral with areas of hemorrhagic necrosis, cavitation of lung parenchyma, resulting in formation of pneumatocele, empyema, or bronchopulmonary fistula.

e. *M. pneumoniae.*
- Smallest self-replicating bacterium; lacks cell wall, dependent on host.
- Binds to ciliated respiratory epithelium and inhibits ciliary action.
- Airways and areas surrounding are filled with infiltrates.
- Causes cellular destruction and inflammatory response.

B. Occurrence.
1. Acute childhood respiratory infections result in 4.5 million deaths/year.
   a. 70% are pneumonia-related deaths.
      - Most often in children with underlying medical conditions.
   b. Bacterial pneumonia less common than viral pneumonia but has highest mortality.
   c. Mortality highest in younger patients.
2. Viral pneumonia.
   a. Peak attack rate between 2–3 years of life.
   b. More common in fall and winter.
      - Fall: Parainfluenza infection-causing croup.
      - Winter: RSV and influenza.
      - Viral pneumonia can be complicated by secondary bacterial infection.
3. Bacterial pneumonia.
   a. More common in children older than 5 years of age.
   b. Occurs in winter to early spring.
   c. Organisms vary according to age of child.
      - *S. pneumoniae.*
        o Children younger than 4 years of age at highest risk.
        o Risk factors: Male > female, daycare attendance, frequent otitis media (3 times in 6 months), frequent URIs (3 infections in 6 months), prematurity, and previous hospitalization for respiratory disease.
        o Period varies by serotype but generally short: 1–3 days.

- *M. pneumoniae.*
  - Leading cause of pneumonia in school-age children, adolescents.
  - Occurs year round, incubation period: 2–3 weeks (range: 1–4 weeks).
  - Rarely severe enough to warrant hospitalization.
- *S. aureus:* Children younger than 2 years of age at highest risk.

C. Clinical manifestations.
 1. Viral pneumonia: Symptoms variable depending on age.
    a. Onset may be acute or gradual but typically progresses more slowly than bacterial infection.
    b. Nasal congestion and coryza.
    c. Lower respiratory symptoms develop insidiously.
    d. Temperature variable depending on causative agent.
    e. Nontoxic appearing.
    f. History of URI symptoms, rhinitis, cough.
    g. Hoarseness, wheezing, rapid/shallow respirations.
 2. Bacterial pneumonia.
    a. *S. pneumoniae.*
       - Infants initially.
         - Mild URI symptoms, unilateral conjunctivitis, or otitis media.
         - Abrupt onset of fever to 104°F. May have seizure due to abrupt spike in temperature.
         - Mild cough; may have diarrhea, vomiting.
       - Infant progress.
         - Restlessness, apprehension.
         - Nasal flaring; rapid, shallow respiration; grunting.
         - Abdominal distention.
         - Cough may be absent.
         - Circumoral cyanosis.
       - Older children and adolescents.
         - Onset abrupt with rigors followed by temperature 102–104°F.
         - Appears ill.
         - Headache.
         - Anorexia, nausea, vomiting, diarrhea, abdominal pain.
         - Dyspnea, pleuritic pain, and cough; cough may be productive.
         - Alternating restlessness and drowsiness.
 3. *M. pneumoniae.*
    a. Slow onset.
    b. Malaise, transient arthritic symptoms.

      c. Persistent dry, hacking cough; sore throat often followed by hoarseness.

      d. Low-grade temperature and chills.

      e. May have ear pain.

D. Physical findings.

  1. Viral pneumonia: Symptoms dependent on causative agent and age of child.

      a. Nontoxic appearing.

      b. Tachypnea, cough, diffuse bilateral wheezing, decreased breath sounds throughout lung fields.

      c. Suprasternal, intercostal, substernal retractions.

      d. Cyanosis.

  2. Bacterial pneumonia.

      a. *S. pneumoniae.*

        • Infants.

          o Tachypnea; nasal flaring, grunting, retractions; diminished breath sounds; crackles, wheezing.

          o Fever.

          o Tachycardia.

          o Palpable liver or spleen secondary to abdominal distention.

          o Air hunger and cyanosis.

        • Older children and adolescents.

          o Diminished breath sounds over affected area of lung.

          o Dullness to percussion over area of consolidation.

          o Increased tactile fremitus over area of consolidation.

          o Cough productive of bloody or rust-tinged sputum.

          o Crackles, wheezing, splinting of respirations on affected side.

          o Fever.

          o Nuchal rigidity and other signs of meningeus may be present if upper lobes are involved.

          o Drowsiness, restlessness.

          o Respiratory distress and hypoxemia are variable or mild without widespread disease or pleural effusion.

  3. *M. pneumoniae.*

      a. Fever.

      b. Diminished breath sounds; coarse, harsh breath sounds.

      c. May have macular rash, erythematous macular rash, urticaria.

      d. Cervical lymphadenopathy.

      e. Conjunctivitis, otitis media.

      f. Arthropathy.

E. Diagnostic tests.
  1. Viral pneumonia.
     a. Definitive diagnosis: Viral isolation/viral antigens in respiratory tract infection.
     b. CXR: Typically shows bilateral, diffuse infiltrates.
     c. WBC: Normal or leukocytosis (not usually 20,000) with lymphocytosis.
  2. Bacterial pneumonia.
     a. No "gold standard" definitive test.
     b. Blood cultures are positive for the causative agent only about 10% of the time.
     c. WBC: Leukocytosis (15,000–40,000) with granulocytosis.
     d. CXR.
        • *S. pneumoniae:* Lobar consolidation; typically single focus but may be multiple foci; "spherical" infiltrate or round pneumonia; right lobes are preferentially affected.
        • *S. aureus:* Bronchopneumonia (multiple, central segmental infiltrates become confluent and diffuse); these infiltrates lead to necrosis, cavitation, pneumatoceles, and abscess formation.
  3. *M. pneumoniae.*
     a. Clinical manifestation and physical exam are essential to diagnosis.
        • Insidious onset, nontoxic.
        • Child older than 5 years of age.
        • Low-grade fever.
     b. *M. pneumoniae* detected by PCR technology.
     c. Cold agglutinins (during acute phase) with titer 1:64 or greater are predictive of *M. pneumoniae.*
     d. WBC: Normal.
F. Differential diagnosis.

Acute bronchiolitis due to other specified organisms, J21.8	Foreign body in other parts of respiratory tract causing asphyxiation, unspecified, initial encounter, T17.800A
Acute nasopharyngitis [common cold], J00	
Acute upper respiratory infection, unspecified, J06.9	Pneumonia due to mycoplasma pneumonia, J15.7
Asthma, J45	Pyothorax with fistula, J86.0
Cystic fibrosis, E84	Viral pneumonia, unspecified, J12.9
Fever of other and unknown origin, R50	

1. Viral pneumonia: URI symptoms and coryza with low-grade fever; bacterial pneumonia: Abrupt onset with high fever; *M. pneumoniae*: Insidious onset and nontoxic appearance.
2. Foreign body aspiration: May be detected on X-ray or by bronchoscopy.
3. Cystic fibrosis: Sweat test is definitive diagnostic test.
4. Asthma: Pattern of symptoms, absence of fever; inspiratory wheezing; prolonged expiratory phase.
5. Aspiration: Swallowing study to determine silent or free aspiration.
6. Tracheoesophageal fistula: Gas-filled bowel on X-ray in an infant with respiratory problems and drooling at birth.
7. Bronchiolitis: Rapid testing for viral antigen.
8. Right lower lobe pneumonia can present as GI process; X-ray can differentiate.
9. Right upper lobe pneumonia can present as meningitis, severity of illness, lumbar puncture.

G. Treatment.
   1. Viral pneumonia.
      a. Supportive care; typically mild illness and can be managed at home; young infant at risk for respiratory fatigue and more severe symptoms.
   2. Bacterial pneumonia.
      a. Dependent on bacteria; dependent on condition of child (oxygenation, hydration status, age: Infants younger than 4–6 months are usually hospitalized).
      b. Acetaminophen for fever and chest pain.
      c. Antibiotic treatment is generally 7–10 days.
      d. Amoxicillin is outpatient drug of choice; alternative choices are clarithromycin for children 6 weeks to 4 years of age; erythromycin for children older than 4 years of age.
      e. With high level of penicillin-resistant pneumococci present in community, consider cefuroxime, amoxicillin-clavulanate (Augmentin), or azithromycin.
   3. *M. pneumoniae*.
      a. Usually mild disease that can be managed at home.
      b. Erythromycin is drug of choice.
      c. Antibiotic treatment is generally 7–10 days.
      d. Acetaminophen for fever.

H. Follow-up.
1. Follow-up X-ray not needed in most cases of community-acquired pneumonia.
   a. Exceptions include severe illness requiring hospitalization, complications such as abscess, empyema, pleural effusion.
   b. May take up to 6 weeks for significant improvement.
2. Daily contact with healthcare provider may be indicated with more serious illness, in children with underlying conditions, and in very young children.
3. Recheck child if no improvement after 48 hours of treatment or if worsening occurs.
4. Follow-up visit at 10–14 days; occasional relapse may occur.
I. Complications.

Bullous erythema multiforme, L51.1	Myelitis, unspecified, G04.91
Disease of pericardium, unspecified, I31.9	Pleural effusion in other conditions classified elsewhere, J91.8
Encephalopathy, unspecified, G93.40	Pneumonia due to mycoplasma pneumonia, J15.7
Guillain-Barré syndrome, G61.0	
Gangrene and necrosis of lung, J85.0	
Methicillin-susceptible *Staphylococcus aureus* infection as the cause of diseases classified elsewhere, B95.61	Pyothorax without fistula, J86.9
	Toxic shock syndrome, A48.3

1. Severe disease requiring hospitalization and ventilatory support.
2. Empyema, pulmonary abscess, pleural effusion, pericarditis.
3. *S. aureus*: Toxic shock syndrome.
4. *M. pneumoniae*: Stevens-Johnson syndrome, transverse myelitis, meningoencephalitis, encephalopathy, Guillain-Barré syndrome.
J. Education.
1. Immunizations are essential to decrease individual morbidity and mortality associated with pneumonia but also to reduce incidence in community. Prevnar 13 is a conjugate vaccine for infants and young children 6 weeks to 5 years of age.
2. Understand symptoms that warrant immediate attention (lethargy, seizure, severe respiratory distress) and symptoms that require follow-up (no improvement 48 hours after starting antibiotics, worsening of respiratory symptoms, signs of dehydration).

3. Need to give antibiotic as prescribed for full course.
4. Careful handwashing, containment of coughs/sneezes reduce spread of disease.
5. *M. pneumoniae*: Common for close household contacts to develop illness.

BIBLIOGRAPHY

Behrman RE, Kliegman R, Jenson HB. *Nelson Textbook of Pediatrics*. 17th ed. Philadelphia, PA: W.B. Saunders; 2004.

Bradley JS, Byington CL, Shah SS, et al. The management of community-acquired pneumonia in infants and children older than 3 months of age: clinical practice guidelines by the Pediatric Infectious Diseases Society and the Infectious Diseases Society of America. *Clin Infect Dis*. 2011;53(7):e25-e76.

Carolan PL. Pediatric bronchitis. Medscape. http://emedicine.medscape.com/article/1001332-overview #a0104. Updated June 18, 2015. Accessed June 30, 2015

Centers for Disease Control and Prevention. Keys facts about seasonal flu vaccine. http://www.cdc.gov/flu /protect/keyfacts.htm. Updated October 22, 2014. Accessed April 10, 2015.

Cherry JD. Clinical practice. Croup. *N Engl J Med*. 2008;358(4):384-391.

Committee On Infectious Diseases; American Academy Pediatrics. Recommendations for prevention and control of influenza in children, 2014–2015. *Pediatrics*. 2014;134(5):e1503-e1519.

Klassen T, Craig WR, Moher D, et al. Nebulized budesonide and oral dexamethasone for treatment of croup: a randomized controlled trial. *J Am Med Assoc*. 1998;279(20):1629-1632.

Long SS, Pickering LK, Prober CG. *Principles and Practice of Pediatric Infectious Diseases*. 2nd ed. Philadelphia, PA: Churchill Livingstone; 2003.

Mathews B, Shah S, Cleveland RH, Lee EY, Bachur RG, Neuman MI. Clinical predictors of pneumonia among children with wheezing. *Pediatrics*. 2009;124(1):e29-e36.

Michael MA. Scope and impact of pediatric asthma. *Nurse Pract*. 2002;27(suppl):3-6.

National Institutes of Health, National Heart, Lung, and Blood Institute. *Expert Panel Report 3: Guidelines for the Diagnosis and Management of Asthma*. Bethesda, MD: National Heart, Lung, and Blood Institute; 2007.

Pickering LK. *Red Book: 2003 Report of the Committee on Infectious Diseases*. 26th ed. Elk Grove Village, IL: American Academy of Pediatrics; 2003.

Ralston SL, Lieberthal AS, Meissner HC, et al. Clinical practice guideline: the diagnosis, management, and prevention of bronchiolitis. *Pediatrics*. 2014;134(5):e1474-e1502.

Snyder J, Fisher D. Pertussis in childhood. *Pediatr Rev*. 2012;33(9):412-420.

Storch G. Rapid diagnostic tests for influenza. *Curr Opin Pediatr*. 2003;15:79.

Taussig LM, Landau LI. *Pediatric Respiratory Medicine*. St. Louis, MO: Mosby; 1999.

Cardiovascular Disorders

Karen M. Corlett and Beth Richardson

I. CHEST PAIN

Acute rheumatic heart disease, unspecified, I01.9

Asthma, J45

Cardiac arrhythmia, unspecified, I49.9

Cardiac murmur, unspecified, R01.1

Cardiomegaly, I51.7

Cardiomyopathy, unspecified, I42.9

Chest pain on breathing, R07.1

Chest pain, unspecified, R07.4

Chronic ischemic heart disease, unspecified, I25.9

Congenital malformation of heart, unspecified, Q24.9

Disease of pericardium, unspecified, I31.9

Dizziness and giddiness, R42

Exercise-induced bronchospasm, J49.990

Gastro-esophageal reflux disease without esophagitis, K21.9

Heart disease, unspecified, I51.9

Heart failure, unspecified, I50.9

Hepatomegaly, not elsewhere classified, R16.0

Intercostal pain, R07.82

Localized swelling, mass and lump, unspecified, R22.9

Marfan's syndrome, unspecified, Q87.40

Mucocutaneous lymph node syndrome [Kawasaki], M30.3

Myocarditis, unspecified, I51.4

Nonrheumatic mitral valve disorders, I34

Obesity, E66

Other pulmonary embolism without acute cor pulmonale, I26.99

Other specified symptoms and signs involving the circulatory and respiratory systems, R09.89

Palpitations, R00.2

Pneumothorax, J93

Supraventricular tachycardia, I47.1

Syncope and collapse, R55

Tachycardia, unspecified, R00.0

Tachypnea, not elsewhere classified, R06.82

Turner syndrome, unspecified, Q96.9

Ventricular tachycardia, I47.2

Viral pneumonia, not otherwise classified, J12

A. Etiology.
 1. Classes of chest pain.
  a. Severe, acute, unremitting chest pain: Refer immediately to pediatrician or urgent/emergent care facility. Rare and most often due to cardiac, pulmonary, or gastrointestinal causes.
  b. Chronic or recurrent chest pain: More likely.
   • Typically patient has had several episodes of chest pain before medical attention is sought.
   • Many times, physical exam may be normal.
   • Patient history is crucial in elucidating etiology of chest pain, although large percentage of chest pain in children will never have etiology determined.
   • Chest pain is distressing to patients, families: Chest pain in adult friends, relatives typically signifies cardiac event, most chest pain in childhood is noncardiac in origin.
   • Thorough history and physical can rule out serious causes for chest pain.
 2. Chest pain, cardiac in origin.
  a. Coronary artery disease.
  b. Congenital heart disease.
  c. Typically have murmur.
  d. Acquired heart disease.
  e. Infectious etiologies.
  f. Cardiomyopathy, pericarditis, Kawasaki disease, rheumatic fever.
  g. Myocardial issues, myocarditis.
  h. Cardiomyopathies.
  i. Dysrhythmias.
  j. Supraventricular or ventricular tachycardias.
 3. Chest pain, noncardiac in origin: Most common.
  a. Musculoskeletal.
  b. Pulmonary.
  c. Gastrointestinal.
  d. Psychogenic.
B. Occurrence.
 1. Few studies of overall incidence of chest pain in pediatric population due to wide range of specialists to whom these patients are referred.
 2. Incidence, particularly in adolescents, is significant.

C. Clinical manifestations.
   1. Chronic or recurrent intermittent chest pain.
      a. Most often occurs in adolescent population.
      b. May or may not limit activities.
      c. Usually chest pain has been long-standing before treatment is sought.
      d. Important to elucidate inciting factors and relieving factors.
         • Relationship of pain to activity varies.
      e. Associated symptoms.
         • Syncope, presyncope, dizziness, palpitations.
      f. Congenital heart disease or previous cardiac surgery is important factor in determining cardiac origin of chest pain; also increases likelihood of dysrhythmia as origin for chest pain.
D. Physical findings.
   1. Most commonly patients will have no significant physical exam findings. Physical exam findings may be clues to origin of chest pain.
   2. Stigmata of certain syndromes: Marfan, Turner.
   3. Cardiac murmur.
   4. Evidence of congestive heart failure.
      a. Tachypnea, increased work of breathing, retractions, flaring, tachycardia, weak peripheral pulses, cool extremities, delayed capillary refill, rales, enlarged liver, easily fatigued, edema.
   5. Obesity: Increased incidence of gastroesophageal reflux (GER).
   6. Reproducible pain with palpation.
   7. Signs of trauma to chest wall.
   8. Decreased breath sounds.
E. Diagnostic tests.
   1. Refer to pediatrician/specialist if chest pain of cardiac origin is suspected; may conduct the following tests as part of evaluation.
   2. Chest X-ray (CXR).
      a. Evaluate for cardiomegaly. May also reveal rib fractures or pneumonia.
   3. Electrocardiogram.
      a. Clue to cardiac origins: Hypertrophied atria or ventricles, long QT syndrome, congenital heart disease, infarcts, dysrhythmias.
   4. Echocardiography.
      a. Structural abnormalities.
      b. Coronary artery anatomy.
      c. Cardiac function.

5. Exercise testing.
   a. ST segment response to exercise.
   b. May provoke dysrhythmias.
   c. May provoke exercise-induced asthma.
6. May reassure patient and parents if normal.

F. Differential diagnosis.

Acute pancreatitis, K85	Myalgia, M79.1
Asthma, J45	Other pulmonary embolism without acute cor pulmonale, I26.99
Calculus of bile duct without cholangitis or cholecystitis, K80.5	
Chest pain on breathing, R07.1	Peptic ulcer, site unspecified, unspecified as acute or chronic, without hemorrhage or perforation, K27.9
Chondrocostal junction syndrome [Tietze], M94.0	
Esophagitis, unspecified, K20.9	
Exercise-induced bronchospasm, J49.990	Pleural condition, unspecified, J94.9
Gastroesophageal reflux disease without esophagitis, K21.9	Pneumothorax, J93
	Precordial pain, R07.2
Hypertrophy of bone, unspecified site, M89.30	Viral pneumonia, not otherwise classified, J12

1. Musculoskeletal.
   a. Costochondritis.
      • Most often at 2nd to 5th costal cartilages.
      • Often reproducible pain with pressure at costochondral junctions.
      • Treated with nonsteroidal anti-inflammatory drugs (NSAIDs).
   b. Slipping rib syndrome.
      • Pain at lower costal margin, often associated with click.
      • Reproducible at times with anterior motion of lower rib.
      • Treated with avoidance of inciting movements.
   c. Trauma (nonaccidental or accidental).
      • Point tenderness at site of trauma.
      • Pain is worse with movement of chest, self-limited.
   d. Muscular pain.
      • History of new physical activity, pain is worse if affected muscles are used.

e. Precordial catch.
- Sharp pain in anterior chest, often when child is bent over.
- Short, intermittent pain, relieved by shallow respirations.
f. Pleural pain.
- Infection affecting intercostal and upper abdominal muscles, intensified with coughing.
- Tender muscles lasting 3–7 days.
- Intense pain separated by pain-free intervals.
2. Pulmonary.
a. Asthma, particularly exercise-induced asthma.
b. Pneumonia.
c. Foreign body aspiration.
d. Pleuritis: Often is remote occurrence to viral infection.
e. Diaphragmatic irritation.
f. Pulmonary embolus: Associated with dyspnea, usually is acute episode.
g. Pneumothorax: Associated with dyspnea, usually is acute episode.
3. Gastrointestinal: Typically localized to substernal area.
a. GER.
b. Related to mealtimes. Exacerbated by supine positioning.
c. Esophagitis.
d. Biliary colic.
e. Acute pancreatitis: Pain radiates to back.
f. Peptic ulcer disease.
4. Psychogenic causes: Often have witnessed episodes of chest pain in family members.
G. Treatment.
1. Musculoskeletal.
a. Analgesics and anti-inflammatories.
b. Avoidance of inciting movements, rest.
2. Pulmonary.
a. Asthma: Trial of bronchodilators, particularly if exercise-induced symptoms.
b. Immediate referral for concern of pulmonary embolus or pneumothorax.
3. Gastrointestinal.
a. GER: H_2 blockers, dietary modifications, weight loss if obesity contributing to symptoms.
b. Referral to specialist if initial medical therapy does not relieve symptoms.

4. Psychogenic.
   a. Frank discussion with patient, family about nonorganic cause of chest pain.
      • Changes in patient's life leading to stress or depression?
      • Assess for secondary gain that pain yields patient.
      • Counseling may be indicated.
   b. Refer to specialist.
5. Cardiac causes.
   a. Refer to specialist.
   b. Coronary artery anomalies, valvular defects: Medical management, surgical repair.
   c. Infectious etiologies.
      • Cardiomyopathy/myocarditis.
      • Treatment of inciting infection if elucidated.
      • Supportive care until recovery of function.
      • Consideration for transplantation if function does not recover.
   d. Kawasaki disease (see later section on page 357).
   e. Myocardial issues.
      • Obstructive cardiomyopathy.
      • Activity restriction.
      • Consideration of medical or surgical therapy.
   f. Dysrhythmias.
      • Identification of dysrhythmia.
      • Antidysrhythmic agents.
      • Ablation of accessory pathways.
H. Follow-up.
   1. Follow up with pediatrician or specialist as indicated.
   2. Support for chronic pain.
   3. Assess for missed diagnosis if pain persists or worsens.
   4. No cause of chest pain may have been identified. Patient, family may require ongoing support, education, particularly if pain continues.
I. Complications.
   1. Misdiagnosis.
   2. Sudden cardiac death rare.
J. Education.
   1. Most often require assurance and education as to noncardiac nature of chest pain and resumption of normal activities.
   2. If cause of chest pain found, education regarding cause and treatment plan.

II. HYPERTENSION

Acute myocardial infarction, I21	Irritability and anger, R45.4
Anorexia, R63.0	Nausea, R11.0
Cerebral infarction due to unspecified occlusion or stenosis of unspecified cerebral artery, I63.50	Obesity, E66
	Other fatigue, R53.83
	Other secondary hypertension, I15.8
Convulsions, unspecified, R56.9	Papilledema associated with increased intracranial pressure, H47.11
Diabetes mellitus, E10-E14	
Disorder of adrenal gland, unspecified, E27.9	Papilledema, unspecified, H47.1
	Systemic lupus erythematosus, organ or system involvement unspecified, M32.10
Disorder of circulatory system, unspecified, I99.9	
Disorder of kidney and ureter, unspecified, N28.9	Thyrotoxicosis, unspecified without thyrotoxic crisis or storm, E05.90
Epistaxis, R04.0	Tuberous sclerosis, Q85.1
Essential (primary) hypertension, I10	Turner syndrome, unspecified, Q96.9
Headache, R51	Vomiting, unspecified, R11.10

A. Etiology.
   1. May be early onset of essential hypertension.
   2. Etiology of adult-onset essential hypertension is unclear and thought to be multifactorial with genetic, familial, environmental factors contributing to development of essential hypertension. Becoming more clear that elevations of blood pressure in childhood are beginnings of adult essential hypertension.
   3. May be a sign of underlying pathology (secondary hypertension).
      a. Renal, cardiac, endocrine diseases.
   4. Related to systemic disease, chronic illness, or medication.
B. Occurrence.
   1. By definition, 5% of children will have hypertension.
   2. Secondary hypertension is more common in children.
C. Clinical manifestations.
   1. Definition is systolic and/or diastolic blood pressure consistently above 95th percentile for age, sex, height taken on 3 separate occasions.
      a. Stage 1 hypertension is 95th to 99th percentile +5 mm Hg and should be repeated on 3 or more separate occasions to confirm.

    b. Stage 2 hypertension is greater than the 99th percentile +5 mm Hg.
- Prompt referral.
- Immediate referral if patient is symptomatic.

    c. Prehypertension now defined as readings between the 90th and 95th percentile, and/or greater than or equal to 120/80 in adolescents.

    d. Check blood pressure in left arm and one lower extremity if hypertension present.

2. Secondary hypertension.

    a. Hypertension secondary to another cause.

    b. Typically more severe elevation of blood pressure.

    c. Younger age.

    d. Severe elevation of blood pressure at any age should trigger an aggressive evaluation to look for an underlying cause.

3. Essential hypertension.

    a. Typically milder elevation in blood pressure, but still > 95th percentile.

    b. Often associated with obesity.

    c. Typically, family history of essential hypertension.

    d. Elevated heart rate is common.

    e. Variable blood pressure measurements on repeated evaluation.

    f. Often no additional findings on history or physical.

    g. For mild elevation of blood pressure in asymptomatic adolescent, it is more likely to be essential hypertension, particularly if positive family history and/or presence of comorbid conditions.

D. Physical findings.

1. Essential hypertension: May be few abnormal physical findings, but patient history is important adjunct to determine whether hypertension is essential or secondary.

    a. Family history of hypertension in first- or second-degree relative; myocardial infarction, stroke, renal vascular diseases, diabetes, obesity.

    b. Obesity in patient.

2. Secondary hypertension: May be physical findings or important clues in patient's history as to possible cause of secondary hypertension.

    a. Neonatal history of invasive umbilical lines.

    b. History of urinary tract infections.

    c. Medication history: OTC, prescribed, and illicit drugs.
- Tobacco, alcohol, diet pills, anabolic steroids, oral contraceptive pills, pseudoephedrine, phenylpropanolamine.

    d. Headaches.

    e. Weight loss (pheochromocytoma, hyperthyroidism).

    f. Overall slowing of growth parameters may indicate underlying chronic disease.

    g. Webbed neck (Turner syndrome associated with coarctation).

    h. Presence of skin lesions (tuberous sclerosis, systemic lupus erythematosus).

    i. Retinal exam: Presence of vascular lesions due to chronic hypertension, papilledema with increased intracranial pressure.

    j. Dysmorphic features: Williams syndrome, Turner syndrome.

    k. Adrenal disorders.

    l. Anorexia, nausea.

    m. Tiredness, irritability.

    n. Epistaxis.

    o. Neurologic symptoms.

      • Headache, nausea, vomiting, anorexia, visual complaints, seizure, papilledema.

E. Diagnostic tests.

  1. Errors in blood pressure measurement are common: Use correct technique, appropriately sized equipment for repeated measurement.

    a. All children > 3 years of age: Blood pressure measured at every pediatric visit.

    b. Appropriate cuff size essential for accurate measurement.

    c. Bladder width of cuff should be 40% of child's arm circumference, bladder should cover 80% or more of circumference of arm.

    d. At least 3 separate measurements to diagnose hypertension.

    e. Measurement should occur after 5 minutes of quiet; child should be seated with back supported and feet on floor.

    f. Auscultation preferred method.

    g. Right arm preferred for measurement.

    h. Ambulatory blood pressure monitoring may be utilized by specialists to more accurately delineate blood pressure readings throughout the day and night.

  2. For all identified as hypertensive:

    a. Serum electrolytes, blood urea nitrogen, and creatinine.

    b. Urinalysis and urine culture.

    c. Complete blood count.

    d. Renal ultrasound.

3. If overweight and prehypertensive and for all hypertensive:
   a. Fasting lipid panel and fasting glucose.
4. Drug screen if concern for use of licit or illicit drugs.
5. Polysomnography if history elucidates snoring.
6. Evaluation for end-organ damage may be ordered by specialists.
   a. Echocardiogram.
   b. Retinal exam.
   c. Plasma renin.
   d. Renovascular imaging.
   e. Plasma and urine steroid and catecholamine levels.

F. Differential diagnosis.

Cushing syndrome, E24	Systemic lupus erythematosus, organ or system involvement unspecified, M32.10
Disorder of kidney and ureter, unspecified, N28.9	
Hypothyroidism, unspecified, E03.9	Tuberous sclerosis, Q85.1
Other secondary hypertension, I15.8	Turner syndrome, unspecified, Q96.9

1. Secondary hypertension.
2. Renal vascular disease, renal parenchymal disease.
3. About 60–80% of secondary hypertension in childhood is due to renal causes.
4. Coarctation of aorta (Turner syndrome).
5. Endocrine and adrenal causes: Hyperthyroidism, Cushing syndrome.
6. Systemic diseases: Systemic lupus erythematosus, tuberous sclerosis.
7. Pharmacologic effect: Steroids, amphetamine or sympathomimetics, oral contraceptives, illicit drugs.
8. CNS manifestations: Increased intracranial pressure, intracranial mass.

G. Treatment.
   1. Treatment goal is to achieve blood pressure < 95th percentile, or < 90th percentile if concurrent conditions present.
   2. Nonpharmacologic treatment first-line therapy.
      a. Weight loss if obese; prevention of obesity if normal weight.
      b. Increase physical activity.
      c. Dietary modifications.
      d. Family-based interventions.

    e. Tobacco cessation; avoid drugs of abuse, particularly cocaine.

    f. Reevaluation of blood pressure.

3. Pharmacologic treatment indicated if symptoms present, target organ damage present, type 1 or 2 diabetes present, or failure of nonpharmacologic treatment with lifestyle modifications.

4. Single-drug therapy preferred. Provider preference since no studies show absolute long-term benefit of any class or drug.

    a. Angiotensin-converting enzyme inhibitors (preferred if diabetes or proteinuria).

    b. Angiotensin-receptor blockers (preferred if diabetes or proteinuria).

    c. Beta blockers (preferred if patient experiences migraine headaches).

    d. Calcium channel blockers (preferred if patient experiences migraine headaches).

    e. Diuretics.

5. Add second class of medication if maximum dose achieved or side effects experienced before blood pressure control achieved.

6. Consider gradual withdrawal of medication if target blood pressure achieved for long period of time.

H. Follow-up.

1. Continued monitoring of blood pressure.

2. Encouragement of and follow-up on lifestyle changes.

3. Refer back to pediatrician or specialist if treatment goals not achieved with lifestyle changes, current medication regime.

I. Complications.

1. End-organ dysfunction.

2. Hypertensive crisis.

J. Education.

1. Essential hypertension.

    a. Chronicity of disease, likely long-term morbidity, end-organ damage if not controlled.

    b. Potential improvements with dietary, lifestyle changes and medications if necessary.

    c. Need for continuous follow-up.

    d. Adherence to medication regime if prescribed.

    e. Encourage patients to return to prescriber if side effects unacceptable because many classes of medications are available for blood pressure control.

    f. Goals of therapy.

2. Suspected or known secondary hypertension.
   a. Thorough evaluation of cause, may be extensive testing.
   b. Follow-up with specialists.
   c. Adherence to treatment or medication regimen.

III. INNOCENT HEART MURMURS

Cardiac murmur, unspecified, R01.1	Other fatigue, R53.83
Clubbing of fingers, R68.3	Other nonrheumatic pulmonary valve disorders, I37.8
Cyanosis, R23.0	
Dyspnea, unspecified, R06.00	Other specified chromosome abnormalities, Q99.8
Edema of unspecified orbit, H05.229	
Generalized hyperhidrosis, R61	Other specified symptoms and signs involving the circulatory and respiratory systems, R09.89
Hepatomegaly, not elsewhere classified, R16.0	
Hypotension, unspecified, I95.9	Shock, unspecified, R57.9
Localized swelling, mass and lump, unspecified, R22.9	Splenomegaly, not elsewhere classified, R16.1
	Tachycardia, unspecified, R00.0

A. Etiology.
   1. Innocent murmur is abnormal heart sound caused by turbulent blood flow not associated with structural heart disease, also called functional or nonorganic murmur.
B. Occurrence.
   1. Cardiac murmurs are noted in 50–70% of children who are asymptomatic.
   2. Vast majority of murmurs heard in infants and children are innocent in nature.
C. Clinical manifestations.
   1. Innocent murmur is typically found on routine physical exam.
   2. Presence of other clinical manifestations: Concern for congenital, acquired heart disease.
   3. Any murmur, innocent or organic, is typically louder with fever, anemia, other high cardiac output states.

D. Physical findings.
  1. Absence of physical findings other than murmur should be expected if innocent murmur is suspected. Innocent murmurs often more prominent during high cardiac output states such as fever, anemia, pregnancy.
  2. Physical exam findings of congenital or acquired heart disease that follow should specifically be evaluated.
     a. Known or suspected syndrome or genetic or chromosomal abnormality.
     b. Failure to grow.
     c. Easily fatigued.
     d. Tachypnea, increased work of breathing, retractions, flaring, grunting.
     e. Diaphoresis, particularly with exertion, feeding in the infant.
     f. Cyanosis, central or peripheral.
     g. Clubbing of digits.
     h. Tachycardia.
     i. Edema, particularly periorbital and facial in infant.
     j. Active precordium.
     k. Palpable thrill.
     l. Weak pulses, delayed capillary refill, hypotension, or other signs of shock.
     m. Differential between upper and lower extremity pulses or blood pressures.
     n. Hepatomegaly or splenomegaly.
     o. Murmur of grade IV (see **Box 26-1**) or higher in intensity.
     p. Diastolic murmur.

Box 26-1 Grading of Cardiac Murmurs

Grade I/VI: Soft, difficult to hear unless room quiet and child cooperative.
Grade II/VI: Soft but heard immediately.
Grade III/VI: Easily heard, moderately loud, no thrill associated.
Grade IV/VI: Loud, can palpate the thrill of turbulent flow on chest wall.
Grade V/VI: Loud, has thrill, able to hear murmur with stethoscope barely off chest wall.
Grade VI/VI: Loud, has thrill, able to hear murmur with stethoscope off chest wall.

3. Careful consideration of murmur description.
   a. Location.
      - Where murmur is heard best, described by location over cardiac structures or location on chest.
      - Most common areas to auscultate innocent murmurs are left upper sternal border and left lower sternal border.
   b. Radiation.
      - Descriptor of where else murmur can be heard.
      - Innocent murmurs rarely radiate to distant parts of chest.
   c. Timing: Where in the cardiac cycle the murmur is heard.
      - Systole: Between S_1 and S_2.
      - Diastole: Between S_2 and S_1.
      - Continuous: Starts in systole, continues into diastole, does not need to continue throughout cardiac cycle but has same sound for duration of murmur.
      - Innocent murmurs are typically systolic; venous hum is continuous murmur. Solely diastolic murmur is never innocent and should be referred.
      - Children with innocent murmurs typically have normal first and second heart sounds (S_1 and S_2) that are audible in addition to murmur. Rapid heart rates of infants, particularly febrile infants, may make it difficult to distinguish between systole and diastole.
   d. Pitch: Sound frequency of murmur. Innocent murmurs typically low to medium in pitch.
   e. Quality: Musical or vibratory in quality.
   f. Intensity: Loudness of the murmur (Box 26-1).
      - Innocent murmurs, typically Grade I–II/VI. Often change in intensity with change in position: Sitting to lying, standing to sitting. May change in intensity from one visit to the next.
      - No clicks or extra sounds if murmur is innocent.
4. Types of innocent murmurs.
   a. Still's murmur.
      - Most common innocent murmur in children; occurs typically in 2- to 6-year olds.
      - Low to medium in pitch, buzzing or vibratory in nature.
      - Short murmur occurring in early systole.
      - Grade I–III/VI.

- Loudest in supine position, diminished by standing.
- Heard best at left lower sternal border.

b. Pulmonary flow murmur.
- Heard in children/adolescents.
- Harsh murmur, blowing, nonmusical.
- Systolic ejection murmur.
- Grade II–III/VI.
- Loudest in supine position, loudest on exhalation.
- Heard best in second to third intercostal space at left sternal border.

c. Peripheral pulmonary arterial stenosis murmur.
- Heard frequently in infants and newborns.
- Medium in pitch.
- Short systolic ejection murmur.
- Grade I–II/VI.
- Often heard best in axillae and over back.
- Turbulence is due to relative smallness of peripheral pulmonary arteries in newborn and angulation of takeoff of right- and left-branch pulmonary arteries from main pulmonary artery.

d. Supraclavicular or brachiocephalic systolic murmur or bruit.
- Heard in children, young adults.
- Low to medium in pitch, harsh.
- Is short, systolic murmur.
- Grade I–III/VI.
- Heard best above clavicles, radiates to neck.
- Heard best in supine, sitting positions; changes with change in neck position.

e. Venous hum.
- Also known as cervical venous hum.
- Continuous murmur.
- Heard over neck, immediately below clavicles.
- Intensity varies, loudness varies with position, activity; best heard in sitting position.
- May disappear when head is turned toward side of murmur.
- Murmur results from turbulence of flow as large veins converge.

E. Diagnostic tests.
1. When murmur is detected, refer to pediatrician or cardiologist to determine significance.

2. Many innocent murmurs do not require further diagnostic tests after thorough history, physical, auscultatory exam.
3. CXR, electrocardiogram, cardiac echocardiography may determine whether murmur is truly innocent.
4. Murmurs associated with structural abnormalities (organic murmurs) may require additional diagnostic evaluation.

F. Differential diagnosis.

Cardiomyopathy, unspecified, I42.9	Mucocutaneous lymph node
Congenital malformation of heart,	syndrome [Kawasaki], M30.3
unspecified, Q24.9	Rheumatic heart disease,
	unspecified, I09.9

1. Congenital heart disease.
2. Cyanotic or acyanotic disease.
3. Acquired heart disease.
4. Cardiomyopathy.
5. Kawasaki disease.
6. Rheumatic heart disease.

G. Treatment.
1. Innocent heart murmurs have no organic cause, no structural abnormality; therefore, no treatment required.
2. Education of patient, family is most important treatment modality.

H. Follow-up.
1. If innocent murmur confirmed, patients may return to usual health maintenance schedule for follow-up visits.
2. If innocent murmur suspected but not yet confirmed as innocent, should return for reevaluation to physician.

I. Complications.
1. None, since no abnormality is present.

J. Education.
1. Crucial for patient, family.
2. Explain murmur as noise.
3. Noise is result of blood flow, no structural problem.
4. No heart disease or abnormality is present.
5. Murmur may change or disappear with time but if persists, still no problem with heart.
6. No activity restrictions required.
7. No treatment required.

IV. KAWASAKI DISEASE

Abdominal and pelvic pain, R10	Ileus, unspecified, K56.7
Abnormal electrocardiogram [ECG] [EKG], R94.31	Jaundice, unspecified, R17
Abnormal results of liver function studies, R94.5	Mucocutaneous lymph node syndrome [Kawasaki], M30.3
Aneurysm of other specified arteries, I72.8	Other disorders of plasma-protein metabolism, not elsewhere classified, E88.09
Arteritis, unspecified, I77.6	Other specified cardiac arrhythmias, I49.8
Cardiomegaly, I51.7	
Conjunctivitis, unspecified, H10.9	Other specified diseases of gallbladder, K82.8
Convulsions, unspecified, R56.9	
Coronary artery aneurysm, I25.41	Other specified disorders of nose and nasal sinuses, J34.8
Cough, R05	Other specified disorders of white blood cells, D72.89
Diarrhea, unspecified, R19.7	
Enlarged lymph nodes, unspecified, R59.9	Pain in unspecified joint, M25.50
Erythematous condition, unspecified, L53.9	Proteinuria, unspecified, R80.9
	Rash and other nonspecific skin eruption, R21
Fever of other and unknown origin, R50	Reye's syndrome, G93.7
Hypertrophy of tongue papillae, K14.3	Vomiting, unspecified, R11.10

A. Etiology.
   1. Syndrome of acute systemic vasculitis of unknown origin.
   2. Affects mostly small- to medium-size arteries, particularly coronary arteries.
   3. Likely of infectious origin or infection-triggered immune disorder.
B. Occurrence.
   1. Most prominent in Japan.
   2. Children of Asian descent more susceptible than Caucasians.
   3. 50% of cases in younger than 2 years of age, 80% of cases in younger than 5 years of age. Peak incidence at 1 year. Rare after 10 years of age.
   4. Boys 1.5 times > girls.
   5. 1–2% of siblings affected.

6. Recurrence rate: 1–3%.
7. More common in winter and early spring.
C. Clinical manifestations.
1. Vasculitis of small- to medium-size arteries, especially coronary arteries. May progress to aneurysm formation in coronary arteries; can lead to thrombosis or scarring, increased risk for myocardial infarction, ischemic heart disease, and sudden death.
D. Physical findings.
1. Fever.
2. Reddened, edematous, indurated palms/soles progressing to desquamation. May be unwilling to walk/use hands to grasp objects.
3. Erythematous rash; most prominent on trunk, groin.
4. Bilateral conjunctival injection; particularly bulbar conjunctiva; nonexudative.
5. Red or peeling lips, strawberry tongue, injected oral, pharyngeal mucosa.
6. Cervical lymphadenopathy.
7. Irritability: Particularly in infants.
8. Evidence of vasculitis in other systems.
    a. Cardiovascular: Murmur, gallop, electrocardiogram changes, cardiomegaly, peripheral arterial aneurysms.
    b. Gastrointestinal: Diarrhea, vomiting, abdominal pain, ileus, jaundice, increased liver enzymes, distention of gallbladder.
    c. Hematologic: Elevated WBC count, elevated platelet count.
    d. Renal: Proteinuria, hypoalbuminemia.
    e. Respiratory: Cough, rhinorrhea.
    f. Joint: Pain, swelling.
    g. CNS: Pleocytosis of cerebral spinal fluid (CSF), seizure.
E. Diagnostic tests.
1. No specific laboratory test to confirm diagnosis.
2. Diagnostic criteria to establish diagnosis.
3. Fever of ≥ 5 days and 4 of the following 5 criteria:
    a. Erythematous, edematous, indurated palms/soles progressing to desquamation later in course.
    b. Polymorphous exanthem.
    c. Bilateral conjunctival injection.
    d. Red or peeling lips, strawberry tongue, injected oral, pharyngeal mucosa.
    e. Cervical lymphadenopathy.
    f. OR: Fever of ≥ 5 days, < 4 of these 5 criteria, and coronary aneurysms documented by echocardiography or cardiac angiography.

4. Kawasaki should be considered in any young child with unexplained fever for ≥ 5 days, leukocytosis, elevated erythromycin sedimentation rate or C-reactive protein, and thrombocytosis.
   a. "Incomplete" Kawasaki, with symptoms inadequate to meet classic criteria is more common in < 1 year of age and adolescents.
   b. Echocardiography may show evidence of coronary arteritis.
F. Differential diagnosis.

Adverse effect of unspecified drugs, medicaments and biological substances, initial encounter, T50.905A	Rheumatic fever without heart involvement, I00
	Streptococcal sepsis, unspecified, A40.9
Bullous erythema multiforme, L51.1	Systemic lupus
Juvenile rheumatoid arthritis, unspecified, of unspecified site, M08.00	erythematosus, organ or system involvement unspecified, M32.10
Measles without complication, B05.9	Toxic shock syndrome, A48.3
Methicillin-susceptible *Staphylococcus aureus* infection as the cause of diseases classified elsewhere, B95.61	Viral infection, unspecified, characterized by skin and mucous membrane lesions, B09
Polyarthritis, unspecified, M13.0	

---

1. Infectious illnesses, particularly streptococcal and staphylococcal infections.
2. Drug reactions or hypersensitivity reactions.
3. Stevens-Johnson syndrome: Erythema, swelling, peeling all advance beyond hands, feet.
4. Other vasculitic diseases.
5. Polyarteritis nodosa, systemic lupus erythematosus.
6. Juvenile idiopathic arthritis: Smaller joints, morning stiffness, fingers involved, joint deformities.
7. Rheumatic fever: Positive antistreptococcal antibody.
8. Viral exanthems: Do not meet all criteria for Kawasaki disease.
9. Measles: Rash more prominent on face and neck.
10. Toxic shock syndrome: Sandpaper rash, more toxic-appearing child, often hypotension with evidence of shock.

G. Treatment.
   1. Referral to pediatrician and specialists.
   2. Hospitalization.
   3. Aspirin.
      a. Used for antipyretic, anti-inflammatory, and antiplatelet effects.
      b. High-dose aspirin for at least 48 hours.
      c. Low-dose aspirin to complete 6–8 weeks of therapy if no coronary artery abnormalities.
      d. Aspirin continued indefinitely if coronary artery aneurysms, second antiplatelet agent may be added.
   4. IV immunoglobulin.
      a. Decreases incidence of coronary artery aneurysms.
      b. Mechanism of protection unknown.
      c. If fever persists > 36 hours after IVIG, repeat IVIG dose.
H. Follow-up.
   1. Pediatric cardiology for echocardiographic evaluation of coronary artery aneurysms. Aneurysms may not develop until after acute stage of illness.
I. Complications.

Acute myocardial infarction, unspecified, I21.9	Heart failure, unspecified, I50.9
Arteritis, unspecified, I77.6	Myocarditis, unspecified, I51.4
Coronary artery aneurysm, I25.41	Other nonrheumatic mitral valve disorders, I34.8
Disease of pericardium, unspecified, I31.9	

   1. Coronary artery aneurysms: Develop in < 20% of individuals, fewer if treated with immunoglobulin.
   2. If coronary artery aneurysms develop, increased risk of coronary artery thrombosis, stenosis, and resultant myocardial infarction.
   3. May also develop valvular heart disease; mitral valve is affected more frequently than aortic valve.
   4. Pericarditis, myocarditis, pericardial effusion, congestive heart failure may occur.
   5. Can have development of vascular aneurysms elsewhere in body.
   6. Can have liver dysfunction from intrahepatic vasculitis.
J. Education.
   1. Serious nature of illness.
   2. Importance of specialty care and follow-up.

3. Possibility of complications after initial phase of illness.
4. Importance of adherence to prescribed medication: Aspirin.
5. Importance of not using aspirin to treat fever in other childhood illnesses: Association with Reye's syndrome.
6. Consider influenza vaccine due to association of Reye's syndrome with flulike illnesses and aspirin.

V. RHEUMATIC FEVER

Acute and subacute infective endocarditis, I33.0	Localized swelling, mass and lump, unspecified, R22.9
Acute rheumatic heart disease, unspecified, I01.9	Myocarditis, unspecified, I51.4
Arteritis, unspecified, I77.6	Other chorea, G25.5
Cardiomegaly, I51.7	Other ill-defined heart diseases, I51.89
Chronic pulmonary edema, J81.1	Pain in joint, M25.5
Disease of pericardium, unspecified, I31.9	Polyarthritis, unspecified, M13.0
Disorder of white blood cells, unspecified, D72.9	Rash and other nonspecific skin eruption, R21
Elevated erythrocyte sedimentation rate, R70.0	Rheumatic fever without heart involvement, I00
Endocarditis, valve unspecified, I38	Streptococcal pharyngitis, J02.0
Erythema marginatum, L53.2	Streptococcus, group A, as the cause of diseases classified elsewhere, B95.0
Fever of other and unknown origin, R50	Tachycardia, unspecified, R00.0
Heart failure, unspecified, I50.9	

A. Etiology.
1. Complication of group A beta-hemolytic streptococcal (GABHS) pharyngitis.
2. Thought to be unique host factors that make certain individuals more susceptible to rheumatic fever after GABHS pharyngitis.
3. Rheumatic fever is classified as collagen vascular disease or connective tissue disease resulting in diffuse vasculitis.

B. Occurrence.
   1. Most common in underdeveloped countries, but there is a resurgence in United States.
   2. Occurs in 2–3% of patients with untreated GABHS.
   3. Rheumatic fever is rare in infants, toddlers. Most cases < 5 years of age.
C. Clinical manifestations.
   1. Inflammation of joints and heart.
   2. Rarely, inflammation of brain and skin.
D. Physical findings.
   1. Migratory polyarthritis.
      a. Occurs in 75% of initial episodes, 50% of recurrent episodes.
      b. Arthritis is typically of larger joints (knees, elbows, wrists, ankles).
      c. Each joint typically affected for < 1 week, often overlap so that > 1 joint is affected at a time.
      d. Joints are painful to touch, red, swollen; painful with movement.
   2. Carditis.
      a. Up to 50% of patients with rheumatic fever have evidence of carditis.
      b. May manifest as myocarditis with poor function, valvular disease with audible murmur, pericarditis with friction rub, or as general symptoms of tachycardia, cardiomegaly, pulmonary edema, or symptoms of congestive heart failure.
   3. Subcutaneous nodule.
      a. Small, hard nodules typically found on elbows, knees, wrists; also felt in occipital area, over vertebrae. Relatively rare finding in rheumatic fever.
   4. Chorea.
      a. Finding of abnormal, involuntary writhing, purposeless movements that extinguish with sleep.
      b. Patients often have uncontrollable facial grimacing.
      c. Often preceding emotional lability thought to be from CNS involvement.
      d. Chorea is often late sign, with latent period of 1–6 months.
   5. Erythema marginatum.
      a. Typical rash of rheumatic fever; painless, does not itch. Spreads peripherally while central clearing, most common on trunk, limbs; face is usually spared.
   6. Low-grade fever.
   7. Painful joints without obvious joint inflammation.

E. Diagnostic tests.
   1. Evidence of previous GABHS.
   2. Modified Jones criteria to make diagnosis.
      a. Major criteria:
         • Carditis.
         • Polyarthritis.
         • Chorea.
         • Erythema marginatum.
         • Subcutaneous nodules.
      b. Minor criteria:
         • Arthralgia.
         • Fever.
         • Elevated acute-phase reactants (erythrocyte sedimentation rate, C-reactive protein, WBC count).
         • Prolonged PR interval.
      c. Diagnosis requires 2 major criteria, or 1 major and 2 minor criteria, and evidence of previous GABHS infection.
      d. Electrocardiogram and echocardiogram for confirmed diagnoses.
F. Differential diagnosis.

Congenital malformation of heart, unspecified, Q24.9	Mucocutaneous lymph node syndrome [Kawasaki], M30.3
Juvenile rheumatoid arthritis, unspecified, of unspecified site, M08.00	Myocarditis, unspecified, I51.4
	Other ill-defined heart diseases, I51.89

   1. Juvenile idiopathic arthritis: Small joints involved, swelling and deformities of joints, morning stiffness, no positive antistreptococcal antibody.
   2. Kawasaki disease.
   3. Congenital heart disease: Murmur without associated symptoms of rheumatic fever.
   4. Infective carditis or myocarditis: Positive viral or bacterial cultures.
G. Treatment.
   1. Prevention: Appropriate diagnosis and treatment of streptococcal pharyngitis.
   2. Referral to pediatrician or specialist if diagnosis suspected.

3. Antibiotics to eradicate streptococcal infection (primary prevention; see **Table 26-1**).
4. Bed rest until fever, symptoms resolve. With carditis, bed rest may be indicated for longer period of time.
5. Aspirin.
   a. If no relief in arthritis with initiation of aspirin therapy, question diagnosis.
   b. Steroids may be considered if no response to aspirin therapy and/or for those with moderate to severe carditis.
6. Secondary prevention (Table 26-1).
   a. To prevent recurrence of rheumatic fever in susceptible individuals.
   b. Antibiotics until 21 years of age and minimum of 5 years if no cardiac involvement.
   c. Antibiotics until 21 years of age and minimum of 10 years if cardiac involvement but no residual cardiac disease.
   d. Antibiotics until 40 years of age and minimum of 10 years if residual valve abnormalities; consider lifelong antibiotic prophylaxis.

H. Follow-up.
   1. With specialist.
   2. Subacute bacterial endocarditis (SBE) prophylaxis if residual valve disease.
I. Complications.

Endocarditis, valve unspecified, I38

---

1. Cardiac involvement.
   a. Valvular heart disease.
2. Recurrence.
   a. Increased risk of recurrence in susceptible hosts.
   b. Cardiac damage is cumulative with each recurrence.
J. Education.
   1. Nature of disease.
   2. Recurrence risk.
   3. Prompt diagnosis and treatment of group A streptococcal pharyngitis.
   4. Cumulative nature of cardiac damage with repeat episodes.
   5. Secondary prevention.
      a. Streptococcal infections do not have to be symptomatic to cause additional cardiac damage.
   6. Importance of continued pediatric subspecialty follow-up and transition to adult healthcare providers when appropriate.
   7. SBE prophylaxis if indicated.

Table 26-1 Primary and Secondary Antibiotic Prophylaxis for Rheumatic Heart Disease

Antibiotic	Dose	Duration	Route
Primary Prevention			
Benzathine penicillin G	< 27 kg: 600,000 units; > 27 kg: 1.2 million units	Once	IM
Penicillin V	< 27 kg: 250 mg 2–3 times/day; > 27 kg, adolescents and adults: 500 mg 2–3 times/day	10 days	Orally
Amoxicillin	50 mg/kg once daily (maximum 1 g)	10 days	Orally
Narrow-spectrum cephalosporin[a]	Variable	10 days	Orally
Clindamycin[a]	20 mg/kg/day in 3 doses (maximum 1.8 g/day)	10 days	Orally
Clarithromycin[a]	15 mg/kg/day in 2 doses (maximum 250 mg bid)	10 days	Orally
Azithromycin[a]	12 mg/kg/dose once daily (maximum 500 mg)	5 days	Orally
Secondary Prevention[b]			
Benzathine penicillin G	< 27 kg: 600,000 units; > 27 kg: 1.2 million units	Once every 4 weeks	IM
Penicillin V	250 mg 2 times daily	Daily	Orally
Sulfadiazine	< 27 kg: 500 mg once daily; > 27 kg: 1000 mg once daily	Daily	Orally
Macrolide or azalide[c]	Variable		Orally

[a] If allergic to penicillin.
[b] See text for duration of therapy.
[c] If allergic to penicillin and sulfadiazine.
Source: Data from Gerber MA, Baltimore RS, Eaton CB, et al. Prevention of rheumatic fever and diagnosis and treatment of acute streptococcal pharyngitis: a scientific statement from the American Heart Association Rheumatic Fever, Endocarditis and Kawasaki Committee of the Council on Cardiovascular Disease in the Young, the Interdisciplinary Council on Functional Genomics and Translational Biology, and the Interdisciplinary Council on Quality of Care and Outcomes Research: endorsed by the American Academy of Pediatrics. *Circulation.* 2009; 119(11):1541-1551.

BIBLIOGRAPHY

Allen HD, Driscoll DJ, Shaddy RE, Feltes TF. *Moss & Adams' Heart Disease in Infants, Children, and Adolescents Including the Fetus and Young Adult.* 8th ed. Philadelphia, PA: Lippincott Williams Wilkins; 2013.

Baker EJ. Non-rheumatic inflammatory disease of the heart. In: Anderson RH, Baker EJ, Penny DJ, et al., eds. *Paediatric Cardiology.* 2nd ed. Philadelphia, PA: Churchill Livingstone; 2010:173-190.

Bragg L, Alvarez A. Endocarditis. *Pediatr Rev.* 2014;35(4):162-167.

Coelho Mota CC, Demarchi Aiello V, Anderson RH. Rheumatic fever. In: Anderson RH, Baker EJ, Penny DJ, et al., eds. *Paediatric Cardiology.* 2nd ed. Philadelphia, PA: Churchill Livingstone; 2010:277-301.

Gerber MA, Baltimore RS, Eaton CB, et al. Prevention of rheumatic fever and diagnosis and treatment of acute *Streptococcal pharyngitis:* a scientific statement from the American Heart Association Rheumatic Fever, Endocarditis, and Kawasaki Disease Committee of the Council on Cardiovascular Disease in the Young, the Interdisciplinary Council on Functional Genomics and Translational Biology, and the Interdisciplinary Council on Quality of Care and Outcomes Research: endorsed by the American Academy of Pediatrics. *Circulation.* 2009;119(11):1541-1551.

National High Blood Pressure Education Program Working Group on High Blood Pressure in Children and Adolescents. The fourth report on the diagnosis, evaluation and treatment of high blood pressure in children and adolescents. *Pediatrics.* 2004;114(2 suppl 4th report):555-576.

Soon MB, Newburger JW. Kawasaki disease. *Pediatr Rev.* 2013;34(4):151-162.

Taketomo CK, Hodding JH, Kraus DM. *Pediatric & Neonatal Dosage Handbook.* 21st ed. Hudson, OH: Lexi-Comp, Inc.; 2015.

Urbina E, Alpert B, Flynn J, et al. Ambulatory blood pressure monitoring in children and adolescents: recommendations for standard assessment: a scientific statement from the American Heart Association Atherosclerosis, Hypertension, and Obesity in Youth Committee of the Council on Cardiovascular Disease in the Young and the Council for High Blood Pressure Research. *Hypertension.* 2008;52:433-451.

Gastrointestinal Disorders

Robin Shannon

I. ABDOMINAL PAIN, ACUTE

Abdominal and pelvic pain, R10	Female pelvic inflammatory disease, unspecified, N73.9
Abdominal hernia with obstruction, without gangrene, unspecified, K46.0	Intussusception, K56.1
Acute pancreatitis, K85	Mittelschmerz, N94.0
Acute pharyngitis, J02	Other specified intestinal infections, A08.8
Appendicitis, unspecified, K37	Ovarian cysts, unspecified, N83.20
Calculus of bile duct without cholangitis or cholecystitis, K80.5	Renal colic, unspecified, N23
Constipation, K59.0	Torsion of testis, unspecified, N44.00
Dysmenorrhea, unspecified, N94.6	Urinary tract infection, site not specified, N39.0
Ectopic pregnancy, unspecified, O00.9	Viral pneumonia, not otherwise classified, J12

A. Etiology.
1. Pain located in abdomen lasting up to several days. Symptom can originate from within or outside gastrointestinal (GI) tract.
2. Pain from visceral (stomach, intestine), parietal (peritoneum), or referred areas.
3. Frequently caused by viral gastroenteritis, urinary tract infection (UTI), constipation.
4. Other possible causes vary by age:
   a. Infant: Colic, gastroenteritis, viral illness, dietary protein allergy, UTI, intussusception, incarcerated hernia, testicular torsion.
   b. Preschool: Gastroenteritis, viral illness, constipation, pharyngitis, UTI, appendicitis, intussusception, pneumonia, trauma.
   c. School age: Gastroenteritis, viral illness, pharyngitis, UTI, constipation, appendicitis, pneumonia, pancreatitis, trauma.

    d. Adolescent: Gastroenteritis, viral illness, UTI, constipation, appendicitis, pancreatitis, cholelithiasis, inflammatory bowel disease (IBD). Female: Mittelschmerz, pelvic inflammatory disease (PID), dysmenorrhea, ectopic pregnancy, ovarian cyst.

B. Occurrence.
    1. Gastroenteritis is the most common medical cause, and appendicitis is the most common surgical cause.

C. Clinical manifestations.
    1. Must take child's age, developmental level into consideration regarding location, duration of pain. Younger children often indicate periumbilical region.
    2. Associated symptoms: Fever, vomiting, diarrhea, cough, anorexia depending on etiology.
    3. Important subjective data should include:
        a. Location, duration, frequency of pain.
        b. Stool frequency, consistency; history of hematochezia or melena.
        c. Vomiting: Frequency, presence of bile or hematemesis.
        d. Symptoms outside GI tract (cough, congestion, dysuria, sore throat, fever, headache).
        e. Medication and diet history.
        f. Sexual activity, vaginal discharge.
        g. Alleviating and aggravating factors.

D. Physical findings.
    1. Weight, temperature, vital signs.
    2. General appearance: Assess degree of discomfort and hydration.
    3. Complete physical exam with attention to following:
        a. Abdominal exam: Ask child to indicate location of pain. Observe for peristaltic waves, distention, guarding. Palpate for masses, stool, hepatosplenomegaly, tenderness. Percuss for rebound tenderness. Have child stand, jump to assess for signs of peritoneal irritation.
        b. Rectal exam: Assess for fissures, erythema.

E. Diagnostic tests.
    1. May include complete blood count (CBC), comprehensive metabolic panel, amylase, lipase, and urinalysis. Consider pregnancy test in postmenarchal girls.
    2. Test stool for occult blood if history dictates.
    3. Chest X-ray (CXR) if pneumonia suspected.
    4. Abdominal X-ray if intestinal obstruction or perforation suspected. Useful to rule out fecal impaction.
    5. Abdominal ultrasound if appendicitis, ovarian cyst, ectopic pregnancy suspected.

F. Differential diagnosis.

Acute pancreatitis, K85

Appendicitis, unspecified, K37

Calculus of bile duct without cholangitis or cholecystitis, K80.5

1. Appendicitis.
   a. Vague periumbilical pain, migrating localized to right lower/middle quadrant.
   b. Often associated with fever, vomiting, anorexia; may see elevated white blood cell (WBC) count.
   c. Involuntary muscle guarding, rebound, signs of peritoneal irritation on abdominal exam. Rovsing sign: Pain in right lower quadrant with palpation of the left side.
   d. Typical signs and symptoms are often not present in children.
2. Constipation, gastroenteritis, intussusception, incarcerated hernia, colic, peptic ulcer.
3. Pancreatitis.
   a. Inflammation of pancreas from infection, medications, trauma, genetic defect, or structural abnormality.
   b. Epigastric pain, often with nausea, vomiting.
   c. Elevated amylase, lipase.
4. Cholelithiasis.
   a. Epigastric or right upper quadrant pain, often radiates to back.
   b. Ultrasound shows stones in gallbladder or bile duct and/or gallbladder wall thickening.

G. Treatment.
1. Appendicitis, cholelithiasis: Surgical consult.
2. Pancreatitis: Possible hospital admission for IV hydration, pain control.
3. Intussusception: Admission for diagnosis and barium enema; incarcerated hernia: Admission for surgery.

H. Follow-up.
1. Telephone contact for any changes/increase in symptoms.
2. Ensure follow-through with any consults that have been requested.

I. Complications.
1. School absence.

J. Education.
1. Reassure if physical exam consistent with nonsurgical abdomen. Parents most often concerned about appendicitis.
2. Review hydration/nutrition needs.
3. Treat fever as needed.

4. Monitor for any changes in symptoms or worrisome signs such as hematochezia, hematemesis, increased or newly localized pain.
5. Education otherwise depends on final diagnosis.

II. ABDOMINAL PAIN, CHRONIC: CHILDHOOD FUNCTIONAL ABDOMINAL PAIN (FAP)

Abdominal and pelvic pain, R10

A. Diagnostic criteria: Must experience *all* of the following symptoms at least once per week for at least 2 months prior to diagnosis:
   1. Episodic or continuous abdominal pain.
   2. Insufficient criteria for other functional GI disorders.
   3. No evidence of an inflammatory, anatomic, metabolic, or neoplastic process that explains the symptoms.
B. Functional abdominal pain syndrome (FAP-S) includes all of the above plus one or more of the following at least 25% of the time:
   1. Some loss of daily functioning.
   2. Additional somatic symptoms such as headache or difficulty sleeping.
C. Etiology.
   1. A functional disorder is classically defined as the absence of specific structural, infectious, inflammatory, or biochemical abnormalities as cause of pain. Using the "biopsychosocial model," it is thought to be due to an interaction of psychological factors and altered gut physiology via the brain–gut axis.
   2. Genetics and environment may play a role in early life. Psychological factors such as coping skills, social support, and stress, along with physiology, including postinfectious states, can influence the enteric nervous system (ENS) and central nervous systems (CNS), which can lead to functional GI disorders in susceptible individuals.
D. Occurrence.
   1. Equal incidence among males and females until age 10 years; then female-to-male ratio is 1.5:1.0. Most common between 8 and 15 years of age.
E. Clinical manifestations.
   1. Periumbilical or generalized abdominal pain lasts from 1 hour to 3 hours.
   2. Occurs daily or intermittently (at least once per week) over at least 8-week period.
   3. May be associated with nausea, fatigue, headache, pallor.
   4. Patient may assume fetal position, grimace/cry during episode.
   5. Pain does not wake child from sleep.
   6. Patient may have school absence, withdraw from social/extracurricular activities.

      7. No weight loss or growth delay.

      8. Not associated with fever, vomiting, melena, or hematochezia.

      9. Important subjective data to obtain:

          a. Description of normal elimination pattern; alleviating or aggravating factors.

          b. Dietary history, medications.

          c. Psychosocial stressors, parent/caregiver usual reaction to the pain.

          d. Sleep habits.

F. Physical findings.

      1. Weight/height: Plot on growth curve and compare with previous.

      2. Perform thorough physical exam at first visit with attention to following:

          a. Abdominal exam: Ask patient to indicate location of pain. Assess for tenderness, masses, hepatosplenomegaly.

          b. Rectal exam: Inspect for erythema, fissures, skin tags. Perform digital exam if constipation suspected.

      3. Tanner staging.

G. Diagnostic tests.

      1. No diagnostic test to make diagnosis of FAP.

      2. Consider screening laboratories:

          a. Urinalysis, urine culture.

          b. CBC, erythrocyte sedimentation rate (ESR), and/or CRP, comprehensive metabolic panel, amylase, lipase. Screen for celiac disease with tissue transglutaminase IgA and total serum IgA.

          c. Stool for occult blood; if indicated stool for ova and parasite, giardia antigen.

          d. Consider lactose breath hydrogen test to rule out lactose intolerance.

H. Differential diagnosis.

Abdominal tenderness, unspecified site, R10.819	Irritable bowel syndrome without diarrhea, K58.9
Abnormal weight loss, R63.4	Melena, K92.1
Acute upper respiratory infection, unspecified, J06.9	Noninfective enteritis and colitis, K50–K52
Constipation, K59.0	Other disorders of intestinal carbo-
Crohn's disease, unspecified, without complications, K50.90	hydrate absorption, E74.39
	Residual hemorrhoidal skin tags,
Diarrhea, unspecified, R19.7	K64.4
Intestinal parasitism, unspecified, B82.9	Ulcerative colitis, unspecified, without complications, K51.90

1. Irritable bowel syndrome (IBS).
2. Infection: UTI, intestinal parasite.
3. Lactose intolerance: Positive lactose breath test or okay after no lactose in diet after 2-week trial.
4. Constipation.
5. IBD (Crohn's disease, ulcerative colitis): Associated with melena, hematochezia, and/or diarrhea. Possible weight loss, growth delay. Physical exam may reveal abdominal tenderness, multiple anal fissures/skin tags, possible joint symptoms. Refer to pediatric gastroenterologist.

I. Treatment.
1. Most valuable treatment is establishment of therapeutic relationship with patient and family. Discuss possibility of FAP at first visit.
2. Can do trial of lactose-reduced diet. Eliminate caffeine.
3. Increase fiber in the diet: May regulate intestinal motility. American Academy of Pediatrics (AAP) recommends: Child's age + 5 = grams of fiber/day minimum.
4. Counseling: Self-hypnosis, biofeedback.
5. Symptom diary.
6. Sleep hygiene: Poor-quality sleep may contribute to FAP.

J. Follow-up.
1. Arrange for clinic visit about 1 month after diagnosis of FAP.
2. Telephone contact for any changes in symptoms.

K. Complications.
1. School absence or avoidance, decreased participation in extracurricular activities.
2. Interference with peer relationships.

L. Education.
1. If physical exam normal, reassure family that it is unlikely any specific cause will be found.
2. Acknowledge pain is real, not fabricated.
3. Insist on return to normal daily activities, school participation.
4. Educate family about reaction to the pain: May be altered reaction to pain or secondary gain if too much attention is given to symptom.
5. Discuss prognosis: Pain may persist for months or years.

III. COLIC

Renal colic, unspecified, N23

  A. Often defined by "rule of 3": Crying for $\geq$ 3 hours a day on $\geq$ 3 days a week in the first 3 months of life in otherwise healthy infant. Diagnostic criteria: Must include all the following in infants from birth to 4 months of age:

     1. Paroxysms of irritability, fussing, or crying that starts and stops without obvious cause.

     2. Episodes lasting 3 or more hours/day and occurring at least 3 days/week for at least 1 week.

     3. No failure to thrive.

  B. Etiology.

     1. Unknown, probably multifactorial.

     2. There is no proof that it is caused by pain in the abdomen or other body part.

  C. Occurrence.

     1. Most studies estimate incidence rates of up to 25% of infants. Equal incidence among males and females, all socioeconomic levels, breastfed versus bottle-fed.

  D. Clinical manifestations.

     1. Inconsolable crying for 3 or more hours per day, often clustering in afternoon or evening. Episodes seem to have a clear beginning and end.

     2. Associated symptoms may include pain facies/grimacing, clenched fists, taut/distended abdomen, drawing legs up to abdomen, flatus.

     3. Crying often described as more intense than normal crying.

     4. Ask parents to describe quality, frequency, duration, timing of crying.

     5. Ask about any other symptoms such as vomiting, regurgitation.

     6. Detailed diet history, including mother if breastfeeding.

     7. Frequency, consistency of stool, hematochezia.

     8. Alleviating or aggravating factors.

     9. Medications given to baby or that breastfeeding mother is taking.

    10. Ask about coping skills of caregivers and opportunity for respite.

  E. Physical findings.

     1. Weight/length/head circumference, temperature, vital signs.

     2. Complete physical exam.

     3. Check baby for evidence of incarcerated hernia, testicular torsion, hair tourniquet.

     4. Observe caregiver and infant: Assess caregiver's anxiety, coping skills.

  F. Diagnostic tests.

     1. No test to diagnose colic: Made by history and physical exam.

G. Differential diagnosis.

Abdominal hernia with obstruction, without gangrene, unspecified, K46.0	Gastroesophageal reflux disease without esophagitis, K21.9
	Malabsorption due to intolerance,
Constipation, K59.0	not elsewhere classified, K90.4
Feeding difficulties, R63.3	Torsion of testis, unspecified, N44.00

1. Inappropriate feeding: Assess infant's intake by history.
2. Milk protein intolerance or allergy: Usually associated with vomiting/ diarrhea. May have history of hematochezia.
3. Constipation: Hard or dry stools regardless of frequency.
4. Incarcerated hernia.
5. Parental stress tension, poor coping.
6. Testicular torsion: Testis tender, cord thickened/shortened.
7. Gastroesophageal reflux (GER).

H. Treatment.
1. Consider 2-week trial of hypoallergenic formula or removing cow's milk protein from breastfeeding mother's diet. Avoid sorbitol-containing fruit juices.
2. Encourage continued breastfeeding; trial of caffeine elimination from mother's diet.
3. Swaddling of infant, rhythmic movement, gentle massage, warm baths.
4. "White noise" such as soft music.
5. Avoid overstimulation. Avoid exposure to tobacco smoke.
6. Counsel parents: Alleviate guilt about cause of colic, need for respite. Reassure them: Infant is not in pain. Acknowledge importance of problem, discuss prognosis.

I. Follow-up.
1. Frequent clinic and/or telephone Follow-up may be necessary to assess any formula changes, parental coping skills.
2. Plan to see baby 2 weeks after initial diagnosis.

J. Complications.
1. Poor parental coping skills.
2. Disruption of maternal–infant relationship.
3. Child abuse.

K. Education.
1. Discuss normal crying patterns. Infants cry more in first 3 months of life than at any other time. Crying increases at 2 weeks and usually peaks in second month, with gradual decline thereafter. Pattern of crying different in all babies.

2. Explain that taut/distended abdomen and flatus are probably result of, not cause of, crying. Reassure them that infant not in pain.
3. Alleviate parental guilt and discuss range of emotions may be experiencing.
4. Stress need for respite: Suggest parents leave baby with reliable caregiver for a few hours. Infant may sense tension in parents if do not allow themselves a break.
5. Trial a of hypoallergenic formula may be indicated, but multiple formula changes are not warranted and should be discouraged. There is minimal, if any, evidence that lactose intolerance plays a role.

IV. CONSTIPATION

Child sexual abuse, suspected, initial encounter, T76.22XA	Malabsorption due to intolerance, not elsewhere classified, K90.4
Constipation, K59.0	Nutritional deficiency, unspecified, E63.9
Cystic fibrosis, E84	
Ectopic anus, Q43.5	Obesity, E66
Hirschsprung's disease, Q43.1	Protein-calorie malnutrition, unspecified, E46
Hypercalcemia, E83.52	
Hypothyroidism, unspecified, E03.9	Stenosis of anus and rectum, K62.4

A. Delayed or difficult defecation for 2 weeks; passage of hard and/or dry stools.
B. Etiology.
   1. Functional: Most common, no underlying pathology.
      a. Diet low in fiber/fluids; sudden change in diet (e.g., formula/breast to cow's milk).
      b. Lack of exercise, obesity.
      c. Stool withholding secondary to painful defecation ("pain-retention cycle").
      d. Family history.
   2. Outlet dysfunction: Hirschsprung's disease, anterior ectopic anus, tethered spinal cord (secondary to occult spinal dysraphism), anal stenosis.
   3. Metabolic/GI: Celiac disease, hypothyroidism, hypercalcemia.
   4. Other: Cystic fibrosis, malnutrition, sexual abuse, cow's milk protein intolerance (infants), medications (e.g., narcotics).
C. Occurrence.
   1. Accounts for about 3% of visits to general pediatrics, 25% to pediatric gastroenterology.

D. Clinical manifestations.
1. Hard bowel movements (BMs), usually infrequent. May be dry, small (incomplete evacuation).
   a. Size, consistency, frequency of BMs: Ask when change in stool became apparent.
   b. Stool-withholding symptoms (hides for BM, crosses legs, dances around).
   c. Blood associated with stool.
   d. Fecal soiling in underwear of previously toilet-trained child.
   e. Did child pass meconium within first 48 hours of life?
   f. What treatments have been instituted thus far?
2. Associated symptoms: Abdominal pain/distention, poor appetite, irritability.
3. Other important questions: Diet history, any changes? Child on any medications? Child toilet trained? Any possibility of sexual abuse?
E. Physical findings.
1. Height/weight: Plot on growth curve.
2. Complete physical exam with attention to:
   a. Abdomen: Assess for fecal masses, particularly in lower quadrants. Assess for distention, tenderness.
   b. Anus: Assess for placement, fissures, erythema. Digital exam to assess anal tone, quality of stool present. Observe for soiling at anal opening.
   c. Lower back: Assess for tuft of hair over lumbar sacral area or deep sacral dimple above gluteal crease. Assess for deviated gluteal crease.
   d. Assess muscle tone throughout, deep tendon reflexes (DTRs).
F. Diagnostic tests.
1. Testing not usually necessary.
2. Abdominal flat-plate X-ray to assess fecal load only if diagnosis is in question/to tailor disimpaction. Avoid X-rays when possible.
3. X-ray of lumbar/sacral (L/S) spine: Assess for occult spinal dysraphism if abnormality on L/S spine area and/or history of lower extremity weakness. If abnormal: MRI.
4. Labs only if red flags in history/physical exam: Serum electrolytes, calcium, lead level, thyroid function (TSH, free T4). Celiac screen (total serum IgA and tissue transglutaminase IgA) and sweat test if poor growth.
5. Unprepped barium enema: If history of delayed passage of meconium, to assess for transition zone associated with Hirschsprung's disease. This can miss short-segment Hirschsprung's in older infants and children.

G. Differential diagnosis.

Child sexual abuse, suspected, initial encounter, T76.22XA	Malabsorption due to intolerance, not elsewhere classified, K90.4
Constipation, K59.0	Nonorganic encopresis, F98.1
Ectopic anus, Q43.5	Other constipation, K59.09
Hirschsprung's disease, Q43.1	Stenosis of anus and rectum, K62.4

1. Vast majority have functional constipation, diagnosis by history and physical exam.
2. Infant dyschezia (functional): At least 10 minutes of crying and straining before passage of soft stools in healthy infant younger than 6 months of age. Reassure, self-limited.
3. Encopresis: Constipation with fecal soiling.
4. Hirschsprung's disease: Absence of ganglion nerve cells in colon to varying degrees. Usually have history of delayed passage of meconium ($>$ 48 hours after birth). May have thin caliber stools, abdominal distention, failure to thrive. No stool in rectal vault on digital exam.
5. Structural: Anterior ectopic anus, anal stenosis.
6. Sexual abuse.
7. Side effect of drugs such as narcotics.
8. Cow's milk protein intolerance: Anal irritation/fissures, subsequent stool retention.

H. Treatment.
1. Stool softeners: Most children will benefit from stool softener as first-line treatment. May be needed for longer than 2 weeks.
   a. Lactulose/sorbitol: 1 mL/kg/dose bid, maximum 30 mL bid. Must be ingested quickly. May mix in beverage. Good choice for infants who don't respond to dietary management. May cause gassiness.
   b. Polyethylene glycol/PEG 3350 (Miralax, Glycolax): Starting dose of 0.4 grams/kg/day. Adjust dose according to clinical response. Stir powder well to dissolve; excellent palatability and acceptance. Titrate dose to achieve soft stools.
   c. Mineral oil: Never give to infants younger than 1 year or patients at risk for aspiration (e.g., neurologically impaired). Difficult to regulate dose, start with 1–3 mL/kg/day, totaling no more than 90 mL/day. Rarely used.
   d. Milk of magnesia: 1–3 mL/kg/day (400 mg/5mL). Avoid in infants. For children 2–5 years: 0.4–1.2 grams/day; 6–11 years: 1.2–2.4 grams/day; 12–18 years: 2.4–4.8 grams/day divided 1–2 times/day.

2. Laxatives/cathartics: Used for disimpaction only, usually over period of 1–3 days.
   a. Magnesium citrate: Older than 2 years: < 6 years: 2–4 ml/kg/day; 6–12 years: 100–150 ml/day; ≥ 12 years: 120–300 ml/day.
   b. Senna: 2–6 years: 2.5–5 mg, 1–2 times/day; 6–12 years: 7.5–10 mg/day.
   c. Bisacodyl: 3–10 years: 5 mg/day; > 10 years: 5–10 mg/day.
3. Enemas/suppositories: For disimpaction only, over 1–3 days.
   a. Glycerin suppository: For children younger than 2 years.
   b. Bisacodyl suppository: Older than 2 years: 0.5–1 suppository/day.
   c. Pediatric fleet enema: Older than 2 years: 1–2 times/day for 1–3 days.
4. A normal fiber diet is recommended in children with constipation: AAP recommends age + 5 g fiber/day. Infants: Prune or pear juice good choice for stool softening. Evidence does not support the use of fiber supplements and extra fluid intake in functional constipation.
5. Toilet training, not yet trained: Delay until constipation resolved. Trained: Encourage scheduled time on toilet bid following meal, for 5–10 minutes. Provide footstool.
6. Positive reinforcement for toilet sitting, successful passage of stool.

I. Follow-up.
   1. Close telephone contact after disimpaction, to monitor response to stool softeners.
   2. Refer to pediatric gastroenterology if patient unresponsive to treatment, red flags in history, or abnormal test results.
   3. Refer to pediatric surgery if Hirschsprung's disease/anal abnormalities concerns.

J. Complications.

Anal fissure, unspecified, K60.2

Nonorganic encopresis, F98.1

---

1. Encopresis.
2. Anal fissure (treat with stool-softening agents, diet, topical cream, e.g., Anusol).
3. Delayed toilet training.

K. Education.
   1. Reassure family if history and physical consistent with functional constipation. Explain pain-retention cycle.
   2. Reassure that stool softeners are not habit forming and are necessary part of breaking pain-retention cycle. Stool softeners are often given daily for a minimum of several weeks.

3. Parents may report child unable to have BM despite effort; explain that what appears to be straining may be child's attempt to withhold stool to avoid pain.
4. Avoid chronic use of laxatives, enemas, suppositories.
5. School-age children frequently avoid using bathroom at school for BM.
6. Explain normal defecation patterns: Not necessary to have BM every day; goal is passage of soft, comfortable stools in good quantities.
7. Instruct family to call if soiling occurs or if child not responding to treatment.

V. DIARRHEA, ACUTE

Diarrhea, unspecified, R19.7

A. Noticeable or sudden increase in frequency and fluid content of stools; usually infectious, self-limited lasting less than 3 weeks. Diarrhea is a symptom, can result from disorders involving digestive, absorptive, secretory functions of intestine.
B. Etiology.
   1. Infectious: Intestinal.
      a. Viral: Rotavirus, adenovirus, Norwalk.
      b. Bacterial: Salmonella, shigella, *Clostridium difficile*, *Escherichia coli* 0157:H7.
      c. Parasite: Giardia, cryptosporidium.
   2. Infectious: Outside GI tract: May be concurrent symptom of systemic illness.
   3. Dietary, medications, toxic ingestion.
   4. Other: Intussusception, hemolytic uremic syndrome (HUS), appendicitis, UTI.
C. Occurrence.
   1. Common symptom in children.
   2. Most commonly caused by infection in older infants/children.
   3. Dietary changes or indiscretions common in early infancy.
D. Clinical manifestations.
   1. Increased frequency, fluid content of stools.
      a. Frequency, consistency of diarrhea?
      b. Hematochezia, melena, mucus, or pus in stool.
      c. Any fecal incontinence in toilet-trained child?
      d. Anyone else in family/school or daycare have diarrhea?

2. Possible associated symptoms: Abdominal pain or cramping, fever, vomiting.
3. Systemic illness: Are there signs of illness outside the GI tract?
4. Medication history: Recent antibiotics? OTC diarrhea remedies? Others?
5. Travel history.
6. Toxic ingestions?
7. Complete diet history: Type, quantity of fluids; appetite; new/contaminated foods.
8. Urine output.

E. Physical findings.
1. Height, weight, temperature, vital signs.
2. Complete physical exam with attention to following:
   a. Abdomen: Assess bowel sounds, tenderness, organomegaly, masses, distention.
   b. Rectal: Observe for stool around anus, erythema, fissures.
3. Assess hydration: Activity level, irritability; degree of thirst; degree of dehydration (**Table 27-1**) and signs/symptoms of dehydration (**Table 27-2**).

F. Diagnostic tests.
1. If patient appears nontoxic, mild/no dehydration: None; most episodes isonatremic.
2. Moderate to severe dehydration: Serum electrolytes.
3. Test stool for occult blood (**Table 27-3**).
4. When testing for *C. difficile*, ask for *C. difficile* toxin B PCR.
5. Not usually necessary to check for parasites unless diarrhea becomes chronic.
6. Test for rotavirus in stool if infant has moderate to severe symptoms.
7. Stool for *E. coli* 0157:H7 is ordered separately.
8. Stool culture in febrile children with bloody diarrhea, check for *C. difficile* if recent antibiotic use.

Table 27-1 Assessment of Degree of Dehydration

	Mild	Moderate	Severe
Infant	5	10	15
Adolescent	3	6	9
Infant/young children	Thirsty, alert, possibly restless	Thirsty, restless, or lethargic	Drowsy, limp, cold, sweaty
Older child	Thirsty, alert, restless	Thirsty, usually alert	Usually apprehensive, cold, sweaty

Table 27-2 Signs and Symptoms of Dehydration

	Mild	Moderate	Severe
Tachycardia	−	+	+
Palpable pulses	Normal	Weak	Decreased
Blood pressure	Normal	Orthostatic hypotension	Hypotension
Skin turgor	Normal	Slight decreased	Decreased
Mucous membranes	Moist	Dry	Dry
Fontanel	Normal	Normal to slightly depressed	Sunken
Urine output	Normal	Decreased	Oliguria, anuria
Tears	+	+/−	Absent

Abbreviations: +, present; +/−, may or may not be present; −, not present.

Table 27-3 Diagnostic Testing for Diarrhea

Symptom	Stool C&S	Stool C. difficile	Stool O&P/giardia Serum electrolytes	CBC w/ diff
Well appearance	−	−	−	−	−
Toxic	+	−	−	+	+
Melena, K92.1	+	+	−	−	+
Blood in stool, history of antibiotics	+	+	−	−	+
Abnormal weight loss, R63.4	−	−	−	+	+

Abbreviations: −, not present; +, present; +/−, may or may not be present; C&S, culture and sensitivity; CBC, complete blood count; diff, differential; O&P, ova and parasite.

G. Differential diagnosis.

Acute gastroenteropathy due to Norwalk agent, A08.11	Giardiasis [lambliasis], A07.1
Adenoviral enteritis, A08.2	Other specified intestinal infections, A08.8
Allergic and dietetic gastroenteritis and colitis, K52.2	Poisoning by unspecified systemic antibiotic,
Bacterial intestinal infection, unspecified, A04.9	accidental (unintentional), initial encounter, T36.91XA
Cryptosporidiosis, A07.2	Rotaviral enteritis, A08.0
Diarrhea, unspecified, R19.7	Salmonella infection, unspecified, A02.9
Enterocolitis due to *Clostridium difficile*, A04.7	Shigellosis, unspecified, A03.9
Escherichia coli [E. coli] as the cause of diseases classified to other chapters, B96.2	Toxic gastroenteritis and colitis, K52.1

1. Viral: Most common GI infectious cause: Rotavirus, adenovirus, Norwalk.
2. Bacterial.
   a. Salmonella: Foodborne. Most resolve in 5–7 days without treatment. Fever, diarrhea +/− blood, abdominal cramping for 4–7 days.
   b. Shigella: Foodborne, usually during warmer months. Sudden high fever, abdominal cramps, nausea, vomiting, diarrhea with blood, mucus, pus. Usually self-limited. Dehydration common.
   c. Enterotoxigenic *Escherichia coli* (ETEC): Bloody diarrhea. Most common form of traveler's diarrhea. *E. coli* 0157:H7 is the toxin-producing strain and the cause of most cases of HUS.
   d. *C. difficile*: Found frequently in stool of healthy infants, role as etiologic agent in these cases controversial. In pathologic cases, diarrhea can occur within days or up to 8 weeks after antibiotic use or any drugs that alter GI flora. Watery diarrhea, +/− blood. Fecal–oral route. Common in hospitals.
3. Parasitic.
   a. Giardia: Waterborne, foodborne. Diarrhea, bloating, abdominal cramping, nausea. Temporary lactase deficiency. Often self-limited. Outbreaks can occur in daycare and long-term care facilities.
   b. Cryptosporidium: Mild diarrhea, usually self-limited.
4. Dietary.
   a. Increase in fluids with high osmotic load: Fruit juices, sports drinks, or any sugared beverages can cause temporary osmotic diarrhea in otherwise healthy infant/child.
   b. Introduction of new food: Possible allergic response.

    5. Antibiotic induced.

    6. Toxic ingestions.

    7. Systemic illness: May have history of upper respiratory infection (URI) or other illness.

H. Treatment.

    1. Viral: Self-limited, supportive care (see rehydration guidelines below).

    2. Bacterial.

       a. Salmonella: Supportive.

       b. Shigella: Supportive, can be self-limited. Antimicrobial treatment for children in hospitals, daycare centers, institutions, and those with severe symptoms. Antibiotic resistance increasing: Consult health department or MD for selection of appropriate antibiotic in your community.

       c. *E. coli* 0157:H7: Supportive.

       d. *C. difficile*: Metronidazole (20–30 mg/kg/day divided tid for 10–14 days) oral.

    3. Parasite.

       a. Giardia: Metronidazole (5–10 mg/kg/dose tid for 7–10 days) or nitazoxanide (Alinia) for children 1–11 years; 12–47 months: 5 mL (100 mg) bid for 3 days; 4–11 years: 10 mL bid for 3 days; 12 and older: 500 mg (1 tab) bid for 3 days, oral.

       b. Cryptosporidium: Supportive in immunocompetent patients; if therapy required: Nitazoxanide.

    4. Rehydration.

       a. Mild dehydration: Oral replacement solution (ORS) 50 mL/kg (5 teaspoons/pound) over 4 hours. Once repletion completed, ORS continued for ongoing diarrhea losses.

       b. Moderate dehydration: ORS 100 mL/kg + replacement of stool losses over 4 hours, reassess hourly.

       c. Severe dehydration: IV fluid: Normal saline (0.9% saline); consult MD; transfer to tertiary care facility.

       d. No dehydration: Continue to feed age-appropriate diet, including milk.

    5. Dietary.

       a. Remove possible offending/allergenic foods.

       b. No fruit juice, sports drinks, other sugared beverages.

       c. Feed full diet: Restricting food deprives gut of nutrients needed for healing.

       d. Continue to breast/formula feed, can alternate with ORS.

       e. Eliminate dairy only if known giardia infection or if symptoms severe.

       f. With dehydrated patient: Refeed age-appropriate diet as soon as rehydrated.

    6. Antidiarrheal medication/bismuth: Avoid; not advised for children.

I. Follow-up.
   1. Telephone: Instruct parent to call and arrange for immediate clinic visit if not improving, new symptoms develop, signs of dehydration.
   2. Return to clinic next day with mild–moderate dehydration.
   3. Referral to MD or local ED for moderate–severe dehydration or lack of response to treatment.
   4. Repeat stool studies after treatment for *C. difficile*, giardia if symptoms persist.
J. Complications.

Diarrhea, unspecified, R19.7	Protein-calorie malnutrition,
Escherichia coli [E. coli] as the cause of	unspecified, E46
diseases classified to other chapters, B96.2	Shigellosis, unspecified, A03.9
Hemolytic-uremic syndrome, D59.3	Volume depletion, E86

   1. Dehydration, malnutrition.
   2. Chronic diarrhea may develop, especially if restricted diet/inappropriate fluids.
   3. Hemolytic uremic syndrome (*E. coli*), bacteremia (shigella).
K. Education.
   1. Reassure: Most cases viral, self-limited.
   2. Review proper hygiene, handwashing techniques, handling of soiled objects. Alcohol-based hand sanitizers are not effective for *C. difficile*.
   3. Review dehydration signs/symptoms: Instruct parent when to call.
   4. Review dietary instructions: Explain that restricting diet may prolong diarrhea. Appropriate beverage selection essential.
   5. Skin care: Prevent diaper rash with effective barrier ointment.

VI. ENCOPRESIS

Abdominal and pelvic pain, R10	Child sexual abuse, suspected, initial
Abdominal distension (gaseous), R14.0	encounter, T76.22XA
Anorexia, R63.0	Nonorganic encopresis, F98.1

A. Fecal incontinence in clothing usually after toilet training completed. Vast majority caused by chronic, functional constipation (retentive encopresis).
B. Etiology.
   1. Chronic, functional constipation. Stool accumulates in rectum, which subsequently leaks out through anus. Soiling is not volitional/intentional.

2. Underlying pathology is rare: Tethered spinal cord (secondary to occult spinal dysraphism), prior anal–rectal surgery, Hirschsprung's disease, ectopic anus.

C. Occurrence.

1. Stool incontinence, usually during day, of varying quantities.
2. Soiling often has soft consistency, and parents misinterpret this as diarrhea, child "can't make it to the bathroom in time."
3. Parents commonly believe this is volitional or result of laziness.
4. Important questions to ask:
   a. Age of toilet training? Was process difficult?
   b. Frequency, consistency, size/amount of BM on toilet. Any blood? What time of day does it usually occur?
   c. Does child hide soiled clothing?
   d. How has family dealt with problem?
5. Associated symptoms may include abdominal pain, abdominal distention, poor appetite, school avoidance.
6. Ask about history of UTI and enuresis.
7. Any possibility of sexual abuse?

D. Clinical manifestations.

1. Common pediatric problem: Boys affected more than girls.

E. Physical findings.

1. Abdomen may appear distended or full. Dull on percussion. Stool may be palpable in lower quadrants (smooth, movable mass).
2. Anus may appear erythematous with stool around exterior. Observe for fissures. Digital exam may reveal decreased tone, copious stool in vault of varying consistency. Check for position of anus, anal wink.
3. Assess back for signs of occult spinal dysraphism: Sacral dimple or hair tuft above gluteal crease, deviated gluteal crease.
4. Assess muscle tone throughout, DTRs.

F. Diagnostic tests.

1. Rarely necessary.
2. Abdominal flat-plate X-ray can be useful to assess fecal load, tailor disimpaction. However, good physical exam and history often eliminates need for X-ray.
3. MRI of lumbosacral spine if concern for tethered spinal cord.

G. Differential diagnosis.

Constipation, K59.0	Nonorganic encopresis, F98.1
Dorsopathy, unspecified, M53.9	Nonorganic enuresis, F98.0

       1. Majority of cases are from functional constipation.

       2. Tethered spinal cord: Can result in both fecal and urinary incontinence.

H. Treatment.

       1. All children with encopresis must first start with disimpaction ("clean out"). Soiling will not resolve without this. Depending on amount of stool on X-ray exam, can give oral cathartics at bedtime for 1–3 nights in row and up to 1 Fleet enema bid for 1–3 days in row.

       2. After clean out, child immediately starts daily stool softening.

       3. Keep track of BMs, soiling episodes on calendar.

       4. High-fiber diet.

       5. Toilet retraining: Child to sit on toilet after meals 2–3 times/day, work up to 5–10 minutes. Provide footstool. Ask child to "try" to have BM, to "practice," not expected to produce BM each time.

       6. Positive reinforcement only. No punishment for soiling. Soiling should be cleaned up swiftly with child's assistance and little attention paid to it.

       7. Education of the underlying pathophysiology is essential for treatment.

I. Follow-up.

       1. Encourage telephone contact. If continues to soil, may need further clean out.

       2. Follow up in clinic about 1 month after diagnosis.

       3. May need abdominal X-ray if results of clean out are in doubt.

       4. Referral if patient not responding to treatment once compliance has been assured.

J. Complications.

Nonorganic enuresis, F98.0

Urinary tract infection, site not specified, N39.0

       1. Low self-esteem/shame.

       2. Child abuse.

       3. School avoidance.

       4. UTI (due to proximity of stool in clothing to urinary tract).

       5. Enuresis.

K. Education.

       1. Stress to parents that child has not had control over soiling episodes.

       2. Relieve parental guilt over prior negative reinforcement.

       3. Explain to parent and child why soiling occurs, discuss normal defecation.

       4. Treatment will take at least 6 months. Parents are advised to be diligent about daily stool softening, toilet training during this time.

       5. Reassure about functional nature of chronic constipation.

       6. Advise parent to speak with school about problem so child will have better access to restroom at school, may need to provide written request.

VII. GASTROESOPHAGEAL REFLUX DISEASE (GERD)

Gastroesophageal reflux disease without esophagitis, K21.9

A. Passive passage of stomach contents into esophagus. GER is a normal physiologic process that can occur in healthy individuals. GERD refers to pathologic degree of GER, causing symptoms.

B. Etiology.
   1. Infants (up to 18 months).
      a. Very common in infants, may be result of immaturity of lower esophageal sphincter (LES).
      b. Position of LES and feeding techniques may induce GER.
      c. GERD probably multifactorial.
   2. Children/adolescents.
      a. Probably multifactorial, exact cause not known.
      b. May be malfunctioning LES: Inappropriate relaxation.
      c. Environmental/dietary influences may induce GER.

C. Occurrence.
   1. About 50% of infants have recurrent vomiting in first 3 months, 67% of 4-month-olds, 5% of 10- to 12-month-olds.
   2. Increased incidence among premature babies, neurologically impaired children.

D. Clinical manifestations.
   1. Infants: Recurrent vomiting, regurgitation ("spit up"); usually effortless.
   2. Important questions to ask for affected infants:
      a. Type, quantity, frequency of feedings? How positioned during, after feeding?
      b. Quality, quantity, timing of emesis? Does baby cry/grimace with emesis?
      c. History of apnea?
   3. Children: Regurgitation (reswallowed/spit up), possible vomiting, nausea, epigastric abdominal pain. Pain may be poorly localized. Can have any/all of these symptoms.
   4. Important questions to ask for affected children:
      a. Frequency, timing of symptoms, including regurgitation with/ without emesis.
      b. Abdominal pain: Location, timing, frequency, quality.
      c. Any specific foods that provoke symptoms?
      d. Complete diet history, including type and amount of beverages.
      e. Any dysphagia, food lodging, chronic throat clearing, dental decay?

    5. For all age groups:

       a. History of hematemesis, melena, asthma, recurrent pneumonia, otitis media, sinusitis?

       b. Any decrease in appetite, poor weight gain, weight loss?

E. Physical findings.

    1. Height, weight: Plot on growth curve.

    2. Full physical exam with attention to following:

       a. Abdomen: Assess for tenderness, particularly over epigastrium.

       b. Rectal exam: Obtain stool to test for occult blood.

       c. Mouth: Assess for dental caries, enamel erosion.

F. Diagnostic tests.

    1. Upper GI series: Only to rule out anatomic abnormalities. Not used to make diagnosis of GERD. Presence of GER on upper GI is common in all people. Must order in infants if forceful vomiting; in older children with frank vomiting, dysphagia.

    2. Stool for occult blood: If positive, may indicate esophagitis.

    3. Other tests by pediatric GI specialist if referral necessary (endoscopy, pH probe).

G. Differential diagnosis.

Adult hypertrophic pyloric stenosis, K31.1	Gastroesophageal reflux disease without esophagitis, K21.9
Gastritis, unspecified, without bleeding, K29.70	Polyphagia, R63.2

    1. GER: Normal physiologic event. Infants with regurgitation who are otherwise well, growing normally, without pain.

    2. GERD: Infants who, in addition to emesis, have irritability during feeds, poor feeding/growth, recurrent lung problems. May be related to apnea. May have one or all of these symptoms. Recurrent GER symptoms in children older than 18 months is almost always considered pathologic (GERD).

    3. Overfeeding; cow's milk protein allergy.

    4. Pyloric stenosis.

    5. Gastritis.

H. Treatment.

    1. Conservative management, infants: For GER, as adjunct to medical therapy in GERD:

       a. Smaller, more frequent feedings. Increase burping opportunities.

       b. Hold upright after feeds; do not place infant in car seat after feedings.

    c. Consider change to commercially available prethickened formula (Enfamil AR). Consider 2-week trial of extensively hydrolyzed infant formula (hypoallergenic).

    d. Can add 1 teaspoon/ounce of cereal to bottle. Cross-cut nipple for easier flow.

    e. Elevate head of crib mattress. No extra bedding in crib. No prone positioning.

2. Conservative management, children: Essential component along with medications.

    a. Smaller, more frequent meals. No skipping meals.

    b. Avoid caffeine, carbonated drinks; fatty, fried foods; citrus; chocolate; peppermint.

    c. Avoid or correct obesity.

    d. Avoid tobacco and alcohol.

    e. Elevate head of bed; no eating within 2 hours of bedtime.

3. Medical management.

    a. Histamine-2 blockers (H2 blockers): Ranitidine (Zantac), famotidine (Pepcid).

    b. Proton pump inhibitors (PPI): Can try after 2-week trial of H2 blockers if no response. Must give about 30 minutes before breakfast, do not skip meal.

      • Lansoprazole (Prevacid): Approved for use in children.

      • Omeprazole (Prilosec).

      • OTC antacids: Not for long-term use. Only for temporary relief.

4. Surgery: Fundoplication. Reserved for severe GERD that failed medical management.

I. Follow-up.

1. Telephone contact after 2 weeks on H2 blocker or PPI.

2. Return to clinic for increased symptoms, new symptoms.

3. Refer to pediatric GI specialist if symptoms severe/no response to initial treatments, lifestyle changes.

J. Complications.

Acute serous otitis media, H65.0	Failure to thrive (child), R62.51
Chronic sinusitis, unspecified, J32.9	Nutritional deficiency, unspecified, E63.9
Esophagitis, unspecified, K20.9	Pneumonitis due to inhalation of food and vomit, J69.0

1. Esophagitis, stricture formation.
2. Failure to thrive, nutritional deficits.
3. Recurrent aspiration pneumonia.
4. May be related to recurrent otitis media, sinusitis.

K. Education.
1. In otherwise healthy infant with normal growth, reassure parent: GER is common, most outgrow by first birthday.
2. Children: Prognosis usually very good but unlikely to "outgrow."
3. Take medication exactly as prescribed. If helpful, medicate minimum of 2 months before discontinuing or stepping down therapy from PPI to H2 blocker.
4. Nutritional guidance: Avoid overfeeding, review all dietary restrictions/ history at each visit.

VIII. HERNIA, INGUINAL

Abdominal distension (gaseous), R14.0	Unilateral inguinal hernia, without obstruction or gangrene, not specified as recurrent, K40.90
Abdominal tenderness, unspecified site, R10.819	
Intra-abdominal and pelvic swelling, mass and lump, unspecified site, R19.00	Vomiting, unspecified, R11.10

A. Protrusion of abdominal organ, usually bowel, into inguinal canal.
B. Etiology.
1. Indirect: Bowel protrudes through deep inguinal ring through inguinal canal lateral to inferior epigastric artery.
2. Direct: Bowel protrudes between interior epigastric artery and edge of rectus muscle.
3. Incarcerated: Hernia that cannot be returned or reduced by manipulation. Can become strangulated.
C. Occurrence.
1. Most common surgical condition in children.
2. 60% are on right side; left 30%; bilateral 10%.
3. Most common type is indirect (approximately 99%).
4. Approximately 50% present before 1 year of age, most seen in first 6 months.
5. Ratio of boys to girls, 4:1. Incidence approximately 10–20 in every 1000 live births.
6. Higher incidence in premature babies, positive family history, cystic fibrosis, undescended testes, hypospadias, congenital dislocation of hip, and congenital abdominal wall defects.

D. Clinical manifestations.
1. Bulge in inguinal region may extend to scrotum. Especially noticeable during crying/straining.
2. History of intermittent groin, labial/scrotal swelling.
3. Parents are usually first to notice.
4. Hernia reduces spontaneously when relaxed/sleeping.
5. Important questions to ask:
   a. When was swelling/bulge first noticed? How often/when does it occur?
   b. Does infant/child appear uncomfortable with it?
   c. Any signs of intestinal obstruction such as vomiting, abdominal distention?
E. Physical findings.
1. Bulge at level of internal/external ring.
2. Scrotal/labial swelling.
3. Do not place finger in inguinal canal, done only for adult hernia exam.
4. In supine position, with legs and arms extended over head: Wait for cry, which will increase intra-abdominal pressure. Should demonstrate bulge over external ring/scrotal swelling.
5. Have older children stand.
6. Palpate testes before palpation of inguinal bulge (retractile testes are common in infants and young children, can be mistaken for hernia).
7. Abdominal exam: Assess for distention, masses, tenderness.
8. If swelling not apparent during exam, check for thickening of spermatic cord (silk sign) by palpating spermatic cord over pubic tubercle. Rubbing together area feels like silk.
F. Diagnostic tests.
1. All girls with inguinal hernia should have rectal exam by experienced examiner; may need to order pelvic ultrasound.
2. Diagnosis otherwise made by history and physical exam.
G. Differential diagnosis.

Hydrocele, unspecified, N43.3

Unilateral inguinal hernia, with obstruction, without gangrene, not specified as recurrent, K40.30

---

1. Inguinal hernia: Scrotal swelling varies during day, increase in size with crying/straining.
2. Incarcerated inguinal hernia: Usually associated with discomfort, positive/negative abdominal distention. Bulge persists.

3. Hydrocele: Circumscribed fluid collection in scrotum; swelling does not change in size throughout day, gradually disappears over first year of life. Transillumination of scrotum cannot distinguish between hydrocele, inguinal hernia.

H. Treatment.

1. Surgery: Inguinal hernia does not resolve spontaneously, surgery usually elective shortly after diagnosis.

2. Supports/trusses are not indicated, may be hazardous.

I. Follow-up.

1. Referral to pediatric surgeon when diagnosis of inguinal hernia made.

J. Complications.

Abdominal hernia with obstruction, without gangrene, unspecified, K46.0	Unilateral inguinal hernia, with obstruction, without gangrene, not specified as recurrent, K40.30
Other noninflammatory disorders of ovary, fallopian tube, and broad ligament, N83.8	Vascular disorders of male genital organs, N50.1

1. Incarcerated hernia: Immediate referral for reduction under sedation.

2. Strangulated incarcerated hernia: Blood supply compromised: Surgical emergency.

3. Ischemia/infarction of testis: Can occur in boys with undescended testicles, inguinal hernia.

4. Ovary/fallopian tube infarction.

K. Education.

1. Uncomplicated indirect inguinal hernia: Review signs, symptoms of incarcerated/strangulated hernia with family: Abdominal distention, vomiting, pain, persistent bulge that does not reduce.

2. Family understands importance of following through with surgical appointments.

3. Operative repair necessary within first year of life due to increased incidence of incarceration after that time.

IX. HERNIA, UMBILICAL

Abdominal and pelvic pain, R10	Umbilical hernia without obstruction or gangrene, K42.9
Abdominal distension (gaseous), R14.0	

A. Protrusion of part of intestine at umbilicus; defect is at abdominal wall, protruding bowel covered with skin, subcutaneous tissue.

B. Etiology.
   1. Due to weakness/incomplete closure of umbilical ring.

C. Occurrence.
   1. Increased incidence among African American infants, low-birth-weight infants, females.

D. Clinical manifestations.
   1. Soft mass covered by skin that protrudes from umbilicus, usually with increased intra-abdominal pressure (crying/straining) or may be more persistent (ask parent about fluctuations in mass size/presence).
   2. Size of defect varies from 1 cm in diameter to 5 cm.
   3. Usually disappears spontaneously by 1 year of age. Larger hernias may resolve spontaneously by 5–6 years of age unless defect 2 cm.

E. Physical findings.
   1. Examine infant in supine position.
   2. Abdomen will reveal soft protrusion through umbilicus, usually easy to reduce through fibrous umbilical ring. Assess for abdominal distention.
   3. Increased size may be visible with crying. Observe for signs of pain.

F. Diagnostic tests.
   1. None.

G. Differential diagnosis.

Umbilical hernia with obstruction, without gangrene, K42.0

---

   1. Strangulated umbilical hernia (very rare): May show signs of intestinal obstruction such as pain, vomiting, persistent umbilical bulge that will not reduce.

H. Treatment.
   1. Most resolve spontaneously.
   2. Surgery reserved for hernias after 3–4 years of age, those causing symptoms (become strangulated), those becoming progressively larger after 1–2 years of age.

I. Follow-up.
   1. Assess hernia routinely at all visits. Immediate return if signs of incarceration.

J. Complications.

Umbilical hernia with obstruction, without gangrene, K42.0

---

   1. Incarceration: Very rare.

K. Education.
1. Instruct parent not to tape or bind umbilicus and on signs, symptoms of incarceration.
2. Reassure most resolve spontaneously.

X. INTUSSUSCEPTION

Abdominal and pelvic pain, R10	Other fatigue, R53.83
Intussusception, K56.1	Shock, unspecified, R57.9
Melena, K92.1	Vomiting, unspecified, R11.10

A. Prolapse or "telescoping" of one part of intestine into lumen of adjoining intestine.
B. Etiology.
1. Can follow infections such as gastroenteritis, otitis media, URI, adenovirus.
2. About 10% have "lead point" such as Meckel's diverticulum, polyp, duplication.
3. May be alteration in intestinal peristalsis that provokes condition.
C. Occurrence.
1. Most common cause of intestinal obstruction 3 months to 6 years of age.
2. 60% occur in infants younger than 1 year, 80% by 2 years. Rare in neonates.
3. Incidence 1–4 in every 1000 live births.
4. Male-to-female ratio is 4:1.
5. Peaks in spring and fall.
D. Clinical manifestations.
1. Sudden onset severe abdominal pain, usually periumbilical/lower abdomen, in previously well child.
2. Pain colicky, paroxysmal occurring at frequent intervals.
3. Child may appear well between episodes of pain at first.
4. During pain, child flexes legs, pulls knees toward abdomen, cries.
5. Vomiting common.
6. Stools may appear normal in first few hours, after which little or no stool.
7. Blood per rectum can occur within first 12 hours or up to 2 days after symptoms start. May be mixed with mucus described as "currant jelly stool."
8. If symptoms unrecognized, may progress to lethargy, bilious vomiting, shock.

E. Physical findings.
1. Weight, temperature, vital signs.
2. Assess overall affect and activity level, observe during pain episode.
3. Abdomen may be distended. Guarding during exam if having pain. About 70% may have palpable, ill-defined ("sausage-shaped") mass, may be mildly tender.
4. Rectal exam may reveal bloody mucus.
F. Diagnostic tests.
1. Diagnosis usually made by history and physical exam.
2. Barium enema: May show filling defect.
3. Abdominal ultrasound can also detect intussusception.
G. Differential diagnosis.

Allergic purpura, D69.0

Meckel's diverticulum (displaced, hypertrophic), Q43.0

Noninfective gastroenteritis and colitis, unspecified, K52.9

---

1. Gastroenteritis.
2. Meckel's diverticulum: Painless, rectal bleeding from congenital appendage of ileum.
3. Henoch-Schönlein purpura: Associated with joint symptoms, purpura rash.
H. Treatment.
1. Barium enema: Hydrostatic/"air contrast" used to diagnose, treat intussusception.
2. Untreated, condition almost always fatal.
3. 10% recurrence rate after reduction by barium enema.
4. Intussusception secondary to "lead point" from Meckel's diverticulum or polyp requires surgery.
I. Follow-up.
1. Immediate referral to tertiary care facility.
2. Telephone or clinic follow-up after reduction.
J. Complications.

Volume depletion, E86

---

1. Dehydration, bowel necrosis, death.
K. Education.
1. Reassure parent that vast majority of cases have no specific lead point and are successfully treated with barium enema.
2. Counsel family to call immediately if any signs of abdominal pain, rectal bleeding following reduction.

XI. IRRITABLE BOWEL SYNDROME (IBS)

Abdominal and pelvic pain, R10	Irritable bowel syndrome without
Abdominal distension (gaseous), R14.0	diarrhea, K58.9
	Nausea, R11.0
Anal fissure, unspecified, K60.2	Other specified diseases of liver, K76.89
Constipation, K59.0	Rectal fistula, K60.4
Diarrhea, unspecified, R19.7	Residual hemorrhoidal skin tags, K64.4

A. Functional bowel disorder characterized by abdominal pain and changes in bowel function. Diagnostic criteria (fulfilled at least once/week for at least 2 months prior to diagnosis): Must include both of the following:
  1. Abdominal discomfort or pain associated with 2 or more of the following at least 25% of the time:
    a. Improvement with defecation.
    b. Onset associated with change in frequency of stool.
    c. Onset associated with change in appearance of stool.
  2. No evidence of an inflammatory, anatomic, metabolic, or neoplastic process that explains the patient's symptoms.
B. Etiology.
  1. Thought to be combination of visceral hypersensitivity and possibly altered gut motility. May be due to alterations in ENS and relationship to CNS.
  2. Stress/anxiety may induce/worsen symptoms but probably not root cause.
  3. May be preceded by episode of viral gastroenteritis or past history of constipation.
C. Occurrence.
  1. Common cause of recurrent abdominal pain in older children and adolescents.
  2. Estimated that about 6% of middle school students and 14% of high school students may fit criteria.
D. Clinical manifestations.
  1. Abdominal pain/discomfort, usually lower abdomen or periumbilical; relieved by defecation/onset associated with change in frequency/appearance of stool.
  2. Otherwise well, without evidence of underlying structural/metabolic abnormalities.
  3. BMs may be predominantly loose, constipated, or fluctuate between the two.
  4. May pass mucus with stool.

5. Stool urgency, especially in morning; occasional feeling of incomplete defecation.
6. Abdominal bloating/distention, especially later in day.
7. Important questions to ask:
    a. Location, timing, frequency, duration, quality of pain.
    b. BM frequency, consistency, size. Straining? Mucus or blood? Stool urgency?
    c. Does BM relieve abdominal pain? Anything that helps or aggravates symptoms?
    d. Is patient on medications? Any OTC remedies?
    e. Sensation of abdominal bloating? What time of day?
8. Complete diet history including beverages. Any weight loss?
9. May have functional dyspepsia symptoms such as nausea. No vomiting.
10. Red flags in history indicating diagnosis other than IBS include growth failure, weight loss, joint symptoms, vomiting, blood in stool, fever, family history of IBD (Crohn's or ulcerative colitis), dysphagia.

E. Physical findings.
    1. Height, weight, temperature, vital signs.
    2. Complete physical exam with attention to:
        a. Abdomen: Assess for tenderness, masses, stool, hepatosplenomegaly.
        b. Rectal: Assess for fissures, skin tags, fistula.

F. Diagnostic tests.
    1. No test to diagnose IBS.
    2. Screening studies usually necessary to be sure no underlying pathology.
        a. Stool for occult blood, ova and parasite, giardia antigen.
        b. CBC, ESR.
        c. Consider lactose breath hydrogen test to rule out lactose intolerance.

G. Differential diagnosis.

Abdominal pain, unspecified, R10.9	Gastroesophageal reflux disease without esophagitis, K21.9
Constipation, K59.0	Noninfective enteritis and colitis, K50–K52
Crohn's disease, unspecified, without complications, K50.90	Ulcerative colitis, unspecified, without complications, K51.90

1. Constipation, GER.
2. Lactose intolerance: Decreased lactase enzyme in small intestine causes malabsorption, subsequent diarrhea, abdominal pain, gas if excessive lactose ingested.

3. IBD: Crohn's disease, ulcerative colitis: Usually associated with growth delay/weight loss, anemia, diarrhea with/without blood, possibly joint pain, mouth ulcerations. Physical exam may reveal abnormal appearance to anus, abdominal tenderness.

H. Treatment.

1. There is currently a lack of high-quality evidence on the effectiveness of dietary interventions.

2. High-fiber diet, consider starting fiber supplement (OTC). AAP recommends: Child's age +5 grams of fiber/day.

3. Regular meals, avoid caffeine.

4. Ensure adequate rest and exercise. Discuss sleep hygiene.

5. Bloating/loose stools: Reduce sorbitol and fructose in diet.

6. Predominantly constipation: Add stool softener such as MiraLax, milk of magnesia.

7. Cognitive–behavioral therapy, such as relaxation and biofeedback.

8. Pharmacologic treatment reserved for continuing symptoms usually monitored by MD. Low-dose tricyclic antidepressants used with some success, probably due to effect on ENS. Antispasmodics used, but little data at this time to support their use. Studies using probiotics inconclusive and ongoing at this time.

I. Follow-up.

1. Return to clinic for any change/worsening of symptoms.

2. Refer to counselor as needed for relaxation therapy or biofeedback.

3. Refer to pediatric GI specialist if red flags or if treatment not successful.

J. Complications.

1. School absence/avoidance.

K. Education.

1. Discuss IBS at first visit. Explain that although diagnosis of exclusion, real diagnosis.

2. Reassure if history consistent with IBS and physical exam and screening studies are negative, further testing not necessary.

3. Discuss ENS and possible reasons for symptoms of IBS.

4. Explain importance of regular meals and exercise; both can help control symptoms.

5. Fiber supplementation may take 8 weeks to make difference.

6. Identify psychologic triggers such as family upset/school difficulties.

7. Insist on regular school attendance.

XII. PYLORIC STENOSIS (PS)

Abnormal weight loss, R63.4	Volume depletion, E86
Adult hypertrophic pyloric stenosis, K31.1	Vomiting, unspecified, R11.10
Other disorders of electrolyte and fluid balance, not elsewhere classified, E87.8	Visible peristalsis, R19.2

A. Gastric obstruction at pylorus muscle.
B. Etiology.
   1. Unknown.
C. Occurrence.
   1. Most common form of nonbilious vomiting in infants.
   2. Usually in infants after 2–3 weeks of age, up to 5 months of age.
   3. About 3 per every 1000 live births in United States.
   4. Male-to-female ratio = 4:1, especially firstborn males.
   5. Caucasians > African Americans.
   6. Increased incidence if mother had PS as infant (20% of her male offspring, 10% of female offspring will develop PS).
   7. Can be associated with other congenital defects (e.g., tracheoesophageal fistula).
D. Clinical manifestations.
   1. Nonbilious vomiting. Vomiting progressively projectile, immediately after feeding.
   2. Can occur intermittently or with every feeding.
   3. Infant hungry after emesis.
   4. As condition worsens, increased fluid losses, electrolyte imbalance, weight loss.
E. Physical findings.
   1. Length, weight, temperature, vital signs.
   2. Assess overall hydration, activity level, signs of hunger.
   3. Abdomen: May palpate firm mass, approximately 2 cm in length, olive shaped. Usually to right of umbilicus in upper abdomen, toward midepigastrium. Easier to palpate after vomiting. Mass may not be palpable in early PS.
   4. Visible peristalsis may occur after feeding.
F. Diagnostic tests.
   1. Abdominal ultrasound confirms majority of cases.
G. Differential diagnosis.

Gastroesophageal reflux disease without esophagitis, K21.9	Noninfective gastroenteritis and colitis, unspecified, K52.9
Metabolic disorder, unspecified, E88.9	Polyphagia, R63.2

    1. GERD.

    2. Gastroenteritis.

    3. Inborn errors of metabolism.

    4. Overfeeding.

  H. Treatment.

    1. Admit patient for rehydration/electrolyte management with referral to pediatric surgery (pyloromyotomy).

  I. Follow-up.

    1. Posthospitalization office visit to ensure infant regaining weight, tolerating feeds.

    2. Follow up with surgical team.

  J. Complications.

Abnormal weight loss, R63.4

Failure to thrive (child), R62.51

Volume depletion, E86

---

    1. Dehydration.

    2. Failure to thrive.

    3. Weight loss.

  K. Education.

    1. Reassure that infants do very well after surgical correction.

    2. Infant may resume normal feeding within 1–2 days postoperatively.

XIII. PEPTIC ULCER DISEASE (PUD)

Abdominal and pelvic pain, R10	Melena, K92.1
Gastrointestinal hemorrhage, unspecified, K92.2	Peptic ulcer, site unspecified, unspecified as acute or chronic, without hemorrhage or perforation, K27.9
Hematemesis, K92.0	
Iron deficiency anemia, unspecified, D50.9	Personal history of peptic ulcer disease, Z87.11
Irritability and anger, R45.4	Vomiting, unspecified, R11.10

  A. Erosion or ulceration of gastroduodenal mucosa.

  B. Etiology.

    1. Imbalance between cytotoxic and cytoprotective factors.

      a. Cytotoxic: Acid, pepsin, medications, infection.

      b. Cytoprotective: Gastric mucous layer provides mechanical barrier.

2. Primary PUD: Mainly caused by *Helicobacter pylori* infection in adults.
   a. Route of transmission unknown, may be fecal–oral, acquired early in life.
   b. Can cause gastritis positive/negative peptic ulcer, usually in older than 10 years of age.
3. Secondary PUD: Physiologic stress (burns, trauma), medications (NSAIDs, aspirin, corticosteroids), caustic ingestion (including alcohol), viral infections, Zollinger-Ellison syndrome, eosinophilic gastroenteritis (allergic inflammation), Crohn's disease.

C. Occurrence.
1. *H. pylori.*
   a. Increased risk for acquiring infection in developing countries, poor socioeconomic conditions, overcrowding.
   b. Possible ethnic/genetic predisposition: Higher rate among Asians, African Americans, Hispanics.
   c. Less common in children, but may acquire infection in childhood that is asymptomatic until later.
   d. Among most common bacterial infections in humans. Debate ongoing as to whether it may be normal flora in some individuals.

D. Clinical manifestations.
1. Neonates (up to 1 month): Usually present with GI hemorrhage/perforation (rare).
2. Infants to 2 years: Vomiting, irritability, poor growth, GI hemorrhage.
3. Preschool: Periumbilical pain, often postprandial, vomiting, GI hemorrhage.
4. School age and older: Epigastric abdominal pain that may awaken child from sleep. Acute/chronic GI blood loss (hematemesis, hematochezia, melena) may occur along with iron-deficiency anemia.
5. Family history of PUD.
6. Difficult to distinguish from other GI disorders such as GERD.
7. Obtain full diet and medication history.
8. Location, frequency, quality, duration, timing of pain. Does it wake child from sleep?
9. Any regurgitation or vomiting? Hematemesis, coffee ground–like emesis?
10. Frequency, consistency of stools. Any melena or hematochezia?

E. Physical findings.
1. Height, weight: Plot on growth curve and compare with previous.
2. Temperature, vital signs.
3. Full physical exam with attention to following:
   a. HEENT: Assess for dental caries, enamel erosion.
   b. Abdomen: Assess for tenderness, masses, hepatosplenomegaly.
   c. Rectal: Perform digital exam. Assess for fissures.

F. Diagnostic tests.
   1. Physical exam: CBC (anemia); comprehensive metabolic panel, amylase, lipase; urinalysis and urine culture.
   2. Test stool for occult blood.
   3. Upper GI series: To assess anatomy in child with vomiting. Little value in diagnosing ulcers or gastritis in children.
   4. *H. pylori* serology: Unreliable in children, not recommended. *H. pylori* stool antigen: Fairly reliable for diagnosis of current infection but should not be used for initial decision for treatment.
   5. Endoscopy with biopsies (test of choice) to diagnose *H. pylori* and PUD.
G. Differential diagnosis.

Crohn's disease, unspecified, without complications, K50.90

Helicobacter pylori [H. pylori] as the cause of diseases classified elsewhere, B96.81

Peptic ulcer, site unspecified, unspecified as acute or chronic, without hemorrhage or perforation, K27.9

---

   1. *H. pylori* infections: Reliable diagnosis in children by upper endoscopy.
   2. Secondary PUD:
      a. Medication: History of NSAID, aspirin, corticosteroid use, and others.
      b. Trauma/stress PUD: History of burns, trauma, surgery.
      c. Caustic ingestion/ETOH.
      d. Crohn's disease: History may include growth problems, diarrhea, blood in stool.
H. Treatment.
   1. *H. pylori*: 14 days of amoxicillin and Biaxin (clarithromycin) and at least 1 month of PPI (e.g., Prevacid [lansoprazole]).
   2. Secondary PUD.
      a. Discontinue offending medication/caustic substance. If on corticosteroids to treat another disease, may wean or give acid-reducing medicine until therapy complete.
      b. Gastritis/PUD can be treated first with H2 blocker (Zantac [ranitidine], Pepcid [famotidine]). If no response in 7–14 days, can increase therapy to PPI.
      c. History of upper GI bleed, melena, hematochezia requires referral to tertiary care facility/consultation of MD before therapy.
      d. Treat iron-deficiency anemia.
I. Follow-up.
   1. *H. pylori*: Follow-up testing (repeat endoscopy) for patients symptomatic after treatment. Other methods can be unreliable or not approved

for children. Stool antigen test can be offered to determine if infection eradicated but must be done after patient off PPIs and antibiotics for at least 2–4 weeks.

   2. Return to clinic 1 month after treatment started for nonspecific/suspected PUD.
   3. Immediate return for any worsening symptoms.
J. Complications.

Chronic or unspecified gastric ulcer with both hemorrhage and perforation, K25.6	*Helicobacter pylori [H. pylori]* as the cause of diseases classified elsewhere, B96.81
Gastrointestinal hemorrhage, unspecified, K92.2	Iron-deficiency anemia, unspecified, D50.9 Malignant neoplasm of stomach, unspecified, C16.9

   1. *H. pylori* (chronic colonization carries theoretical risk of developing gastric cancer).
   2. Massive GI bleed/perforation.
   3. Chronic iron-deficiency anemia.
K. Education.
   1. *H. pylori* not common in children, communicability low. Increased risk among household contacts of others with this infection.
   2. Explain that because differentiating between GERD and PUD is difficult, if no response to treatment with acid-reducing medication, endoscopy may be necessary.
   3. Employ conservative management for symptoms, such as dietary restrictions.

XIV. PINWORMS (ENTEROBIASIS)

Enterobiasis, B80	Insomnia, unspecified, G47.00
Erythematous condition, unspecified, L53.9	Other specified diseases of anus and rectum, K62.89

A. Etiology.
   1. Humans only known hosts for this obligate parasite; ingest embryonated eggs, which hatch in stomach. Larvae migrate to cecum area where mature into adult worms.
   2. Adult worms are about 1 cm in length. Females migrate by night to perianal region to deposit eggs.

   3. Ova mature after approximately 6 hours. Larvae viable for about 20 days.
   4. Eggs carried under fingernails, transmitted directly to another human or deposited in environment (dust, bed clothes) where others come in contact. Autoinfection/reinfection common; highly communicable.
B. Occurrence.
   1. Highest prevalence in children 5–14 years of age.
   2. Increased incidence in crowded living conditions, among family members of infected patients, in institutions.
C. Clinical manifestations.
   1. Anal pruritus, especially nocturnal (most likely from female pinworm depositing eggs).
   2. Sleeplessness.
   3. Perianal irritation/erythema may occur (most likely from scratching).
D. Physical findings.
   1. Child should appear well. Physical exam normal or nonspecific perianal irritation.
E. Diagnostic tests.
   1. Cellophane tape test.
      a. Adult worms sometimes visualized in evening around anus using flashlight: White, thread-like moving worm.
      b. Essentially diagnostic, specimen rarely required.
F. Differential diagnosis.

Erythematous condition, unspecified, L53.9

Streptococcal sepsis, unspecified, A40.9

---

   1. Perianal streptococcal infection: Anal erythema, pain. No pruritus.
G. Treatment.
   1. Vermox: Children older than 2 years, adults: 100 mg (chew, crush, swallow). Repeat in 2 weeks.
   2. Consider simultaneous treatment for household contacts (except pregnant women and children younger than 2 years).
H. Follow-up.
   1. As needed, not usually necessary.
   2. Consult with MD for patients younger than 2 years.
I. Complications.

Other specified diseases of anus and rectum, K62.89

---

   1. Perianal irritation/discomfort; secondary bacterial infection from scratching.

2. Rarely affects ectopic sites (i.e., female genital tract, appendix, peritoneal cavity, liver, spleen).
J. Education.
  1. Teach parent proper technique for obtaining specimen if needed.
    a. Use only clear cellophane tape. Spread buttocks early in morning, before toileting, or at night and apply tape sticky side down to perianal area.
    b. Place tape sticky side down on clear glass slide.
    c. Teach proper precautions for handling communicable specimen.
  2. Infection highly contagious and reinfection is common.
  3. Discuss strategies to avoid reinfection.
    a. Keep fingernails very short. Frequent handwashing, especially with toileting.
    b. Wash bedclothes, underwear daily; handle with precaution. Bathe daily.
    c. Discourage child from scratching anus and from placing fingers in mouth.
  4. Infections are spread only human to human. Cannot be spread by pets.
  5. Eggs are viable in environment for several days or longer.
  6. Discuss importance of second dose of medication at 2 weeks.
  7. Reassure about benign nature of the infection.
  8. Treatment side effects include abdominal pain, diarrhea.

XV. VIRAL GASTROENTERITIS

Abdominal and pelvic pain, R10	Myalgia, M79.1
Diarrhea, unspecified, R19.7	Other specified intestinal infections, A08.8
Fever of other and unknown origin, R50	Volume depletion, E86
Headache, R51	Vomiting, unspecified, R11.10

A. Viral infection of GI tract.
B. Etiology.
  1. Caused by several viruses, mainly:
    a. Rotavirus: Highly contagious, incubation period 1–3 days. Spread by fecal–oral route. Most common viral cause.
    b. Adenovirus: Second most common cause, mainly children younger than 2 years. Incubation period: 8–10 days.
    c. Norwalk group: Mainly older children, adults. Main cause of viral gastroenteritis epidemics. Highly contagious, fecal–oral route. From contaminated food, water, or person to person.

    2. Osmotic diarrhea usually results from carbohydrate malabsorption, increased fluid/salts in intestines.

C. Occurrence.

    1. Rotavirus most common cause of severe, dehydrating diarrhea in infants/ young children. Occurs mainly during winter months.

    2. Adenovirus can occur year-round, slight increase in summer months.

    3. Norwalk can occur year-round.

D. Clinical manifestations.

    1. Watery diarrhea most common symptom. Vomiting and fever common.

    2. Rotavirus may cause severe, watery diarrhea for 5–7 days.

    3. Adenovirus diarrhea may last for 1–2 weeks with/without vomiting at onset. May be associated with low-grade fever.

    4. Norwalk may cause acute-onset vomiting, abdominal cramps, diarrhea for 1–2 days. Vomiting main symptom in children; can have fever, headache, muscle aches.

    5. Pertinent history to obtain:

        a. Onset of symptoms, sudden? Any sick contacts? Fever history?

        b. Stools: Consistency, frequency, quantity, history of melena/ hematochezia.

        c. Vomiting: Frequency, quantity, quality. Contain bile or blood?

        d. Abdominal pain, cramping: Frequency, duration, relation to stools.

        e. Complete diet and medication history.

E. Physical findings.

    1. Weight, temperature, vital signs.

    2. Assess hydration status and level of activity.

    3. Complete physical exam with attention to abdomen (tenderness, guarding, masses) and rectal area (perianal irritation, diaper rash from diarrhea).

F. Diagnostic tests.

    1. Not usually necessary.

    2. Rotavirus/adenovirus diagnosed using commercially available kit.

    3. If dehydrated: Serum electrolytes.

G. Differential diagnosis.

Giardiasis [lambliasis], A07.1

Other specified bacterial agents as the cause of diseases classified elsewhere, B96.89

---

    1. Parasite infection (giardia, campylobacter).

    2. Bacterial infection.

H. Treatment.
   1. Supportive care: Prevent/correct dehydration.
I. Follow-up.
   1. Return to clinic if any increased symptoms or signs of dehydration.
J. Complications.

Diaper dermatitis, L22
Volume depletion, E86

   1. Dehydration.
   2. Diaper rash.
K. Education.
   1. Reassure family about self-limited nature of viral gastroenteritis.
   2. Review signs/symptoms of dehydration with family.
   3. Discuss communicability, precautions (handwashing, handling of soiled objects).

XVI. VOMITING, ACUTE

Abdominal and pelvic pain, R10	Melena, K92.1
Diarrhea, unspecified, R19.7	Pain in unspecified joint, M25.50
Dysuria, R30.0	Vomiting, unspecified, R11.10
Headache, R51	

A. Forceful expulsion of stomach contents through mouth. Highly coordinated reflex; can be symptom of disease within or outside GI tract.
B. Etiology.
   1. Common symptom of infection such as gastroenteritis. Can also be from infection outside GI tract such as UTI, otitis media, other systemic infections.
   2. Different from regurgitation-type emesis (nonforceful), common sign of GERD.
   3. Additional etiologies vary by age:
      a. Infant: Overfeeding, mechanical obstruction (pyloric stenosis, malrotation, volvulus), necrotizing enterocolitis, Hirschsprung's disease, intussusception, cow's milk protein allergy.
      b. Child: Appendicitis, sinusitis, toxic ingestions, gastritis, mechanical obstruction (foreign body, malrotation).
      c. Adolescent: Appendicitis, sinusitis, toxic ingestion, IBD, migraine, pregnancy, bulimia.

C. Occurrence.
   1. Common pediatric symptom.
   2. Infection is one of most common medical causes of nonbilious vomiting in first year of life, usually acute gastroenteritis.
D. Clinical manifestations.
   1. Usually forceful, may be preceded by nausea, increased salivation, retching.
      a. Describe vomiting and symptoms preceding it.
      b. How often is child vomiting? When did it first begin?
      c. Any bile staining or hematemesis?
      d. How soon after oral intake does vomiting occur?
   2. Ask about possible associated symptoms:
      a. Fever? How is it treated? Any headache, body aches, joint pain?
      b. Describe stools; any diarrhea? Any melena or hematochezia?
      c. Is child continuing to urinate? Any dysuria or frequency?
      d. Any URI symptoms, cough, ear, throat pain? Abdominal pain?
   3. Diet history:
      a. Type, quantity of fluids, foods.
      b. History of ingestion of contaminated food?
      c. Medications/drugs or toxic ingestion history?
      d. Exposure to others with similar symptoms?
E. Physical findings.
   1. Weight, compare with previous measurements.
   2. Temperature, vital signs.
   3. Assess level of activity; does child appear ill?
   4. Complete physical exam with attention to:
      a. Abdomen: Assess for distention, guarding, tenderness, masses.
      b. Hydration status.
      c. Rectal exam: Observe for any abnormalities, digital exam may be necessary to check for occult blood.
      d. CNS: Assess fontanel. Assess for irritability, nuchal rigidity, Brudzinski and Kernig's signs, funduscopic exam.
F. Diagnostic tests.
   1. If child appears ill, dehydrated: Serum electrolytes, CBC.
   2. If bilious vomiting, consider upper GI series to rule out mechanical obstruction.
   3. Projectile vomiting in infant younger than 5 months: Abdominal ultrasound to rule out pyloric stenosis.
   4. Abdominal flat-plate X-ray: If ingested radiopaque foreign body/bezoar suspected.
   5. Urinalysis with specific gravity.
   6. Other tests to be determined by history, physical exam.

G. Differential diagnosis.

Acute upper respiratory infection, unspecified, J06.9	Poisoning by unspecified drugs, medicaments and biological substances, accidental (unintentional), initial encounter, T50.901A
Adult hypertrophic pyloric stenosis, K31.1	
Hirschsprung's disease, Q43.1	
Metabolic disorder, unspecified, E88.9	Polyphagia, R63.2
Migraine, unspecified, not intractable, without status migrainosus, G43.909	Urinary tract infection, site not specified, N39.0
Noninfective enteritis and colitis, K50–K52	Viral pneumonia, not otherwise classified, J12
Other specified intestinal infections, A08.8	Vomiting of pregnancy, unspecified, O21.9

1. Infection: Usually associated with fever/all ages: Viral gastroenteritis, UTI, pneumonia, upper respiratory tract infections (otitis media, sinusitis, pharyngitis).
2. Mechanical: Pyloric stenosis, infants, malrotation/volvulus (infants, children: Bilious vomiting, abdominal pain, anorexia), foreign body ingestion or bezoar (children), Hirschsprung's disease (infants: Delayed passage of meconium, constipation).
3. Metabolic: Inborn errors of metabolism (infants, rare).
4. CNS: Migraine (children, adolescents: Headache, photophobia, family history common), brain tumor (rare), labyrinthitis.
5. Medication overdose, reaction, toxic ingestion (including lead).
6. Overfeeding (infants): Normal physical exam, review feeding techniques.
7. Pregnancy: Consider in postmenarchal girls.
8. Bulimia.
9. IBD (child, adolescent): Crohn's disease, ulcerative colitis. Hematochezia, melena, abdominal pain, diarrhea, weight loss, anemia.

H. Treatment.
1. Treat, prevent dehydration.
    a. Mild–moderate dehydration: Oral rehydrate solution 5 mL every 1–5 minutes plus replacement of estimated volume of emesis. Mild dehydration: Goal 50 mL/kg + losses over 4 hours. Moderate: 100 mL/kg + losses over 4 hours, reassess hourly.
    b. Severe dehydration: Emergency department or admission for IV fluids. Start with normal saline or lactated Ringer's solution at 10–20 mL/kg over 1 hour.

    2. As vomiting decreases, offer larger amounts of ORS at less frequent intervals.

    3. After rehydration, other fluids including milk, food may be reintroduced.

    4. Antiemetic medications are generally not warranted/recommended.

I. Follow-up.

    1. No/mild dehydration: Telephone next day.

    2. Moderate dehydration: See patient next day.

    3. Immediate return if increased symptoms, signs of dehydration.

    4. Severe dehydration requires visit following discharge from emergency department/hospital.

J. Complications.

Gastroesophageal laceration-hemorrhage syndrome, K22.6

Volume depletion, E86

---

    1. Dehydration.

    2. Mallory-Weiss tear (linear tear at gastroesophageal junction from repeated vomiting): Fresh red blood in emesis after multiple episodes of vomiting.

    3. Other complications depend on etiology.

K. Education.

    1. Most cases of acute vomiting are from viral gastroenteritis.

    2. Can be successfully treated at home if no signs of or mild dehydration.

    3. Review dehydration signs/symptoms with family, reassure most cases self-limited.

    4. Repeated vomiting can induce reflux of bile into stomach, resulting in bile staining.

BIBLIOGRAPHY

Aiken JJ, Oldham KT. Inguinal hernias. In: Kliegman RM, Stanton BF, St. Geme J, Schor N, Behrman RE, eds. *Nelson Textbook of Pediatrics.* 19th ed. Philadelphia, PA: Saunders; 2011:1362-1368.

Bhutta ZA. Acute gastroenteritis in children. In: Kliegman RM, Stanton BF, St. Geme J, Schor N, Behrman RE, eds. *Nelson Textbook of Pediatrics.* 19th ed. Philadelphia, PA: Saunders; 2011:1323-1339.

Blanchard SS, Czinn SJ. Peptic ulcer disease in children. In: Kliegman RM, Stanton BF, St. Geme J, Schor N, Behrman RE, eds. *Nelson Textbook of Pediatrics.* 19th ed. Philadelphia, PA: Saunders; 2011:1291-1294.

Hyman P, Milla PJ, Bennings MA, Davidson GP, Fleisher DF, Taminiau J. Childhood functional gastrointestinal disorders: neonate/toddler. *Gastroenterology.* 2006;130(5):1519-1526.

Ishimine P. Abdominal pain, acute. In: Zorc JJ, Alpern ER, Brown L, Clark BJ, Marino BS, Mollen CM, eds. *Schwartz's Clinical Handbook of Pediatrics.* 4th ed. Philadelphia, PA: Lippincott Williams and Wilkins; 2008:117-129.

King C, Glass R, Bresee JS, et al. Managing acute gastroenteritis among children: oral rehydration, maintenance, and nutritional therapy. *MMWR Recomm Rep.* 2003;52(16):1-16.

Koletzko S, Jones NL, Goodman KJ, et al. Evidence-based guidelines from ESPGHAN and NASPGHAN for *Helicobacter pylori* infection in children. *J Pediatr Gastroenterol Nutr.* 2011;53(2):230-243.

Liacouras CA. Vomiting. In: Zorc JJ, Alpern ER, Brown L, Clark BJ, Marino BS, Mollen CM, eds. *Schwartz's Clinical Handbook of Pediatrics.* 4th ed. Philadelphia, PA: Lippincott Williams and Wilkins; 2008:240-248.

Rasquin A, DiLorenzo C, Forbes D, et al. Childhood functional gastrointestinal disorders: child/adolescent. *Gastroenterology.* 2006;130(5):1527-1537.

Scholl J, Allen PJ. A primary care approach to functional abdominal pain. *Pediatr Nurs.* 2007;33(3):247-254, 257-259.

Tabbers MM, DiLorenzo C, Berger MY, et al. Evaluation and treatment of functional constipation in infants and children: evidence-based recommendations from ESPGHAN and NASPGHAN. *J Pediatr Gastroenterol Nutr.* 2014;58(2):258-274.

Vandenplas Y, Rudolph CD, Di Lorenzo C, et al. Pediatric gastroesophageal reflux clinical practice guidelines: joint recommendations of the North American Society for Pediatric Gastroenterology, Hepatology, and Nutrition (NASPGHAN) and the European Society for Pediatric Gastroenterology, Hepatology, and Nutrition (ESPGHAN). *J Pediatr Gastroenterol Nutr.* 2009;49(4):498-547.

Vernacchio L, Vezina RM, Mitchell AA, Lesko SM, Plaut AG, Acheson DW. Characteristics of persistent diarrhea in a community-based cohort of young US children. *J Pediatr Gastroenterol Nutr .* 2006;43(1):52-58.

Wiley CC. Diarrhea, acute. In: Zorc JJ, Alpern ER, Brown L, Clark BJ, Marino BS, Mollen CM, eds. *Schwartz's Clinical Handbook of Pediatrics.* 4th ed. Philadelphia, PA: Lippincott Williams and Wilkins; 2008:323-332.

Hunter AK, Liacouras CA. Pyloric stenosis and other congenital anomalies of the stomach. In: Kliegman RM, Stanton BF, St. Geme J, Schor N, Behrman RE, eds. *Nelson Textbook of Pediatrics.* 19th ed. Philadelphia, PA: Saunders; 2011:1274-1276.

Young RJ, Philichi L, eds. *Clinical Handbook of Pediatric Gastroenterology.* 2nd ed. St. Louis, MO: Quality Medical Publishing; 2015.

Genitourinary Disorders

Shelly J. King

I. MALE GENITALIA DISORDERS

Absence and aplasia of testis, Q55.0	Disorder of male genital organs,
Cardiogenic shock, R57.0	unspecified, N50.9
Congenital adrenogenital disorders	Hypospadias, unspecified, Q54.9
associated with enzyme	Indeterminate sex, unspecified, Q56.4
deficiency, E25.0	Retractile testis, Q55.22

A. Cryptorchidism.
B. Etiology/incidence.
   1. Cryptorchid testes can be absent, undescended, ectopic.
   2. Can be result of chromosomal, hormonal, anatomic factors.
   3. Majority (about 80%): Palpable, are undescended or ectopic testes. Retractile testes: Also palpable, sometimes misdiagnosed as undescended. Nonpalpable (20%) can be intra-abdominal, inguinal, absent testes.
C. Occurrence.
   1. Most common male congenital anomaly, affects nearly 3–5% of term infants and approximately 30% of premature males. In 10% of cases, it is bilateral.
D. Clinical manifestations.
   1. Risk of cryptorchidism increases in premature infant.
   2. Bilateral nonpalpable testes or cryptorchid testes associated with hypospadias should be evaluated at birth for life-threatening intersex conditions such as congenital adrenal hyperplasia.
   3. Parents may note retractile testicles in scrotum intermittently, especially after warm bath. Retractile testes are associated with an overactive cremasteric reflex. When examined, they can be placed in the scrotum and will remain there for a short time after released. If they retract immediately, they should be considered undescended.
   4. In case of absent testicle, contralateral testicle may be larger than expected.

E. Physical findings.
1. Often helpful to have child in cross-legged sitting position for exam.
2. Retractile testes can be placed into scrotum, remain there for short period.
3. Nonpalpable testes may be ectopic, found in femoral or perineal regions.
4. Scrotum may be flat/underdeveloped on affected side.
5. Larger-than-expected testicle may represent absent or nonfunctioning testicle on contralateral side.

F. Diagnostic tests.
1. Unilateral or bilateral palpable testes: No diagnostic testing indicated.
2. Bilateral nonpalpable testes or unilateral nonpalpable testes associated with phallic abnormality: Evaluate with karyotype, endocrine testing, and appropriate radiographic studies. Imaging not usually necessary, occasionally used to evaluate the very obese child when adequate exam cannot be performed.
   a. Human chorionic gonadotropin (hCG) stimulation test differentiates between anorchia and undescended testicles.
   b. hCG can stimulate testosterone production in functioning testes and can also result in testicular descent.

G. Differential diagnosis.

| Indeterminate sex, unspecified, Q56.4 |
| Retractile testis, Q55.22 |

1. Retractile testes.
2. Intersex conditions.

H. Treatment.
1. If at 6 months of age testes remain undescended, intervention is necessary.
   a. Type of treatment depends on testes's location, patient's age, association with other anomalies.
   b. Reasons for treatment: Reduced fertility, risk of tumor formation, trauma, torsion, repair of commonly associated defects such as inguinal hernia, psychological factors related to body image.
2. Placing testes into scrotum does not decrease risk of testicular cancer but does provide easy exam for early detection. Risk of testes cancer in cryptorchid male is 1 in 2000, highest risk between ages 17 and 25 years.
3. Orchiopexy or open surgery fixes testicle in scrotum and repairs hernia if needed. Laparoscopy can be used to locate nonpalpable testes or blind-ending vessels. There is also laparoscopic approach to orchiopexy.
4. Hormone administration is not as successful as surgical approach but a good option in high-risk patients and/or patients who have testes found in high scrotum or at external inguinal ring.

I. Follow-up.
1. After surgery, examine incisions at 2–4 weeks, 4–6 months postop.
2. Hormonal therapy: Examine at 1 month, 6 months posttreatment (higher risk of reascension).
3. Yearly exam important; patient should be taught self-exam at puberty. Can be performed by local medical provider or pediatric urologist.
   a. Asymmetry of testes needs further evaluation.
4. Retractile testes are rarely problematic, should be evaluated annually for possible ascension; increased risk in patients with anomalies of the central nervous system.

J. Complications.

Atrophy of testis, N50.0

1. Testicular atrophy is rated most serious complication of orchiopexy.

K. Education.
1. All males need to be taught self-scrotal exam at puberty. Especially important with history of undescended testicle due to 40% increased risk of cancer. Most common tumor is seminoma.
2. Prior to puberty, annual exam should be done. Scrotal pain needs to be evaluated immediately to rule out risk of testicular torsion, trauma, epididymitis, torsed testicular appendage. Postpubertal males should be taught to perform testicular self-exam monthly and report any changes immediately.

II. HYDROCELE

Abdominal hernia, unspecified, without obstruction or gangrene, K46.9	Indeterminate sex, unspecified, Q56.4
Hydrocele, unspecified, N43.3	Other specified disorders of male genital organs, N50.8

A. Etiology.
1. Occurs when processus vaginalis (channel that allows testicle to move from abdomen to scrotum during development) remains patent.
2. Difference between hernia and hydrocele is size of patent processus vaginalis and its contents.
   a. Narrow channel only allows fluid from peritoneal cavity to pass, resulting in hydrocele.
   b. Inguinal hernia: Much wider, can allow both fluid and intestinal contents to pass.

B. Occurrence.
1. About 80% of infants are born with patent processus vaginalis; by end of first month of life, decreases to about 60%.
2. By 18–24 months of age, only 20–30% remain.
3. Rare in females: 6 males to 1 female.
C. Clinical manifestations.
1. Females: Rare, usually presents with soft bulge in labia or inguinal canal.
   a. Bulge can represent ovary or hernia.
   b. Intersex conditions (especially testicular feminization): Evaluate in female.
2. Males: Parents complain of scrotal swelling in one or both sides. Can be continuous or intermittent; size can fluctuate.
   a. Parent may describe bluish hue to scrotum, often small in size in morning and growing larger during day as fluid accumulates.
   b. History is very important because may not be present at time of exam.
D. Physical findings.
1. Hydroceles typically transilluminate with penlight to scrotum.
2. Palpate testicle; if testicle cannot be palpated, can be seen by transillumination. If testes not seen or palpated, need scrotal ultrasound to differentiate.
3. Classified as communicating (patent processus vaginalis) or noncommunicating. Almost all congenital hydroceles are communicating. Noncommunicating hydroceles do not fluctuate in size.
4. Condition rarely painful unless associated with hernia that becomes incarcerated.
E. Diagnostic tests.
1. If any concern regarding testes, ultrasound imaging is indicated.
F. Differential diagnosis.

Epididymitis, N45.1	Undescended testicle, unspecified, Q53.9
Retractile testis, Q55.22	Unilateral inguinal hernia, without obstruction or gangrene, not specified as recurrent, K40.90

1. Inguinal hernia.
2. Epididymitis.
3. Retractile testes.
4. Ectopic testes.
5. Absent testes.

G. Treatment.
1. Generally safe to watch hydroceles until 18–24 months. After that age, spontaneous resolution is uncommon.
2. Earlier surgical intervention is indicated if hydrocele is large or associated with hernia secondary to increased risk of incarceration. Any abnormality of testes requires evaluation by scrotal ultrasound and could lead to earlier surgical intervention.
H. Follow-up.
1. Child younger than 18 months of age should be examined every 6 months. If no change, no intervention indicated until 18–24 months.
2. If hydrocelectomy is performed, see patient 4 weeks postop to evaluate incision and scrotum. If exam is normal, can return to routine annual exam with healthcare provider.
I. Complications.

Abdominal hernia, unspecified, with obstruction, without gangrene, K46.0

Atrophy of testis, N50.0

Hydrocele, unspecified, N43.3

---

1. Complications from hydroceles are rare.
2. Risk of incarcerated hernia in patients with wide patent processus vaginalis.
3. Postoperative complications are rare; include recurrent hydrocele, testicular atrophy, lysis of vas deferens.
J. Education.
1. Although hydroceles and hernias are not really associated with increased risk of testicular cancer, discuss importance of self-scrotal exam.
2. Teach parents importance of regular exam during observation period.
3. If any scrotal pain, child needs to be seen immediately.

III. EPIDIDYMITIS

Chlamydial infection, unspecified, A74.9	Exstrophy of urinary bladder, unspecified, Q64.10
Congenital absence, atresia and stenosis of large intestine, part unspecified, Q42.9	Gonococcal infection, A54
Disorder of male genital organs, unspecified, N50.9	Neuromuscular dysfunction of bladder, unspecified, N31.9
Dysuria, R30.0	Torsion of testis, unspecified, N44.00
Epididymitis, N45.1	Urethral discharge, unspecified, R36.9

A. Etiology.
1. Epididymitis refers to edema, irritation of epididymis or lining of testicle.
2. Can occur from infectious/inflammatory cause.
3. Can be difficult to distinguish epididymitis from testicular torsion because both can be quite painful.
4. Can be sexually acquired; *Neisseria gonorrhoeae* and chlamydia are common pathogens.
5. Can be related to genitourinary abnormalities or urethra manipulation.
6. Rarely associated with heavy lifting or straining that results in efflux of urine into vas deferens. Urinalysis should be obtained; if infectious, then bacterial epididymitis can occur; if not, chemical inflammation develops.
B. Occurrence.
1. Rare in children before puberty unless child has genitourinary abnormality. Most common cause of the acute scrotum. Incidence ranges from 0.8 to 1.2 cases for every 1000 persons per year.
2. More commonly occurs in sexually active adolescents.
C. Clinical manifestations.
1. Most likely to occur in postpubertal male and very young males.
2. Those with imperforate anus, exstrophy, neurogenic bladder, any conditions requiring intermittent catheterization are more prone to this type of infection.
D. Physical findings.
1. Include sexual history in postpubertal male.
2. Urethral discharge may be present.
3. Often slow onset of pain that continues to become more severe.
4. May have dysuria and see blood or discharge in urine.
5. Physical exam yields swollen and inflamed scrotum.
6. May complain of tenderness along epididymis.
7. If testicle is tender and swollen, may also have orchitis.
8. Up to 33% may be febrile.
E. Diagnostic tests.
1. Urine culture and urinalysis may be positive or negative for bacteria. If positive (2–6% of cases), then X-ray evaluation by voiding cystourethrogram (VCUG) and renal-bladder ultrasound is indicated.
2. Scrotal ultrasound with Doppler flow is useful in differentiating epididymitis from testicular torsion. Ultrasound will show enlarged epididymis with increased blood flow unless edema is so severe it results in ischemia. May also show enlarged testicle with increased low flow in orchitis.

F. Differential diagnosis.

Allergic purpura, D69.0	Torsion of testis, unspecified, N44.00
Epididymitis, N45.1	Urinary tract infection, site not specified, N39.0

1. Testicular torsion.
2. Chemical epididymitis.
3. Bacterial epididymitis.
4. Torsion of testicular appendage.
5. Urinary tract infection (UTI).

G. Treatment.
1. Start 2 weeks of appropriate broad-spectrum antibiotic while cultures are pending. If necessary, change appropriately when cultures are final.
   a. Children not sexually active: Cephalexin: 40 mg/kg/day in 2 divided doses. Can also use:
      • Ampicillin: 50 mg/kg bid.
      • Trimethoprim-sulfamethoxazole (TMP-SMX): Older than 2 months of age: 4 mg/kg and 20 mg/kg bid.
      • Ciprofloxacin: 15 mg/kg bid postpuberty. The safety of quinolone antimicrobial use in children remains a concern and must be considered. Some clinical situations (such as complicated UTI or pyelonephritis) have been FDA approved; others may warrant off-label use.
2. Ibuprofen for several days will help decrease inflammation, pain.
3. Scrotal support and elevating scrotum will help resolve edema.
4. Limited activity for 2–3 days.
5. Application of heat/cold compresses helps reduce pain and edema.
6. If pain and edema are severe or not responding to treatment, consider IV antibiotics. Prolonged infection can result in damage to epididymis.
7. Identified STI should be treated with appropriate antibiotic regimen.

H. Follow-up.
1. If pain increases, see patient immediately.
2. If condition is resolving, follow up in 2 weeks with repeat ultrasonography.
3. If positive urine cultures, a VCUG and renal-bladder ultrasound should be done. Increased likelihood of genitourinary abnormalities in males with positive urine cultures. Prophylactic antibiotics should be given until radiographic evaluation is complete (see UTI section on page 424).

I. Complications.
   1. Possible damage to vas deferens, epididymis with recurrent or untreated infection.
J. Education.
   1. Preventive education especially when epididymitis is associated with sexually transmitted infections (STIs).
   2. Signs/symptoms of testicular torsion and acute scrotum indicate need for immediate attention by medical professional.
   3. Genitourinary abnormalities can be associated with urinary infections, so follow up with necessary testing.

IV. HYPOSPADIAS/CHORDEE

Disorder of male genital organs, unspecified, N50.9	Other specified disorders of penis, N48.89
Hypospadias, unspecified, Q54.9	

A. Etiology/incidence.
   1. Cause of hypospadias is unknown; genetic link is suspected (many families with multiple occurrences).
   2. Hypospadias is a congenital anomaly in which urethral meatus is ectopic; it is located on the undersurface of the penis any place between the glans and the scrotum.
   3. Spectrum defect ranging from mild to severe, depending on degree of chordee (bend of penis), location of urethral opening. Mild forms can be found during newborn circumcision; stop circumcision—foreskin used to repair defect.
B. Occurrence.
   1. Occurs in 1 of every 250 males in United States; incidence increased to 1 of every 100 if immediate family history.
C. Clinical manifestations.
   1. Difficult for older child to stand to urinate.
   2. If associated with chordee, future intercourse may be difficult.
   3. Parental anxiety/guilt common with genital malformation.
D. Physical findings.
   1. Urethral opening lies on undersurface of penis.
   2. Degrees of hypospadias: Distal shaft refers to opening being closest to natural location.
      a. As opening gets closer to scrotum, condition becomes more severe.

   b. Referred to as midshaft, penoscrotal (located at penoscrotal junction), and perineal (located just beneath scrotum).
   3. Chordee or bend of penis is present in 35% of cases.
   4. Foreskin typically seen only on dorsal side of penis, gives "hooded" appearance.
   5. Penile glans has spade like appearance and cleft/blind-ending pit may be seen at location where meatus would normally reside.
   6. Cryptorchidism associated 7–9% of cases.
E. Diagnostic tests.
   1. Rarely necessary with hypospadias.
   2. Early referral to experienced pediatric urologist important: Allay fears about child's masculinity, opportunity to assess for intersex disorders (uncommon but considered with severe hypospadias and hypospadias associated with cryptorchidism).
   3. Karyotype and endocrine evaluation to rule out disorders of sexual differentiation may be indicated with severe hypospadias and cryptorchidism.
   4. In some of the more extensive cases, urinary tract will need to be evaluated.
F. Differential diagnosis.

Indeterminate sex, unspecified, Q56.4
_____

   1. Intersex disorders.
G. Treatment.
   1. Referral to pediatric urologist as soon after birth as possible (reassure parents after surgical intervention child's potency/fertility no longer affected; makes it easier to discuss problem with other family members).
   2. More than 200 surgical techniques described for hypospadias repair.
      a. Goals same in each repair; cosmetically normal-appearing penis, straight with urethral meatus at tip. Repairs are performed in healthy males as early as 6 months of age.
      b. Patient should be able to stand to void.
      c. Selected cases may require preadministration of testosterone to enhance blood supply to genitalia.
      d. Most surgery is done on outpatient basis.
      e. Many approaches to postoperative dressing. Absorbable sutures are used in repairs, will not need to be removed.
      f. Stent may be left through urethra to drain bladder while urethra heals. Nonabsorbable suture may be used to hold stent in place, will need to be removed about 1 week postop.

H. Follow-up.
   1. See in 1 week to inspect incision, remove any dressings, stent if necessary.
   2. See again 2–3 months later, after majority of edema is resolved, to ensure penis is straight, meatus is widely open.
   3. Some surgeons schedule visit after toilet training to visualize normal voiding stream; others see child after puberty to discuss surgery, alleviate fears, and rare late complications.
   4. If ever difficulty voiding or UTI, patient should be seen immediately by pediatric urologist.
I. Complications.

Injury of unspecified intra-abdominal organ, S36.9	Urethral diverticulum, N36.1
	Urethral fistula, N36.0
Other specified disorders of penis, N48.89	Urethral stricture, unspecified, N35.9

   1. Experienced hypospadiac surgeon is important to minimize complications.
   2. Rate of complication varies according to severity of defect.
      a. Early postoperative complications: Uncommon but include wound infection, urethrocutaneous fistula, hematoma.
      b. Late complications: Urethral stricture, meatal stenosis residual chordee, urethral diverticulum.
      c. If secondary procedure necessary, not performed until tissues well healed—approximately 6 months after initial repair.
J. Education.
   1. Important to educate newborn-care providers not to circumcise if any penile defects: Foreskin is used for repair.
   2. Understanding defect and its correction can alleviate parental fears. Reassure them child's masculinity not affected; structural problem that can be corrected surgically.
   3. Patient must understand potential for complications. Any difficulty voiding or UTI need follow-up with pediatric urologist.

V. FEMALE GENITALIA DISORDERS

Condition, unspecified, associated with female genital organs and menstrual cycle, N94.9	Fusion of labia, Q95.5
	Urge incontinence, N39.41
Dysuria, R30.0	

A. Etiology.
1. Labial adhesions are fusion of labia minora, occur as result of vulvar irritation, lack of estrogen.
2. Possible causes: Chronic inflammation, irritation secondary to infection, trauma, incontinence.
B. Occurrence.
1. Primarily in girls 3 months to 6 years of age.
C. Clinical manifestations.
1. Dysuria and incontinence are common complaints when efflux of urine is blocked and urine is trapped behind adhesions.
2. Toilet-trained girls may complain of postvoid dribbling. Maternal estrogens seem to prevent adhesions in newborns.
D. Physical findings.
1. Labial adhesions appear as thin film that begins posteriorly and advance anteriorly.
2. In more severe cases, cannot see vaginal introitus or urethral meatus.
3. Presence of scarring that deviates from midline or more dense adhesions should raise question of repeat trauma/sexual abuse.
E. Diagnostic tests.
1. None.
F. Differential diagnosis.

Child sexual abuse, suspected, initial encounter, T76.22XA

Indeterminate sex, unspecified, Q56.4

---

1. Intersex conditions.
2. Sexual abuse.
G. Treatment.
1. Majority requires no treatment, resolves spontaneously.
   a. Keep child clean and dry to prevent irritation and superficial infection.
2. More significant adhesions that present with dysuria and postvoid dribbling can be treated with hormone cream, betamethasone 0.05% cream, or lysis of adhesions.
   a. Premarin cream: 0.625 mg applied with gentle pressure to the translucent midline twice a day for 10–14 days.
   b. Betamethasone cream 0.05% bid can be used up to 4 weeks.
3. Lysis of thinned adhesions can be done in office after EMLA cream application.
4. More dense-appearing adhesions or those that have been broken down previously may be done more effectively and with less trauma in operat-

ing room. Critical to prevent readherence by applying barrier cream to previously attached tissues twice a day for 8–12 weeks.

H. Follow-up.

1. No treatment: Follow up with each well-child check, may become more severe with time (best obtained by urethral catheterization).

2. If complaints of dysuria: Careful collection of urine specimen is important; it is difficult to collect valid specimen by voiding when adhesions are present (catheterization preferred).

3. Posttreatment: See patient 4–6 weeks later to ensure no reoccurrence.

I. Complications.

Urinary tract infection, site not specified, N39.0

---

1. Biggest risk is reoccurrence due to poor parental compliance with barrier cream placement after adhesions have been lysed.

2. If painful voiding, child may delay voiding, empty more poorly, resulting in true UTIs.

3. Prolonged use of estrogen can result in development of secondary sex characteristics.

J. Education.

1. Importance of post treatment management must be stressed to parents; most important in preventing further problems with adhesions. Sometimes difficult for parents, especially if child complains of discomfort when medication is applied.

2. Child should learn to void with legs widely separated to facilitate good bladder emptying and to keep labia separated during voiding.

3. If urine specimen necessary, take care to avoid contamination; done best by catheterization.

4. Parents understand length of Premarin treatment; possible side effects of prolonged or repeated use.

VI. PEDIATRIC URINARY TRACT INFECTIONS

Abdominal pain, unspecified, R10.9	Frequency of micturition, R35.0
Constipation, K59.0	Irritability and anger, R45.4
Diarrhea, unspecified, R19.7	Nausea, R11.0
Dysuria, R30.0	Urge incontinence, N39.41
Feeding difficulties, R63.3	Urinary tract infection, site not specified, N39.0
Fever of other and unknown origin, R50	Vomiting, unspecified, R11.10

A. Etiology.
   1. Periurethral bacteria infect bladder, ureter, kidney. *Escherichia coli* most frequently identified pathogen.
B. Occurrence.
   1. Fairly common: 2.4% of children yearly, majority are ascending.
   2. Up to 6 months of age, more common in males than females, incidence of 2 cases per 100 live births. Uncircumcised males less than 6 months old have a tenfold increased risk for UTI development.
   3. After 1 year of age, much more common in females.
   4. Approximately 3% of toilet-trained females will develop infection.
      a. Of children who develop infection, 15% will develop infection-related renal scarring.
      b. Of those, 10–20% will have hypertension.
C. Clinical manifestations.
   1. Symptoms of UTI in infants often difficult to recognize.
   2. Usually generalized illness with fever, irritability, poor feeding, vomiting, diarrhea. Suspect when no other source for fever or illness.
   3. Older children complain of dysuria, suprapubic/urethral pain, urinary frequency, incontinence. Can also have fever, flank pain, nausea, vomiting if kidney is involved.
   4. Foul-smelling urine, constipation (commonly associated, obtain stool history).
D. Physical findings.
   1. Perform thorough exam.
   2. May detect renal mass in infants with gross anatomic abnormalities such as obstruction or mass.
   3. Costal-vertebral angle (CVA) tenderness seen while palpating flank of older children.
   4. If dysuria is primary concern, perineal exam may show external irritation related to incontinence, vaginal voiding, labial adhesions.
   5. Sometimes treated as UTIs: Vaginitis and pinworms sometimes mistaken (because often present with dysuria).
   6. Vaginal discharge: Culture if present; may have suprapubic tenderness.
   7. Males: Scrotal exam to rule out epididymitis, especially in older males who may be sexually active.
      a. Look for urethral discharge; culture if present.
      b. UTIs younger than 6 months of age are very uncommon, need evaluation.
      c. Abdominal exam may also yield large stool burden; constipation very common in children with UTIs.

E. Diagnostic tests.
1. Collecting urine specimen is very important in documenting infection. Four techniques for obtaining a specimen are listed in **Table 28-1**.
2. X-ray evaluation: Infants, febrile UTIs, males, recurrent UTIs, children who are not toilet trained. Important that true infection is documented by catheterized culture when deciding what additional evaluation is indicated.
3. Multiple guidelines for evaluation of UTI in children exist today; it is important that the provider consider evaluation carefully.
   a. The UK National Institute for Health and Clinical Excellence (NICE) and the American Academy of Pediatrics (AAP) have guidelines that

Table 28-1 Techniques for Obtaining a Specimen

Techniques	Use for Specimen	Drawbacks
Bagged specimen (baggy attached to perineum)	Helpful in ruling out UTI	If positive, catheter specimen needs to be obtained (false positives: 90%, especially if left on for 20 minutes)
Clean-catch midstream	Better collection; provides results of multiple organisms of small colony counts that are suggestive of contamination	Difficult for children (parents have a hard time cleaning, separating labia in girls); urine often hits perineum before reaching the cup
Catheterized specimen	Most widely accepted technique for determining true UTIs	Some offices not set up to catheterize children
Urinalysis	Provides information on leukocytes and nitrates (positive leukocytes and nitrites are highly predictive of infection), urine culture should be sent to assess colony count, pathogens present, appropriate antibiotic treatment	
Suprapubic aspirate	Most reliable	Rarely utilized because of anxiety associated with placing needle through abdominal wall and into bladder; can be threatening to child, parent/care provider

are widely accepted by experts in pediatric urology. The seriousness of the illness and atypical infection are important factors in determining the evaluation. Renal ultrasound should be done promptly if the child is not responding to therapy. If ultrasound abnormal, then VCUG or DMSA should be considered.

b. Obstructions of urinary tract seen in 5–10%; 21–57% have vesicoureteral reflux.

- If tests are negative, no additional evaluation necessary unless further problems arise (if continued febrile UTI, refer to pediatric urologist).
- If tests are positive, refer to pediatric urologist for evaluation, consultation, and treatment.

4. In case of significantly ill, febrile child, serum chemistries can identify elevation in creatinine or blood urea nitrogen (BUN), may implicate urinary tract. Complete blood count (CBC) with elevated white blood cell (WBC) count can indicate bacterial infection.

F. Differential diagnosis (see **Table 28-2**).

G. Treatment.

1. Goals: Prevent renal damage, urosepsis, recurrent infections.

a. How goals are accomplished varies according to severity and age of patient.

Table 28-2 Urinary Tract Infections

Febrile UTIs	Afebrile UTIs
Obstructive and reflux uropathy, unspecified, N13.9	Disorder of the skin and subcutaneous tissue, unspecified, L98.9
Vesicoureteral-reflux-associated uropathy, N13.7	Other specified inflammation of vagina and vulva, N76.8
Disorder of kidney and ureter, unspecified, N28.9	Other specified noninflammatory disorders of vulva and perineum, N90.89
Urinary tract infection, site not specified, N39.0	Enterobiasis, B80
Female pelvic inflammatory disease, unspecified, N73.9	Hematuria, unspecified, R31.9
Sexually transmitted infections	Disorder of calcium metabolism, unspecified, E83.50

2. Hospitalization should be considered for infants who appear systemically ill or are less than 3 months of age.

   a. Parenteral broad-spectrum antibiotics, such as third-generation cephalosporins, and/or aminoglycosides can be used. If appropriate, oral therapy with cephalosporins, quinolones, TMP-SMX, or amoxicillin with clavulonic acid are also options. Therapy should last for 7–14 days and is based on the antimicrobial susceptibility of the isolated uropathogen.

   b. Some situations can be managed with outpatient therapy:
      - Parenteral ceftriaxone if child is taking fluids well, parents are reliable enough to contact provider if condition changes.
      - Some older children can be managed as outpatients with cephalosporins, penicillins, sulfonamides. Antibiotic treatment is 7–14 days.
      - Parent involvement is very important when managing patients outside hospital; provider must have confidence in family.

   c. Continue parenteral treatment until culture, sensitivity returns, and clinical picture is improving, then place child on appropriate oral antimicrobial.

   d. Quinolones are approved for complicated pediatric UTI/pyelonephritis management, but there is still concern for the safety of use in children. Some clinical situations may warrant limited off-label use.

   e. Nitrofurantoin is not a good antimicrobial in a systemically ill patient, does not attain high serum concentrations.

3. Lower tract or bladder infections are referred to as uncomplicated UTI.

   a. Children: 3- to 5-day course of oral antimicrobials.

   b. Nitrofurantoin: Good option, provides high urinary concentration (other agents used: Sulfonamides, cephalosporins, penicillins).

   c. Antibiotic prophylaxis is indicated when there is sufficient concern for recurrence of infection that may result in renal injury. Prophylaxis may be continued if vesicoureteral reflux, urinary tract obstruction, immunosuppression, recurrent UTIs, or less than 6 months of age.
      - Nitrofurantoin: 1.2–2.4 mg/kg or TMP-SMX 2 mg/kg of trimethoprim once a day are common choices.
      - Cephalosporins (such as cephalexin) or ampicillin: 25% treatment dose daily.

- Nitrofurantoin: Do not use until older than 1 month of age.
- TMP-SMX: Do not use until older than 2 months of age.
- Both Keflex and ampicillin can be used in newborns.
  d. Treatment must also include good oral intake of fluids, encouraging toilet-trained patient to void more frequently.
  e. If associated constipation, this must also be addressed.
- Alters normal voiding habits.
- Provides good medium for microbial growth.
- Bowel/bladder dysfunction (poor emptying of bowel and bladder) is hallmark of UTIs in toilet-trained patients.
  f. Educate parent in treatment of problem.
- Urination on timed schedule usually every 2 hours with techniques for relaxation of external urinary sphincter.
- Voiding to completion with each attempt is vital to preventing further infections. Have child sit comfortably on the toilet with legs widely separated and feet supported on a footstool if they don't reach the floor. Some children sit backward on the toilet.
- Stool softeners are often necessary while working on dietary measures to prevent constipation.
  g. Perineal irritation.
- Scented soaps, bubble baths may irritate urethra, cause burning that results in disrupted urinary stream, poor emptying of bladder; discontinue in patients with recurrent UTIs.
- Covering perineum with barrier cream helps prevent burning caused from irritation, especially with incontinence associated with infection.
- Vulvovaginitis can be treated with baking soda sitz bath (3 tablespoons) in a shallow tub bath daily for 1 week. Educate to void with leg widely separated to prevent vaginal trapping of urine and associated perineal irritation.

H. Follow-up.
   1. Follow-up culture to prove infection has resolved.
   2. If X-ray evaluation is positive or if infections are recurrent: Urology consult, preferably with pediatric urology group. Specialist can do postvoid ultrasound/other treatments to help patient learn to empty more effectively, correct any structural abnormalities if necessary.
   3. More thorough education of problems associated with infection will help family and provider.

I. Complications.

Disorder of kidney and ureter, unspecified, N28.9	Other chronic cystitis without hematuria, N30.20
Essential (primary) hypertension, I10	Urge incontinence, N39.41
Other chronic cystitis with hematuria, N30.21	

1. Serious risks, warrants effective management.
   a. Renal scarring, loss of renal function are most serious complications.
   b. Hypertension can result from renal scaring.
   c. Chronic cystitis can result in poor functional use of bladder, sometimes incontinence.
J. Education.
   1. Understand signs/symptoms of UTIs and need for treatment/evaluation.
   2. Importance of daily antibiotic and/or stool softener (if prescribed); easy to forget to take medication.
   3. Understand bowel/bladder dysfunction and its treatment, primarily need to empty bladder frequently to completion, to avoid constipation.
   4. Follow-up critical in management of UTIs due to risk of renal sequelae.

VII. HEMATURIA

Allergic purpura, D69.0	Hemolytic-uremic syndrome, D59.3
Alport syndrome, Q87.81	Nephritic syndrome, unspecified, with unspecified morphologic changes, N05.9
Congenital malformation, unspecified, Q89.9	Other symptoms and signs involving the urinary system, R39
Disorder of calcium metabolism, unspecified, E83.50	Systemic lupus erythematosus, organ or system involvement unspecified, M32.10
Disorder resulting from impaired renal tubular function, unspecified, N25.9	Urinary calculus, unspecified, N20.9
Glomerular disorders in diseases classified elsewhere, N08	Urinary tract infection, site not specified, N39.0
Hematuria, unspecified, R31.9	

A. Etiology/incidence.
   1. Gross hematuria (blood visible to naked eye) can originate from upper/lower urinary tract.
   2. Causes: Variable; include trauma, UTI, calculi, disorders of renal parenchyma, glomerulonephritis, Alport syndrome, hypercalciuria, benign

exercise-induced hematuria, anatomic abnormalities, hemolytic uremic syndrome, sickle cell nephropathy, Henoch-Schönlein purpura, Goodpasture disease, lupus erythematosus, medication toxicity/chemotherapy, urethralgia, viral bladder infections, STIs (in postpubertal child).
B. Occurrence.
1. Common in children (unlike adults): Rarely associated with neoplasm (1%).
2. Microscopic hematuria found on routine health exam by dipstick urinalysis in 0.5–2% of school-age children.
C. Clinical manifestations.
1. History important in determining diagnosis.
a. Urinary frequency, fever, dysuria may indicate infection, most common cause of blood in school-age child's urine.
b. May describe recent trauma.
c. Blood in other sites (i.e., sputum/stools) may indicate blood dyscrasia.
2. Family history: Familial diseases such as hypercalciuria, Alport syndrome, calculi, structural anomalies.
3. Hemolytic uremic syndrome, one of most common causes of acute renal failure in children: Preceded by gastroenteritis, bloody diarrhea.
a. Question child regarding any joint pain, edema, tenderness.
b. Any recent cold, upper respiratory symptoms? Sore throat/skin infection present?
4. Acute nephritic syndrome: Associated with gross hematuria, edema, hypertension, renal insufficiency.
a. Post-streptococcal glomerulonephritis occurs 7–14 days after onset of strep infection.
b. Winter months: Commonly associated with strep pharyngitis.
c. Summer months: More likely to be skin infections.
5. When bleeding occurs, urine color is important.
a. Brown/cola-colored urine: More likely from kidney.
b. Red/pink urine: More likely from bladder.
c. Red blood spotting at end of urinary stream/in underwear: Most likely from urethra.
D. Physical findings.
1. Full-body exam to look for:
a. Abdominal or renal mass.
b. Presence of abdominal, CVA tenderness.
2. Check child's underwear for blood, perineum for signs of trauma.
3. Assess joints for edema, inflammation, tenderness.
4. Edema of face, hands, or feet.
5. Assess for signs of upper respiratory infection, pharyngitis, or other illness.

E. Diagnostic tests.
 1. Urinalysis may reveal infection or proteinuria.
 2. Laboratory analysis: Formal urinalysis, culture if thought to be infection; urine calcium/creatinine ratio; urine protein/creatinine ratio.
 3. Serum studies: CBC with differential and platelet count, complete metabolic panel, anti-streptolysin enzyme (ASO) or streptozyme, antinuclear antibody (ANA) and C3.
 4. Skin or throat cultures when appropriate.
 5. Sickle cell screen in all African American patients.
 6. Coagulation studies with history of bleeding from other sites.
 7. Cystoscopy: Only if persistent gross hematuria.
 8. Renal-bladder ultrasound.
F. Differential diagnosis.

Hematuria, unspecified, R31.9

Hypercalcemia, E83.52

---

 1. Pseudohematuria.
 2. Idiopathic hypercalcemia.
 3. Extrarenal hematuria.
 4. Exercise-induced hematuria.
G. Treatment.
 1. Systemically ill child with gross hematuria: Admit while being evaluated.
 2. If elevated ASO and low C3 (hypocomplementemia), refer to nephrologist to rule out/treat nephritis.
 3. If abnormal ultrasound, referral to urologist to determine presence of structural anomalies.
 4. With UTIs, refer to urologist and consider VCUG.
 5. Abnormal ANA results, elevated ANA: Consult rheumatology, nephrology; commonly associated with positive crithidia/DNA (ds) antibody may indicate lupus erythematosus.
 6. Other blood dyscrasias: Consult hematology.
 7. Elevated serum creatinine, hypertension, peripheral edema, abnormal calcium/creatinine ratio, protein/creatinine ratio: Refer to nephrologist. Renal biopsy/cystoscopy may be necessary to diagnose.
 8. Urethralgia: Hallmarked by blood at end of urinary stream or in underwear, can persist without negative consequence in child for years. Treatment is controversial: Some use antibiotics, but have not been proved effective.
 9. If child develops hypertension or proteinuria, refer to nephrologist. Renal biopsy may be indicated.

10. If chlamydia or gonorrhea is suspected:
    a. Younger than 9 years of age: Erythromycin 50 mg/kg/day qid (max 2 g/day).
    b. 9–15 years of age: Ceftriaxone 250 mg IM single dose followed by 7 days of doxycycline 200 mg/day bid.
    c. Older than 15 years of age: Azithromycin 1 g in 1 dose.
H. Follow-up.
    1. Determined by disease, usually done by appropriate specialist.
    2. Urethralgia without significant symptoms and benign familial hematuria without proteinuria and hypertension: Monitor by checking urine and blood pressure every 6–12 months.
I. Complications.

Kidney failure, unspecified, N19

Other disorders of electrolyte and fluid balance, not elsewhere classified, E87.8

1. Renal failure.
2. Significant electrolyte imbalance.
3. Follow-up with specialist very important for children with these complications.
J. Education.
    1. Parents must understand importance of having studies done and follow up with specialists.
    2. If medications prescribed, how and when to give and possible side effects.
    3. Know signs/symptoms of progressive renal disease: Edema, hypertension, increasing blood in urine, proteinuria, UTI, lethargy, pallor.

VIII. PROTEINURIA

Calculus of bile duct without cholangitis or cholecystitis without obstruction, K80.50

Disorder of urinary system, unspecified, N39.9

Effect of reduced temperature, unspecified, T69.9

Essential (primary) hypertension, I10

Fever of other and unknown origin, R50

Generalized edema, R60.1

Hematuria, unspecified, R31.9

Nephritic syndrome, unspecified, with unspecified morphologic changes, N05.9

Other forms of acute ischaemic heart disease, I24.8

Polycystic kidney, unspecified, Q61.3

Proteinuria, unspecified, R80.9

Tubulo-interstitial nephritis, not specified as acute or chronic, N12

A. Etiology.
1. Renal insufficiency often associated with proteinuria.
2. Diagnosed by random urinalysis on well-child checkup or associated with serious illness.
3. Common causes of proteinuria include chronic pyelonephritis, renal scarring, febrile illness, glomerulonephritis, exercise induced, idiopathic, orthostatic, polycystic kidney disease, acute tubular necrosis, cold exposure, congestive heart disease, obstructive uropathy, pregnancy, drug induced, trauma.

B. Occurrence.
1. Positive screening by dipstick: Approximately 10% of 8- to 15-year-olds.
   a. Dipstick finding considered positive if it is 1+ (30 mg/dL). False positives can occur with concentrated urine specimens; if specific gravity is 1.015, dipstick finding for protein needs to be higher than 2+.
2. If in doubt, look for other symptoms: Hypertension, edema, hematuria.
3. Always best to confirm lower range and asymptomatic results by rechecking/confirming by protein-to-calcium ratio.

C. Clinical manifestations.
1. Varies with diagnosis.
2. Glomerulonephritis presents with hematuria and proteinuria.
   a. Decreased glomerular filtration rate can result in sodium and water retention, oliguria, circulatory overload, edema, hypertension.
   b. Chronic glomerulonephritis results in failure to thrive, slow growth, fatigue.
3. Postural or orthostatic proteinuria: Usually discovered on well-child check.
   a. Usually older than 8 years of age and totally asymptomatic.
   b. Exercise-induced proteinuria is seen after vigorous exercise, resolves with 48 hours rest.
   c. Febrile proteinuria resolves as temperature returns to normal.
4. Henoch-Schönlein purpura nephritis (a systemic vasculitis) presents with abdominal cramping, purpuric rash, joint pain.
   a. Bloody diarrhea occurs in 50% of patients.
   b. Hemolytic uremic syndrome, systemic lupus erythematosus can also present with purpura, inflammatory bowel.
   c. Known history of renal disease or strong family history of renal compromise.

D. Physical findings.
1. Urinalysis shows proteinuria ranging from trace to 4+, microscopic/gross hematuria.

2. May be associated with infection indicated by elevated urine WBC, nitrites.
3. Blood pressure may be elevated.
4. Edema (especially periorbital) may be present.
5. Patient complains of joint pain, stiffness. Joints swollen, inflamed on exam.
6. Complaints of dysuria or frequency: Signs of infection, CVA tenderness, flank pain may indicate obstruction or pyelonephritis.

E. Diagnostic tests.
    1. In nonacute setting: Obtain protein-to-creatinine ratio.
        a. If > 0.2, repeat; if still elevated, obtain 12- or 24-hour urine.
        b. Supine and upright collection obtained to rule out orthostatic proteinuria. Nonpathologic proteinuria associated with posture, fever, or exercise usually yields results < 1 g/24 hours.
        c. Renal-bladder ultrasound (additional radiographic evaluation if ultrasound abnormal).
    2. Pathologic proteinuria results from glomerular, tubular disorders of kidney.
        a. Protein-to-creatinine ratio is > 0.2, 24-hour urine results are = 3 g of protein in 24 hours.
        b. Renal ultrasound can show infectious or obstructive nephropathy.
        c. Complete metabolic panel, CBC with differential and platelets, ASO, C3, ANA help sort out the immunologic from the nephrologic causes.
        d. Throat and/or skin cultures can identify post-streptococcal glomerulonephritis.

F. Differential diagnosis.
    1. See *Etiology*.

G. Treatment.
    1. Treatment is dependent on type and severity of proteinuria; obstructive uropathy can be repaired surgically.
    2. Infectious uropathy: Treat with antibiotics.
    3. Associated hypertension: May need short- or long-term treatment.
    4. Urgent nephrology referral with edema and hypertension.
    5. Systemically ill patients require hospitalization to determine cause.
    6. If creatinine-to-protein ratio is > 0.2, refer to nephrology for further evaluation.

H. Follow-up.
    1. Follow-up may be lifelong depending on cause.
    2. Recheck asymptomatic proteinuria annually by dipstick analysis and blood pressure: If either is abnormal, referral or additional evaluation needed.

I. Complications.

Acute kidney failure, unspecified, N17.9
Failure to thrive (child), R62.51
Essential (primary) hypertension, I10

    1. Failure to thrive, renal failure, hypertension.

J. Education.

    1. Know signs/symptoms of progressive disease process.

    2. Ensure routine urinalysis remains part of well-child check so early evaluation and treatment can be done.

    3. Follow nonpathologic proteinuria annually.

    4. Close observation for pathologic proteinuria.

BIBLIOGRAPHY

Behrman RE, Kliegman R, Jenson HB, eds. *Nelson Textbook of Pediatrics.* 17th ed. Philadelphia, PA: W.B. Saunders; 2004.

Brandström P, Esbjörner E, Herthelius M, et al. The Swedish Reflux trial in children: I. Study design and study population characteristics. *J Urol.* 2010;184(1):274-279.

Cabana MD. *The 5-Minute Pediatric Consult Standard.* 7th ed. Philadelphia, PA: Wolters Kluwer; 2015.

Gearhart JP, Rink RC, Mouriquand PDE, eds. *Pediatric Urology.* 2nd ed. Philadelphia, PA: W.B. Saunders; 2010.

Gomelia LG. *The 5-Minute Urology Consult.* 2nd ed. Philadelphia, PA: Wolters Kluwer; 2010.

Johnson KB, Oski FA, eds. *Oski's Essential Pediatrics.* Philadelphia, PA: Lippincott-Raven; 1997.

Koyle MA, Shifrin D. Issues in febrile urinary tract infection management. *Pediatr Clin North Am.* 2012;59(4):909-922.

McDougal WS, Wein AJ, Kavoussi LR, et al., eds. *Campbell-Walsh Urology.* 10th ed. Philadelphia, PA: Elsevier; 2012.

Montini G, Tullus K, Hewitt I. Febrile urinary tract infections in children. *N Engl J Med.* 2011;365(3):239-250.

National Institute for Health and Care Excellence (NICE). Urinary tract infection in children: diagnosis, treatment and long-term management. NICE Clinical Guideline 54. http://guidance.nice.org.uk/CG054. Published August 2007. Accessed August 15, 2015.

Newman TB. The new American Academy of Pediatrics urinary tract infection guideline. *Pediatrics.* 2011;128(3):572-575.

O'Neill JA Jr, Grosfeld JL, Fonkalsrud EW, Coran AG, Caldamone AA, eds. *Principles of Pediatric Surgery.* 2nd ed. St. Louis, MO: Mosby; 2004.

Rajimwale A, Williams A, Shenoy M, et al. Critical analysis of the NICE guidelines on UTI in children: a perspective from the UK. *Dialogues in Pediatric Urology.* 2011;32:7-9.

RIVUR Trial Investigators, Hoberman A, Greenfield SP, et al. Antimicrobial prophylaxis for children with vesicoureteral reflux. *N Engl J Med.* 2014;370(25):2367-2376.

Roberts KB, Subcommittee on Urinary Tract Infection, Steering Committee on Quality Improvement and Management. Urinary tract infection: clinical practice guideline for the diagnosis and management of the initial UTI in febrile infants and children 2 to 24 months. *Pediatrics.* 2011;128(3):595-610.

Salo J, Ikaheimo R, Tapiainen T, Uhari M. Childhood urinary tract infections as a cause of chronic kidney disease. *Pediatrics.* 2011;128(5):840-847.

Gynecologic Disorders

Mary Lou C. Rosenblatt and Meg Moorman

I. AMENORRHEA

Amenorrhea, unspecified, N91.2	Intrauterine synechiae, N85.6
Benign neoplasm of unspecified adrenal gland, D35.00	Noninflammatory disorder of ovary, fallopian tube and broad ligament, unspecified, N83.9
Congenital malformation of female genitalia, unspecified, Q52.9	Oophoritis, unspecified, N70.92
Congenital malformation of male genital organ, unspecified, Q55.9	Other disorders of pituitary gland, E23.6
	Other ovarian dysfunction, E28.8
Disorder of adrenal gland, unspecified, E27.9	Polycystic ovarian syndrome, E28.2
	Pregnant state, incidental, Z33.1
Ectopic pregnancy, O00	Thyrotoxicosis, unspecified without thyrotoxic crisis or storm, E05.90
Hypothyroidism, unspecified, E03.9	

A. Primary: No episodes of spontaneous uterine bleeding by 15 in the presence of normal growth and secondary sexual characteristics by age 15. Evaluate for delayed puberty if no secondary sex characteristics by 1 year.

B. Secondary: After onset of menarche, absence of uterine bleeding for 6 months or time equal to 3 previous menstrual cycles. Regular monthly cycles not often seen until 1–2 years after menarche. Because evaluation of amenorrhea applies to all amenorrhea, not necessary to categorize workup as primary or secondary.

C. Etiology.
   1. External genital anomaly: Androgen insensitivity (46,XY).
   2. Internal genital anomaly:
      a. Vaginal agenesis.
      b. Imperforate hymen.
      c. Transverse vaginal septum.

        d. Agenesis of the cervix.

        e. Agenesis of the uterus.

        f. Gonadal dysgenesis.

   3. Hypogonadotropic hypogonadism:

        a. Stress.

        b. Weight loss or gain.

- Obesity.
- Eating disorders: May be related to the role of leptin deficiency.
- Competitive athletics.
- Familial (ask ages of menarche for mother, sisters).
- Drugs (phenothiazines, oral contraceptives, medroxyprogesterone acetate [Depo Provera], illicit drugs).
- Environmental changes (such as going away to college).

   4. Pregnancy is most common cause of secondary amenorrhea.

   5. Central nervous system (CNS) tumor.

   6. Pituitary gland infarct, irradiation, surgery.

   7. Adrenal gland tumor, disease.

   8. Chronic diseases.

   9. Hypo- or hyperthyroidism.

   10. Autoimmune oophoritis.

   11. Ovarian failure, tumor, irradiation, or surgery.

   12. Polycystic ovary syndrome (PCOS).

   13. Asherman's syndrome (history of uterine surgery).

   14. Endometrial ablation if patient has had prior endometrial ablation performed.

D. Occurrence.

   1. Primary: 3 out of 1000 girls have menarche after 15.5 years.

   2. Secondary: Most common reason is pregnancy. Also consider stress, weight changes, eating disorders.

        a. 8–10% of 14- to 18-year-olds report missing 3 consecutive menses in past year.

E. Clinical manifestations.

   1. May have no signs or, depending on cause, may be specific signs, such as wide-spaced nipples, web neck, short stature of Turner syndrome, obesity, acanthosis nigricans of PCOS, or wasting of anorexia.

   2. Evaluate galactorrhea/amenorrhea for prolactinoma and empty sella syndrome.

F. Physical findings.

   1. Physical exam to rule out nonreproductive system problems.

2. Plot height and weight looking for Turner syndrome, obesity, anorexia; explain need for genital exam.
3. On external exam check for patent hymen.
4. A cotton Q-tip can determine the length of the vagina.
5. A one-finger, vaginal–abdominal or rectal–abdominal exam may determine the presence of a cervix and uterus.
6. Estrogenized vaginal mucosa is pink.
7. A pelvic exam for sexually active teens to identify normal organ structure. Clitoromegaly is seen in the presence of excess androgens.

G. Diagnostic tests.
1. Testing indicated in stepwise progression based on history and physical exam.
2. If any concern about sexual activity, obtain pregnancy test. Keep in mind admitting sexual activity may be difficult for some teens.
   a. Negative pregnancy test: Follow stepwise progression again, starting with thyroid-stimulating hormone (TSH) and prolactin, and follicle-stimulating hormone (FSH).
   b. Obtain past medical history, risk factors, medications, and symptoms.
   c. Physical exam: Height, weight, and calculation of body mass index (BMI). Look for hirsutism, acne, stria, acanthosis nigricans, vitiligo, and bruises. Examine breasts for galactorrhea. Vulvovaginal exam should be done looking for signs of estrogen deficiency. Parotid gland swelling and dental enamel erosion may indicate eating disorder.
   d. Pelvic ultrasound to look at pelvic structures may be needed. May order endometrial thickness measurement.
   e. Vaginal maturation index can be obtained to evaluate estrogenization of vagina.
   f. Progestational challenge checks endogenous estrogen levels and competency of outflow tract.

H. Differential diagnosis.
1. See *Etiology*.

I. Treatment.
1. Cause of amenorrhea determines treatment.

J. Follow-up.
1. Determined by the cause and treatment.
2. Referral may be needed in cases of anatomic or chromosomal abnormality, CNS tumor, eating disorder, or specialized management.

K. Complications.

Female infertility, unspecified, N97.9

---

1. Infertility may result from some causes of amenorrhea, making it important to listen to patient's questions and concerns and to offer emotional support.
L. Education.
   1. Offer information relevant to the cause and treatment of the individual's diagnosis.

II. CHLAMYDIAL INFECTION

Abdominal tenderness, unspecified site, R10.819

Chlamydial infection, unspecified, A74.9

Epididymitis, N45.1

Hypertrophic elongation of cervix uteri, N88.4

Inflammatory disease of cervix uteri, N72

Nonspecific urethritis, N34.1

Other specified noninflammatory disorders of vagina, N89.8

Salpingitis, unspecified, N70.91

Urethral discharge, unspecified, R36.9

A. Etiology.
   1. An obligate intracellular bacterial agent with at least 18 serologic variants.
B. Occurrence.
   1. Most common sexually transmitted infection (STI) in United States with high rates among sexually active adolescents.
C. Clinical manifestations.
   1. Causes urethritis, cervicitis, epididymitis, salpingitis, perihepatitis, endometritis, reactive arthritis.
   2. Can lead to acute and chronic pelvic inflammatory disease (PID).
   3. Incubation varies; about 1 week.
D. Physical findings.
   1. May be no symptoms for males or females.
   2. Females: Mucopurulent vaginal discharge, hypertrophic cervical ectopy, abdominal tenderness.
   3. Males: Penile discharge, abdominal tenderness, testicular tenderness.
   4. If having rectal intercourse, males and females may contract chlamydia rectally and experience rectal pain, discharge, or bleeding.

E. Diagnostic tests.
  1. Tissue culture.
  2. Nucleic acid amplification: Highly sensitive from cervical, urethral, rectal, vaginal swabs, oropharyngeal or urine.
F. Differential diagnosis.

Gonococcal infection, A54

  1. Other STIs, such as gonorrhea.
G. Treatment.
  1. Recommended regimens:
    a. Azithromycin 1 g one dose PO, OR
    b. Doxycycline 100 mg PO bid for 7 days.
    c. See Centers for Disease Control and Prevention (CDC) guidelines (see Bibliography) for alternative regimens or treatment guidelines for PID. To maximize adherence, medications for chlamydia should be administered on site, and the patient should be directly observed taking the first dose. Persons treated for chlamydial infections should abstain from sexual intercourse for 7 days until completion of medication to minimize transmission to sex partners.
H. Follow-up.
  1. Rescreen 3–4 months after treatment in high-risk population. In pregnant patients, retesting should be done 3 weeks after completion of therapy to ensure therapeutic cure. Testing at < 3 weeks after completion of therapy can yield a false-positive result and is not recommended. Those diagnosed with chlamydia should also be tested for other STIs like HIV, GC, and syphilis.
I. Complications.

Ectopic pregnancy, unspecified, O00.9	Female pelvic inflammatory disease, unspecified, N73.9
Female infertility, unspecified, N97.9	Pelvic and perineal pain, R10.2

  1. PID.
  2. Ectopic pregnancy.
  3. Infertility.
  4. Chronic pelvic pain.
J. Education.
  1. Abstain from sexual intercourse until 7 days after single-dose treatment or completion of 7-day regimen.

2. Sex partner(s) need treatment.
3. Inform about risks associated with untreated infection to motivate completion of treatment.
4. Avoid multiple partners.
5. Educate about safer sex: Use condoms during all intercourse, limit number of sexual partners, carefully screen any potential partner.

III. DYSMENORRHEA

Abdominal and pelvic pain, R10	Nausea, R11.0
Diarrhea, unspecified, R19.7	Nervousness, R45.0
Dizziness and giddiness, R42	Other symptoms and signs involving
Dysmenorrhea, unspecified, N94.6	the musculoskeletal system, R29.898
Headache, R51	Vomiting, unspecified, R11.10

A. Primary: Pain associated with menstrual cycle without organic source.
B. Secondary: Menstrual pain due to organic disease.
C. Etiology.
   1. Primary: Elevated prostaglandins, prostaglandin levels are higher in women with ovulatory cycles.
   2. Secondary: Due to pelvic pathology such as infection, structural abnormalities, endometriosis.
D. Occurrence.
   1. 60% of teens report pain with menses; 10–14% of those miss school days due to pain.
E. Clinical manifestations.
   1. Primary: May begin 6–36 months after menarche.
      a. Lower abdominal pain; may radiate to thighs or back.
      b. Nausea, vomiting, diarrhea, dizziness, nervousness, headache, fatigue may accompany.
      c. Commonly pain starts within 1–4 hours of onset of menses, lasts 1–2 days. Pain may begin before menses and last 2–4 days.
   2. Secondary: Pain with menses and associated symptoms. History should include sexual history, gastrointestinal and genitourinary systems history.
F. Physical findings.
   1. Primary: Normal physical exam.
   2. Patients with STIs may have purulent cervical discharge, cervical motion tenderness, uterine tenderness, adnexal tenderness. Mass in adnexa

could be cyst, ectopic pregnancy, tubo-ovarian abscess. Tender/nodular cul-de-sac may be found with endometriosis.

G. Diagnostic tests.
   1. For sexually active teens: Pelvic exam to rule out STIs, gonorrhea and chlamydia tests, pregnancy test (if menses are irregular/missed).
   2. Urinalysis if urinary symptoms.
H. Differential diagnosis.

Acute cystitis without hematuria, N30.00	Inflammatory disease of cervix uteri, N72
	Noninfective enteritis and colitis, K50-K52
Chlamydial infection, unspecified, A74.9	Nonspecific urethritis, N34.1
	Other congenital malformations of
Constipation, K59.0	uterus, Q51.818
Dyspareunia, N94.1	Ovarian cysts, unspecified, N83.20
Endometriosis, unspecified, N80.9	Postoperative adhesions of vagina, N99.2
Female pelvic inflammatory disease, unspecified, N73.9	Tubulo-interstitial nephritis, not specified as acute or chronic, N12
Gonococcal infection, A54	

1. Cervicitis or PID caused by agents such as gonorrhea, chlamydia.
2. Cystitis, pyelonephritis.
3. Inflammatory bowel disease.
4. Constipation.
5. Endometriosis: Not common in adolescents but may be significant in adolescents with chronic pelvic pain. Pain may occur before and after menses, may include dyspareunia, pain on defecation, abnormal uterine bleeding.
6. Uterine malformation.
7. Ovarian cysts.
8. Postsurgical adhesions.

I. Treatment.
   1. Primary: Nonsteroidal anti-inflammatory drugs (NSAIDs), oral contraceptives.
   2. Secondary: Treat identified cause.
J. Follow-up.
   1. If standard treatments such as NSAIDs or oral contraceptives do not relieve pain or if etiology is complex, refer to gynecologist.
   2. When infections are the cause, treat and follow up per protocol.
      a. PID: Inpatient or outpatient therapy, monitor for medication compliance.
      b. Gonorrhea or chlamydia: Rescreen every 3–4 months.

K. Complications.

Dysmenorrhea, unspecified, N94.6

1. Primary dysmenorrhea should improve with either NSAID or oral contraceptive therapy. If not, consider other causes.
2. Secondary dysmenorrhea: May have complications based on diagnosis (e.g., teens with PID may suffer from infertility, adhesions, or ectopic pregnancy).

L. Education.
1. Take anti-inflammatory agents with food; start as soon as symptoms occur.
2. Hormonal contraception is useful when contraception is needed. Teach sexually active teens about safer sex.
3. When infection is cause, partners need to be treated.

IV. GENITAL HERPES

Anogenital herpesviral infection, unspecified, A60.9	Vulvar cyst, N90.7
Other specified conditions associated with female genital organs and menstrual cycle, N94.89	

A. Etiology.
1. Recurrent lifelong infection, 2 types: Herpes simplex virus type 1 (HSV-1) and herpes simplex virus type 2 (HSV-2).
2. HSV-2 causes most genital HSV infection, but increasing numbers of genital HSV are caused by HSV-1.

B. Occurrence.
1. 50 million persons in United States have genital HSV infection, with 776,000 new cases reported in 2008.

C. Clinical manifestations.
1. Vesicular or ulcerative lesions of male or female genitalia.
2. Infection can be more severe in immunocompromised individuals.
3. Infections caused by direct contact.
4. Incubation period: 2 days to 2 weeks. Virus persists for life in latent form.
5. Recurrent infections shed virus for 3–4 days rather than 1–2 weeks in primary infection.

D. Physical findings.
1. Vesicular or ulcerative lesions of male or female genitalia.

E. Diagnostic tests.
1. HSV culture provides best sensitivity when lesions are cultured before they begin to heal. Cell culture and PCR are the preferred tests for diagnosis of genital ulcers or mucocutaneous lesions. Failure to identify HSV by culture does not indicate the absence of HSV due to the intermittent shedding of the virus. The use of Pap tests for detection of HSV is insensitive and should not be relied upon.
2. Type-specific and nonspecific antibodies to HSV develop in weeks after infection and persist indefinitely, but do not differentiate between genital and orolabial infections. Serologic type-specific glycoprotein G2 (HSV-2) and G-1 (HSV-1) are type-specific glycoproteins.
F. Differential diagnosis.

Abrasion of unspecified external genital organs, female, initial encounter, S30.816A	Other specified follicular disorders, L73.8
Candidiasis, unspecified, B37.9	Primary genital syphilis, A51.0
Multiple injuries, unspecified, T07	
Other early congenital syphilis, symptomatic, A50.09	Viral wart, unspecified, B07.9

1. Folliculitis.
2. Chancre of syphilis, warts, candidal inflammation, excoriation.
G. Treatment.
1. Primary infection: Oral acyclovir therapy begun within 6 days of onset of infection can decrease viral shedding by 3–5 days. Subsequent severity/frequency of recurrences not affected by treatment. Topical antiviral drugs not recommended.
   a. Recommended regimens:
   - Acyclovir 400 mg PO tid for 7–10 days, OR
   - Acyclovir 200 mg PO 5 times per day for 7–10 days, OR
   - Valacyclovir 1 g PO bid for 7–10 days, OR
   - Famciclovir 250 mg PO tid for 7–10 days.
2. Recurrent infections: Acyclovir therapy started within 2 days of onset of recurrence may shorten clinical course by 1 day. Provide prescription so immediate therapy can begin in case of recurrence.
   a. Recommended regimens:
   - Acyclovir 400 mg PO tid for 5 days, OR
   - Acyclovir 800 mg PO bid for 5 days, OR
   - Acyclovir 800 mg PO tid for 2 days, OR

- Valacyclovir 500 mg PO bid for 3 days, OR
- Valacyclovir 1 g PO qd for 5 days, OR
- Famciclovir 125 mg PO bid for 5 days, OR
- Famciclovir 1000 mg orally bid for 1 day, OR
- Famiciclovir 500 mg once, followed by 250 mg bid for 2 days.

3. Suppressive therapy for recurrent infections (6 episodes per year): Can benefit from daily therapy. Acyclovir: Safety and effectiveness for 6 years; valacyclovir or famciclovir for 1 year. Because outbreaks diminish in frequency over time, periodic discontinuation of therapy (i.e., yearly) may be helpful in reassessing need for therapy.

   a. Recommended regimens:
- Acyclovir 400 mg PO bid, OR
- Valacyclovir 500 mg PO daily, OR
- Valacyclovir 1 g PO for one day, OR
- Famiciclovir 250 mg orally twice a day.

H. Follow-up.
   1. Follow patient's emotional adjustment to having HSV.
   2. Test for other STIs.

I. Complications.

Anogenital herpesviral infection, unspecified, A60.9

Calcinosis cutis, L94.2/Other general symptoms and signs, R68.89

Viral wart, unspecified, B07.9

---

1. Daily medication may not suppress recurrent outbreaks.
2. Immune-suppressed patients may have prolonged/severe outbreaks requiring IV therapy.
3. Transmission to neonate from infected mother is highest among women who acquire genital HSV near time of delivery.

J. Education.
   1. Psychological burden may be great. Counseling includes supportive groups, CDC website, written materials. If depression is identified, refer to mental health provider.
   2. Latex condoms may reduce transmission if used correctly.
   3. Patients should refrain from sexual contact if lesions are present.
   4. Sexual partners should be notified by patient.
   5. Sexual transmission may occur with asymptomatic viral shedding.
   6. Explain risk of neonatal infection to male and female patients; they should inform provider during pregnancy.

V. GENITAL WARTS

Anogenital (venereal) warts, A63.0   Other viral warts, B07.8

A. Etiology.
   1. 90% of anogenital warts are caused by human papilloma viruses (HPV) types 6 or 11, which are nononcogenic. HPVs are DNA viruses and include 100 types; 30 types can infect genital tract.
   2. Types 16, 18, and 45 are associated with cervical cancer.
B. Occurrence.
   1. HPV is so common that almost everyone will be infected at some point in their lives with this virus, but most will not know they have been infected.
   2. HPV causes about 9000 cancers in men each year and about 17,000 cases in women.
C. Clinical manifestations.
   1. May have no symptoms.
   2. When present, warts are epithelial tumors of skin/mucous membrane.
   3. Immunocompromised individuals may have larger quantity of warts.
   4. Incubation unknown; likely ranges from 3 months to several years.
   5. May regress spontaneously or may persist for years.
D. Physical findings.
   1. Skin-colored lesions with cauliflower-like surface may be several millimeters to several centimeters wide; may be painless or itch, burn, bleed; can be found on vagina, cervix, vulva, penis, anus, perianal area, scrotum.
E. Diagnostic tests.
   1. Anogenital warts are usually made by visual inspection and can be confirmed by a biopsy if lesions are atypical and pigmented, bleeding, ulcerated, or fixed to underlying tissue. For those who are immunocompromised, as in HIV-infected persons, a biopsy should be considered.
   2. HPV DNA testing for anogenital wards is not recommended because the results do not confirm the diagnosis, nor does it assist with management of the warts.
   3. Some providers use 3–5% acetic acid applied to a suspicious wart to see if it turns the affected area white in detection of HPV-infected genital mucosa. It is not, however, type specific and should not be used for diagnosis and treatment planning.

F. Differential diagnosis.

Anogenital (venereal) warts, A63.0

Condyloma latum, A51.31

Molluscum contagiosum, B08.1

---

1. Molluscum contagiosum.
2. Condyloma lata (syphilis).
3. Pink, pearly penile papules.

G. Treatment.
1. Recommended regimens.
    a. Patient applied:
        - Imiquimod 3.75% or 5% cream, OR
        - Podofilox 0.5% solution or gel, OR
        - Sinecatechins 15% ointment.
    b. Provider administered:
        - Cryotherapy with liquid nitrogen or cryoprobe, OR
        - Surgical removal either by tangential scissor excision or tangential shave excision, curettage, laser or electrosurgery, OR
        - Trichloroacetic acid (TCA) or bichloroacetic acid (BCA) 80–90% solution.

H. Follow-up.
1. Women with genital warts do not need Pap tests more often than others.

I. Complications.
1. Genital warts that are left untreated may go away, stay, or increase in size and number. Genital warts do not turn into cancer, and the type of HPV that causes genital warts is different from the kind that causes cancer. Recurrences common due to reactivation of virus. May persist for life. Duration of contagiousness unknown.
2. Local treatment can damage normal surrounding skin.

J. Education.
1. Females: Women with genital warts do not need Pap tests more frequently than those without warts.
2. Screen for other STIs.
3. Partners should be informed and may want to consider being screened for other STIs
4. Teach safer sex. Condoms may lower transmission of genital warts, but HPV can infect areas not covered by the condom and may not prevent HPV transmission.

K. Vaccinations.
1. Cervarix (bivalent) vaccine contains HPV types 16 and 18 (which cause 70% of cervical cancers).

2. Gardasil (quadrivalent) vaccine contains HPV types 6, 11, 16, and 18 (which cause 90% of genital warts).

3. Either vaccine can be administered to girls aged 11–12 years, or the series of vaccines can be started at age 9 years. They can also be administered to women ages 13–26 who have not started or completed the vaccine. It is most beneficial if given before onset of sexual activity. Gardasil can be used in males aged 13–21 to prevent genital warts. Vaccination is recommended routinely for both men who have sex with men (MSM) and immunocompromised persons aged 22–26 years. Both vaccines are administered in a 3-series injection schedule over a 6-month period. Providers should consider a 15-minute waiting period for vaccine recipients following the first injection. After injection 1 is given, the second is given 1–2 months later, then at 6 months after the first injection for a total of 3 injections. Women should still receive routine cervical cancer screening after receiving the vaccine.

VI. GONORRHEA

Gonococcal infection, A54

A. Etiology.
   1. *Neisseria gonorrhoeae* is Gram-negative, oxidase-positive diplococcus.
B. Occurrence.
   1. 820,000 new cases of gonorrhea per year in the United States.
   2. Women aged < 25 are at the highest risk of gonococcal infections.
   3. Coinfection with chlamydia is common.
C. Clinical manifestations.
   1. Males tend to have symptomatic infections of urethra.
   2. Females may have cervicitis, PID, perihepatitis, bartholinitis.
   3. Rectal and pharyngeal infections may be asymptomatic.
   4. Disseminated infections occur in up to 3% of untreated persons.
      a. Bacteremia causes arthritis-dermatitis syndrome.
      b. More common in females infected within 1 week of menstrual period.
   5. Incubation is 2–7 days.
D. Physical findings.
   1. May be no symptoms.
   2. Males may experience penile discharge, dysuria.
   3. Females may have vaginal discharge, abdominal pain.

E. Diagnostic tests.

1. Culture is excellent but may require special handling. Culture requires specimen from female endocervical or male urethral swab.
2. Nucleic acid amplification test (NAAT) is highly sensitive; may be used with mucosal discharge/urine. Must read product inserts and specimen types for NAAT. In cases of treatment failure, clinician should perform a culture and antimicrobial susceptibility test.
3. Gram stain showing Gram-negative intracellular diplococci is most useful in acutely ill patients.

F. Differential diagnosis.

Abdominal and pelvic pain, R10	Other specified noninflammatory
Chlamydial infection, unspecified,	disorders of vagina, N89.8
A74.9	Urethral discharge, unspecified,
Dysuria, R30.0	R36.9

1. Chlamydia may cause similar symptoms.
2. Non-gonococcal urethritis (NGU): 40% of cases caused by chlamydia; 20–30% caused by *Ureaplasma urealyticum*; and 30–40% uncertain but may include HSV, *Trichomonas vaginalis*, *Escherichia coli*, and others.

G. Treatment.

1. Recommended regimens for uncomplicated gonococcal infections of cervix, urethra, rectum:
   a. Combination therapy with ceftriaxone 250 mg intramuscularly PLUS azithromycin 1 g orally as a single dose.
   b. If ceftriaxone is not available, may use cefixime 400 mg po PLUS azithromycin 1 g PO.
   c. For those allergic to cephalosporins, CDC recommends a single 2 g dose of azithromycin orally.
2. Note: Any treatment failures should be reported to the CDC through local or state public health officials within 24 hours.

H. Follow-up.

1. Test of cure for uncomplicated gonococcal infection not indicated.
2. Persistent infection may be due to reinfected or untreated coinfection with chlamydia.
3. Persons with pharyngeal gonorrhea who are treated with an alternative regimen should return 14 days after treatment for a test of cure.
4. Sex partners should be referred for evaluation and treatment if they have had sexual contact with a partner within 60 days before patient's onset of symptoms or gonorrhea diagnosis.

I. Complications.

Ectopic pregnancy, unspecified, O00.9	Gonococcal infection of kidney and ureter, A54.21
Female infertility, unspecified, N97.9	
Female pelvic inflammatory disease, unspecified, N73.9	Salpingitis and oophoritis, unspecified, N70.93

    1. PID.
    2. Tubal scarring.
    3. Infertility.
    4. Ectopic pregnancy.
    5. Hematogenous spread causing skin and joint syndrome.

J. Education.
    1. Partners need to be evaluated and treated.
    2. Encourage use of condom.
    3. Screen for other STIs (chlamydia, HIV, syphilis, hepatitis B).

VII. SYPHILIS

Disorder of the skin and subcutaneous tissue, unspecified, L98.9	Other early congenital syphilis, symptomatic, A50.09
Early syphilis, latent, A51.5	Other fatigue, R53.83
Enlarged lymph nodes, unspecified, R59.9	Primary genital syphilis, A51.0
Fever of other and unknown origin, R50	Rash and other nonspecific skin eruption, R21
Headache, R51/Vascular headache, not elsewhere classified, G44.	Syphilis, unspecified, A53.9

A. Etiology.
    1. Person-to-person transmission of spirochete, *Treponema pallidum*.
    2. Incubation is 10–90 days.

B. Occurrence.
    1. Rare in much of industrialized world but problem in large U.S. urban areas and the rural South.

C. Clinical manifestations.
 1. Primary: Painless, indurated ulcers (chancres) at site of inoculation, within 3 weeks of exposure.
 2. Secondary: 1–2 months later, generalized maculopapular rash (includes palms and soles), fever, malaise, headache, lymphadenopathy.
 3. Hypertrophic, papular lesions (condyloma lata) in moist areas of vulva or anus.
 4. Latent: Seroreactivity but no clinical manifestations of syphilis, may last years.
   a. Early latent: Acquired in last year.
   b. Late latent: Acquired more than 1 year ago or unknown duration.
 5. Tertiary: May be many years after acquiring infection; features major organ damage.
 6. Neurosyphilis: CNS disease can occur during any stage of syphilis; examine cerebrospinal fluid in patients with neurologic involvement.
D. Physical findings.
 1. Primary: Chancre at site of inoculation, painless ulcer.
 2. Secondary: Maculopapular rash, generalized, including palms/soles, condyloma lata.
 3. Neurosyphilis: Abnormal neurologic exam.
E. Diagnostic tests.
 1. Positive dark-field exam is definitive for syphilis from lesion exudate or tissue but may not be readily available.
 2. Nontreponemal tests (VDRL, RPR) are quantitative, testing activity, treatment response. Same lab should measure subsequent tests to ensure reliability. Tests may become negative 2 years after treatment.
 3. Treponemal tests (FTA-ABS, TP-PA) or EIAs must confirm nontreponemal test.
 4. Tests usually positive for life. Other spirochetal disease causes positive test (yaws, pinta, leptospirosis, rat-bite fever, Lyme disease).
F. Differential diagnosis.

Pityriasis rosea, L42

---

 1. Rash of secondary syphilis can be confused with pityriasis rosea, making blood evaluation important for sexually active adolescents diagnosed with pityriasis.
G. Treatment.
 1. Recommended regimen for adults.
   a. Primary and secondary.

- Penicillin G benzathine, 2.4 million units IM single dose (preferred), OR
- If penicillin allergic, not pregnant: Doxycycline 100 mg PO bid for 14 days, OR tetracycline 500 mg PO qid for 14 days.
  b. Early latent, late latent, latency of unknown duration, tertiary or neurosyphilis, HIV-positive, and pregnant patients, refer to CDC guidelines for treatment.
  c. All persons who are positive for primary and secondary syphilis should be tested for HIV infection.
H. Follow-up.
  1. Clinical and serologic evaluation should be performed at 6 and 12 months after treatment, or more frequently if follow-up is uncertain. Serologic response by titer should be compared to titer at time of treatment. If there is a failure in nontreponemal test titers to decline fourfold within the first 6–12 months, treatment may be considered a failure. These persons should receive additional clinical and serologic follow-up.
I. Complications.

Asymptomatic human immunodeficiency virus [HIV] infection status, Z21`	Other congenital malformations of uterus and cervix, Q51.8
Human immunodeficiency virus [HIV] disease, B20–B24	Stillbirth, P95
Hydrops fetalis not due to hemolytic disease, P83.2	Syphilis, unspecified, A53.9

  1. Untreated syphilis causes damage to most body organs over time, infects partners.
  2. Coinfection with HIV, other STIs.
  3. Infected pregnant women pass along syphilis to fetus, resulting in stillbirth, hydrops fetalis, or prematurity. Infants may suffer numerous complications.
  4. Jarisch-Herxheimer reaction (acute, febrile reaction with headache myalgia) may occur in first 24 hours after treatment (occurs most with patients being treated for early syphilis). Antipyretics may be used but may not prevent this reaction.
J. Education.
  1. Sexual partners must be treated. Public health department finds contacts anonymously.
  2. HIV status should be checked. If negative, recheck in 3 months.
  3. Safer sex counseling.

VIII. TRICHOMONIASIS

Other specified noninflammatory disorders of vagina, N89.8	Trichomonal vulvovaginitis, A59.0

A. Etiology.
   1. *Trichomonas vaginalis* is a flagellated protozoan.
B. Occurrence.
   1. Primarily sexually transmitted, may coexist with other STIs.
C. Clinical manifestations.
   1. Most males have no symptoms.
   2. Females may have profuse, pruritic, malodorous, yellow-green vaginal discharge or no symptoms at all.
   3. Incubation period: 4–28 days.
D. Physical findings.
   1. Females: Frothy white, yellow-green vaginal discharge with erythematous vaginal mucosa and friable "strawberry cervix."
E. Diagnostic tests.
   1. On wet mount, trichomonad has jerky motion and lashing flagella.
   2. NAATs may detect a prevalence 3–5 times higher than a wet mount. OSOM Trichomonas Rapid Test by Sekisui Diagnostics may also confirm trichamonas, and the OSOM Trichomonas Rapid Test provides results in 10 minutes.
F. Differential diagnosis.

Candidiasis, unspecified, B37.9	Gonococcal infection, A54
Candidiasis of vulva and vagina, B37.3	Pruritus, unspecified, L29.9
Chlamydial infection, unspecified, A74.9	

   1. Other STIs such as gonorrhea and chlamydia could be cause of discharge.
   2. Monilia could be cause of pruritus.
G. Treatment.
   1. Recommended regimen: Metronidazole 2 g dose PO in a single dose, OR
   2. Tinidazole 2 g orally in a single dose, OR
   3. Alternative regimen: Metronidazole 500 mg PO bid for 7 days.
H. Follow-up.
   1. None needed unless discharge persists.

I. Complications.
1. If no response to initial treatment, may repeat metronidazole 1 g bid for 7 days OR 2 g daily for 3–5 days. If treatment failure occurs twice with metronidazole 2 g single dose, treat with metronidazole 500 PO bid for 7 days OR or tinidazole 2 g PO for 5 days.
2. In rare cases where infection persists despite treatment of patient and partner, CDC may be helpful in looking at resistance of organism.
J. Education.
1. Concurrent treatment of all partners for symptomatic relief and prevention is recommended, and abstinence from unprotected sex is advised until completion of therapy.
2. Patients should abstain from sex until they and any partners are treated and asymptomatic.
3. Safer sex counseling.
4. Screen for other STIs.
5. Because of the high rate of reinfection among women, retesting for trichamonas should be done within 3 months of initial treatment. Not enough data exists to recommend retreatment in men. NAAT testing can be done 2 weeks after treatment.
6. Patient should avoid alcohol consumption while being treated with nitromidazoles and should continue abstinence for 24 hours after completion of medication. This is to avoid a disulfiram-like reaction (flushing, pulsating headache, violent vomiting, restlessness).

IX. BACTERIAL VAGINOSIS (BV)

| Acute vaginitis, N76.0 | Other specified noninflammatory |
| Other inflammation of vagina and vulva, N76 | disorders of vagina, N89.8 |

A. Etiology.
1. BV is a syndrome found in sexually active females caused by changes in vaginal flora and is more common among women with female partners. Normal vaginal ecosystem is disrupted by increases in *Gardnerella vaginalis, Mycoplasma, Ureaplasma* species, and anaerobic bacteria, as well as a marked decrease in lactobacillus species.
2. Incubation is unknown.
B. Occurrence.
1. Common, may occur with other infections.
2. Although not proved to be sexually transmitted, it is uncommon in sexually inexperienced females.

C. Clinical manifestations.
  1. May have no symptoms.
  2. White, homogenous, adherent vaginal discharge with fishy odor.
D. Physical findings.
  1. White, malodorous vaginal discharge.
  2. Not associated with abdominal pain or pruritus.
E. Diagnostic tests.
  1. Three of following four criteria establish diagnosis:
      a. Homogenous, white, adherent vaginal discharge.
      b. Vaginal fluid pH 4.5 or more.
      c. Fishy odor before or after adding 10% KOH (whiff test).
      d. Clue cells (squamous vaginal epithelial cells covered with bacteria, causing granular appearance) on microscopic exam.
F. Differential diagnosis.

Candidiasis of vulva and vagina, B37.3	Generalized edema, R60.1
Candidiasis, unspecified, B37.9	Gonococcal infection, A54
Chlamydial infection, unspecified, A74.9	Other specified noninflammatory disorders of vagina, N89.8
Erythematous condition, unspecified, L53.9	Pruritus, unspecified, L29.9

  1. Characterized by white, thick, pruritic discharge with pH 4.5; pseudohyphae are seen under microscope when 10% KOH is added. Candida also causes erythema and edema of vulva-vagina.
  2. Rule out other STIs.
G. Treatment.
  1. Treatment is recommended for women who are symptomatic. Other benefits of treatment include reduction in risk of acquiring *N. gonorrhoeae*, HIV, and *C. trachomatis*.
  2. Recommended regimens:
      a. Metronidazole 500 mg PO bid for 7 days, OR
      b. Metronidazole gel 0.75%, one full applicator (5 g) intravaginally, once a day for 5 days, OR
      c. Clindamycin cream 2%, one applicator intravaginally at bedtime for 7 days.
H. Follow-up.
  1. Recurrence is common.

I. Complications.

Asymptomatic human immunodeficiency virus [HIV] infection status, Z21	Preterm labor with preterm delivery, unspecified trimester, not applicable or unspecified, O60.10X0
Endometritis following delivery, O86.12	Preterm labor without delivery, second trimester, O60.02
Female pelvic inflammatory disease, unspecified, N73.9	Preterm labor without delivery, third trimester, O60.03
Human immunodeficiency virus [HIV] disease, B20–B24	Puerperal sepsis, O85

  1. May be risk factor for PID, HIV, preterm labor, postpartum endometritis.
J. Education.
  1. Women should refrain from sexual activity during treatment regimen. Douching may increase risk of return of BV.
  2. Not clearly sexually transmitted.
  3. Routine treatment of sex partners is not recommended.

X. VULVOVAGINAL CANDIDIASIS (VVC)

Acute vaginitis, N76.0 Candidiasis, unspecified, B37.9	Other specified noninflammatory disorders of vagina, N89.8

A. Etiology.
  1. Usually caused by *Candida albicans* or other Candida types of yeast.
B. Occurrence.
  1. 75% of women have at least 1 episode of VVC.
C. Clinical manifestations.
  1. Pruritus.
  2. Dyspareunia.
  3. Vaginal soreness.
  4. White, thick vaginal discharge.
D. Physical findings.
  1. Vulvar redness and edema.
  2. Thick, curdy white discharge.
E. Diagnostic tests.
  1. Vaginal pH of < 4.5.
  2. Wet mount with 10% KOH with budding yeast, hyphae, or pseudohyphae upon microscopic exam.
  3. Positive yeast culture.

F.   Differential diagnosis: BV, STIs.

Gonorrhoea complicating pregnancy, childbirth and the puerperium, O98.2

Nonspecific urethritis, N34.1

Trichomoniasis, unspecified, A59.9

G.   Recommended treatment regimen.
   1.   Butoconazole 2% cream, 5 g intravaginally in a single application, OR
   2.   Clotrimazole 1% cream 5 g intravaginally qd for 7–14 days, OR
   3.   Clotrimazole 2% cream 5 g intravaginally qd for 3 days, OR
   4.   Miconazole 2% cream 5 g intravaginally qd for 7 days, OR
   5.   Miconazole 4% cream 5 g intravaginally qd for 3 days, OR
   6.   Miconazole 100 mg vaginal suppository 1 suppository qd for 7 days, OR
   7.   Oral agent: Fluconazole 150 mg PO in a single dose.
H.   Follow-up.
   1.   Women only need to follow up if symptoms persist.
I.   Education.
   1.   VVC is not usually acquired through sexual intercourse, and partner does not need to be treated.
   2.   Recurrent frequent infections warrant screening patient for HIV and diabetes.

BIBLIOGRAPHY

Joffe A. Amenorrhea. In: Hoekelman RA, Adam HM, Nelson NM, Weitzman ML, Wilson MH, eds. *Primary Pediatric Care.* 4th ed. St. Louis, MO: Mosby; 2001:975-977.

Neinstein LS, ed. *Adolescent Health Care: A Practical Guide.* 4th ed. Philadelphia, PA: Lippincott Williams & Wilkins; 2002.

Peipert JF. Clinical practice. Genital chlamydial infections. *N Engl J Med.* 2003;349(25):2424-2430.

Pickering LK, ed. *Red Book: 2003 Report of the Committee on Infectious Disease.* 26th ed. Elk Grove Village, IL: American Academy of Pediatrics; 2003.

Sanfillippo JS, Muram D, Dewhurst J, Lee PA, eds. *Pediatric and Adolescent Gynecology.* 2nd ed. Philadelphia, PA: W.B. Saunders; 2001.

Speroff L, Glass RH, Kase NG, Seifer DB. *Clinical Gynecologic Endocrinology and Infertility.* 6th ed. Philadelphia, PA: Lippincott Williams & Wilkins; 2001.

Welt CK, Barbieri RL. Etiology, diagnosis, and treatment of secondary amenorrhea. UpToDate. http://www.uptodate.com/contents/etiology-diagnosis-and-treatment-of-primary-amenorrhea. Updated April 13, 2015. Accessed June 10, 2015.

White, CD. Amenorrhea – primary. MedlinePlus. http://www.nlm.nih.gov/medlineplus/ency/article/001218.htm. Accessed June 15, 2015.

Workowski KA, Berman S; Centers for Disease Control and Prevention. Sexually transmitted diseases treatment guidelines, 2010. *MMWR Recomm Rep.* 2010;59(No. RR-12):1-110.

Workowski KA, Bolan G. *Sexually Transmitted Diseases Treatment Guidelines, 2014.* http://www.cdc.gov/std/treatment/2014/2014-std-guidelines-peer-reviewers-08-20-2014.pdf. Accessed June 8, 2015.

Endocrine Disorders

Linda S. Gilman

I. HYPERTHYROIDISM

Abnormal weight loss, R63.4

Agranulocytosis, D70

Amenorrhea, unspecified, N91.2

Autoimmune thyroiditis, E06.3

Cardiomegaly, I51.7

Cough, R05

Edema of unspecified orbit, H05.229

Exophthalmic conditions, H05.2

Eyelid retraction unspecified eye, unspecified lid, H02.539

Fever of other and unknown origin, R50

Flushing, R23.2

Generalized edema, R60.1

Generalized hyperhidrosis [sweating], R61

Heat fatigue, transient, initial encounter, T67.6XXA

Hypothyroidism, unspecified, E03.9

Insomnia, unspecified, G47.00

Nontoxic goiter, unspecified, E04.9

Other general symptoms and signs, R68.89

Other specified symptoms and signs involving the circulatory and respiratory systems, R09.89

Other visual disturbances, H53.8

Palpitations, R00.2

Rash and other nonspecific skin eruption, R21

Shortness of breath, R06.02

Tachycardia, unspecified, R00.0

Thyrotoxicosis, unspecified without thyrotoxic crisis or storm, E05.90

Thyrotoxicosis with diffuse goitre, E05.0

Tremor, unspecified, R25.1

Visual loss, unspecified, H54.7

A. Clinical syndrome resulting from excessive exposure of body tissues to action of thyroid hormone.

B. Etiology.

1. Hyperthyroidism in childhood, with few exceptions, is due to autoimmune response to thyroid-stimulating hormone (TSH) receptors on the thyroid cell membrane, resulting in excessive synthesis and secretion of thyroid hormone. This tissue response causes a condition known as Graves' disease. Graves' disease is a common cause of hyperthyroidism in children.

2. Increases as adolescence approaches.
3. No specific etiology known.

C. Occurrence.

1. Approximately 5% of all patients are younger than 15 years old.
   a. Peak incidence is between 10 and 15 years of age.
   b. Five times higher in girls than boys.
   c. May be present at birth if mother thyrotoxic during pregnancy.
2. Symptoms develop gradually; time between onset and diagnosis may be 6–12 months and longer in prepubertal children compared with adolescents.

D. Clinical manifestations.

1. Insomnia.
2. Heat intolerance followed by diaphoresis.
3. Weight loss, voracious appetite without weight gain.
4. Increased sweating, palpitations, tachycardia.
5. Muscle weakness and fatigue.
6. Light menses or amenorrhea.
7. Hyperactive GI tract with vomiting or frequent stooling.
8. Tremors, nervousness, irritability, hyperactivity, emotional lability.
9. Schoolwork suffers.
10. Breathlessness.
11. Blurred vision.

E. Physical findings.

1. Enlarged thyroid, thyroid bruits, thrills.
2. Thinning of hair.
3. Proptosis, exophthalmia, noticeable lid lag, lid retraction, periorbital edema.
4. Diffuse enlarged goiter.
5. Fast heart rate, cardiac enlargement, widening pulse pressure, heart palpitations.
6. Trembling hands, tremor of finger with extended arm.
7. Staring gaze, loss of visual acuity.
8. Flushed moist skin, excessive sweating.
9. Pedal edema.
10. Palmar erythema.
11. Increased deep tendon reflexes.
12. Hypercalcemia osteoporosis.

F. Diagnostic tests.

1. TSH produced by pituitary gland.
2. Thyroid hormones (T3, T4).

    3. Iodine thyroid scan.

    4. Antithyroid antibodies test.

G. Differential diagnosis.

Benign neoplasm of pituitary gland, D53.2

    1. Pituitary tumor.

H. Treatment/management.

    1. Refer to endocrinologist.

    2. Antithyroid agents:

       a. Methimazole (Tapazole): To induce remission.

       b. Propylthiouracil (PTU): To induce remission.

       c. Propranolol (Inderal): To decrease adrenergic hyperresponsiveness symptoms.

    3. Subtotal thyroidectomy.

    4. Radioactive iodine (131-iodine).

I. Follow-up.

    1. Monitor for adverse side effects of antithyroid drugs such as skin reactions, leukopenia, agranulocytosis.

    2. Most serious side effect: Agranulocytosis, usually occurs in first 3 months of therapy.

    3. Report rash, fever, chills, cough that does not resolve in 1 week.

    4. When patient is euthyroid as determined by lab tests of TSH and T4, a 6-month follow-up should be instituted to assess for risk of relapse.

J. Complications.

Agranulocytosis, D70	Nephritic syndrome with unspecified morphologic changes, unspecified, N05.9
Arteritis, unspecified, I77.6	
Hepatic failure, unspecified without coma, K72.90	Systemic lupus erythematosus, organ or system involvement unspecified, M32.10
Inflammatory liver disease, unspecified, K75.9	Thyrotoxicosis, unspecified with thyrotoxic crisis or storm, E05.91

    1. Toxic reaction with drug therapy, most severe: Hypersensitivity, agranulocytosis, hepatitis, hepatic failure, lupus-like syndrome, glomerulonephritis, vasculitis of skin, thyroid storm, or thyrotoxicosis.

K. Education.

    1. Initial adjustment to therapy: Stress need to report side effects of therapy.

    2. Compliance to treatment: Do not miss doses; if dose is missed, take missed dose as soon as possible.

    3. Side effects of medication.

4. If after several weeks of therapy, symptoms, continue, may need increased dose of antithyroid medication.
5. Watch for potential complication of Graves' disease, such as thyroid storm, cardiac arrhythmia, and cardiac failure.

II. HYPOTHYROIDISM

Abdominal distension (gaseous), R14.0

Abnormal weight gain, R63.5

Ataxia, unspecified, R27.0

Autoimmune thyroiditis, E06.3

Congenital iodine-deficiency syndrome, unspecified, E00.9

Constipation, K59.0

Delayed puberty, E30.0

Disturbances in tooth eruption, K00.6

Dysphagia, unspecified, R13.10

Effusion, unspecified ankle, M25.473

Feeding difficulties, R63.3

Headache, R51

Hypoglycaemia, unspecified, E16.2

Hypothermia, not associated with low environmental temperature, R68.0

Hypothyroidism, unspecified, E03.9

Jaundice, unspecified, R17

Major depressive disorder, single episode, unspecified, F32.9

Nontoxic goiter, unspecified, E04.9

Other fatigue, R53.83

Other general symptoms and signs, R68.89

Other hair color and hair shaft abnormalities, L67.8

Other heavy for gestational age newborn, P08.1

Other visual disturbances, H53.8

Other voice and resonance disorders, R49.8

Precocious puberty, E30.1

Short stature (child), R62.52

Sleep apnea, unspecified, G47.30

Sleep disorders, G47

Slow fetal growth, unspecified, P05.9

Unspecified intellectual disabilities, F79

A. Condition resulting from deficient production of thyroid hormone or defect in hormonal receptor activity.
B. Etiology.
   1. Hypothyroidism may be congenital or acquired.
      a. Congenital hypothyroidism.
         • Most commonly from inadequate production of thyroid hormone due to agenesis, dysplasia, ectopy of thyroid, or autosomal

recessive defects in thyroid hormone synthesis and defects in other enzymatic steps in T4 synthesis and release.
- Most common preventable cause of mental retardation.
   b. Acquired hypothyroidism most commonly caused by autoimmune destruction (Hashimoto thyroiditis).

C. Occurrence.
   1. One case per 3500 persons for congenital hypothyroidism.
   2. Acquired hypothyroidism: 6% of age 12- to 19-year-olds have evidence of autoimmune disease.
      a. Depending on diagnostic criteria, may be as high as 10% in young females. Higher incidence in females (2:1).
      b. Congenital if untreated condition results in profound growth failure, developmental cognitive delay (cretinism).
      c. When untreated in older children: Growth failure, slow metabolism, impaired memory.

D. Clinical manifestations.
   1. Congenital.
      a. Constipation.
      b. Hypotonia.
      c. Hypoglycemia.
      d. Hypothermia.
      e. Poor feeding.
      f. Hoarse cry, noisy respirations.
      g. Large for gestation.
   2. Acquired.
      a. Asymptomatic goiter.
      b. Hoarseness, dysphagia.
      c. Mild weight gain.
      d. Slow growth/delayed osseous maturation.
      e. Lethargy, sleep disturbance/sleep apnea.
      f. Cold intolerance.
      g. Constipation.
      h. Sexual pseudoprecocity.
      i. Headaches.
      j. Depression.

E. Physical findings.
   1. Congenital.
      a. Large for gestation infant.
      b. Hypotonia, puffy face.

      c. Wide anterior, posterior fontanel.

      d. Prolonged jaundice.

      e. Abdominal distention.

      f. Feeding difficulties/slowed gastric motility.

  2. Acquired.

      a. Visual problems.

      b. Precocious puberty (young children).

      c. Dry skin.

      d. Slowed pulse.

      e. Delayed puberty.

      f. Coarse, sparse hair.

      g. Delayed dentition.

      h. Ankle and feet swelling.

      i. Short stature.

F. Diagnostic tests.

  1. Newborn screen for T4: If low, then TSH drawn for definitive testing.

  2. Serum thyrotropin concentration/TSH.

  3. T4 and T3.

  4. Serum antithyroid globulin antibodies.

  5. Antithyroid peroxidase.

  6. Radionucleotide studies.

  7. Radioisotope-based thyroid scanning.

G. Differential diagnosis.

Congenital iodine-deficiency syndrome, E00	Other specified disorders of adrenal gland, E27.8
Diabetes mellitus, E10-E14	Precocious puberty, E30.1
Disorder of kidney and ureter, unspecified, N28.9	Protein-calorie malnutrition, unspecified, E46
Hypopituitarism, E23.0	Short stature (child), R62.52
Irritable bowel syndrome without diarrhea, K58.9	Turner's syndrome, unspecified, Q96.9

  1. Endemic goiter/nutritional iodine deficiency.

  2. Chromosomal abnormalities such as Turner syndrome.

  3. Precocious puberty in young child.

  4. Familial short stature.

  5. Constitutional growth delay.

  6. Growth hormone deficiency.

  7. Chronic bowel syndrome.

8. Renal disease.
9. Malnutrition/gluten-induced enteropathy.
10. Cortisol excess.
11. Diabetes mellitus.

H. Treatment.
1. Levothyroxine (Levothroid, Levoxyl, Synthroid), a synthetic drug identical to human T4, is preferred thyroid hormone replacement.
2. Neonates: Initial doses 10–15 mcg/kg PO every morning before meals. Dosage titrated on basis of thyroid function tests every 3 months until 2 years of age. Desired T4 range: 10–15 mcg/dL.
3. Children: 2–6 years of age: 5 mcg/kg PO every morning before meals; 6–12 years of age: 4–5 mcg/kg PO every morning before meals.
4. Adolescents: 100–150 mcg PO every morning before meals.
5. With age, levothyroxine dose decreases on weight basis.

I. Follow-up.
1. Monitor for behavior change, school performance.
2. Monitor serum TSH 2–3 months after change in dosage.
3. Monitor for symptoms of hypothyroidism, hyperthyroidism.

J. Complications.
1. Noncompliance with treatment protocol.

K. Education.
1. Educate parents on signs/symptoms of hypothyroidism and hyperthyroidism.
2. Allow child to take responsibility for own care as soon as old enough (9–10 years of age).
3. Educate parents to be aware that initial treatment may sometimes cause temporary behavior problems as well as poorer school achievement, and the child may not be restored to full growth potential.
4. Goal of treatment is to restore child to normal growth and development.

III. SHORT STATURE

Hypopituitarism, E23.0	Turner's syndrome, unspecified, Q96.9
Short stature (child), R62.52	

A. Generally accepted definition is stature below third percentile, or two standard deviations (SD) below mean, for age and sex.
B. Etiology.
1. Familial short stature.
2. Constitutional growth delay.
3. Growth hormone deficiency.
4. Chromosomal disorder/Turner syndrome.

C. Occurrence.
1. Growth hormone deficiency estimated 10,000 to 15,000 children in United States.
2. Turner syndrome: 1 in 2500 female births.
3. About 1 million children in United States have height more than 2 SD below mean for age.

D. Clinical manifestations.
1. Familial short stature.
   a. Growth pattern remains in its centile channel for height and weight.
   b. Family history of short stature, normal birth length/weight, normal growth rate with predicted adult height of third percentile.
   c. Normal bone age and no abnormalities in laboratory studies.
2. Constitutional growth delay.
   a. Bone age lower than chronological age.
   b. Family history reveals short stature in childhood, delayed puberty, eventual normal stature for family genetics.
3. Growth hormone deficiency.
   a. Small child with immature face, chubby body build.
   b. Rate of growth of all body parts is slow.
4. Chromosomal disorder/Turner syndrome:
   a. Short stature.
   b. Pubertal delay.

E. Physical findings.
1. Familial short stature.
   a. Clinical/laboratory findings: No evidence of systemic disease or endocrine insufficiency.
   b. Annual growth rate within normal limits, growth at or below but progressing parallel to third percentile.
2. Constitutional growth delay.
   a. Child growing at normal or near normal rate, annual growth rate of 5 cm/year, small for age.
   b. Delayed skeletal maturity.
   c. Normal thyroid and growth hormone levels.
3. Growth hormone deficiency.
   a. Typical child with growth hormone deficiency is short, slightly overweight.
   b. When present at birth, infant may have hypoglycemia, prolonged unexplained jaundice.
4. Chromosomal disorder/Turner syndrome.
   a. Short stature, short neck, webbing of neck, low posterior hairline, shield chest, wide carrying angle, short 4th and 5th metacarpals, narrow high-arched palate, epicanthal folds, nail dysplasia, clinodactyly.

F. Diagnostic tests.
  1. Detailed history, physical, and depending on findings, the following tests:
     a. X-ray of left hand and wrist to assess skeletal maturity.
     b. Urinalysis to assess ability to acidify and concentrate urine.
     c. Blood tests to include:
        - Urea nitrogen.
        - Creatinine.
        - CO_2.
        - Electrolytes.
        - Calcium.
        - Phosphorus.
        - Alkaline phosphatase.
        - T3, T4.
        - TSH.
        - Erythrocyte sedimentation rate (ESR).
        - Somatomedin C/1GF-1.
        - Complete blood count (CBC).
     d. Female patients: Karyotype for abnormalities of X chromosome.
     e. X-ray of skull: Sella turcica size, abnormality of sella area.
G. Differential diagnosis.

Anorexia, R63.0	Nutritional deficiency, unspecified, E63.9
Celiac disease, K90.0	
Diabetes mellitus, E10-E14	Other specified disorders of adrenal gland, E27.8
Disorder of pituitary gland, unspecified, E23.7	Short stature (child), R62.52
Heart disease, unspecified, I51.9	Short stature due to endocrine disorder, E34.3
Nephritic syndrome with unspecified morphologic changes, unspecified, N05.9	Slow fetal growth, unspecified, P05.9
Noninfective enteritis and colitis, K50-K52	

  1. Intrauterine growth retardation.
  2. Skeletal dysplasia.
  3. Nutritional deficiencies/second-generation anorexia.
  4. Intestinal/gluten-induced enteropathy (celiac disease).
  5. Chronic inflammatory bowel disease.
  6. Renal disease.
  7. Cardiac disease.
  8. Diabetes mellitus.

9. Psychosocial dwarfism, endocrine short stature, pituitary dwarfism.
10. Cortisol excess.
H. Treatment.
1. Refer to pediatric endocrinologist for diagnosis and treatment.
2. Growth hormone is continued as long as potential for growth exists and child is responding to therapy; can expect to reach normal adult height.
I. Follow-up.
1. Monitor growth patterns in response to medications.
2. Awareness of therapy, including expected response and possible adverse reactions.
J. Complications.

Abnormal level of blood mineral, R79.0

Osteochondropathy, unspecified of unspecified site, M93.90

1. Growth hormone administration: Hyperglycemia, increased incidence of slipped capital femoral epiphysis.
K. Education.
1. Provide guidance for physical, psychologic, social development.
2. Assist short children and their families with ways to cope with living in bigger world.

IV. DIABETES MELLITUS

Abnormal weight loss, R63.4	Other abnormal glucose, R73.09
Acetonuria, R82.4	Other fatigue, R53.83
Anhedonia, R45.84	Other polyuria, R35.8
Candidiasis of vulva and vagina, B37.3	Other visual disturbances, H53.8
Cerebral edema, G93.6	
Convulsions, unspecified, R56.9	Polydipsia, R63.1
Diabetes mellitus, E10-E14	Polyphagia, R63.2
Dyspnea, unspecified, R06.00	Psychosis not due to a substance or known physiological condition, unspecified, F29
Essential (primary) hypertension, I10	
Flushing, R23.2	Type 2 diabetes mellitus with other specified complication, E11.69
Glycosuria, R81	
Headache, R51	
Nocturia, R35.1	Volume depletion, E86
Nonorganic enuresis, F98.0	Vomiting, unspecified, R11.10

A. Type 1 diabetes: Metabolic syndrome (autoimmune disease) characterized by glucose intolerance, causing hypoglycemia/lack of pancreatic hormone (insulin). Insulin is an essential hormone that allows glucose to enter insulin-dependent tissue such as skeletal muscle, liver, and fat cells. Lack of available insulin results in catabolism and development of diabetic ketoacidosis.

B. Etiology.
   1. Beta cell mass in islets of Langerhans of pancreas is gradually destroyed in genetically susceptible child.
   2. Triggers, such as environmental, dietary, viral, bacterial, or chemical, that induce T-cell–mediated beta cell injury and production of humoral auto-antibodies.
   3. Pancreatic islet cell antibodies are found in 70–85% of newly diagnosed diabetes mellitus. Degree of beta cell destruction determined by first-phase insulin response during testing for glucose tolerance.

C. Occurrence.
   1. Annual incidence in United States is about 11.7–17.8/100,000 per year for child population.
   2. Peak ages for presentation of diabetes mellitus: 5–7 years of age, at time of puberty; however, present in growing number of children between 1 and 2 years of age.

D. Clinical manifestations.
   1. Polydipsia, polyphagia, enuresis in toilet-trained child.
   2. Polyuria, nocturia.
   3. Blurred vision.
   4. Weight loss, vomiting.
   5. Fatigue, decrease in activity.
   6. Cerebral edema in diabetic ketoacidosis warning signs:
      a. Headache.
      b. Lethargy.
      c. Incontinence.
      d. Seizures.
      e. Pupillary changes.
      f. Decreasing heart rate.
      g. Increasing blood pressure.
   7. Cerebral edema occurs in 1–5% of those with diabetic ketoacidosis.

E. Physical findings.
   1. Ketonuria, ketonemia, glucosuria.
   2. Vomiting.
   3. Dehydration.
   4. Slow, labored breathing, flushed face and cheeks.

    5. Mental confusion, lethargy.
    6. Fruity odor to breath.
    7. High blood glucose levels.
    8. Monilial vaginitis in adolescent females.
F. Diagnostic tests.
    1. Fasting plasma glucose, casual plasma glucose.
    2. Urine for ketones and glucose.
    3. Electrolytes and pH.
    4. Blood urea nitrogen.
    5. CBC.
G. Differential diagnosis.

Hypoglycaemia, unspecified, E16.2	Other gastritis without bleeding, K29.60
Localized swelling, mass and lump, head, R22.0	Sepsis, unspecified organism, A41.9

    1. Hypoglycemia.
    2. Salicylate intoxication.
    3. Sepsis.
    4. Intracranial lesions.
H. Treatment.
    1. Multidisciplinary approach involving family with pediatric endocrinologist, PNP, diabetic nurse educator, social worker, nutritionist.
    2. Educate child and family in stabilizing blood sugars, diabetes management. Due to complexity of illness, management requires incorporation into daily life.
    3. Treatment replaces insulin that child is unable to produce—the cornerstone of management.
    4. Insulin dosage is tailored to child's blood glucose and HbA1c levels (**Table 30-1**). Diabetic control: Based on HbA1c levels, clinical symptoms. HbA1c levels provide information on glycemic control during past 60 days.
    5. Insulin is categorized by peak of onset.
    6. Various insulin injection devices available.
I. Follow-up.
    1. Review medical, nutritional, insulin therapy, daily blood glucose monitoring (**Table 30-2**).
    2. Follow up every 3 months to review management plans, physical/psychosocial needs (**Table 30-3**).

Table 30-1 HbA1c and Glycemic Targets

	Premeal (mg/dL [mmol/L])	Postmeal (mg/dL [mmol/L])	HbA1c
Infants, toddlers	< 7.5 to 8.5	100 to 180 (5.6 to 10)	< 200 (11.1)
School age children	< 8.0	70 or 80 to 150 (3.9 or 4.4 to 8.3)	< 200 (11.1)
Teens	< 7.5	70 to 140 or 150 (3.9 to 7.7 or 8.3)	< 180 (10)

Source: Kaufman FR. Type 1 diabetes mellitus. *Pediatr Rev.* 2003;24(9):291-300. Reproduced with permission by the AAP.

Table 30-2 Principal Adjustments in Basic or Set Insulin Dose

Rapid-, short-, intermediate-, or long-acting insulin is adjusted after a pattern has been identified over 3–7 days.

Increase or decrease by 0.5, 1.0, 1.5, or 2.0 units (10% of dose).

Time of Test	Change This Insulin
2 or 3 Insulin Injections	
Before breakfast	Evening intermediate- or long-acting
Before lunch	Morning rapid- or short-acting
Before dinner	Morning intermediate- or long-acting
Before bedtime	Evening rapid- or short-acting
In the night	Evening intermediate- or long-acting
Multiple Insulin Injections (same as above except:)	
Before dinner	Lunch rapid- or short-acting
Insulin Pump	
Change bolus dose if blood glucose abnormal	< 2–3 hours after the meal
Change basal dose if blood glucose abnormal	> 3 hours after the meal

Recheck to be sure the changes made return blood glucose levels to the target range.

Source: Kaufman FR. Type 1 diabetes mellitus. *Pediatr Rev.* 2003;24(9):291-300. Reproduced with permission by the AAP.

Table 30-3 The Outpatient Visit for Patients with Diabetes

Physical Examination	Frequency Recommendations
Weight, height, body mass index (BMI)	Every 3 months/assess changes in percentile
Sexual maturity rating stage	Every 3 months/note pubertal progression
Blood pressure	Every 3 months/target < 90th percentile for age
Eye	Dilated funduscopic examination every 12 months after 5 years of diabetes
Thyroid	Every 3 months/presence of goiter, signs of thyroid dysfunction
Abdomen	Every 3 months/presence of hepatomegaly, fullness, signs of malabsorption, inflammation
Foot, peripheral pulses	Every 3 months inspection/after 12 years of age, thorough
Skin, joints, injection sites	Every 3 months/injection sites, joint mobility, lesions associated with diabetes
Neurologic	Every 12 months/signs of autonomic changes, pain, neuropathy
Laboratory test	Frequency
HbA1c	Every 3 months
Microalbuminuria	Every 12 months after puberty or after 5 years of diabetes
Urinalysis, creatinine	At presentation and with signs of renal problems
Fasting lipid profile	After stabilization at diagnosis and every few years
Thyroid function tests, including antithyroid antibodies	Every 12 months
Celiac screen	At time of diagnosis; if symptoms, at puberty
Islet antibodies	At diagnosis

Source: Kaufman FR. Type 1 diabetes mellitus. *Pediatr Rev.* 2003;24(9):291-300. Reproduced with permission by the AAP.

J. Complications.

Background retinopathy, unspecified, H35.00	Type 2 diabetes mellitus with other specified complication, E11.69
Candidiasis, unspecified, B37.9	
Eating disorders, F50	Unspecified nephritic syndrome with unspecified morphologic changes, N05.9
Type 1 diabetes mellitus with diabetic polyneuropathy, E10.42	

1. Ketoacidosis.
2. Vaginal yeast infections.
3. Retinopathy.
4. Nephropathy.
5. Neuropathy.
6. Lipid profile.
7. Eating disorders.

K. Education.
1. Prevention of diabetic ketoacidosis.
2. Knowledge of onsets of action, peak action, duration of action of five types of insulin (**Table 30-4**).
3. Recognition of hypoglycemia and hyperglycemia.
4. Management of hypoglycemia: Evening protein or fat snack to prevent hypoglycemia.
5. Prevention of long-term complications.
6. Role of exercise in management: Exercise improves glucose utilization.
7. Insulin therapy and monitoring of glucose levels.
8. Meal planning, nutrition: Eat meals and snacks within 1 hour of usual time.
9. School issues and coping skills.
10. Monitoring weight: Maintain ideal body weight.

V. TYPE 2 DIABETES

Acanthosis nigricans, L83	Obesity, E66
Acute vaginitis, N76.0	Other lack of expected normal physiological development, R62.8
Diabetes mellitus, E10-E14	
Dysuria, R30.0	
Essential (primary) hypertension, I10	Other polyuria, R35.8
Family history of diabetes mellitus, Z83.3	Polydipsia, R63.1
Lipoprotein deficiency, E78.6	Sleep apnea, unspecified, G47.30

Table 30-4 Onset of Action, Peak Action, and Duration of Action in Five Types of Insulin

Insulin Preparation	Duration of Action (hours)	Maximal Duration (hours)	Onset of Action (hours)	Peak Action (hours)
Rapid-Acting				
Lispro	¼–½	1–2	3–5	4–6
Aspart	¼–½	1–2	3–6	5–8
Short-Acting				
Regular	½–1	2–4	3–6	6–8
Intermediate-Acting				
NPH (isophane)	2–4	8–10	10–18	14–20
Lente (zinc suspension)	2–4	8–12	12–20	14–22
Long-Acting				
Ultralente (extended zinc suspension)	6–10	10–16	18–20	20–24
Basal Glargine	1–2	None	19–24	24

Source: Kaufman FR. Type 1 diabetes mellitus. *Pediatr Rev.* 2003;24(9):291-300. Reproduced with permission by the AAP.

A. Chronic metabolic disorder characterized by insulin resistance.
B. Etiology.
   1. Most common clinical factor for type 2 diabetes is obesity/body mass index (BMI) > 85% for age and sex.
C. Occurrence.
   1. Female-to-male ratio is 1.7:1 regardless of race. Youths between 8–19 years of age.
D. Clinical findings.
   1. Obesity.
   2. Polyuria.
   3. Polydipsia and weight loss.
   4. Vaginal infection as chief complaint.

    5. Dysuria.

    6. Family history.

    7. Sedentary lifestyle, sleep apnea.

E. Physical findings.

    1. Obesity.

    2. Acanthosis nigricans: Darkened thick, velvety pigmentation in skin folds.

    3. Hypertension.

    4. Dyslipidemia.

    5. Vaginal infection.

F. Diagnostic tests.

    1. Clinical impression with urinalysis.

    2. Plasma insulin.

    3. C-peptide concentrations.

    4. Autoantibodies to islet cell.

    5. Glutamic acid decarboxylase and tyrosine phosphatase helpful in distinguishing between type 1 and type 2 diabetes.

    6. Androgen levels.

    7. Serum testosterone levels.

G. Differential diagnosis.

Type 1 diabetes mellitus without complications, E10.9

---

    1. Type 1 diabetes.

    2. Polycystic ovarian syndrome.

H. Treatment.

    1. Whenever possible, manage child with multidisciplinary team.

    2. Treat underlying cause of disorder: Obesity.

    3. Increasing physical activity/moderate exercise is of primary importance.

    4. Diet should aim for gradual, sustained weight loss (eat smaller portions, lower caloric foods).

    5. Treat hypertension if it exists.

    6. May consider treatment with metformin to help decrease hepatic glucose production and absorption and to lower the blood sugar.

I. Follow-up.

    1. Routine health visits including dilated eye exam, foot exams, blood pressure, lipids, albuminuria.

    2. Assistance with lifestyle changes.

J. Complications.

Type 1 diabetes mellitus with ketoacidosis without coma, E10.10

---

    1. Type 1 diabetes, ketoacidosis.

K. Education.
   1. Lifestyle changes: Most important, challenging issues.
   2. Near normalization of blood glucose and glycohemoglobin.
   3. Control lipids.
   4. Set outcome goals of mutual agreement.
   5. Review medication usage and insulin or oral medication if prescribed.

VI. STEROID USE WITH ATHLETES

Abnormal weight gain, R63.5	Hirsutism, L68.0
Acne vulgaris, L70.0	Irregular menstruation, unspecified, N92.6
Alopecia areata, L63	
Atrophy of breast, N64.2	Jaundice, unspecified, R17
Atrophy of testis, N50.0	Major depressive disorder, single episode, unspecified, F32.9
Decreased libido, R68.82	
Disturbances of skin sensation, unspecified, R20.9	Other persistent mood [affective] disorders, F34.8
Enlarged prostate without lower urinary tract symptoms, N40.0	Other voice and resonance disorders, R49.8
Essential (primary) hypertension, I10	Priapism, unspecified, N48.30
Female infertility associated with anovulation, N97.0	Pure hypercholesterolemia, E78.0
	Seborrheic dermatitis, unspecified, L21.9
Generalized edema, R60.1	Strain of unspecified Achilles tendon, initial encounter, S86.019A
Headache, R51	

A. Anabolic, androgenic steroids: Synthetic hormones used to develop bulk, muscle strength.
B. Etiology.
   1. Administration of or use by competing athletes for sole intention of increasing performance in artificial, unfair manner.
   2. Anabolic and androgenic steroids mimic action of hormones normally present.
   3. Anabolic compounds stimulate building of muscle.
   4. Androgenic compounds stimulate development of masculine characteristics.
   5. Steroids refer to class of drugs; known as performance-enhancing drugs.

6. In males, testosterone is produced by testes and adrenal gland.
7. In females, testosterone is produced only by adrenal gland; much less testosterone than males.

C. Occurrence.
1. The prevalence of self-reported use of anabolic steroids in adolescence has ranged from 5 to 11% of males and up to 2.5% of females.
2. Athletes in nonschool sports as well as nonathletes have been shown to represent a significant portion of the user population.

D. Clinical manifestations.
1. Improbable gains in lean body mass, muscle bulk, definition.
2. Behavioral changes/mood swings.
3. Advanced stages of acne on chest and back.
4. Headaches.
5. Depressed libido.
6. Early male baldness.
7. Sustained penile erection/priapism.
8. Deepening voice with laryngeal changes.
9. Abnormal menses.
10. Inhibition of ovulation.
11. Depression, aggressiveness/combativeness.

E. Physical findings.
1. Yellowing of eyes/jaundice.
2. Oily skin.
3. Water retention in tissue.
4. Unexplained weight gain or loss.
5. Breast development in males.
6. Testicular atrophy.
7. Seborrhea.
8. Hypertension.
9. Increased total cholesterol.
10. Prostate hypertrophy.
11. Weakened tendons resulting in tearing or rupture.
12. Damage to growth plate at end of bones, permanently stunting growth.
13. Baldness/alopecia.
14. Clitoral enlargement.
15. Hirsutism.
16. Breast atrophy in females.
17. Acne.

F. Diagnostic tests.
  1. Urine for steroids.
  2. Electrolytes.
  3. Alkaline phosphatase.
  4. Serum glutamic oxaloacetic transaminase (SGOT), serum glutamic pyruvic transaminase (SGPT).
  5. Liver enzymes.
  6. Cholesterol profile.
  7. CBC.
G. Differential diagnosis.

Bipolar affective disorder, F31

Disorder of pituitary gland, unspecified, E23.7

Localized swelling, mass and lump, neck, R22.1

  1. Bipolar disease.
  2. Brain tumor.
  3. Pituitary gland dysfunction.
H. Treatment.
  1. Discontinuance of steroids, psychologic counseling.
  2. Have an informed discussion of the desired effects and possible risks of anabolic steroids.
  3. Advise normal laboratory tests will not guarantee freedom from future complications.
I. Follow-up.
  1. Emphasize benefits of proper training and nutrition.
  2. Provide effective role models for athlete.
  3. Evaluate hypertension, lipids.
J. Complications.

Atherosclerotic heart disease, I25.1

Other specified diseases of liver, K76.89

  1. Anabolic steroid psychologic addiction (addiction syndrome).
  2. Epiphyseal plate closure if adolescent continues to grow while taking steroids.
  3. Liver tumors.
  4. Risk of coronary heart disease directly related to low-density lipoprotein.
K. Education.
  1. Risks of steroid use; long-term health effects of continued use.

VII. POLYCYSTIC OVARIAN SYNDROME/DISEASE

A. Etiology.
   1. Endocrine disorder characterized by symptoms of obesity, amenorrhea, hirsutism, polycystic ovaries, and excessive androgen production. Etiology unknown; however, there is strong support for a genetic component.
B. Occurrence.
   1. High during adolescence and prevalence ranges from 8 to 26% of females age 12–45 years.
C. Clinical manifestation.
   1. Obesity.
   2. Hirsutism.
   3. Acne.
   4. Menstrual irregularities.
   5. Acanthosis nigricans suggesting insulin resistance.
D. Physical findings.
   1. Obesity/weight above 95% for age and sex.
   2. Hyperpigmentation of skin/neck, axillae, skin folds, and vulva.
   3. Acne.
   4. Dysfunctional bleeding/delayed menarche or amenorrhea.
E. Diagnostic tests.
   1. Serum testosterone levels free and total.
   2. Fasting insulin levels.
   3. Ultrasound of ovaries "pearl necklace appearance."
   4. LH and FSH levels.
   5. DHEA-S.
   6. 17 hydroxy-progesterone level.
   7. T3, T4.
   8. Triglycerides and cholesterol levels.
   9. Glucose tolerance.
   10. Serum cortisol level.
F. Differential diagnosis.
   1. Type 2 diabetes.
   2. Pituitary thalamus disorder.
   3. Thyroid disease.
   4. Adrenal cortex disease.
   5. Ovarian dysfunction.
G. Treatment.

1. Referral to endocrinologist.
2. Regulate menses with oral contraceptive. Oral contraceptives such as norgestimate/ethinyl estradiol (Ortho-Cyclen) and norgestimate ethinyl estradio (Ortho Tri-Cyclen) help regulate menses, help with hirsutism, reduce acne, increase bone density, reduce follicular activity, and reduce ovarian and endometrial cancer risk. Oral contraceptives act by suppressing plasma androgens and inhibit ovarian function. If the patient cannot tolerate oral contraceptives, the next therapy would be medroxyprogesterone acetate (Depo Provera) for irregular menses.
3. Stabilize or reduce body weight/manage lifestyle changes.
4. Spironolactone (Aldactone) in daily doses of 50–2000 mg orally. Acts by binding at sites of androgen receptors and inhibiting testosterone biosynthesis.
5. Cosmetic treatment for unwanted hair: Either laser or electrolysis.
6. Acne treated with clindamycin (Cleocin) or other antibacterial medications as indicated.
7. Insulin resistance may be treated with glucophage (Metformin).
8. Cholesterol- and triglyceride-lowering drugs as indicated.

H. Follow-up.
   1. Monitor for prevention of long-term health problems such as cardiovascular disease.
   2. Lifestyle modification such as diet and exercise for obesity.

I. Complications.
   1. Hypertension.
   2. Hyperlipidemia.
   3. Hyperinsulinemia.
   4. Endometrial hyperplasia.
   5. Type 2 diabetes mellitus.

BIBLIOGRAPHY

Alemzadeh R, Wyatt DT. Diabetes mellitus in children. In: Kliegman RM, Behrman RE, Jenson HB, Stanton BF, eds. *Nelson Textbook of Pediatrics*. 18th ed. Philadelphia, PA: W.B. Saunders; 2007:2404-2431.

Barron AM, Falsetti D. Polycystic ovary syndrome in adolescents. A hormonal barrage and metabolic upheaval. *Adv Nurse Pract*. 2008;16(3):49-50, 52, 54.

Bauer AJ. Approach to the pediatric patient with Graves' disease: when is definitive therapy warranted? *J Clin Endocrinol Metab*. 2011;96(3):580-588.

Cohen P, Rogol AD, Deal CL, et al. Consensus statement on the diagnosis and treatment of children with idiopathic short stature: a summary of the Growth Hormone Research Society, the Lawson Wilkins Pediatric Endocrine Society, and the European Society for Paediatric Endocrinology Workshop. *J Clin Endocrinol Metab*. 2008;93(11):4210-4217.

Congeni J, Miller S. Supplements and drugs used to enhance athletic performance. *Pediatr Clin North Am.* 2002;49(2):435-461.

Diaz A, Lipman Diaz EG. Hypothyroidism. *Pediatr Rev.* 2014;35(8):336-347.

Gibson M, Huddleston HG. Polycystic ovary syndrome and hirsutism. In: Kliegman RM, Stanton BF, St. Geme J, Schor NF, Behrman RE, eds. *Nelson Textbook of Pediatrics.* 19th ed. Philadelphia, PA: W.B. Saunders; 2011:1870.

Greydanus DE, Patel DR. Sports doping in adolescent: the Faustian conundrum of Hors de Combat. *Pediatr Clin North Am.* 2010;57(30):729-750.

Gunder LM, Haddow S. Laboratory evaluation of thyroid function. *The Clinical Advisor.* 2009;12(12):26-32.

Ho J, Loh CTF, Pacaud D, Leung AKC. Type 1 diabetes mellitus in children and adolescents: part 1, overview and diagnosis. *Consultant for Pediatricians.* 2010;9(2):55-57.

Kaufman FR. Type 1 diabetes mellitus. *Pediatr Rev.* 2003;24(9):291-300.

Klein J, Vuguin P, Hyman S. Cushing syndrome. *Pediatr Rev.* 2014;35(9):405-407.

Lee L, Sanders RA. Metabolic syndrome. *Pediatr Rev.* 2012;33(10):459-466.

Leung AKC. Thyroid disorders in adolescents: autoimmune versus biochemical hyperthyroidism. *Consultant for Pediatrics.* 2012;11(9):268-270.

Osipoff JN ,Wilson TA. Consultant with the specialist: thyroid nodules. *Pediatr Rev.* 2012;33(2):75-81.

Wong K, Potter A, Mulvaney S, Russell WE, Schlundt DG, Rothman RL. Pediatric endocrinologist's management of children with type 2 diabetes. *Diabetes Care.* 2010;33(3):512-514.

Yawn V. Polycystic ovarian syndrome. *Adv NPs PAs.* 2012;3(12):11-14.

Musculoskeletal Disorders

Miki M. Patterson

I. INJURIES: SPRAIN, STRAIN, OVERUSE

Dislocation, sprain and strain of unspecified body region, T14.3	Sprain and strain of ankle, S93.4
	Sprain and strain of wrist, S63.5
Injury, unspecified, T14.90	Sprain of unspecified part of unspecified
Other injury of unspecified body region, T14.8	wrist and hand, initial encounter, S63.90XA

A. Etiology.
   1. Damage or disruption to tendon (attaches muscle to bone), ligament (attaches bone to bone) from overstretching, exertion, repetitive application of excessive forces.
B. Occurrence.
   1. Wrist, finger, ankle sprains are common among children.
C. Clinical manifestations.
   1. Limp or pain with extremity or joint use.
   2. Felt tearing or heard a "pop" during activity or with trauma.
D. Physical findings.
   1. Pain, tenderness to palpation, swelling, discoloration (ecchymosis or erythema).
E. Diagnostic tests.
   1. Radiograph in two planes to ensure no fracture and to assess bony relationships. May need views of unaffected side to compare ossification centers and normal alignment.
   2. Physical exam: Stress joints to varus, valgus, anterior, posterior. If a "give" is felt (e.g., at a knee or ankle joint "opening up"), refer patient to orthopedist. Palpation over physis should be pain free.

F. Differential diagnosis.

Dislocation, sprain and strain of unspecified body region, T14.3	Other injury of unspecified body region, T14.8
Injury, unspecified, T14.90	Other symptoms and signs involving the nervous system, R29.818

1. Fracture, dislocation, ligament tears, neurologic deficit, vascular condition.

G. Treatment.
1. Protect, Rest, Ice, Compression, Elevation (PRICE) and medication for pain as needed:
   a. *Protect:* With splint/brace or relief of weight bearing with crutches.
   b. *Rest:* Do not use extremity.
   c. *Ice:* Apply ice immediately for 10–20 minutes, then every 3–4 hours for the first 24–48 hours.
   d. *Compression:* With ACE wrap; do not pull tightly when wrapping; compression will decrease amount of blood allowed to seep from injured tissues and decrease range of motion at joint.
   e. *Elevation:* Above level of heart will decrease swelling accumulating from gravity.
   f. Identify and alter factors that contributed to overuse.
   g. May continue to do activities that do not cause pain.
   h. Pain relievers such as ibuprofen or narcotic, if needed.

H. Follow-up.
1. Return in 1 week to ensure resolution of majority of pain, swelling, and return of function.
2. Pain and swelling after 2 weeks requires further workup.

I. Complications.

Multiple injuries, unspecified, T07
Other early complications of trauma, initial encounter, T79.8XXA

1. Missed fracture.
2. *Caution:* Salter fractures (through the growth plate) may not be visible on X-ray; if physis is tender, treat as fracture (**Figure 31-1**).
3. Compartment syndrome.
4. Skin breakdown (presents as burning sensation under brace or splint; results from ischemia of tissue; pressure should be relieved immediately).

Figure 31-1 Salter I fracture. Note the increased width compared to the distal tibial physis.

Source: Courtesy of Miki Patterson.

J. Education.
1. Teach family to call immediately for any burning or worsening of pain, neurovascular changes such as paresthesias (numbness or tingling), pallor, paralysis, pulselessness, cyanosis—these 4 Ps are signs of compartment syndrome.
   a. Considered a surgical *emergency*.
   b. Most important: Worsening pain and tightness.
   c. Compartment syndrome is accumulation of pressure in tissues not relieved with elevation.
   d. Most common areas: Calves, forearms, hands, feet.
2. Range of motion, stretching should be pain free before beginning strengthening rehabilitation exercises, then gradual return to regular activity.

II. INJURIES: FRACTURE, DISLOCATION

Dislocation, sprain and strain of unspecified body region, T14.3	Other disorder of circulatory system, I99.8
Erythematous condition, unspecified, L53.9	Other injury of unspecified body region, T14.8

A. Etiology.
   1. Damage/disruption to bone or joint, respectively, from trauma, exertion, overuse.
   2. Most common causes: Child abuse and neglect, sports, falls, motor vehicle or pedestrian/bicycle events.
B. Occurrence.
   1. All age groups can be affected.
   2. Fractures are most common presentation of child abuse; 70% of fractures in children younger than 6 months are inflicted.
   3. Fractures suggestive of nonaccidental trauma in children: Metaphyseal, rib (seen in 5–20% of abused children), scapular/distal clavicle/night stick (mid-shaft ulna), vertebral fracture or subluxation, fingers in nonambulating child, humerus (except supracondylar) in those younger than 3 years of age, bilateral/multiple fractures in different stages of healing as well as complex skull.
C. Clinical manifestations.
   1. Felt tearing or heard "pop" or "crack."
   2. Most affect function.
   3. Findings suspect for abuse:
      a. Fracture in child younger than 1 year of age.
      b. Unknown or unwitnessed injury.
      c. Delay in seeking medical attention.
      d. Changing story of how injury occurred.
      e. Fracture does not fit mechanism described (e.g., twisting an extremity will result in spiral fracture, whereas direct blow produces transverse fracture).
D. Physical findings.
   1. Pain, point tenderness, swelling, ecchymosis or erythema, loss of function, obvious deformity.
E. Diagnostic tests.
   1. Radiographs in two planes: AP and lateral or both obliques.
   2. May require computed tomography (CT) scan or MRI for complex injuries (i.e., pelvis or spine).
F. Differential diagnosis.

Injury, unspecified, T14.90

   1. Sprain.

G. Treatment.
1. Protect with immobilization/splinting, compression, ice, elevation.
2. Do not use extremity.
3. Pain medication (typically narcotic) such as acetaminophen (Tylenol) with codeine at 1 mg/kg of body weight every 4–6 hours for small children or hydrocodone (Vicodin), oxycodone (Percocet), or morphine by weight for those > 100 pounds.
4. Dislocation and displaced fractures refer stat to orthopedist. Oral medication should not be used if surgical intervention is an imminent possibility.

H. Follow-up.
1. Should be per orthopedist.
2. Many will not allow use of extremity for a period of time while healing.
3. Muscles will spasm around fracture to try to pull bone ends together for healing.
4. Fractures without fixation move for 10–14 days after injury while granulation occurs (even in casts).
5. Frequent X-rays may be needed to ensure alignment of fractures.
6. In 2–6 weeks: Callus develops, bone ends become "sticky," pain is reduced.
7. Consolidation begins at 3 weeks in infants, may take 3–6 months in older children, adults.
8. Weight bearing, casting, splinting, bracing, or full use are all related to fracture configuration, healing, patient specifics.
9. Remodeling of bone that occurs in children younger than 8 years of age allows acceptance of angulated fractures.
10. Increased circulation to fractured bone causes some overgrowth (basis for 1-cm overlap of fractured femurs in young children).

I. Complications.

Abnormalities of gait and mobility, unspecified, R26.9
Multiple injuries, unspecified T07
Other early complications of trauma, initial encounter, T79.8XXA

1. Compartment syndrome.
2. Loss of alignment.
3. Shortening, angulation, delayed, or nonunion of fracture.
4. Skin breakdown.
5. Neurovascular problems.
6. Infection.
7. Missed abuse.

J. Education.
   1. Same as for sprains.
   2. Family should seek medical attention for neurovascular changes or pain inside cast/splint/brace.

III. BACK PAIN

Dorsalgia, unspecified, M54.9	Scoliosis, M41

A. Etiology.
   1. See *Differential Diagnosis* below.
B. Occurrence.
   1. Most common in preadolescent and adolescent.
C. Clinical manifestations.
   1. Complaint of back pain, sometimes night pain (red flag), with/without numbness or tingling.
D. Physical findings.
   1. May or may not have:
      a. Deformity of spine.
      b. Pain with motion.
      c. Positive straight leg raise sign.
      d. Tight hamstrings (unable to sit upright with legs extended straight out in front).
      e. Neurologic changes or skin lesions.
E. Diagnostic tests.
   1. Radiographs: AP and lateral thoracolumbar and/or lumbosacral spine.
   2. Other testing as exam or history indicates (e.g., bone scan, MRI, labs: Complete blood count (CBC) with differential, erythrocyte sedimentation rate [ESR], antinuclear antibodies [ANA], rheumatoid factor, or human leukocyte antigen B27 [HLA-B27]).
F. Differential diagnosis.

Ankylosing spondylitis of unspecified sites in spine, M45.9	Other intervertebral disc degeneration, lumbosacral region, M5.37
Benign neoplasm of bone and articular cartilage, unspecified, D16.9	Other psoriatic arthropathy, L40.59
Congenital spondylolisthesis, Q76.2	Reiter's disease, unspecified site, M02.30
Discitis, unspecified, site unspecified, M46.40	
Dysmenorrhea, unspecified, N94.6	Renal tubulo-interstitial disease, unspecified, N15.9
Kyphosis, unspecified, site unspecified, M40.209	Scoliosis, M41
Noninfective enteritis and colitis, K50-K52	Sickle-cell disorders, D57

Figure 31-2 (a) Spondylolisthesis (slipped forward) L-5 on S-1 with (b) spondylolysis (fractured).

Source: Courtesy of Miki Patterson.

1. Overuse (heavy backpacks).
2. Fracture, spondylolysis (defect or separation of pars interarticularis), and spondylolisthesis (anterior slippage of vertebral body) typically occur at L-5 (**Figure 31-2**).
3. Scheuermann's kyphosis (anterior wedging > 5° of 3 or more adjacent vertebrae).
4. Scoliosis (see later discussion).
5. Degenerative disk disease, infection, discitis.

6. Inflammatory conditions, such as ankylosis spondylitis, psoriatic arthritis, inflammatory bowel disease, Reiter's syndrome (hallmark sign is morning stiffness).
7. Neoplastic such as osteoid osteoma (hallmark sign is night pain or constant pain independent of motion).
8. Other: Sickle cell crisis, functional illness, referred pain such as kidney infection or menstrual cramping.

G. Treatment.
1. Depends on diagnosis: Rest, nonsteroidal anti-inflammatory drugs (NSAIDs), stretching, abdominal strengthening, proper posture and backpack use, or referral to orthopedist.

H. Follow-up.
1. Symptoms should improve in 2 weeks for overuse or strains.

I. Complications.
1. Missed diagnosis (see *Differential Diagnosis*).

J. Education.
1. Demonstrate exercises to help ensure that they are done correctly.
2. Work with family on medication schedule.
3. If symptoms persist or new symptoms occur, call healthcare provider.

IV. SCOLIOSIS

Congenital malformation, unspecified, Q89.9

A. Abnormal lateral curvature of spine, typically with vertebral rotation.
B. Etiology.
1. Idiopathic: 90% (most common), unknown etiology, familiar pattern has been noted.
C. Occurrence.
1. Idiopathic: 3–5% in adolescents screened; males = females.
2. 0.6% require treatment; however, females are treated more often (1%) than males (0.1%).
D. Clinical manifestations.
1. Does not typically cause back pain (< 14%).
E. Physical findings.
1. Difficulty with fitting clothes.
2. S- or C-shape curve of spine.
3. Prominent: Scapular, ribcage, paraspinal musculature (especially on forward bend test) or breast.
4. Asymmetric waistline or shoulder level.
5. Plumb line dropped from C-7 does not correlate with gluteal crease.

F. Diagnostic tests.
   1. Inspection with minimal clothing.
   2. Radiographs: Scoliosis series, which is standing postero-anterior (PA) and lateral views of entire spine on one cassette.
G. Differential diagnosis.

Cerebral palsy, unspecified, G80.9	Myopathy, unspecified, G72.9
Fracture, unspecified, of sacrum, initial encounter for closed fracture, S32.10XA	Neurofibromatosis, unspecified, Q85.00
Fracture, unspecified, of unspecified lumbar vertebra, initial encounter for closed fracture, S32.009A	Other acute paralytic poliomyelitis, A80.39
Fracture, unspecified, of unspecified thoracic vertebra, initial encounter for closed fracture, S22.009A	Sacral spina bifida without hydrocephalus, Q05.8
Muscular dystrophy, G71.0	

   1. Congenital: Embryonic malformation.
   2. Paralytic: Polio, muscular dystrophy, cerebral palsy, spina bifida, myopathies, neurofibromatosis.
   3. Traumatic: Fracture of vertebrae.
   4. Hysterical: Rare, nonstructural, result of emotional disturbance.
H. Treatment.
   1. Orthopedic referral all curves > 10°.
   2. Orthopedic treatment for curves 10–20° observation.
   3. Curves 20–40°: Bracing (controversial) to prevent further curvature.
   4. Curves > 40°: Surgical intervention, posterior spinal fusion with segmental instrumentation occasionally requires anterior release.
I. Follow-up.
   1. Per orthopedics: Until skeletal maturity (about 1 year after menstruation for girls).
J. Complications.

Low back pain, M54.5

   1. Progressive untreated scoliosis may result in significant deformity, cardiopulmonary compromise, debilitating lumbar back pain.
K. Education.
   1. If braces and/or exercises ordered, ensure compliance.
   2. Bracing helps delay progression of curve.

3. Frequent skin inspection necessary with brace use.
4. Continue usual activities if pain free in brace.

V. HIP PAIN

Pain in unspecified hip, M25.559

A. Differential diagnosis.
1. Infection: Septic arthritis, osteomyelitis, Lyme disease, psoas abscess, appendicitis.
2. Inflammatory: Transient synovitis, systemic arthritis, juvenile rheumatoid arthritis (JRA), Kawasaki disease, idiopathic chondrolysis.
3. Orthopedic conditions: Legg-Calvé-Perthes disease, avascular necrosis (AVN), slipped capital femoral epiphysis (SCFE), stress fracture, apophyseal injuries, trochanteric bursitis, muscular strain.
4. Neoplastic: Osteoid osteoma, leukemia, solid tumor primary, pigmented villonodular synovitis (PVNS), or sickle cell crisis pain.

VI. SEPTIC HIP/SEPTIC ARTHRITIS

Appendicitis, unspecified, K37

Arthropathies, M00-M25

Benign neoplasm of bone and articular cartilage, unspecified, D16.9

Cutaneous abscess, furuncle and carbuncle of limb, L02.4

Fever of other and unknown origin, R50

Hypertrophy of bone, unspecified site, M89.30

Idiopathic aseptic necrosis of unspecified bone, M87.00

Infective myositis, M60

Injury, unspecified, T14.90

Juvenile rheumatoid arthritis, unspecified, of unspecified site M08.00

Leukemia, unspecified not having achieved remission, C95.90

Lyme disease, unspecified, A69.20

Mucocutaneous lymph node syndrome [Kawasaki], M30.3

Osteomyelitis, unspecified, M86.9

Other juvenile osteochondrosis of hip and pelvis, unspecified leg, M91.80

Pain in unspecified hip, M25.559

Pyogenic arthritis, unspecified, M00.9

Sickle-cell disorders, D57

Slipped upper femoral epiphysis (nontraumatic), unspecified, unspecified hip, M93.003

Synovitis and tenosynovitis, M65

Trochanteric bursitis, unspecified hip, M70.60

Villonodular synovitis (pigmented), unspecified site, M12.20

A. Infection in joint; hip joint is infected often, second only to knee in children.
B. Etiology.
   1. Bacterial infection spread hematogenously or from osteomyelitis of the femoral head.
   2. Most common organisms are *Staphylococcus* and *Streptococcus*.
C. Occurrence.
   1. Males = females; infancy to 6 years.
D. Clinical manifestations.
   1. Hip pain.
   2. Refusal to bear weight.
   3. Fever.
   4. Ill-appearing child with extreme pain and resistance to hip motion. Infection builds up pressure in hip capsule and can impede blood flow.
E. Physical findings.
   1. Fever > 37°C, typically lie with hip flexed and externally rotated.
   2. Infants may be irritable with pseudoparalysis of lower extremity.
F. Diagnostic tests.
   1. Elevate white blood cells (WBC) and ESR.
   2. Ultrasound or radiographs demonstrate widening of joint space.
   3. Diagnosis confirmed with CT or ultrasound-guided aspiration.
G. Differential diagnosis.

Cutaneous abscess, furuncle and carbuncle of limb, L02.4

   1. Septic sacroiliac joint.
H. Treatment.
   1. Emergent referral to hospital for surgical drainage of hip joint.
   2. Intravenous antibiotics tailored to culture results.
   3. Make sure child receives nothing by mouth (NPO).
I. Follow-up.
   1. Per orthopedics, usually 1–2 weeks postop and 3–6 months to follow hip maturity.
J. Complications.

Joint derangement, unspecified, M24.9

Osteomyelitis, unspecified, M86.9

Sepsis, unspecified organism, A41.9

   1. Septicemia, osteomyelitis, joint destruction.
K. Education.
   1. Prepare family for child's hospitalization and treatment with IV antibiotics.

VII. DEVELOPMENTALLY DISLOCATED HIP

Dislocation of hip, S73.0	Other specified congenital deformities of
Newborn (suspected to be) affected by	hip, Q65.89
breech delivery and extraction, P03.0	

A. Broad spectrum of hip dysplasia regarding dislocated or dislocatable or subluxing femoral head in relation to acetabulum at birth or early development.
B. Etiology.
   1. Genetic, intrauterine position, postnatal positioning.
C. Occurrence.
   1. Most common hip disorder in children.
   2. 1 in 100 infants have hip instability at birth, and true dislocation is seen in 1 of 1000 births.
   3. Ratio: 6 female: 1 male.
   4. Left hip > right.
   5. Higher frequency in firstborn children.
D. Clinical manifestations.
   1. Breech birth commonly associated with this condition.
   2. Difficulty diapering (abducting leg).
   3. Older children may have awkward Trendelenburg gait, leg length discrepancy, pain with ambulation.
E. Physical findings.
   1. Difficult in infants due to variety of levels of hip dysplasia.
   2. Unequal thigh skin creases/gluteal folds.
   3. Limited abduction.
   4. Positive Barlow maneuver (to see if dislocatable with femur flexed and midline: Adduct 10° gentle pressure posterior feel click with telescoping; **Figure 31-3**).
   5. Positive Ortolani maneuver (abducting hip, feel it clunk back into place; **Figure 31-4**).
   6. Galeazzi test (prone with knees flexed and heels at buttock): Positive when knee heights are different (**Figure 31-5**).
F. Diagnostic tests.

Congenital malformation, unspecified, Q89.9	Unequal limb length (acquired), unspecified femur, M21.759
Cutaneous abscess, furuncle and carbuncle of limb, L02.4	Unequal limb length (acquired), unspecified tibia and fibula, M21.769
Immobility syndrome (paraplegic), M62.3	

Figure 31-3 Barlow maneuver: Knees flexed and brought to midline with gentle downward pressure to see if hip "clunks" out posteriorly.

Figure 31-4 Ortolani maneuver: Abduct hip while pushing up posteriorly with fingers trying to pop hip into the socket. A click is a positive finding.

Figure 31-5 Positive Galeazzi test. Note the knee height difference.

1. Ultrasound of hips. Radiographs less helpful because femoral heads have not ossified.
G. Differential diagnosis.
   1. Congenital anomalies, arthrogryposis, septic hip, leg length discrepancy.
H. Treatment.
   1. Refer to orthopedist.
   2. Treatment goal: Reduce femoral head to anatomic position.
   3. May need Pavlik harness, hip spica cast, or surgical intervention.
I. Follow-up.
   1. Reexamine hips each visit.
J. Complications.

Abnormalities of gait and mobility, unspecified, R26.9	Scoliosis, M41
Low back pain, M54.5	Spondylosis without myelopathy or radiculopathy, site unspecified, M47.819
Other specified congenital deformities of hip, Q65.89	

1. Delayed treatment affects normal growth of hip joint.
2. If untreated: Residual dysplasia, limited range of motion, unstable gait, pain, functional scoliosis, low back pain, early degenerated changes.
K. Education.
   1. Report any range-of-motion or neurovascular changes.
   2. Important to hold and cuddle baby even in braces and casts.

VIII. TRANSIENT SYNOVITIS

Fever of other and unknown origin, R50	Urinary tract infection, site not specified, N39.0
Synovitis and tenosynovitis, M65	

A. Etiology.
   1. Unknown theory of posttraumatic or allergic cause.
   2. Infection frequently assumed because 32–50% follow upper respiratory tract infection.
B. Occurrence.
   1. 0.2–3% of children 3–8 years of age; 6:1 male-to-female ratio.
C. Clinical manifestations.
   1. Pain and limp.
D. Physical findings.
   1. Symptoms present < 1 week to 1 month.
   2. Fever absent or low grade. Do not appear severely ill.
E. Diagnostic tests.
   1. Negative CBC and ESR.
   2. Ultrasound positive: Effusion.
F. Differential diagnosis.

Lyme disease, unspecified, A69.20	Other juvenile osteochondrosis of hip and pelvis, unspecified leg, M91.80
Osteomyelitis, unspecified, M86.9	Pyogenic arthritis, unspecified, M00.9

   1. Septic arthritis *must* be ruled out. Osteomyelitis, Legg-Calvé-Perthes disease.
G. Treatment.
   1. Conservative.
   2. NSAIDs, rest, return to activity as tolerated.
H. Follow-up.
   1. If concerned, follow up in 1–2 days to be sure symptoms are resolving.
I. Complications.

Other juvenile osteochondrosis of hip and pelvis, unspecified leg, M91.80
Pyogenic arthritis, unspecified, M00.9

   1. Missed septic arthritis (rare).
   2. 1–2% may develop Legg-Calvé-Perthes disease.
J. Education.
   1. Any fever > 101.1°F(38.4°C) or ill appearance of child should prompt reexamination.

IX. HIP PAIN: LEGG-CALVÉ-PERTHES DISEASE

Other juvenile osteochondrosis of hip and pelvis, unspecified leg, M91.80	Pain in unspecified hip, M25.559 Synovitis and tenosynovitis, M65

A. Idiopathic AVN of femoral head in children.

B. Etiology.

   1. Unknown cause of avascularity; however, multiple theories include trauma, transient synovitis, systemic abnormalities, vascular disturbances from intraosseous venous hypertension and venous obstruction.

C. Occurrence.

   1. 1 in 1200 in general population.

   2. 4:1 male-to-female ratio.

   3. Typically 4–8 years of age.

   4. Bilateral in only 15%; reported to be associated with attention-deficit/hyperactivity disorder (ADHD).

D. Clinical manifestations.

   1. Pain of groin, medial thigh, or knee.

E. Physical findings.

   1. Pain with weight bearing.

   2. Limited internal rotation or abduction of hip.

   3. Muscle spasm may have atrophy of thigh, calf, or buttock from disuse.

   4. Leg length inequality.

F. Diagnostic tests.

   1. Radiographs: AP pelvis and frog lateral hips.

   2. Initial X-rays may be normal; may need CT to see early changes.

   3. Four stages:

      a. Initial: Interruption of blood supply, "crescent sign" areas of hyper- and hypodense appearance of femoral head.

      b. Fragmentation: Epiphysis appears fragmented.

      c. Reossification: Normal bone density returns, deformity becomes apparent.

      d. Healed: Healing complete, residual deformity common.

G. Differential diagnosis.

Cutaneous abscess, furuncle and carbuncle of limb, L02.4 Fracture, unspecified, of unspecified patella, initial encounter for closed fracture, S82.009A	Lyme disease, unspecified, A69.20 Slipped upper femoral epiphysis (nontraumatic), unspecified, unspecified hip, M93.003 Synovitis and tenosynovitis, M65

1. Knee problem, fracture.
2. Transient synovitis.
3. Septic hip, SCFE.
4. Neuromuscular condition.

H. Treatment.
    1. Refer to orthopedist.
    2. Goal: Prevent femoral head deformity, alter growth disturbances.
    3. Generally try to unload femoral head while allowing motion.
    4. Abduction brace and bed rest, home traction with progressive abduction of legs.
    5. Surgical adductor release or derotational femoral or pelvic osteotomies and spica body cast occasionally needed.

I. Follow-up.
    1. Per orthopedics.
    2. Patients will be followed long term, bed rest with traction, bracing, and surgery performed as indicated.

J. Complications.

Abnormalities of gait and mobility, unspecified, R26.9

Spondylosis without myelopathy or radiculopathy, site unspecified, M47.819

1. May not show on initial films.
2. Delayed treatment affects normal growth of hip joint.
3. Residual deformities (coax magna), limited range of motion, unstable gait, pain, early degenerated changes seen with treated and untreated.

K. Education.
    1. Progressive until body replaces "dead" femoral head with new bone; younger it occurs, longer body has to replace collapsing bone and remodel femoral head.
    2. No pressure should be put on rebuilding bone but should be able to move in joint for shaping.

X. HIP PAIN: SLIPPED CAPITAL FEMORAL EPIPHYSIS

Slipped upper femoral epiphysis (nontraumatic), unspecified, unspecified hip, M93.003

A. Femoral neck "slips" (displaces anteriorly) at physis (growth plate), leaving femoral head behind in acetabulum (**Figure 31-6**).

B. Etiology.
    1. Unknown; however, suspect multifactorial cause, biomechanical, obesity, endocrine, metabolic, trauma, genetics, and other causes (e.g., kidney disorders or radiation).

Figure 31-6 Slipped capital femoral epiphysis. Note the appearance of ice cream falling off the cone.

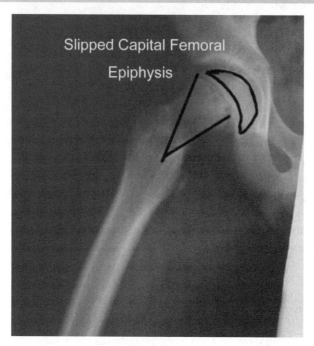

Source: Courtesy of Miki Patterson.

    C. Occurrence.
        1. Most common hip disorder of adolescents, 3 of 100,000 are 8–17 years of age.
        2. Males (10–17 years of age) affected 2–3 times more often than females (8–15 years of age).
        3. Left hip most often affected; bilateral 25–70%.
    D. Clinical manifestations.
        1. Hip, groin, medial thigh, knee pain; sometimes for months.
        2. May be brought on by very minor trauma (chronic/acute or acute on chronic).
        3. Antalgic gait (limp to keep weight off painful extremity) or inability to bear weight.
    E. Physical findings.
        1. Range of motion may be limited depending on severity of slip, may have limited internal rotation and abduction of the hip.

F. Diagnostic tests.
  1. Radiographs AP pelvis and true lateral (not frog lateral because may cause more femoral head displacement).
G. Differential diagnosis.

Appendicitis, unspecified, K37	Pain in unspecified hip, M25.559
Lyme disease, unspecified, A69.20	Torsion of testis, unspecified, N44.00

  1. Knee problem.
  2. Infection.
  3. Inflammation.
  4. Referred pain such as appendicitis, testicular torsion.
  5. Other orthopedic conditions or malignancy.
H. Treatment.
  1. Immediate referral to orthopedist.
  2. *Do not* allow further weight bearing because femoral head can "slip" further.
  3. Surgical intervention with "pinning" by screw(s) to fuse physis between femoral head and neck.
I. Follow-up.
  1. Orthopedics typically allow partial weight bearing with crutches for 6–8 weeks.
  2. Return in 2 weeks for wound check, staple removal.
  3. Follow healing clinically and radiographically for several months/years.
J. Complications.

Hypertrophy of bone, unspecified site, M89.30	Malunion of fracture, M84.0
Idiopathic aseptic necrosis of unspecified bone, M87.00	Spondylosis without myelopathy or radiculopathy, site unspecified, M47.819

  1. Missed on X-ray 25% of time.
  2. AVN.
  3. Chondrolysis (acute hylan cartilage necrosis).
  4. Loss of range of motion.
  5. Limb shortening.
  6. Early degenerative changes.
  7. Malunion.
K. Education.
  1. High incidence of recurrence of other hip.
  2. Parents or child should report any similar findings and be seen immediately.

XI. KNEE PAIN: OSGOOD-SCHLATTER DISEASE

Pain in unspecified knee, M25.569	Juvenile osteochondrosis of tibia and fibula, unspecified leg, M92.50

A. Painful swelling of tibial tubercle, caused by traction and resulting in apophysitis.
B. Etiology.
   1. Overuse by chronic repetitive knee flexion.
C. Occurrence.
   1. 11–14 years of age during rapid growth.
   2. Males > females, but ratio changing with increased female participation in sports.
   3. Frequently bilateral.
D. Clinical manifestations.
   1. Pain with running, jumping, kneeling. Resolves/fades with rest.
E. Physical findings.
   1. Pain in anterior knee; warmth, swelling, and tenderness over tibial tubercle, especially with resistive knee extension (kicking motion) or squatting.
F. Diagnostic tests.
   1. Radiographs of knee: AP and lateral and 10° obliques to rule out tumor or fracture.
   2. Classic prominent tibial tubercle above physis (**Figure 31-7**).
G. Differential diagnosis.

Fracture, unspecified, of unspecified patella initial encounter for closed fracture, S82.009A

Lyme disease, unspecified, A69.20

   1. Lyme disease.
   2. Tumor.
   3. Fracture.
   4. Sinding-Larsen-Johansson syndrome (apophysitis of distal pole of patella).
H. Treatment.
   1. Limit activities, especially sports; ice after activity.
   2. Hamstring and quadriceps stretching and strengthening.
   3. Knee immobilizer or cylinder casting for brief periods to manage severe pain.
   4. Ibuprofen.
I. Follow-up.
   1. Teach patients, families to decrease activity; wear knee immobilizer when painful.
   2. Follow up until skeletal maturity seen in closure of physis or growth plate.

Figure 31-7 Osgood-Schlatter disease: Apophysitis of the tibial tubercle.

Source: Courtesy of Miki Patterson.

J. Complications.

Acquired deformity of musculoskeletal system, unspecified, M95.9

Osteochondrosis (juvenile) of tibial tubercle, M92.5

Unspecified fracture of shaft of right tibia, initial encounter for closed fracture, S82.201A

1. Enlargement of tibial tubercle (bony prominence).
2. Pain may continue into adulthood.
3. Fracture of tibial tubercle.
4. Premature closure of apophysis causing recurvatum deformity.

K. Education.
1. "Bump" made because body thinks there is injury to bone, which is being pulled apart at growth plate by patella; tendon bump will *not* go away.

2. Continued use while painful typically increases size of "bump"; this is cosmetically unappealing for most and may interfere with kneeling. Condition ceases to exacerbate on skeletal maturity.

XII. PHYSIOLOGIC GENU VARUM (BOW LEGS)

Varus deformity, not elsewhere classified, unspecified knee, M21.169

A. Etiology.
  1. Physiologic genu varum or bowing is part of normal development.
B. Occurrence.
  1. Most common cause of bow legs in toddlers.
  2. Varum is greatest at 6 months of age, may progress to neutral by 18–24 months of age.
  3. Adult physiologic valgus (knock knee): About 8°, typically reached by 5–6 years of age.
C. Clinical manifestations.
  1. Pain-free bowing appearance to legs of toddler.
D. Physical findings.
  1. Gentle curve to entire leg.
  2. Normal knee flexion, extension without pain.
  3. Normal progression: 15° genu varum at birth (**Figure 31-8**); 0° (straight) 18–24 months; 10–12° genu valgum (knock knees) at 30 months to 4 years; 0° (straight) to 4–6° genu valgum normal at 4–6 years.
E. Diagnostic tests.
  1. Radiographic bowing of entire limb, no acute angulation seen (Figure 31-8).
  2. Medial proximal tibial physeal changes suggestive of pathology (Blount's disease), refer to orthopedist.
F. Differential diagnosis.

Achondroplasia, Q77.4	Osteogenesis imperfect, Q78.0
Disorder of kidney and ureter, unspecified, N28.9	Osteomyelitis, unspecified, M86.9
Juvenile osteochondrosis of tibia and fibula, unspecified leg, M92.50	Other injury of unspecified body region, T14.8
	Rickets, active, E55.0

  1. Blount's, vitamin D–resistant rickets, renal failure, chondrodysplasia, achondroplasia, osteogenesis imperfecta, osteomyelitis, neoplasm, fracture.

Figure 31-8 Physiologic genu varum. Normal "beaking" of distal femur and proximal tibial metaphysis.

Source: Courtesy of Miki Patterson.

G. Treatment.
   1. Generally resolve spontaneously.
   2. Refer to orthopedics for obvious asymmetry, clear progressive deformity, or if associated with pain.
   3. Osteotomy and correction of angulation may be performed using internal or external fixation devices.
H. Follow-up.
   1. Return visits every 3–6 months.
I. Complications.

Juvenile osteochondrosis of tibia and fibula, unspecified leg [Blount's, tibial vara], M92.50

1. Tibial vara or Blount's disease (abrupt deformity medial proximal tibia).
2. May be seen in children younger than 5 years of age but more common in adolescents.
3. Females > males.
4. Bilateral 80% of time.
5. Higher incidence in obese and African American children.
6. Will not correct with age.

J. Education.
1. Reassurance of normal finding.
2. Encourage child not to sleep or sit with legs tucked underneath; position might delay spontaneous correction.

XIII. IN-TOEING: METATARSUS ADDUCTUS

Congenital metatarsus (primus) varus, Q66.2

A. Etiology.
1. Unknown, theory of intrauterine position.
B. Occurrence.
1. Most common childhood foot problem.
2. 1 in 5000 births.
3. 1:20 in sibling.
4. Males, twins, preterm infants have higher incidence.
5. Seen first year of life; left > right, often bilateral.
C. Clinical manifestations.
1. Medial deviation of forefoot on hindfoot, in-toeing gait.
D. Physical findings.
1. C-shaped foot.
E. Diagnostic tests.
1. No radiographs needed for infants.
2. Children older than 4 years of age should have standing foot films, 3 views.
F. Differential diagnosis.

Abnormal involuntary movements, unspecified, R25.9

Congenital talipes equinovarus, Q66.0

1. Spastic anterior tibialis.
2. Talipes equinovarus (clubbed foot).

G. Treatment.
   1. Most will correct with normal use.
   2. Severe deformity: Refer to orthopedist for stretching, serial casting of flexible conditions; surgical intervention is rare.
H. Follow-up.
   1. Per orthopedics until deformity is corrected.
   2. Serial casting may be done weekly. Have parents remove semirigid cast night before appointment. Teach to stretch, then apply new cast with orthopedist holding position.
I. Complications.
   1. Cast/skin complications.
   2. Neurovascular problems.
   3. Incorrect position, especially if cast slips and toes are no longer visible (common with infants).
J. Education.
   1. Most resolve spontaneously.
   2. Return to orthopedist if circulation problems, irritability (e.g., suspect cast is bothering child), or if child kicks cast off.

XIV. IN-TOEING: TIBIAL TORSION

Acquired deformity, unspecified, of unspecified lower leg, M21.969

A. Etiology.
   1. Normal development in utero, genetic influence.
B. Occurrence.
   1. Birth 0–20° internal tibial rotation normal: 90% correct with growth, adults achieve 0–20° of external rotation.
C. Clinical manifestations.
   1. Curved appearance to tibia or in-toeing or out-toeing gait.
   2. If knees are pointing forward, feet may point either in (internal tibial torsion) or out (external tibial torsion); becomes less noticeable with running.
D. Physical findings.
   1. Thigh-foot angle (**Figure 31-9**). Child prone with knee bent at 90° angle of imaginary line drawn down thigh and middle of foot. Normal 0–30° external.

Figure 31-9 Thigh-foot angle. A line drawn along the axis of the femur bisects the foot.

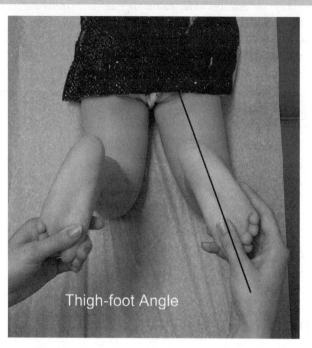

Thigh-foot Angle

Source: Courtesy of Miki Patterson.

2. Foot progression angle is angle of foot compared to line extended in front of ambulating child. Best observed from directly behind patient (**Figure 31-10**).
E. Diagnostic tests.
1. None if younger than 8 years of age and symmetrical pain-free appearance.
2. If needed, standing leg length X-ray (scanogram) done on long cassette.
F. Differential diagnosis.

Other reduction defects of unspecified lower limb, Q72.899

1. Developmental dysplasia of hip, neuromuscular conditions.
G. Treatment.
1. Observation.
2. None unless unilateral or severe or remains after age 8 years.
3. Tibial osteotomy rare but may be performed for severe cases.

Figure 31-10 Foot progression angle: Normal variations.

20° External

5° External

Source: Courtesy of Miki Patterson.

H. Follow-up.
   1. If persists at 8 years of age, refer to orthopedist.
I. Complications.
   1. Rare and related to surgical intervention.
J. Education.
   1. Reassurance and handouts.
   2. Despite grandparents' (or older relatives'/caregivers') insistence, braces are not effective. Studies show same improvement or correction through normal growth without braces.
   3. Many athletic children, adults have tibial torsion; does not result in any increased incidence of arthritis or interfere with activity.

XV. IN-TOEING: FEMORAL ANTEVERSION

Other specified congenital deformities of hip, Q65.89

A. Etiology.
  1. Normal and appears when child begins walking, causing ligaments to get looser; thus hips are allowed more internal rotation, especially in children 2–6 years of age.
B. Occurrence.
  1. Normal in 2- to 4-year-olds, usually corrects spontaneously by 8 years of age.
C. Clinical manifestations.
  1. In-toeing gait.
  2. Children tend to "W" sit pain free.
D. Physical findings.
  1. Knees and toes point inward when standing.
  2. Able to internally rotate hips up to 90°.
E. Diagnostic tests.
  1. None.
F. Differential diagnosis.

Other specified acquired deformities of unspecified limb, M21.80

Other specified congenital deformities of hip, Q65.89

---

  1. Tibial torsion, hip dysplasia.
G. Treatment.
  1. Discourage "W" sitting.
  2. Observation unless functional deformity after 8 years old.
  3. Refer to orthopedist for unilateral, severe, or painful deformity.
  4. Surgical intervention with femoral derotational osteotomy.
H. Follow-up.
  1. Yearly if not progressive.
I. Complications.
  1. None unless surgical intervention.
J. Education.
  1. Normal, child will grow out of it. Braces or shoe modification are ineffective.

XVI. FOOT PROBLEMS: TALIPES EQUINOVARUS (CLUBBED FOOT)

Congenital talipes equinovarus, Q66.0

A. Rigid fixed foot deformity with inverted heel, forefoot adduction, and down-facing toes.

B. Etiology.
1. Unknown; possibly genetic, mechanical, chemical embryologic insults.
C. Occurrence.
1. Age: Newborn.
2. 2:1 males to females.
3. 1.24 in every 1000 live births.
4. Increased incidence in families where parents/siblings have same disorder.
D. Clinical manifestations.
1. Tight Achilles tendon, joint capsule, medial ligaments.
2. Short angulated talus, thin atrophic muscles.
E. Physical findings.
1. Small foot and calf, with rigid equinus deformed foot with heel in varus.
2. Prominent crease in arch of foot.
3. Adducted forefoot.
F. Diagnostic tests.
1. Clinical exam of newborn; radiographs are of little use.
G. Differential diagnosis.

Immobility syndrome (paraplegic), M62.3

Other specified congenital deformities of feet, Q66.89

Spastic hemiplegia affecting unspecified side, G81.10

1. "Positional clubbed foot," arthrogryposis, spastic hemiplegia, calcaneovalgus.
H. Treatment.
1. Refer to orthopedist. Serial casting and surgical intervention may be necessary.
I. Follow-up.
1. Per orthopedist.
2. Treatment soon after birth: Weekly visits for manipulation and casting by orthopedist experienced in this form of treatment.
3. If rigid deformity, surgical intervention may be necessary; may entail heel cord and joint capsule releases and casting typically at 6 months of age.
4. Casting or braces may be used for a period of time; follow-up is ongoing because deformity may recur until about age 7 years.
J. Complications.

Unequal limb length (acquired), unspecified femur, M21.759

Unequal limb length (acquired), unspecified tibia and fibula, M21.769

1. Progressive deformity, leg length discrepancy, surgical complications.

K. Education.
  1. Affected foot will always be smaller but may function near normal after correction.

XVII. PES PLANUS: FLAT FOOT

Flat foot [pes planus] (acquired), unspecified foot, M21.40

A. Etiology.
  1. Flexible normal (asymptomatic) genetic etiology or rigid (symptomatic) tarsal coalition (fusion of calcaneus with talus or navicular) common cause.
B. Occurrence.
  1. Normal occurrence younger than 2 years of age due to medial fat pad. Rigid is rare.
C. Clinical manifestations.
  1. Flat foot while standing; normal arch that returns while sitting and hanging over exam table is flexible pes planus.
  2. Bilateral.
  3. Hereditary expression.
  4. May cause some discomfort for older children.
D. Physical findings.
  1. Loss of normal plantar arch while standing.
  2. Limited subtalar joint motion for rigid pes planus.
  3. Look at parents' feet!
E. Diagnostic tests.
  1. If rigid: Radiographs, three standing views of both feet, CT or MRI looking for coalition.
F. Differential diagnosis.

Arthropathy, unspecified, M12.9
Fracture, unspecified, of unspecified foot, initial encounter for closed fracture, S92.909A
Immobility syndrome (paraplegic), M62.3

  1. Overuse.
  2. Arthrogryposis.
  3. Neuromuscular condition.
  4. Arthritis.

      5. Infection.

      6. Trauma/fracture.

  G. Treatment.

      1. Refer rigid pes planus to orthopedist, orthotics may decrease symptoms of older child with flexible pes planus.

      2. Apply before sling.

  H. Follow-up.

      1. May require further workup or referral if not pain free after 1 month.

  I. Complications.

      1. None known.

  J. Education.

      1. Proper shoe wear. Sneakers with built-in arch preferred.

XVIII. NURSEMAID'S ELBOW: RADIAL HEAD SUBLUXATION

Sprain and strain of elbow, S53.4

  A. Etiology.

      1. Traction along axis of extended pronated arm resulting in radial head subluxation with annular ligament displacement.

      2. Typically "pulling" child's hand/arm to prevent from falling or pulling away or swinging child by arms.

  B. Occurrence.

      1. Most common elbow injury of children age 1–4 years.

      2. Female > males.

      3. Left > right.

  C. Clinical manifestations.

      1. Will not use arm.

      2. Holds arm close to body with elbow slightly flexed and pronated (palm down).

  D. Physical findings.

      1. Restricted supination of elbow.

      2. Typically nontender or swollen; however, exhibits distress if tries moving elbow.

  E. Diagnostic tests.

      1. Radiographs AP and lateral of elbow if questionable success of reduction. **Note:** Many times these are reduced when arm is rotated to get lateral X-ray.

Figure 31-11 Reduction maneuver for "nursemaid's elbow." Flex elbow to 90°, fully pronate wrist (palm down), then with gentle pressure over radial head supinate the wrist (palm up).

F. Differential diagnosis.

Fracture of upper end of ulna, S52.0

    1. Fracture.

G. Treatment.

    1. Reduction maneuver.

        a. Child in parent's lap.

        b. Flex child's elbow to 90° with gentle pressure of thumb over radial head.

        c. Fully or "hyper" pronate wrist, then fully supinate wrist; typically click will be felt and child will stop resisting (**Figure 31-11**).

    2. Sling and refer to orthopedist if child fails to use arm.

H. Follow-up.

    1. Call or visit to ensure child is using arm normally within 1 week.

I. Complications.

    1. Unreduced radius.

J. Education.

    1. Teach parents mechanism of injury to prevent reoccurrence (30–40%).

XIX. GROWING PAINS

Symptoms and signs, unspecified, involving the musculoskeletal system, R29.91

   A. Etiology.
      1. Unknown theory of periosteal irritation.
   B. Occurrence.
      1. Peak in 3–5 and 8- to 12-year-olds.
   C. Clinical manifestations.
      1. Muscular pain (not joint): Thighs, calves, behind knee.
      2. Typically late afternoon, early evening after physically active day.
      3. Can wake child from sleep.
   D. Physical findings.
      1. None.
   E. Diagnostic tests.
      1. Only if suspicious, X-ray to exclude fracture/lesion.
   F. Differential diagnosis.
      1. Diagnosis of exclusion:
         a. No fever.
         b. Not in joint.
         c. No swelling, erythema, warmth.
         d. No trauma.
         e. No weight loss, rashes, unusual fatigue or behavior.
   G. Treatment.
      1. Massage, heat, acetaminophen/ibuprofen.
   H. Follow-up.
      1. Follow up if lasts > 24 hours at time.
      2. Follow up if child does not respond to medications and massage.
   I. Complications.
      1. None.
   J. Education.
      1. Normal, may come and go; child is not "faking."

XX. COSTOCHONDRITIS

Chondrocostal junction syndrome [Tietze], M94.0

   A. Etiology.
      1. Diagnosis of exclusion.

Figure 31-12 "Crowing rooster." Elbows are pulled back and up to expand chest. A positive test is when pain is reproduced with this maneuver.

Source: Courtesy of Miki Patterson.

    B. Occurrence.
       1. Unknown.
    C. Clinical manifestations.
       1. Insidious and persistent lasting hours to days.
       2. Worse with position change and deep breathing. May be diffuse or localized. Common after repetitive new activity of upper trunk and arms.
    D. Physical findings.
       1. Skin lesions, chest wall syndrome tests, "crowing rooster," "horizontal arm flexion," "hooking maneuver" diagnostic: If pain is reproduced, test is positive (**Figure 31-12**).
       2. Chest expansion test (tape measure around chest at fourth intercostal level max)—exhale then inhale = 5 cm excursion; < 2.5 cm abnormal.
    E. Treatment.
       1. NSAIDs, rest.
    F. Diagnostic tests.
       1. Radiographs of chest to rule out fracture or tumor.
       2. CT, bone scan (most sensitive to rule out arthropathies, tumors, infection).
       3. ESR, ANA, rheumatoid factor purpose to rule out: Cardiopulmonary, abdominal sources associated with rheumatologic condition or assess structure of chest wall.

G. Differential diagnosis.

Ankylosing spondylitis of unspecified sites in spine, M45.9

Myalgia, M79.1

1. Cardiopulmonary.
2. Esophagus, head, neck, and interior chest wall.
3. Ankylosing spondylitis.
4. Sternoclavicular hyperostosis.
5. Infection.
6. Fibromyalgia.

H. Follow-up.
1. Within 2 weeks to document resolution of symptoms.

I. Complications.
1. Missed diagnosis.

J. Education.
1. Call for changes in symptoms.

XXI. OSTEOPOROSIS

Osteoporosis, unspecified, M81.9

A. Etiology.
1. Bony calcium deficit from various causes, including lack of intake while prepubertal, absorption or metabolic origin.

B. Occurrence.
1. Disease of childhood with severe adulthood complications.

C. Clinical manifestations.
1. Majority (50–66%) of total body calcium is deposited to bone by end of puberty.
2. Earlier in females than males.
3. Highest velocity of increased bone mineral content within 9–12 months of menarche.

D. Physical findings.
1. Stress fractures, fractures with minimal trauma or no findings in childhood.

E. Diagnostic tests.
1. Lack of calcium in past 3-day diet history.
2. Poor dietary habits.
3. High suspicion in lactose-intolerant or anorectic children.

F. Differential diagnosis.
1. None.
G. Treatment.
1. Increase dietary calcium intake or supplementation.
H. Follow-up.
1. Continue to assess calcium intake, stress importance to prepubertal/pubescent children.
I. Complications.

Kyphosis, unspecified, site unspecified, M40.209

Other injury of unspecified body region, T14.8

Spondylosis without myelopathy or radiculopathy, site unspecified, M47.819

---

1. Fractures.
2. Dowager's hump (kyphosis).
3. Early adulthood degenerative joint changes.
J. Education.
1. Three servings of milk, cheese, yogurt daily: 1200 mg of calcium.

BIBLIOGRAPHY

American Academy of Pediatrics Committee on Quality Improvement, Subcommittee on Developmental Dysplasia of the Hip. Clinical practice guideline: early detection of developmental dysplasia of the hip. *Pediatrics.* 2000;105(4):896-905.

Clark MC. Approach to child with a limp; 2013. UpToDate. http://www.uptodate.com/contents/approach-to-the-child-with-a-limp. Updated July 30, 2014. Accessed May 15, 2015.

Flynn JM, Mehta S. An evidence-based approach to the evaluation and management of hip pain in children. *Pediatr Case Rev.* 2002;2(1):26-32.

Kleposki RW, Abel K, Sehgal K. Common pediatric hip diseases in primary care. *Clinical Advisor.* 2010;13(6):21-26.

Lincoln TL, Suen PW. Common rotational variations in children, *J Am Acad Orthop Surg.* 2003;11(5): 312-320.

Proulx AM, Zryd TW. Costochondritis: diagnosis and treatment. *Am Fam Physician.* 2009;80(6):617-620.

Rosenfeld SB. Developmental dysplasia of the hip: clinical features and diagnosis. UpToDate. http://www.uptodate.com/contents/developmental-dysplasia-of-the-hip-clinical-features-and-diagnosis. Updated April 14, 2015. Accessed May 15, 2015.

Smalley MJ. Pediatric and congenital disorders. In: Schoenly L, ed. *Core Curriculum for Orthopaedic Nursing.* 7th ed. Chicago, IL: National Association of Orthopaedic Nurses; 2013:263-316.

Staheli LT. *Fundamentals of Pediatric Orthopedics.* 4th ed. Philadelphia, PA: Lippincott Williams & Wilkins; 2008.

Neurologic Disorders

Kristin Miller

I. MENINGITIS

A. Inflammation of the protective membranes covering the brain and spinal cord, collectively called the meninges, usually due to the spread of infection.

Attention-deficit hyperactivity disorder, unspecified type, F90.9	Other symptoms and signs involving the nervous system, R29.818
Convulsions, unspecified, R56.9	Papilloedema, unspecified, H47.1
Fever of other and unknown origin, R5	Somnolence, R40.0
	Stupor, R40.1
Headache, R51	Torticollis, M43.6
Meningitis, unspecified, G03.9	Vomiting, unspecified, R11.10

B. Etiology.
   1. Infectious.
      a. Viral infections—most common cause, usually termed *aseptic meningitis* when no bacterial cause can be found.
      • Enteroviruses (90%).
      • Herpes simplex virus type 2.
      • Varicella zoster virus.
      b. Bacterial.
      • Newborns to 3 months of age.
         o Group B streptococci.
         o *Escherichia coli.*
         o Listeria monocytogenes.
      • Older children.
         o *Neisseria meningitidis.*
         o Streptococcus pneumonia.
         o *Haemophilus influenzae* type B, especially in countries that do not offer vaccinations.

519

    c. Parasitic.
- *Angiostrongylus cantonensis.*
- *Gnathostoma spinigerum.*

  2. Noninfectious.

    a. Cancer.

    b. Drugs.
- Nonsteroidal anti-inflammatory drugs (NSAIDs).
- Antibiotics.
- Intravenous immunoglobulin.

    c. Inflammatory conditions.
- Sarcoidosis.
- Systemic lupus erythematous.
- Vasculitis.

C. Occurrence.

  1. Viruses more likely in late summer and fall.

  2. Bacterial: 3 per 100,000.

  3. Viral: 10.9 per 100,000.

  4. Increased risk with crowding and prolonged exposure such as daycare, military, college dorms, and those with compromised immune systems.

  5. Age—most cases occur in children younger than 5 years, but decreased incidence with increased vaccination rates.

  6. Race—higher incidence in African Americans than Caucasians.

  7. Sex—viral 3 times more likely in males than females.

D. Clinical manifestations.

  1. General population.

    a. Classic triad of severe headache, nuchal rigidity, high fever.

    b. Altered mental status.
- Confusion.
- Extreme irritability.
- Sleepiness
- Abnormal cry.
- Seizures.

    c. Sensitivity to light.

E. Physical findings.

  1. Signs in newborns.

    a. Constant cry.

    b. Excessive sleepiness or irritability.

    c. Poor feeding.

    d. Bulging fontanel (increased intracranial pressure [ICP]).

      e. Stiffness of body and/or neck.

      f. Difficult to comfort, cries harder when picked up.

  2. Positive Kernig's sign or Brudzinski's sign.

F. Diagnostic tests.

  1. Lumbar puncture (LP)—definitive test for diagnosis; will see low glucose, increased white blood cells (WBC), increased protein; culture and Gram stain should be done.

  2. Complete blood count (CBC), blood culture, C-reactive protein, polymerase chain reaction (PCR), erythrocyte sedimentation rate (ESR).

  3. CT or MRI before LP since LP contraindicated with tumor, abscess, or increased ICP; MRI often done later to assess complications/sequelae.

G. Differential diagnosis.

Extradural and subdural abscess, unspecified, G06.2	Intracranial abscess and granuloma, G06.0
Injury of head, unspecified, initial encounter, S09.90XA	Myelitis, unspecified, G04.91
	Other disorders of brain, G93

H. Treatment.

  1. Viral.

      a. Supportive care—bed rest, fluids, analgesics.

      b. Antiviral drugs—acyclovir for herpes simplex and varicella zoster.

      c. May need to be admitted to monitor ICP or complications.

  2. Bacterial.

      a. Early intervention with antibiotics critical.

      b. Always treat with antibiotic for most commonly known pathogens until diagnosis confirmed.

      c. May need to be admitted to manage ICP, complications, administration of IV fluids and antibiotics.

      d. Birth to 6 weeks—ampicillin and third-generation cephalosporin (cefotaxime or ceftriaxone).

      e. Older than 6 weeks—vancomycin and third-generation cephalosporin.

      f. Prophylactic treatment of contacts with patients with *Neisseria meningitidis*—sulfadiazine or rifampin.

I. Complications.

  1. Increased ICP.

  2. Deafness—may be prevented with prophylactic steroids.

  3. Hydrocephalus.

  4. Seizures.

    5. Venous or cerebral infarction.

    6. Cranial nerve palsies.

    7. Up to 70% sustain sequelae from bacterial meningitis.

    8. Most children with nonherpetic viral meningitis recover completely.

J. Follow-up.

    1. Frequent visits when cared for at home.

    2. Immediately for any decline in neurological condition or respiratory distress.

    3. Shortly after hospitalization to follow neurological status and assess pain for treatment of any sequelae.

K. Education.

    1. Importance of prevention via immunizations.

    2. Handwashing and infection-control measures, especially in crowded locations.

    3. Prophylaxis for certain exposures.

    4. Support and coordination of comprehensive services may be needed.

II. ENCEPHALITIS

A. Inflammation of the brain due to a viral infection.

Convulsions, unspecified, R56.9	Psychosis, unspecified, not due to a substance or known physiological condition, F29
Headache, R51	Somnolence, R40.0
Meningitis, unspecified, G03.9	Stupor, R40.1
Myelitis, unspecified, G04.91	Torticollis, M43.6
Other fatigue, R53.83	Vomiting, unspecified, R11.10

B. Etiology.

    1. Primary form: Direct viral infection of the brain and spinal cord.

    2. Secondary form: Viral infection that first occurs elsewhere in the body and travels to the brain.

    3. Exposure to viruses through:

        a. Breathing in respiratory droplets from infected person.

        b. Contaminated food or drink.

        c. Insect bites or animal bites (rabies).

        d. Specific viruses:

            • Arboviruses—most common cause, carried by mosquitoes or ticks.

            • Enteroviruses—coxsackievirus, echovirus, poliovirus.

- Others: Herpes simplex encephalitis (most common and worst prognosis—10–40% mortality).
- Eastern equine: 70–90% mortality.
- Western equine.
- St. Louis encephalitis: 30% mortality.
- West Nile.
- California and Venezuela equine.

4. Allergic reaction to vaccinations (extremely rare).
5. Effects of cancer and treatments.
6. Autoimmune or immune response problems (immunocompromised, HIV).

C. Occurrence.
  1. Seasonal: More common summer and fall.
  2. Age: More prevalent or severe in young children and elderly.
  3. Higher in those with weakened immune system.
  4. Geographic: Higher in areas where mosquito-borne viruses are common.
  5. Outdoor activities increase risk.

D. Clinical manifestations.
  1. Headache.
  2. Nausea.
  3. Lethargy.
  4. Behavioral changes—confusion, disorientation, irritability, personality changes.
  5. Joint pain, stiff neck.

E. Physical findings.
  1. Fever.
  2. Positive Brudzinski's sign or Kernig's sign.
  3. Abnormal reflexes.
  4. Rash.
  5. Emergency symptoms:
     a. Low level of consciousness (LOC), poor responsiveness.
     b. Muscle weakness or paralysis.
     c. Seizure.
     d. Sudden change in mental functions.
     e. Bulging fontanel.

F. Diagnostic tests.
  1. LP with CSF exam may show hemorrhagic component and increase WBC.
  2. Electroencephalogram (EEG)—periodic sharp waves at 2- to 3-second intervals on a background of diffuse or lateralized slowing if characteristic but nonspecific.
  3. MRI—often abnormal, showing limited or massive areas of inflammation and necrosis.

4. PCR and blood antibodies—can show positive DNA for viruses.
5. CBC, toxicology screen.
G. Differential diagnosis.

Convulsions, unspecified, R56.9	Nontraumatic intracranial hemorrhage, unspecified, I62.9
Demyelinating disease of central nervous system, unspecified, G37.9	Other specified disorders involving the immune mechanism, not elsewhere classified, D89.89
Malignant neoplasm of brain, unspecified, C71.9	Poisoning by unspecified drugs, medicaments and biological substances, undetermined, initial encounter, T50.904

H. Treatment.
1. Antiviral medications.
   a. Acyclovir—herpes encephalitis or varicella zoster virus.
   b. Ganciclovir—cytomegalovirus (CMV).
2. Antibiotics if bacterial cause.
3. Seizure medications as needed.
4. Steroids to reduce swelling.
5. Acetaminophen for fever and headache.
6. Rest and fluids.
I. Complications.
1. Acute phase lasts 1–2 weeks, may take several months to fully recover.
2. Permanent brain damage can occur in severe cases—can affect hearing, memory, muscle control, sensation, speech, vision.
3. Outcomes vary—high recovery (Rocky Mountain spotted fever), high morbidity (herpes encephalitis) definite mortality, especially if untreated (rabies).
J. Follow-up.
1. Emergency for sudden fever or other symptoms of encephalitis.
2. Call for decline in neurological condition.
3. 2–4 weeks to assess for sequelae.
K. Education.
1. Importance of vaccinations: Measles-mumps-rubella (MMR), varicella, meningococcal.
2. Immunizations specific for foreign travel.
3. Take steps to prevent genital herpes.
4. Avoidance of mosquitoes.
   a. Apply DEET products, not on face, hands, or infants younger than 2 months.

        b. Remove sources of standing water.

        c. Wear long-sleeve shirts and pants when outside, especially at dusk.

    5. Avoidance of ticks.

        a. Avoid woods, clear brush in yard, and keep grass mowed.

        b. Inspect body after return inside.

        c. Avoid contact with vector/host animals.

    6. Thoroughly cook meat and wash fruits/vegetables, especially in endemic areas.

III. HEAD INJURY

A. Any trauma that leads to injury to scalp, skull, or brain.

Fracture of skull and facial bones, S02	Psychosis, unspecified, not due to a substance or known physiological condition, F29
Injury of head, unspecified, initial encounter, S09.90XA	
Nausea, R11.0	Somnolence, R40.0
Other symptoms and signs involving the nervous system, R29.818	Stupor, R40.1
	Vomiting, unspecified, R11.10

B. Etiology.

    1. Trauma from motor vehicle accident (MVA), physical assaults, falls, accidents at home, work, outdoors, or while playing sports.

    2. Common causes include biking, skating, skateboarding, and contact sports.

    3. Types.

        a. Closed head—did not break the skull, more common.

        b. Penetrating or open—break in skull where objects enter brain (50% mortality rate).

        c. Focal brain injury—acute epidural, subdural, or subarachnoid hemorrhage.

C. Occurrence.

    1. 1.7 million people sustain traumatic brain injury (TBI) annually. Majority are concussions or other forms of mild TBI.

    2. Contributes to substantial number of deaths and causes of permanent disability.

    3. Range from mild with brief change in mental status or consciousness to severe with extended period of unconsciousness.

    4. Falls cause 50% of TBI in children age 0 to 14 years.

    5. Strike by moving or stationary object causes 25% of TBI in children ages 0 to 14 years.

    6. Males more often sustain TBI (59%).

    7. High-risk age groups—0 to 4 years and 15 to 19 years.

D. Clinical manifestations.

    1. Occur immediately or over several hours to days.

    2. Minor head injury symptoms:

        a. Headache.

        b. Dizziness.

        c. Impaired concentration, thinking, and memory.

        d. Blurred vision.

        e. Distractibility.

        f. Noise sensitive.

        g. Depression.

        h. Anxiety.

    3. Severe head injury symptoms:

        a. Impaired hearing, smell, taste, or vision.

        b. Irritability, personality changes, unusual behavior.

        c. Severe headache.

E. Physical findings.

    1. Minor head injuries.

        a. Unsteadiness.

        b. Fatigue.

        c. Irritability.

    2. Severe head injuries.

        a. Changes in or unequal pupils.

        b. Convulsions.

        c. Fracture in skull or face, bruising of face, swelling at site of injury.

        d. Inability to move one or more limbs.

        e. Loss of consciousness, confusion, drowsiness.

        f. Restlessness, clumsiness, lack of coordination.

        g. Stiff neck or vomiting.

F. Diagnostic tests.

    1. Important to obtain history of exact details of injury.

    2. Glasgow Coma Scale.

    3. Head CT to identify significant contusion, hemorrhage, and swelling.

    4. Skull and cervical plain films to evaluate skull or neck trauma.

    5. Angiogram to evaluate blood vessels in cases of bleeding.

    6. Certain cases may require CBC, comprehensive metabolic panel (CMP), blood alcohol level, drug screen, prothrombin time (PT), partial thromboplastin time (PTT), fibrinogen.

G. Differential diagnosis.

Convulsions, unspecified, R56.9	Myelitis, unspecified, G04.91
Bacterial meningitis, unspecified, G00.9	Poisoning by unspecified
Malignant neoplasm of brain, unspecified, C71.9	drugs, medicaments and biological substances,
Migraine, unspecified, not intractable, without status migrainosus, G43.909	undetermined, initial encounter, T50.90

H. Treatment.
1. Mild head injury—treated at home as long as someone available to monitor.
2. Acetaminophen for pain. No aspirin or ibuprofen due to increased risk of bleeding.
3. *Do not:*
   a. Wash head wound that is deep or profusely bleeding.
   b. Remove any object sticking out of wound.
   c. Move the person unless absolutely necessary.
   d. Shake the person to arouse.
   e. Remove helmet if you suspect a serious head injury.
   f. Pick up a fallen child with any sign of head injury.
4. Apply ice to reduce swelling.
5. Roll on side if vomiting.
6. Cover bleeding area with clean cloth, only press firmly if no concern for skull fracture.
7. Always treat as if spinal injury if patient unconscious, keep head midline and immobile.
8. Maintain airway and vital signs, CPR if needed.
9. Admit to hospital for severe injury, monitor for progression of symptoms or concern for increased ICP.

I. Complications.
1. Increased ICP.
2. Surgery to remove objects, control hemorrhage, or decompress brain.
3. Seizures.
4. Resulting focal deficits.
   a. Weakness, aphasia, personality and intellectual changes, depression, anxiety, aggression, loss or change in: Sensations, hearing, vision, taste, smell, speech, or language.
5. Paralysis.
6. Chronic headaches.

J. Follow-up.
1. Seek care immediately for:
   a. Vomiting more than once.
   b. Confusion.
   c. Drowsiness, unable to awaken.
   d. Weakness or inability to walk.
   e. Severe headache.
   f. Severe head trauma or fall from more than height of the person.
   g. LOC for > 1 minute.
   h. Stops breathing.
   i. Severe head or facial bleeding.
2. Follow up in 1 week after injury and every few weeks to monitor for and manage any sequelae.

K. Education.
1. Wear helmets for biking, skating, and other similar sports.
2. Wear proper sports equipment, and make sure in good condition.
3. Wear seat belts, use age-appropriate car seats.
4. Prevent falls by child-proofing home—stairs, bathtubs, rugs, furniture.
5. Be visible and obey traffic laws when biking.
6. Safe areas to play.
7. Know signs and symptoms of head injury/concussion, and know when to seek medical care.

IV. CONCUSSION

A. Alteration in mental status after a blow to the head, loss of consciousness may or may not occur.

Concussion without loss of consciousness, initial encounter, S06.0X0A	Psychosis, unspecified, not due to a substance or known physiological condition, F29
Dizziness and giddiness, R42	Postconcussional syndrome, F07.81
Injury of head, unspecified, initial encounter, S09.90XA	Somnolence, R40.0
	Stupor, R40.1

B. Etiology.
1. Type of TBI caused from: Bump, blow, or jolt to the head.
2. Blow to body can cause head and brain to move rapidly back and forth, resulting in head injury.

3. Results from falls, MVA, and players that collide with each other, ground, or obstacles.

C. Occurrence.

1. 135,000 sports- and recreation-related TBIs come to emergency departments (EDs) each year (includes concussions in children age 5–18 years).
2. Athletes who have had a concussion are at increased risk for another.
3. Children and teens are more likely to get a concussion and take longer to recover than adults.
4. More than 2 million concussions happen per year, 85% never diagnosed.
5. 50% of football players may experience one concussion per year.

D. Clinical manifestations.

1. Hallmark signs—confusion and amnesia that may occur immediately or several minutes after injury occurs.
2. Early (minutes and hours) symptoms experienced:
   a. Headache.
   b. Dizziness or vertigo.
   c. Lack of awareness of surroundings.
   d. Nausea or vomiting.
3. Late (days to weeks) symptoms experienced:
   a. Persistent low-grade headache.
   b. Light-headedness.
   c. Poor attention and concentration.
   d. Memory dysfunction.
   e. Easy fatigability.
   f. Irritability and low frustration tolerance.
   g. Intolerance to bright light or loud noises.
   h. Anxiety or depressed mood.

E. Physical findings.

1. Vacant stare.
2. Delayed verbal and motor responses.
3. Confusion and inability to maintain focus.
4. Disorientation.
5. Slurred or incoherent speech.
6. Incoordination.
7. Memory deficits.
8. Emotional.
9. Any period of unconsciousness.

F. Diagnostic tests.

1. Sideline/immediate evaluation.
   a. ABCs: Airway, Breathing, Circulation checks if unconscious.
   b. Orientation—to time, place, person, and situation.

    c. Concentration—digits backward, months of year in reverse.

    d. Memory—recall 3 words or objects, details of contest, names.

    e. Neurological tests.
- Pupils, coordination, sensation.

2. Head CT—for loss of consciousness.

3. Immediate postconcussion assessment and cognitive testing (ImPACT) to assess cognitive functioning, done soon after concussion and before return to activities.

G. Differential diagnosis.

Convulsions, unspecified, R56.9	Transient alteration of awareness, R40.4
Migraine, unspecified, not intractable, without status migrainosus, G43.909	Transient cerebral ischemic attack, unspecified, G45.9

H. Treatment.

1. Remove from contest.

2. Monitor for progressive neurological changes.

3. ED for loss of consciousness.

4. When to return to play: Need to be asymptomatic with normal neurological assessment at rest and with exertion. Must be cleared by health professional before return to play.

I. Complications.

1. Seizures.

2. Second impact syndrome—repeat concussion that occurs before the brain recovers from the first, can slow recovery or increase likelihood of long-term problems, including brain damage, brain swelling, and even death.

3. Depression—not being able to participate in their sport.

4. Rare case for development of blood clot on brain.

5. Headaches.

J. Follow-up.

1. Repeat ImPACT testing.

2. Call or go to ED for:

    a. Unequal pupils.

    b. Drowsy and cannot awaken.

    c. Worsening headache.

    d. Weakness, numbness.

    e. Repeated vomiting.

    f. Seizure.

    g. Slurred speech.

    h. Increased confusion.

      i. Unable to recognize people or places.

      j. LOC.

K. Education.

   1. Use protective equipment that fits properly and is well maintained.

   2. Practice safe playing techniques/good sportsmanship.

   3. Know signs and symptoms of concussion, when to sit out and when to return.

V. STATUS EPILEPTICUS

A. 30 minutes or more of continuous seizure activity or a series of seizures without return to full consciousness between seizures.

Generalized idiopathic epilepsy and epileptic syndromes, not intractable, with status epilepticus, G40.301

Somnolence, R40.0

Stupor, R40.1

B. Etiology.

   1. Idiopathic.

   2. Central nervous system (CNS) neoplasms, stroke, infections, electrolyte abnormalities, trauma, metabolic disorders, toxic ingestion, hypoxic insult.

   3. History of epilepsy.

   4. Noncompliance with antiepileptic medications.

   5. History of injury—MVA, fall.

C. Occurrence.

   1. 50,000—200,000 cases per year.

   2. Mortality rate 20%, mostly from underlying case of brain injury.

   3. Can occur in all age groups, more in elderly.

   4. Males and females affected equally.

D. Physical findings.

   1. Absence status.

      a. Confusion, lethargy.

      b. EEG with continuous or intermittent but frequent spikes and slow wave discharges.

   2. Focal motor status.

      a. Continuous jerking of restricted muscle groups.

   3. Complex partial status.

      a. Confused, dazed, automatisms often present.

      b. Most often series of seizures, remaining confused between seizures.

      4. Generalized tonic-clonic status.

         a. Continuous convulsions or repetitive convulsions without resolution of postictal depression between episodes.

  E. Diagnostic tests.

      1. EEG.

      2. Head CT initially, may do MRI later if warranted.

      3. CMP (focus on glucose, Na+, Ca++), toxicology screen, WBC.

      4. LP if CNS infection in differential.

  F. Differential diagnosis.

Bacterial meningitis, unspecified, G00.9	Hyponatremia, E87.1
Cerebral infarction due to unspecified occlusion or stenosis of unspecified cerebral artery, I63.50	Myelitis, unspecified, G04.91
Hypoglycaemia, unspecified, E16.2	Nontraumatic subarachnoid hemorrhage, unspecified, I60.9

  G. Treatment.

      1. Maintain vital signs and ABCs.

      2. Administer DIASTAT AcuDial after 5 minutes of seizure activity. Call 911 if seizure continues.

      3. Ativan IV: 0.1 mg/kg at 2 mg/min.

      4. Diazepam IV: 0.3–0.5 mg/kg at 2 mg/min.

      5. Fosphenytoin, phenobarbital, phenytoin (Dilantin), divalproex sodium (Depakote IV). Monitor for respiratory depression.

      6. Correct any abnormal laboratory findings.

      7. Treat any underlying infection.

  H. Complications.

      1. Respiratory failure.

      2. Aspiration.

      3. Hypotension.

      4. Acidosis.

      5. Hyperthermia.

  I. Follow-up.

      1. Coordinate with specialists for any associated injuries or complications.

      2. See neurologist in 2 weeks.

      3. Start maintenance antiepileptic medication, call for any side effects or further seizures.

  J. Education.

      1. Know signs and symptoms and when and how to give DIASTAT AcuDial.

2. Medication information and compliance.
3. Avoidance of any seizure triggers: Sleep deprivation, alcohol.
4. Seizure safety: No tub baths unsupervised, monitor closely with swimming, helmets appropriate for sports, no driving until seizure free for 6 months, what to do during a seizure—lay on side on ground, do not put anything in mouth, time event, and keep safe.

VI. CONFUSIONAL MIGRAINE

A. Characterized by a typical migraine aura, headache, and confusion.

Headache, R51	Psychosis, unspecified, not due to a substance or known physiological condition, F29
Irritability and anger, R45.4	
Other migraine, not intractable, without status migrainosus, G43.809	

B. Etiology.
   1. Idiopathic.
   2. Triggered by head trauma.
C. Occurrence.
   1. Rare, only 5% of migraine patients.
   2. Single attacks are most common, multiple attacks are rare.
   3. May evolve into typical migraine episodes.
D. Clinical manifestations.
   1. Inattention.
   2. Distractibility.
E. Physical findings.
   1. Impaired speech and motor activities.
   2. Can last 10 minutes to 20 hours. A more profound, disturbed LOC may lead to migraine stupor, which can last from hours to up to 5 days.
   3. Confusional state is usually followed by sleep.
F. Diagnostic tests.
   1. Complete neurological exam.
   2. MRI and MRA to evaluate arteries within the brain.
   3. History may include family history, history of trauma, and classic symptoms.

G. Differential diagnosis.

Localization-related (focal) (partial) symptomatic epilepsy and epileptic syndromes with complex partial seizures, not intractable, without status epilepticus, G40.209 Metabolic encephalopathy, G93.41	Poisoning by unspecified drugs, medicaments and biological substances, accidental (unintentional), initial encounter, T50.901A Psychosis, unspecified, not due to a substance or known physiological condition, F29 Viral encephalitis, unspecified, A86

H. Treatment.
1. Sleep.
2. Typical migraine-abortive medications.
I. Follow-up.
1. Reoccurrence of episodes.
2. Change in neurological status (resulting from any head trauma).
J. Education.
1. Avoidance of migraine triggers.
2. Keep a headache/episode diary.
3. Limit use of over-the-counter analgesics.
4. Keep a regular schedule: Meals, sleep, hydration, exercise, and minimize stress.

VII. MIGRAINES

A. Episodic headache disorder characterized by various combinations of neurological, gastrointestinal, psychophysiological, and autonomic changes.

Benign paroxysmal vertigo, bilateral, H81.13	Motion sickness, initial encounter, T75.3XXA
Dizziness and giddiness, R42	Nausea with vomiting, unspecified, R11.2
Headache, R51	Other visual disturbances, H53.8
Irritability and anger, R45.4	Psychosis, unspecified, not due to a substance or known physiological condition, F29
Migraine with aura [classical migraine], G43.1	
Migraine, unspecified, not intractable, without status migrainosus, G43.909	Visual discomfort, unspecified, H53.149
	Vomiting, unspecified, R11.10

B. Etiology.
   1. Generally inherited disorder, 70–80% familial.
   2. Leading hypothesis for origin—neurovascular disturbance triggered by multiple stimuli and affecting serotonin transmission in the CNS.
   3. Episodic brain malfunction—a CNS disorder of primarily the brain and nerves, and secondarily of the blood vessels. Malfunction is caused in part by changes in the level of circulating neurotransmitters and involves serotonin in particular.
   4. Head trauma.
   5. Illness and infection.
   6. Environmental and emotional factors.
   7. Certain foods and beverages.
C. Occurrence.
   1. Mean age of onset is 7.2 years for boys and 10.9 years for girls.
   2. 3% of children age 3–7 years.
   3. 4–11% for children age 7–11 years.
   4. 8–23% for children age 11–15+ years.
   5. Risk factors:
      a. Children who have a family history of headaches or migraines.
      b. Boys before they reach puberty.
      c. Girls after they reach puberty.
      d. Children over age 10 years.
D. Clinical manifestations.
   1. Pounding or throbbing head pain. In children, pain usually affects the front or both sides of the head. In adolescents, pain usually affects one side of head.
   2. Pallor or paleness of skin.
   3. Irritability.
   4. Phonophobia or sensitivity to sound.
   5. Photophobia or sensitivity to light.
   6. Loss of appetite.
   7. Nausea and/or vomiting, abdominal pain.
   8. Dizziness.
E. Physical findings.
   1. May have none if not experiencing migraine at time of exam.
   2. Due to pain, may see increase in heart rate or blood pressure.
   3. Look of discomfort in facial expressions and demeanor.
   4. Wanting to lie down in quiet, dark room.
F. Diagnostic tests.
   1. Most important aspect of diagnosing migraine is the headache history.
      a. Description of current and previous headaches, when started.
      b. Headache frequency, duration, and associated symptoms.

      c. What medications have been taken and are currently being taken.

      d. Family and medical history.

      e. Pain location, quality, and severity—how disabling?

      f. Social history—psychological symptoms.

      g. Precipitating factors.

  2. Complete neurological exam—including fundoscopic exam to rule out papilledema.

  3. Head CT.

      a. Recent/new onset.

      b. Evolution or change in headaches.

  4. Head MRI.

      a. Papilledema present.

      b. Focal neurological signs—abnormal exam, hemiparesis.

      c. Complicated migraine—examine blood vessels that supply the brain.

  5. Evaluation as needed if concern for infectious cause.

      a. LP if concern for increased ICP/papilledema present; generally need to do head MRI prior to LP.

G. Differential diagnosis.

Benign intracranial hypertension, G93.2	Nontraumatic intracranial hemorrhage, unspecified, I62.9
Cerebral infarction due to unspecified occlusion or stenosis of unspecified cerebral artery, I63.50	Other specified disorders of brain, G93.8
Chronic sinusitis, unspecified, J32.9	Other symptoms and signs involving the nervous system, R29.818
Injury of head, unspecified, initial encounter, S09.90XA	Papilloedema, unspecified, H47.1
Mental disorder, not otherwise specified, F99	Viral meningitis, unspecified, A87.9

H. Treatment.

  1. Treat underlying pathology if present.

      a. Diamox for pseudotumor cerebri.

  2. Goals of treatment.

      a. Reduce attack frequency, severity, and duration.

      b. Improve responsiveness to treatment of acute attacks.

      c. Improve function, reduce disability, and improve quality of life.

  3. Nonpharmacologic treatments.

      a. Relaxation techniques, biofeedback, stress management.

      b. Rest, quiet dark room, applying ice packs to forehead or neck.

    c. Lifestyle/behavioral interventions.
- Maintain routine sleep pattern with adequate sleep hours.
- Regular routines, meal, exercise, school attendance.
- Staying hydrated.
- Avoidance/discontinuation of caffeine.
- Avoidance/discontinuation of overuse of abortive medications.
- Stress reduction.

4. Acute medication treatment.
    a. Medication should not be used more than 2 or, at most, 3 days a week to prevent development of rebound headaches.
    b. Prevents or stops progression of headache.
    c. Use medication as early as possible to prevent escalation and to increase the drug's effectiveness.
    d. Mild to moderate pain: Ibuprofen (NSAIDs with or without caffeine) or acetaminophen (Tylenol).
    e. Moderate to severe pain: Triptans (contraindicated for migraine variant such as hemiplegic or basilar migraine), ergotamine, dihydroergotamine (DHE).
    f. Antiemetics to help relieve pain, nausea, vomiting.
    g. Steroid dose pack to break migraine status, prolonged migraine.

5. Preventive medication treatment.
    a. Use when:
- Recurring migraine that interferes with daily routine despite acute treatment (two or more attacks/month that produce disability and can last up to 3 days or more).
- Failure, contraindication, or side effects from acute medications.
- Overuse of acute medications.
- Frequent headaches (more than 2/week) with risk for rebound headache syndrome.

    b. Medication options:
- Antidepressants: Amitriptyline (Elavil), fluoxetine (Prozac), duloxetine (Cymbalta).
- Beta blockers: Propranolol (Inderal).
- Antihistamines: Cyproheptadine (Periactin) (most effective in toddlers).
- Calcium channel blockers: Verapamil.
- Anticonvulsants: Valproic acid (Depakote), topiramate (Topamax).

I. Follow-up.
   1. Assess medication effectiveness, monitor for any possible side effects.
   2. When abortive medications do not elevate migraine, may need IM or IV abortive medications and fluids such as ketorolac (Toradol) or promethazine (Phenergan).
   3. Any neurological changes or progression in headaches.
J. Complications.
   1. Comorbid anxiety and/or depression.
   2. Medication side effects.
   3. Acute vascular disorder.
   4. High incidence of motion sickness.
   5. Sleep disturbance.
   6. Drop in school performance due to missed days, and inability to concentrate with a headache.
K. Education.
   1. Migraine diagnosis and treatment (medications/possible side effects).
   2. Keep a headache diary, look for headache triggers.
   3. Know symptoms and when to treat headache.
   4. Limit use of abortive medications.
   5. Behavioral modifications, follow routine schedule.
   6. Daily school attendance.
   7. Reduce stress and avoid triggers.
   8. Empower patient and family to be involved and take control of their headaches and treatment.

VIII. TENSION-TYPE HEADACHES

A. Headache that presents with pressure/tightening quality and lacks migraine criteria.

Cervicalgia, M54.2

Headache, R51

Irritability and anger, R45.4

B. Etiology.
   1. Behavioral.
   2. Muscular.
   3. Vascular.
   4. May coexist with otherwise typical migraine headaches.
C. Occurrence.
   1. Most common benign headache disorder.
   2. 10–25% prevalence in childhood and adolescence.

3. Boys and girls tend to suffer equally until age 11 or 12, when female preponderance occurs.
D. Clinical manifestations.
  1. Episodic headaches occur less than 15 days/month.
  2. Chronic headaches occur more than 15 days/month.
  3. Can last 30 minutes to 7 days.
  4. Pain is mild to moderate (not severe).
  5. Pain is bilateral and described as pressing or tightening, may occur in a hat band distribution.
  6. Pain not aggravated by physical activity (unlike migraine).
  7. No nausea or vomiting.
  8. May have photophobia or phonophobia, but not both.
E. Physical findings.
  1. Normal neurological exam, worrisome if abnormal.
  2. May see signs of pain: Facial expressions, demeanor, increased heart rate and blood pressure.
  3. May be misdiagnosed as sinus headache.
F. Diagnostic tests.
  1. Same as migraine.
  2. History/complaints consistent with tension-type headache criteria.
G. Differential diagnosis.

Allergy, unspecified, initial encounter, T78.40XA	Migraine, unspecified, not intractable, without status migrainosus, G43.909
Chronic sinusitis, unspecified, J32.9	Nontraumatic subarachnoid hemorrhage, unspecified, I60.9
Essential (primary) hypertension, I10	Temporomandibular joint disorders (TMJ), K07.6
Glaucoma, unspecified, H40.9	

H. Complications.
  1. Depression.
  2. Poor academic performance, difficulty concentrating, missed school days and other activities.
I. Treatment.
  1. Nonpharmacologic treatments.
    a. Healthy habits.
      • Adequate routine sleep schedule.
      • Balanced meals.
      • Regular exercise.
      • No caffeine.

      b. Psychophysiological therapy.
- Reassurance.
- Counseling.
- Stress management.
- Relaxation therapy.
- Biofeedback.
- Treatment of anxiety and/or depression.

   2. Pharmacotherapy.
      a. Acute treatment—not to be used more than 2 days/week.
- NSAIDs.
- Acetaminophen.

      b. Preventive treatment.
- Amitriptyline (Elavil).
- Selective serotonin reuptake inhibitors (SSRIs).
- Muscle relaxers (tizanidine [Zanaflex]).

J. Follow-up.
   1. Assess medication effectiveness and any possible side effects.
   2. Any neurological change or headache progression.

K. Education.
   1. As with migraines.

IX. COMMON MEDICATIONS TO TREAT HEADACHES IN CHILDREN

A. Preventive:
1. Cyproheptadine (Periactin): 0.25–0.4 mg/kg or 2–4 mg daily bid.
2. Amitriptyline: Start 10 mg at bedtime. Up to 1–2 mg/kg at bedtime.
3. Propranolol (Inderal): 1–2 mg/kg/day up to 4 mg/kg/day bid. Unless using LA form.
4. Tizanidine (Zanaflex): 2–4 mg at bedtime up to 12 mg. Monitor hepatic panel at 1, 3, and 6 months.
5. Valproic acid (Depakote): 10–20 mg/kg bid up to 60 mg/kg.
6. Topiramate (Topamax): Titrate to 50 mg bid.
7. Verapamil: 40 mg tid or SR 120 mg, 180 mg, 240 mg daily.

B. Abortive:
1. Sumatriptan (Imitrex NS): 5–10 mg (1–2 sprays). Oral 25 mg up to 100 mg.
2. Rizatriptan (Maxalt): 5–10 mg tab.
3. Dihydroergotamine mesylate (Migranal): 1 spray each nostril, may repeat in 15 minutes.

4. Zolmitriptan (Zomig): 2.5–5 mg tab; 5 mg NS.
5. Eletriptan (Relpax): 20–40 mg tab.
6. Metoclopramide (Reglan): 0.1–0.2 mg/kg/dose up to 4 times a day.
7. Promethazine (Phenergan): 0.25 mg/kg/dose (max 25 mg) up to 4 times a day.
8. Ibuprofen: 15 mg/kg/dose every 6 hours.
9. Acetaminophen (Tylenol): 10 mg/kg/dose every 4 hours.

X. FEBRILE SEIZURES

A. Seizure in association with a febrile illness in the absence of CNS infection or acute electrolyte imbalance in children older than 3 months of age without a prior afebrile seizure.

Convulsions, unspecified, R56.9	Simple febrile convulsions, R56.00
Fever of other and unknown origin, R50	Somnolence, R40.0
	Stupor, R40.1

B. Etiology.
   1. Benign age-dependent epilepsy syndrome, seizure in early life in presence of fever without intracranial infection.
   2. Genetic disposition—two to three times more common among family members of affected children than general population.
C. Occurrence.
   1. 2–5% of children will have a febrile seizure.
   2. Most common between ages of 6 months and 3 years, with peak incidence at 18 to 24 months of age.
   3. Risk factors.
      a. High peak temperature during illness.
      b. Family history of febrile seizures in a first- or second-degree relative.
      c. Developmental delay.
      d. Neonatal nursery stays longer than 30 days.
      e. Attendance at daycare.
D. Physical findings.
   1. Temperature of at least 39°F.
   2. Simple febrile seizure.
      a. Generalized tonic-clonic movements.
      b. Eyes roll back.

  c. Loss of consciousness.

  d. Last few seconds to minutes (less than 15 minutes).

  e. Postictal depression is brief.

 3. Complex febrile seizures.

  a. Last longer than 15 minutes.

  b. May reoccur within the same day.

  c. Prolonged period of postictal drowsiness or neurological abnormalities.

  d. Focal seizure manifestations.

E. Diagnostic tests.

 1. Simple febrile seizure.

  a. Extensive history taking.

  b. Evaluation for cause of fever, CBC.

  c. LP for infants younger than 6 months of age.

 2. Complex febrile seizure.

  a. CSF evaluation.

  b. Head CT if warranted.

  c. EEG if concerned.

F. Differential diagnosis.

Generalized idiopathic epilepsy and epileptic syndromes, not intractable, without status epilepticus, G40.309	Metabolic disorder, unspecified, E88.9
Meningitis, unspecified, G03.9	Myelitis, unspecified, G04.91
	Sepsis, unspecified organism, A41.9

G. Treatment.

 1. Control fever with antipyretic medication.

 2. Antibiotics appropriate for any bacterial infections.

 3. Treat cause of fever, fluids.

 4. Diazepam rectally or lorazepam (Ativan) IV for seizures lasting longer than 5 minutes.

 5. No need for anticonvulsant medication.

H. Complications.

 1. Rare, no neurological sequelae.

 2. Fewer than 10% of patients experience severe or recurrent attacks.

 3. Likelihood of developing epilepsy less than 5%.

 4. Possible complications if septic nature is cause for fever and seizure.

 5. Risk for reoccurrence.

  a. Neurological or developmental abnormality.

  b. Positive family history.

      c. Onset of febrile seizures before age 1 year.

      d. Low peak temperature at onset of seizure.

      e. Duration of fever.

I. Follow-up.

  1. Any seizure without fever.

  2. As needed for treatment of cause of fever.

J. Education.

  1. Reassurance of the benign nature.

  2. First aid during a seizure.

  3. When to call the doctor or go to the emergency room: Need to find and treat cause of fever to stop seizure that continues past 5 minutes and does not stop with diazepam rectal (DIASTAT).

XI. GENERALIZED SEIZURES

A. Seizure in which the first clinical changes indicate initial involvement of both hemispheres.

Absence epileptic syndrome, not intractable, without status epilepticus, G40.A09	Epilepsy, G40
	Generalized idiopathic epilepsy and epileptic syndromes, not intractable, without status epilepticus, G40.309
Convulsions, unspecified, R56.9	

B. Etiology.

  1. Up to 80% have unclear etiology.

  2. Hereditary.

  3. Perinatal: Infectious, hypoxia, trauma.

  4. Metabolic, toxic, nutritional.

  5. Infectious.

  6. Vascular.

  7. Neoplastic.

C. Occurrence.

  1. Children account for about 15% of all epilepsy cases.

  2. Generalized seizures account for one-third of all epilepsies.

  3. Most often start in childhood or adolescence.

D. Clinical manifestations.

  1. Generalized tonic-clonic (grand mal).

     a. Starts suddenly with stiff muscles (tonic phase) and then rhythmic contractions (clonic phase).

      b. Impaired consciousness.

      c. Loss of bladder control common.

      d. Can last a few minutes.

      e. Postictal phase that can include drowsiness, confusion, and headache.

   2. Atonic seizure (drop attack).

      a. Sudden drop to the floor, head may nod/drop.

      b. Brief episode, loss of consciousness brief.

      c. Injuries are common.

   3. Absence seizures.

      a. Abrupt sudden loss of consciousness with cessation of all motor activity.

      b. Brief periods of staring blankly into space.

      c. Ends abruptly, no postictal state.

      d. Can be induced by hyperventilation.

      e. May see lip smacking, chewing, eye fluttering.

   4. Myoclonic.

      a. Brief contraction of a muscle group.

      b. Can drop objects.

      c. Recovery is immediate and often maintains consciousness.

   5. Infantile spasms.

      a. Clusters of seizures involving flexion jerk of the neck, trunk, and extremities.

      b. Range from subtle head drop or shoulder shrug to more violent action.

      c. Decreased responsiveness may follow spasms.

      d. Spasms are brief, lasting just a few seconds.

E. Physical findings.

   1. Seizure rare to happen in office to observe, can have family video episodes.

   2. May be "normal" between seizures.

   3. Low-grade fever, up to 101°F may occur after seizure.

   4. Injuries possible, especially with atonic seizures.

F. Diagnostic tests.

   1. EEG in awake and sleep states.

   2. MRI if focal spike on EEG or abnormal neuro exam.

   3. May do CMP, CBC if concerned abnormalities might be a cause.

   4. EKG for concern for cardiac disorder (syncope).

   5. Prolonged EEG to catch episodes if warranted.

G. Differential diagnosis.

Apnea, not elsewhere classified, R06.81	Hyperventilation, R06.4
Cardiac arrhythmia, unspecified, I49.9	Migraine, unspecified, not intractable, without status migrainosus, G43.909
Conduct disorder, unspecified, F91.9	Other abnormalities of breathing, R06.89
Convulsions, unspecified, R56.9	Sleep disorders, G47
Dissociative fugue, F44.1	Syncope and collapse, R55

H. Treatment.
1. Anticonvulsant medication.
    a. Absence seizures—ethosuximide (Zarontin), lamotrigine (Lamictal), divalproex (Depakote).
    b. Generalized—divalproex (Depakote), lamotrigine (Lamictal), topiramate (Topamax), levetiracetam (Keppra), felbamate (Felbatol), zonisamide (Zonegran).
    c. Infantile spasms—ACTH, topiramate (Topamax), vigabatrin (Sabril).
2. 70% of patients with epilepsy will gain seizure freedom with medications.
3. Vagal nerve stimulator or ketogenic diet for intractable seizures.
I. Follow-up.
1. Medication management, anticonvulsant therapeutic levels, and possible need for CMP, liver functions, CBC for some medications.
2. Medication side effects.
3. Continued seizures.
J. Complications.
1. High risk for depression in epilepsy patients.
2. Medication side effects.
3. Developmental delay.
4. Anxiety, intellectual underachievement.
K. Education.
1. Seizure/epilepsy etiology and prognosis.
2. Seizure safety.
3. Psychosocial comorbidities.
4. Medication management and possible side effects.
5. Reevaluation parameters.

XII. PARTIAL SEIZURES

A. Seizure, electrical disturbance, arising from one area of the brain; consciousness may or may not be preserved. Can spread to become generalized.

Convulsions, unspecified, R56.9	Localization-related (focal) (partial) symptomatic epilepsy and epileptic syndromes with complex partial seizures, not intractable, without status epilepticus, G40.209
Disorder of the autonomic nervous system, unspecified, G90.9	Localization-related (focal) (partial) symptomatic epilepsy and epileptic syndromes with simple partial seizures, not intractable, without status epilepticus, G40.109

B. Etiology.
   1. Idiopathic (most common in children).
   2. Brain injury/trauma.
   3. Developmental brain abnormality.
   4. Tumors (rare).
   5. Infectious or hypoxic injuries.
C. Occurrence.
   1. Most common type of seizure experienced by people with epilepsy.
   2. Risk factors—developmental and brain abnormalities.
D. Clinical manifestations.
   1. Depends on which part and how much of the brain is affected.
   2. Virtually any movement, sensory, or emotional symptom can occur.
   3. Simple partial.
      a. No loss of consciousness.
      b. Motor signs.
         • Focal nature.
         • Postural.
         • Phonatory (vocalizations or arrest of speech).
         • Eye or truncal deviations.
      c. Somatosensory symptoms.
         • Visual.
         • Auditory.
         • Olfactory.
         • Gustatory.
         • Vertiginous.
      d. Autonomic symptoms.
         • Epigastric sensations.
         • Pallor.

- Sweating.
- Flushing.
- Papillary dilation.
4. Complex partial.
   a. Impairment of consciousness.
   b. Can start as simple and evolve to loss of consciousness.
   c. May also progress to generalized seizure (partial seizure that secondarily generalizes).
E. Physical findings.
   1. Generally none on office exam, unless cause of seizure leaves or is cause of a neurological deficit.
F. Diagnostic tests.
   1. As with generalized seizures, but head MRI warranted.
G. Differential diagnosis.

Abnormal involuntary movements, unspecified, R25.9	Dystonia, unspecified, G24.9
	Generalized idiopathic epilepsy and epileptic syndromes, not intractable,
Convulsions, unspecified R56.9	without status epilepticus, G40.309

H. Treatment.
   1. Anticonvulsant medications.
      a. Oxcarbazepine (Trileptal), or broad-spectrum anticonvulsant medication.
   2. Surgical intervention if intractable to medications.
   3. Vagal nerve stimulator or ketogenic diet.
I. Follow-up.
   1. As with generalized seizures.
J. Complications.
   1. As with generalized seizures.
K. Education.
   1. As with generalized seizures.

XIII. COMMON ANTICONVULSANT MEDICATIONS FOR CHILDREN

A. Divalproex (Depakote): Start 10–20 mg/kg/day given bid, liquid tid; maintenance dose 30–60 mg/kg/day. Monitor CBC with platelets and liver enzymes every 6 months for liver failure, thrombocytopenia.
B. Levetiracetam (Keppra): Start 10–20 mg/kg/day bid; maintenance dose 30–60 mg/kg/day.

C. Lamotrigine (Lamictal): Titrate slowly over 8–12 weeks to starting dose. Risk for Stevens-Johnson syndrome. Maintenance dose 5–15 mg/kg/day bid; lower dose when on enzyme inducer anticonvulsant.

D. Topiramate (Topamax): Start 1 mg/kg/day bid; maintenance 3–9 mg/kg/day. Monitor bicarb for metabolic acidosis.

E. Oxcarbazepine (Trileptal): Start 10 mg/kg/day bid; maintenance 30–60 mg/kg/day.

F. Ethosuximide (Zarontin): Start 10–15 mg/kg/day bid; maintenance dose 15–40 mg/kg/day. Monitor CBC for leucopenia, aplastic anemia.

G. Zonisamide (Zonegran): Start 1–2 mg/kg/day daily or bid; maintenance dose 5–8 mg/kg/day.

XIV. GLOBAL DEVELOPMENTAL DELAY

A. Subset of developmental disabilities defined as significant delay in two or more of the following developmental domains: Gross/fine motor, speech/language, cognition, social/personal, and activities of daily living.

Ataxia, unspecified, R27.0	Other reduction deformities of brain, Q04.3
Delayed milestone in childhood, R62.0	Other specified chromosome abnormalities, Q99.8
Expressive language disorder, F80.1	

B. Etiology.
   1. Genetic abnormalities.
   2. Early environmental deprivation.
   3. Metabolic abnormalities.
   4. Abnormal CNS/brain development.
   5. Idiopathic/unknown.

C. Occurrence.
   1. Developmental disabilities of early onset affect 5–10% of children.
   2. Refers to younger children younger than 5 years of age.
   3. 1–3% of children younger than 5 years of age are affected.

D. Clinical manifestations.
   1. Two standard deviations or more below the mean on age-appropriate standardized norm-referenced testing.

E. Physical findings.
   1. Not walking independently by 18 months of age.
   2. Poor/clumsy fine motor skills.

    3. No two-word sentences by 2 years of age.

    4. Does not follow two-step commands at age 2 years.

    5. Does not know 6 body parts by 2 years of age.

    6. Unable to feed, dress, or do activities of daily living.

    7. May see poor feeding, poor weight gain, dysmorphic features, cardiac or liver, kidney, bowel abnormalities.

F. Diagnostic testing.

    1. Obtain detailed history and examination.

    2. Refer for auditory and ophthalmologic screening.

    3. Consider metabolic studies/T4 if newborn screening not done.

    4. EEG if history suspects seizures.

    5. If close family member with global developmental delay due to a known cause, test for that disorder and obtain cytogenetic screen.

    6. Head MRI.

    7. Lead screen.

    8. Complete metabolic panel.

    9. Lactic acid.

    10. High resolution chromosomes, fragile X, Rett syndrome.

    11. Urine genetic screen.

    12. Microarray if other tests negative.

    13. Mitochondrial testing, muscle biopsy, if suspected and other testing inconclusive or negative.

G. Differential diagnosis.

Atypical autism, F84.1	Encephalopathy, unspecified, G94.30
Cerebral palsy, unspecified, G80.9	Other disorders of brain in diseases classified elsewhere, G94
Chromosomal abnormality, unspecified, Q99.9	Other specified congenital malformation syndromes, not elsewhere classified, Q87.89

H. Treatment.

    1. Therapy—speech, physical, occupational, developmental, and/or nutritional.

    2. Medications as needed for any underlying cause.

    3. Genetic counseling.

I. Follow-up.

    1. Discussion of test results.

    2. For any regression or loss of developmental milestones.

    3. Every 3 months to assess progression/development.

    4. To obtain further recommendations for testing in stepwise approach.

    5. For need for additional resources: Referral to genetics, metabolism, developmental pediatrics, therapies, psychiatry, neurology, and other services as needed.

J. Complications.

    1. Progressive loss of skills or lack of progression if untreated.

    2. Seizures.

    3. Behavioral disturbances.

    4. Some disorders may affect systemic organs/systems.

K. Education.

    1. Explaining test results, possible outcomes, prognosis.

    2. Possible complications.

    3. Medications if needed/treatment plan.

    4. Resources.

    5. Genetic and other counseling.

XV. TOURETTE SYNDROME

A. Neurobiological disorder characterized by tics—involuntary, rapid, sudden movements and/or vocal outbursts that occur repeatedly.

Abnormal involuntary movements, unspecified, R52.9

Combined vocal and multiple motor tic disorder [de la Tourette], F95.2

B. Etiology.

    1. No known cause has yet been established.

    2. Evidence points to abnormal metabolism of dopamine.

    3. Genetic studies indicate that Tourette syndrome is inherited as a dominant gene.

C. Occurrence.

    1. Estimated that 200,000 people in United States are affected—up to 18% of children.

    2. Often undiagnosed or misdiagnosed.

    3. 50% chance of affected parent passing to child.

    4. Sons are 3 to 4 times more likely to be affected than daughters.

    5. Peak severity of symptoms between 8 and 12 years and adolescents.

6. Can occur as early as 2 years of age, mean age of onset 6–7 years.
7. More common in males.
8. Exacerbated by anxiety, excitement, anger, fatigue, tension, stress.
9. Can decrease with relaxation or concentrating on an absorbing task.

D. Clinical manifestations.
   1. Motor tics—involuntary rapid repetitive stereotyped movements of muscle groups.
      a. Simple—involves one muscle group: Eye blinking, facial grimacing, head jerking, shoulder shrugging.
      b. Complex—involves either a cluster of simple movements or more coordinated sequence of movements: Hopping, clapping, tensing arm or neck muscles, touching people or objects.
   2. Vocal tics—transient vocalizations, meaningless sounds or noises or even words or phrases.
      a. Simple vocal tics: Sniffing, humming, clearing throat, coughing, squeaking.
      b. Rare, complex vocal tics:
         • Echolalia—repeating others' words.
         • Palilalia—repeating one's own words.
         • Coprolalia—repeating obscene words.
   3. Symptoms vary in children by type of specific tic and degree of severity.

E. Physical findings.
   1. May or may not see tics exhibited on exam while in office because some children can temporarily suppress them, but still have urge.
   2. May complain of muscle pain due to frequent motor tics.

F. Diagnostic testing.
   1. Based on observing symptoms and evaluating history.
   2. Must meet *Diagnostic and Statistical Manual of Mental Disorders* (DSM–V) criteria:
      a. Both motor and vocal tics must be present at same time.
      b. Tics occur many times a day (usually in bouts) nearly daily or intermittently for more than 1 year without a tic-free period of 3 months or more.
      c. Onset prior to age 18.
      d. Tics are not due to physiological effects of medication or underlying medical condition.

G. Differential diagnosis.

Akathisia, 781	Idiopathic orofacial dystonia, G24.4
Ataxia, unspecified, R27.0	Other specified congenital
Atypical autism, F84.1	malformations, Q89.8
Chorioretinal inflammation, unspecified, bilateral, H30.93	Poisoning by unspecified drugs, medicaments and biological
Convulsions, unspecified, R56.9	substances, accidental (unintentional), initial encounter, T50.901A
Genetic torsion dystonia, G24.1	Stereotyped movement disorders,
Huntington's disease, G10	F98.4

H. Treatment.
   1. None if tics are not disruptive to patient/child.
   2. Teach coping skills and relaxation techniques.
   3. Maintain adequate sleep hours and routine.
   4. Treat with medication if disruptive, causes pain, decreases self-esteem, child is teased, child is frustrated, interferes socially or academically.
      a. Guanfacine (Tenex)—low side effects, but effective only 50% of time.
      b. Clonidine—sedating.
      c. Haloperidol (Haldol).
      d. Risperidone (Risperdal)—can cause weight gain.
      e. Pimozide (Orap)—monitor EKG for prolonged QT interval.
      f. Topiramate (Topamax)—limited studies, but can be effective.
I. Follow-up.
   1. To monitor progression of symptoms to see if they become disruptive.
   2. For education and assessment of comorbidities.
   3. Medication management.
J. Complications.
   1. ADHD: Seen in up to 70% of patients who have tics/Tourette syndrome.
   2. Obsessive compulsive disorder: Seen in up to 50% of patients who have tics/Tourette syndrome.
   3. Depression.
   4. Anxiety.
   5. Muscle pain.
K. Education.
   1. Explanation of tics and Tourette syndrome, no known specific cause and no harm to brain, most often "normal" child and IQ.
   2. Do not criticize child or draw attention to tics.

3. Be sensitive to child's feelings, child unable to fully stop tics.
4. Teach coping skills and relaxation techniques.
5. Most children have tics for only a few months or less.
6. One-third of children will outgrow Tourette syndrome.
7. Discuss possible complications and when to treat.

BIBLIOGRAPHY

American Psychiatric Association. *Diagnostic and Statistical Manual of Mental Disorders*. 5th ed. Arlington, VA: American Psychiatric Association; 2013.

Arizona Sports Concussion Center. Heads up: concussion in youth sports. http://www.azsportsconcussion.com/concussion.php. Accessed July 5, 2015.

Bruun RD, Cohen DJ, Leckman JF. *Guide to the Diagnosis and Treatment of Tourette Syndrome*. 3rd ed. Bayside, NY: Tourette Syndrome Association; 1997.

Centers for Disease Control and Prevention. Injury prevention & control: traumatic brain injury. http://www.cdc.gov/TraumaticBrainInjury/index.html. Updated March 27, 2015. Accessed July 5, 2015.

Cleveland Clinic Children's. Headaches in children and adolescents. http://my.clevelandclinic.org/childrens-hospital/health-info/diseases-conditions/hic-headaches-in-children-and-adolescents. Accessed July 15, 2015.

Devinsky O, Feldmann E, Weinreb HJ, Wilterdink JL. *The Resident's Neurology Book*. Philadelphia, PA: F. A. Davis Company; 1997.

Goldenberg LB. Beyond a single seizure. Identification and treatment of epilepsy. *Adv Nurse Pract*. 2004;12(6):61-65.

Goldstein JL. Evaluating new onset of seizures in children. *Pediatr Ann*. 2004;33(6):368-374.

Heller JL. Head injury–first aid. http://www.nlm.gov/medlineplus/ency/article/000028.htm. Updated January 13, 2014. Accessed July 5, 2014.

Hershey AD, Kabbouche MA, Powers SW. Treatment of pediatric and adolescent migraine. *Pediatr Ann*. 2010;39(7):416-423.

Leung AK, Robson WL. Febrile seizures. *J Pediatr Health Care*. 2007;21(4):250-255.

Lewis D, Ashwal S, Hershey A, et al. Practice parameter: pharmacological treatment of migraine headache in children and adolescents: report of the American Academy of Neurology Quality Standards Subcommittee and the Practice Committee of the Child Neurology Society. *Neurology*. 2004;63(12): 2215-2224.

Mayo Clinic Staff. Encephalitis. http://www.mayoclinic.org/diseases-conditions/encephalitis/basics/symptoms/con-20021917?_ga=1.68960529.1688663537.1439152314. Updated May 15, 2014. Accessed July 5, 2015.

Mayo Clinic Staff. Headaches in children. http://www.mayoclinic.org/diseases-conditions/headaches-in-children/basics/symptoms/con-20034478?_ga=1.124789386.1688663537.1439152314. Updated June 26, 2013. Accessed July 5, 2015.

Mayo Clinic Staff. Meningitis. http://www.mayoclinic.org/diseases-conditions/meningitis/basics/definition/con-20019713?_ga=1.68960529.1688663537.1439152314. Updated March 19, 2013. Accessed July 5, 2015.

Medline Plus. Encephalitis. http://www.nlm.nih.gov/medlineplus/ency/article/001415.htm. Updated August 30, 2014. Accessed September 15, 2014.

Pakalnis A, Yonker M. "Other" headache syndromes in children. *Pediatr Ann*. 2010;39(7):440-446.

Panayiotopoulos C. Idiopathic generalized epilepsies. http://www.epilepsy.com/information/professionals/about-epilepsy-seizures/idiopathic-generalized-epilepsies. Published January 2005. Accessed July 5, 2015.

Saper JR, Silberstein SD, Gordon CD, Hamel RL. *Handbook of Headache Management: A Practical Guide to Diagnosis and Treatment of Head, Neck, and Facial Pain*. Baltimore, MD: Lippincott Williams & Wilkins; 1993.

Schachter SC. Types of seizures. http://www.epilepsy.com/learn/types-seizures. Reviewed November 2013. Accessed July 5, 2014.

Shevell M, Ashwal S, Donley D, et al. Practice parameter: evaluation of the child with global developmental delay: report of the Quality Standards Subcommittee of the American Academy of Neurology and The Practice Committee of the Child Neurology Society. *Neurology*. 2003;60(3):367-380.

Shinnar S, O'Dell C. Febrile seizures. *Pediatr Ann*. 2004;33(6):394-401.

Silberstein SD, Lipton RB. Variants confused with epilepsy. http://www.epilepsy.com/information/professionals /co-existing-disorders/migraine-epilepsy/variants-confused-epilepsy. Reviewed April 2004. Accessed July 5, 2015.

Silberstein SD, Lipton RB, Goadsby PJ. *Headache in Clinical Practice*. 2nd ed. London, UK: Martin Dunitz Ltd; 2002.

Tourette Association of America [homepage]. http://www.tsa-usa.org. Accessed July 3, 2015.

Wedro B. Head injury (brain injury). http://www.emedicinehealth.com/head_injury/article_em.htm. Accessed July 15, 201v5.

Wyllie E, Gupta A, Lachhwani DK, eds. *The Treatment of Epilepsy: Principles and Practice*. 4th ed. Philadelphia, PA: Lippincott Williams & Wilkins; 2006.

Hematologic Disorders

Betsy Atkinson Joyce and Terea Giannetta

I. IRON-DEFICIENCY ANEMIA (IDA)

Anemia, unspecified, D64.9	Irritability and anger, R45.4
Cardiac murmur, unspecified, R01.1	Other fatigue, R53.83
	Pallor, R23.1
Gastrointestinal hemorrhage, unspecified, K92.2	Protein-calorie malnutrition, unspecified, E46
Headache, R51	Splenomegaly, not elsewhere classified, R16.1
Iron deficiency anemia, unspecified, D50.9	Tachycardia, unspecified, R00.0

A. Most common anemia of childhood. Anemia is defined as reduction in red blood cell (RBC) mass or in hemoglobin concentration to a level that is > 2 standard deviations below mean in healthy children. Can be determined in primary care setting by physical examination, important aspects of history, and hemoglobin concentration. Screening should occur routinely around 9 months to 1 year. High-risk infants: Screen earlier, more often.

B. Etiology.
1. Microcytic anemia reflecting defect in production of hemoglobin during erythrocyte maturation, resulting from defect in heme synthesis due to inadequate quantities of iron:
   a. Inadequate supply of iron at birth, inadequate dietary iron.
   b. High demand for iron associated with growth.
   c. Blood loss without replacement.
   d. Impaired absorption associated with diagnoses such as inflammatory bowel disease.
   e. Menstruation, early onset, irregular or prolonged flow patterns.

C. Occurrence.
1. Common between 1 and 3 years of age because of inadequate dietary iron due to cow's milk being major staple in most children's diets.

    2. Lack of adequate iron stores to meet needs for growth.

      a. Affects 7% of children < 2 years of age.

      b. Affects 9–16% of adolescent females.

    3. Lack of adequate iron to meet needs for RBC production.

      a. Affects 3% of children < 2 years of age.

      b. Affects up to 3% of adolescent females and < 1% of adolescent males.

D. Clinical manifestations.

    1. Mild anemia (hemoglobin of 9.5–11): May be asymptomatic; sometimes only minimal symptoms when severe anemia (hemoglobin of ≤ 8–9.5) is present. May only be detected on routine screening or discovered when blood count ordered for another reason.

    2. History of fatigue, irritability, excessive milk intake, headaches.

E. Physical findings.

    1. Mild anemia (normal physical exam).

    2. More severe anemia.

      a. Poor weight gain.

      b. Sclera or palmar pallor.

      c. Splenomegaly: 15% of affected children.

      d. Tachycardia.

      e. Systolic flow murmurs: With progression of the iron deficit.

F. Diagnostic tests.

    1. Hemoglobin concentration (**Table 33-1**).

    2. Complete blood count (CBC).

      a. RBC hypochromic, microcytic.

      b. Mean cell volume (MCV) decreased.

      c. Ratio of MCV/RBC > 13 (Mentzer index).

        • > 13 = IDA.

        • < 13 = thalassemia trait.

    3. Iron studies if need further information.

      a. Serum iron: Decreased.

      b. Total iron-binding capacity (TIBC): Increased.

      c. Ferritin: Decreased.

      d. Percentage of iron saturation: Decreased.

G. Differential diagnosis.

Hereditary sideroblastic anemia, D64.0

Other thalassemias, D56.8

Toxic effect of lead and its compounds, accidental (unintentional), initial encounter, T56.0X1A

---

    1. Thalassemia trait.

    2. Lead poisoning.

Table 33-1 Maximum Hemoglobin Concentration and Hematocrit Values for IDA

Sex/Age, Years	Hemoglobin (g/dL)	Hematocrit (%)
Both Genders		
1 to < 2 years	11.0	32.9
2 to < 5 years	11.1	33.0
5 to < 8 years	11.5	34.5
8 to < 12 years	11.9	35.4
Females		
12 to < 15 years	11.8	35.7
15 to < 18 years	12.0	35.9
≥ 18 years	12.0	35.7
Males		
12 to < 15 years	12.5	37.3
15 to < 18 years	13.3	39.7
≥ 18 years	13.5	39.9

Source: Modified from Centers for Disease Control and Prevention. Recommendations to prevent and control iron deficiency in the United States. *MMWR Recomm Rep.* 1998;47(RR-3):1–29.

H. Diagnosis.
1. Diagnosis of IDA requires laboratory-confirmed evidence of anemia, as well as evidence of low iron stores. Anemia is defined as a hemoglobin level two standard deviations below normal for age and sex (**Table 33-2**).
2. Chronic infection.
3. Sideroblastic anemia.
I. Treatment.
1. Nutritional strategies: Breast and/or formula until age 1 year.
2. Reduce milk to no more than 16–24 oz/day at 1 year of age.
   a. Increase intake of high-iron foods (e.g., dark green vegetables, beans, whole cereals, dried fruit, pork, beef).
   b. Iron therapy for infants and children:
      • Ferrous sulfate: May start as early as 2 months of age in premature infants and 4–6 months for term infants.

Table 33-2 Age-Related Variations in Hemoglobin Level and MCV

| Age | Hemoglobin Level (g per dL [g per L]) | | MCV (µm³ [fL]) | |
	Mean	Diagnostic of Anemia	Mean	Diagnostic of Microcytosis
3 to 6 months	11.5 (115)	9.5 (95)	91 (91)	74 (74)
6 months to 2 years	12.0 (120)	10.5 (105)	78 (78)	70 (70)
2 to 6 years	12.5 (125)	11.5 (115)	81 (81)	75 (75)
6 to 12 years	13.5 (135)	11.5 (115)	86 (86)	77 (77)
12 to 18 years (female)	14.0 (140)	12.0 (120)	90 (90)	78 (78)
12 to 18 years (male)	14.5 (145)	13.0 (130)	88 (88)	78 (78)
20 to 59 years (white men)	NA	13.7 (137)	90 (90)	80 (80)
≥ 60 years (white men)	NA	13.2 (132)	90	80
≥ 20 years (white women)	NA	12.2 (122)	90	80
20 to 59 years (black men)	NA	12.9 (129)	90	80
≥ 60 years (black men)	NA	12.7 (127)	90	80
≥ 20 years (black women)	NA	11.5 (115)	90	80

Abbreviations: MCV, mean corpuscular volume; NA, not available.
Source: Modified with permission from Van Vranken M. Evaluation of microcytosis. *Am Fam Physician.* 2010;82(9):1118.

- o Mild to moderate iron deficiency: Elemental iron 3 mg/kg/day in 1–2 divided doses.
- o Severe iron deficiency: Elemental iron 4–6 mg/kg/day in 2–3 divided doses.
- J. Follow-up.
  1. Recheck hemoglobin in 1 month.
  2. Treat until hemoglobin and hematocrit reach normal ranges. Then give at least 1 month additional treatment to replenish iron stores.
  3. If response not adequate within 1–2 months, consider further diagnostic testing for gastrointestinal (GI) bleeding or other microcytic hypochromic anemias.

K. Complications.

Conduct disorder, unspecified, F91.9	Iron deficiency anemia, unspecified, D50.9
Disorder of psychological development, unspecified, F89	Lack of expected normal physiological development in childhood, unspecified, R62.50
Hypopituitarism, E23.0	

1. Result from long-standing IDA.
   a. Increased susceptibility to infection.
   b. Poor growth.
   c. Developmental delays (lower mental and motor test scores).
   d. Behavioral delays.

L. Education.
   1. Need for balanced diets and foods containing iron.
      a. Cereal, egg yolks, green/yellow vegetables, yellow fruits, red meat, potatoes, tomatoes, raisins.
   2. Amount of milk necessary/day (age dependent).
   3. Information about iron medications:
      a. Give after meals with orange juice to enhance absorption.
      b. Do not give with milk (inhibits absorption of iron).
      c. Give with straw or brush teeth after giving (may stain teeth).
      d. May cause abdominal discomfort, constipation, black stools.
      e. Extremely poisonous if taken in excessive amounts.
      f. Keep out of reach of small children.

II. THALASSEMIA

A. An inherited anemia that can affect both males and females and can be mild or severe. Hemoglobin has two types of protein chains, alpha globin and beta globin, which are needed to properly form the RBC and allow it to then carry enough oxygen. Therefore, one can have either an alpha thalassemia or a beta thalassemia. It occurs most often in people of Italian, Greek, Middle Eastern, Asian, and African descent. Severe form is diagnosed on newborn screening that is done in all states in the U.S. and is a lifelong condition.

B. Etiology.
   1. Alpha thalassemia: Need 4 genes (2 from each parent) to make enough alpha protein chains, located on chromosome 16.

    a. Mild anemia.
- One missing gene, silent carrier, no symptoms but may be microcytic.
- Two missing genes—carrier and mild anemia and microcytosis.

    b. Moderate to severe anemia.
- Three missing genes—hemoglobin H disease.
- Four missing genes—alpha thalassemia major or hydrops fetalis.

  2. Beta thalassemia—need 2 genes (one from each parent) to make enough beta globin protein—located on chromosome 11.

    a. Mild anemia.
- One missing or altered gene—carrier status with microcytosis.

    b. Moderate or severe anemia.
- Two missing or altered genes.
  - o Beta thalassemia intermedia—moderate anemia.
  - o Beta thalassemia major—Cooley's anemia, severe, often blood product dependent.

C. Occurrence.

  1. Family history and ancestry are the two risk factors.

    a. Alpha thalassemias most often affect ancestry origin of Indian, Chinese, Filipino, or Southeast Asian.

    b. Beta thalassemias most often affect ancestry origin of Mediterranean (Greek, Italian, Middle Eastern), Asian, or African.

D. Clinical manifestations.

  1. No symptoms if a silent carrier, as in alpha thalassemia.

  2. May or may not have symptoms with mild anemia—usually fatigue—most often mistaken for IDA.

  3. More severe symptoms with moderate anemia that may include slowed growth and development and physical problems with bones and the spleenomegaly.

  4. Symptoms of severe anemia due to thalassemias occur during the first 2 years of life and include other serious health problems besides the severe anemia.

E. Physical findings.

  1. Mild anemia—normal physical exam.

  2. More severe anemia.

    a. Pale and listless appearance.

    b. Poor appetite.

    c. Dark urine.

    d. Jaundice.

    e. Enlarged spleen, liver, and heart.

    f. Bone problems, especially the bones of the face.

    g. Delayed puberty.

    h. Slowed growth.

 F. Diagnostic tests.

   1. CBC with differential.

   2. Iron tests—to rule out IDA.

   3. Hemoglobin electrophoresis testing.

   4. Genetic studies: Alpha or beta globin gene analysis.

 G. Differential diagnosis.

   1. IDA: May have both IDA and thalassemia, especially in toddlers, so you must correct the iron deficiency before further testing for thalassemia.

   2. Other anemias.

 H. Treatment.

   1. Mild forms need no treatment.

   2. Moderate to severe forms.

    a. Regular blood transfusions—RBCs live 120 days so may need transfusions for severe anemia every 2 to 4 weeks.

    b. Iron chelation therapy—transfusions can lead to a buildup of iron in the blood.

     • Deferoxamine—liquid given slowly under the skin with a pump; takes time and is often painful, and side effects include loss of vision and hearing.

     • Deferasirox—pill taken once a day; side effects include headache, nausea, vomiting, diarrhea, joint pain, and fatigue.

    c. Folic acid supplements—a B vitamin that helps build healthy RBCs.

    d. Bone marrow/stem cell transplant—only cure for thalassemia.

 I. Follow-up.

   1. Well-child physical as indicated.

   2. Vaccines as scheduled.

   3. Follow with hematology providers on routine basis.

 J. Complications.

   1. Heart disease—caused by iron overload from the transfusions.

   2. Heart attack.

   3. Arrhythmias.

   4. Heart failure.

   5. Liver disease—also caused by iron overload and damage to the organ.

   6. Infection—risk of infection higher in persons whose spleen has been removed.

   7. Osteoporosis.

K. Education.
  1. Follow the treatment plan as outlined by the hematology service.
    a. Blood transfusions as needed.
    b. Chelation medications to be taken as prescribed.
    c. Take your folic acid supplements.
  2. Routine maintenance.
    a. Yearly well-child checks (WCC).
      • Height and weight.
      • Test for iron buildup in the liver, heart, and pancreas (MRI with T2* imaging).
      • Vision and hearing tests annually if on chelation treatment.
    b. Monthly CBCs.
    c. Quarterly tests for iron buildup in the blood (ferritin).
  3. Measures to stay healthy.
    a. Healthy eating.
    b. Vaccinations as scheduled, including annual flu vaccine.
    c. Watch for signs of infection.
    d. Wash hands.
    e. Avoid crowds during cold and flu season.
    f. Call clinic/doctor if develop fever.
  4. Support groups—parents and children.

III. LEAD POISONING

Abdominal and pelvic pain, R10	Muscle weakness (generalized), M62.81
Anorexia, R63.0	Other fatigue, R53.83
Convulsions, unspecified, R56.9	Other lack of expected normal physiological development, R62.8
Disturbance of activity and attention, F90.0	Other malaise, R53.81
Headache, R51	Sleep disorders, G47
Irritability, R45.4	Toxic effect of lead and its compounds, accidental (unintentional), initial encounter, T56.0X1A
Lack of coordination, unspecified, R27.9	

A. Most common, widespread environmental health concern, especially for children < 6 years of age. Can cause decrease in gestational weight and age; may increase possibility of stillbirths and miscarriages.

B. Etiology.
1. Increased lead levels in children occur by exposure to deteriorating paint, household dust, bare soil, air, drinking water, food, ceramics, home remedies, hair dyes, other cosmetics. Usually exposure is in child's own home.
2. Manufacture, use, disposal of modern products containing lead results in fine lead particles that release into environment. Lead particles enter air, water, food; also contaminate soil, dust.
3. Lead-containing toys, crayons, soft vinyl lunch boxes.
C. Occurrence.
1. Estimated at least 400,000 children < 6 years of age have too much lead in their bodies.
2. Questions for assessing risk of lead poisoning:
   a. Live in, regularly visit, or have lived in a place with peeling or chipping paint built before 1960?
      - Includes daycare, preschools, homes of babysitters, relatives.
      - Houses with recent, ongoing, planned renovation or remodeling.
   b. Brother or sister, housemate, playmate being followed or treated for lead poisoning (blood level > 15 mcg/dL)?
   c. Live with adult whose job or hobby involves exposure to lead?
      - Ceramics, furniture refinishing; stained glass work; construction workers.
   d. Taking home remedies such as azarcon and greta?
   e. Live near active smelter, battery-recycling plant, other industry likely to release lead into air?
3. Lead toxicity is decreasing in the United States, but approximately 25% of children still live in housing with deteriorating lead-based paint.
D. Clinical manifestations.
1. Many symptoms resemble common childhood complaints: Headache, stomachache, irritability, tiredness, poor appetite.
2. Other subtle symptoms: Poor attention span and memory, sleep disorders.
3. All of these can lead to coma and death because not noticed until brain damage has already occurred. Once organ systems are damaged, damage often irreversible.
E. Physical findings.
1. Weight loss, decreased growth.
2. Muscular weakness (diminished reflexes).
3. Seizures (signs of anemia).
4. Loss of visual motor coordination.
5. Irritability.
6. Constipation, abdominal pain.
7. Learning difficulties/cognitive impairment.

F. Diagnostic tests.
   1. CBC.
   2. Lead blood levels: < 10 mcg/dL. Screening tests as recommended by Centers for Disease Control and Prevention (CDC) (**Table 33-3**).
   3. Free erythrocyte protoporphyrin (FEP): Elevated.
G. Differential diagnosis.

Abdominal and pelvic pain, R10	Convulsions, unspecified, R56.9
Conduct disorder, unspecified, F91.9	Iron deficiency anemia, unspecified, D50.9

   1. Neurologic problems (unexplained seizures, behavioral disorders).
   2. IDA.
   3. Unexplained abdominal pain.
H. Treatment.
   1. Lead blood level determines treatment (Table 33-3).
   2. Alteration in environment; stop unusual exposure to lead.
   3. Good nutrition.
   4. Chelation therapy.
      a. British anti-Lewisite (BAL).
      b. Edetate calcium disodium ($CaNa_2EDTA$).
      c. Dimercaptosuccinic acid (DMSA) or Succimer.
      d. d-Penicillamine.
I. Follow-up.
   1. Follow recommendations in Table 33-3 for rescreening. Treatment time is lengthy: There will be rebound levels as stored lead releases from bones and teeth.
   2. After chelation therapy: Obtain another blood lead level in 10–14 days.
   3. Blood lead level determines subsequent treatment.
J. Complications.

Abnormal finding in specimens from male genital organs, unspecified, R86.9	Hearing loss, unspecified, H91.90
	Hypopituitarism, E23.0
	Intellectual disabilities, unspecified, F79
Coma, unspecified, R40.20	Male infertility, unspecified, N46.9
Convulsions, unspecified, R56.9	Other developmental disorders of scholastic skills, F81.89
Disorder of kidney and ureter, unspecified, N28.9	
Essential (primary) hypertension, I10	Other specified abnormal findings of blood chemistry, R79.89
Female infertility, unspecified, N97.9	Toxic effect: Lead and its compounds, T56.0
Headache, R51	Vomiting, unspecified, R11.10

Table 33-3 Recommended Actions Based on Blood Lead Level

< Reference Value	≥ Reference Value ≤ 45	≥ 45 ≤ 69	≥ 70
Lead education –Dietary –Environmental	Lead education –Dietary –Environmental	Lead education –Dietary –Environmental	Hospitalize and commence chelation therapy (following confirmatory venous blood lead test) in conjunction with consultation from a medical toxicologist or a pediatric environmental health specialty unit
Environmental assessment[a] for pre –1978 housing	Follow-up blood lead monitoring	Follow-up blood lead monitoring	Proceed according to actions for 45–69 µg/dL
Follow-up blood lead monitoring	Complete history and physical exam	Complete history and physical exam	
	Lab work: –Iron status Consider Hemoglobin or hematocrit	Lab work: –Hemoglobin or hematocrit –Iron status –Free erythrocyte protoporphyrin	
	Environmental investigation Lead hazard reduction	Environmental investigation Lead hazard reduction	
	Neurodevelopmental monitoring –Abdominal X-ray (if particulate lead ingestion is suspected) with bowel decontamination if indicated	Neurodevelopmental monitoring Abdominal X-ray with bowel decontamination if indicated Oral Chelation therapy Consider hospitalization if lead-safe environment cannot be assured	

[a] The scope of an "environmental assessment" will vary based on local resources and site conditions. However, this would include at a minimum a visual assessment of paint and housing conditions, but may also include testing of paint, soil, dust, and water and other lead sources. This may also include looking for exposure from imported cosmetics, folk remedies, pottery, food, toys, etc., which may be more important with low level lead exposure.

Source: Reproduced from Centers for Disease Control and Prevention. Centers for Disease Control and Prevention. *Low Level Lead Exposure Harms Children: A Renewed Call for Primary Prevention.* Atlanta, GA: Centers for Disease Control and Prevention; 2012. http://www.cdc.gov/nceh/lead/acclpp/final_document_030712.pdf

1. Lead encephalopathy and toxicity:
   a. Headache, persistent vomiting.
   b. Seizures, coma, death.
   c. Mental retardation, learning disabilities.
   d. Impaired growth.
   e. Hearing loss.
2. Renal disorders: Hypertension, kidney diseases (later in life), elevated blood urea nitrogen (BUN).
3. Reproductive system:
   a. Diminished fertility, abnormal sperm and lower counts, sterility—male and female.
   b. Increased chance of miscarriage.

K. Education.
   1. Prevention.
   2. Advice for families:
      a. If suspect exposure, test child.
      b. Use caution when purchasing older home.
      c. Maintenance to keep old lead-based paint intact.
      d. Watch for lead dust when doing home improvement projects: Protect furniture from lead dust, wet mop work area after projects using detergent.
      e. Wash work clothes separately from family's clothing.
      f. Encourage children to play in sand, grass rather than dirt.
      g. Wash hands, pacifiers before naps, bedtime.
      h. Avoid folk remedies or cosmetics containing lead.
      i. Test water supply for lead.
      j. Wash fruits, vegetables before eating.
      k. Eat healthy diet rich in iron: Helps body to absorb less lead.
      l. Use only cold water from tap for drinking, cooking, making baby formula. Hot water more likely to contain higher levels of lead.

IV. SICKLE CELL DISEASE

Abdominal and pelvic pain, R10	Acute hepatitis E, B17.2
Acquired hemolytic anemia, unspecified, D59.9	Acute stress reaction, F43.0
	Angina pectoris, unspecified, I20.9
Acute delta-(super) infection of hepatitis B carrier, B17.0	Aplastic anemia, unspecified, D61.9
Acute hepatitis C without hepatic coma, B17.10	Background retinopathy, unspecified, H35.00

Cytomegaloviral disease, unspecified, B25.9

Delayed puberty, E30.0

Disease of gallbladder, unspecified, K82.9

Dyspnea, unspecified, R06.00

Fever of other and unknown origin, R50

Gastrojejunal ulcer, unspecified as acute or chronic, without hemorrhage or perforation, K28.9

Headache, R51

Hemoptysis, R04.2

Hepatitis A without hepatic coma, B15.9

Hereditary hemolytic anemia, unspecified, D58.9

Irritability and anger, R45.4

Maxillary hyperplasia, M26.01

Meningitis, unspecified, G03.9

Non-pressure chronic ulcer of unspecified part of unspecified lower leg with unspecified severity, L97.909

Orthopnea, R06.01

Other cerebrovascular disease, I67.89

Other chest pain, R07.89

Other fatigue, R53.83

Other general symptoms and signs, R68.89

Other voice and resonance disorders, R49.8

Pallor, R23.1

Pneumonia, unspecified organism, J18.9

Priapism, unspecified, N48.30

Pulmonary fibrosis, unspecified, J84.10

Respiratory disorders in diseases classified elsewhere, J99

Sickle-cell disorders, D57

Splenomegaly, not elsewhere classified, R16.1

Tachycardia, unspecified, R00.0

Urinary tract infection, site not specified, N39.0

Viral hepatitis B without hepatic coma, unspecified, B19.10

Volume depletion, E86

Vomiting, unspecified, R11.10

A. Group of inherited heme disorders characterized by sickle hemoglobin (HbS); several variants within sickle cell disease. This section aimed at variant that results when one is homozygous for HbS, sometimes referred to as sickle cell anemia (HbSS).
B. Etiology.
1. Due to single defective hemoglobin module inherited as gene from both parents (autosomal-recessive disorder).
2. Abnormal HbS is produced instead of HbA, normal hemoglobin.
3. The abnormal hemoglobin S, when deoxygenated, deforms red cells into sickle shapes that occlude small vessels, slowing blood flow, creating vaso-occlusive crises in blood vessels and in organs such as spleen.
C. Occurrence.
1. Predominantly in African Americans, with about 1 in 400 African Americans affected.
2. Mediterranean or Arabic descendants also found to have HbSS but in fewer numbers.

D. Clinical manifestations.
1. Chronic hemolytic anemia (aplastic crisis, hemolytic crisis, sequestration crisis).
2. Vaso-occlusion resulting in ischemia to tissues.
   a. Painful crisis: From infarcts of muscle, bone, bone marrow, lung, intestines.
   b. Cerebrovascular accident.
   c. Acute chest syndrome.
   d. Chronic lung disease such as pulmonary fibrosis.
   e. Priapism.
   f. Ocular retinopathy.
   g. Gallbladder disease.
   h. Renal.
   i. Cardiomyopathy.
   j. Leg ulcerations.
3. Susceptibility to infection.
4. Growth failure, delayed puberty.
5. Psychologic problems (narcotic addiction, chronic illness, unusual dependence).
E. Physical findings.
1. Depends on which clinical manifestation is presenting.
2. Chronic hemolytic anemia: Pallor/jaundiced skin, tachycardia, fatigue.
3. Susceptibility to infection: Fever, other symptoms related to causative organism or system infected: For example, meningitis; urinary tract infection (UTI); cytomegalovirus (CMV); hepatitis A, B, C, D, E; pneumonia.
4. Vaso-occlusive crisis: Again depends on location of occlusion.
5. Splenomegaly.
6. Maxillary hyperplasia and dental malocclusion result from compensatory bone marrow expansion.
F. Diagnostic tests.
1. Newborn screening for hemoglobinopathies. Electrophoresis on cellulose acetate indicates type of hemoglobin: Fetal (F), normal adult (A), sickle (S), hemoglobin C (C).
2. Repeat testing with abnormal hemoglobin (FS) pattern on newborn screen.
3. CBC with hemoglobin MCV.
G. Differential diagnosis.

Other thalassemias, D56.8

Sickle-cell disorders, D57

---

1. Sickle cell trait (benign), beta-thalassemia anemia.

H. Treatment.
1. Preventive care.
   a. Education of the family, including genetic counseling.
      - Adequate fluid intake.
      - Immediate medical help for fevers.
      - Importance of prophylactic treatment.
   b. Immunizations per the schedule.
2. Pharmaceutical therapies.
   a. Penicillin prophylaxis:
      - 2 months to 3 years of age: Penicillin VK 125 mg PO bid.
      - 3 years to 5+ years of age: Penicillin VK 250 mg PO bid.
   b. Alternative to penicillin: Erythromycin (EES) 20 mg/kg/day divided bid.
   c. Folic acid: 1 mg/day.
   d. Multivitamin once daily.
   e. Hydroxyurea drug therapy.
      - Anti-sickling effect of hydroxyurea can decrease frequency of vaso-occlusive crises.
      - Starting dose: 15 mg/kg/day, increase gradually by 5 mg/kg/day while monitoring for toxicity.
      - Toxicity manifested by falls in neutrophil count to < 2500/mm^3 or platelet count < 80,000/mm^3.
   f. Pain medications: Acetaminophen or nonsteroidal anti-inflammatory drugs (NSAIDs) (mild pain), acetaminophen with codeine (moderate pain), morphine (severe pain).
I. Follow-up.
1. Routine WCC:
   a. Birth to 6 months: Every 2 months, CBC every visit.
   b. 6 months to 2 years: Every 3 months.
      - CBC every 3–6 months.
      - Urinalysis (UA) annually.
      - Ferritin or serum iron and TIBC once at 1–2 years of age.
      - BUN, creatinine, liver function tests (LFTs) once at 1–2 years of age.
      - Influenza vaccine annually.
      - Start folic acid daily at 1 year of age or when retic ct > 3%.
   c. 2–5 years: Visits every 6 months.
      - CBC and UA at least yearly.
      - BUN, creatinine, LFTs every 1–2 years.
      - 23-valent pneumococcal vaccine at 2 years of age, with booster at 5 years.
      - Hearing, vision, purified protein derivative (PPD) per standard practice.

  d. Older than 5 years: Visits every 6–12 months.
- CBC and UA at least annually.
- BUN, creatinine, LFTs every 2–3 years.
- Influenza vaccine yearly.
- Continue folic acid.
- May opt to stop penicillin V if immunization titers indicate adequate protection.

  e. Adolescent: Yearly visits.
- CBC and UA yearly.
- BUN, creatinine, LFTs every 2–3 years.
- Ferritin or serum iron and TIBC at least once.
- Hearing, vision, PPD as per standard practice.
- Influenza vaccine yearly.

 2. Close monitoring by family for complications.

J. Complications.

Acquired hemolytic anemia, unspecified, D59.9	Idiopathic aseptic necrosis of unspecified femur, M87.059
Aplastic anemia, unspecified, D61.9	Iron deficiency anemia, unspecified, D50.9
Background retinopathy, unspecified, H35.00	Kidney failure, unspecified, N19
Calculus of bile duct without cholangitis or cholecystitis, K80.5	Non-pressure chronic ulcer of unspecified part of unspecified lower leg with unspecified severity, L97.909
Disorder of circulatory system, unspecified, I99.9	Other cerebrovascular disease, I67.89
Disorder of kidney and ureter, unspecified, N28.9	Other disorders of lung, J98.4
Fever, unspecified, R50.9	Priapism, unspecified, N48.30
Hb-SS disease with splenic sequestration, D57.02	Respiratory disorders in diseases classified elsewhere, J99
	Serous retinal detachment, unspecified eye, H33.20

 1. Acute and chronic complications (hemolysis, anemia, gallstones) need early recognition, prompt treatment to reduce morbidity and mortality.

 2. Acute events:
  a. Painful vaso-occlusive events.
  b. Febrile events.
  c. Acute chest syndrome.
  d. Splenic sequestration.

       e. Stroke.

       f. Aplastic crisis.

    3. Chronic events:

       a. Avascular necrosis of hips/shoulders.

       b. Priapism.

       c. Chronic lung disease.

       d. Leg ulcers.

       e. Renal dysfunction or renal failure.

       f. Retinopathy and retinal detachment.

K. Education.

    1. When family/patient should seek immediate medical care:

       a. Fevers or persistent low-grade fever.

       b. Pain unrelieved by prescribed oral medications.

       c. Persistent abdominal pain, recurrent emesis.

       d. Dyspnea, pain with breathing, hemoptysis, or feelings of tightness in chest.

       e. Angina, exercise intolerance, or orthopnea.

       f. Visual/speech changes, weakness/numbness in extremities, persistent headaches.

       g. Sustained penile erections unrelieved by prescribed medications.

       h. Increased lethargy, irritability, or pallor.

    2. Factors that may precipitate painful vaso-occlusive crises:

       a. Inadequate rest, emotional stress, fatigue.

       b. Vasoconstrictive drugs, smoking, constrictive clothing.

       c. Dehydration, strenuous physical exercise.

       d. Extreme hot/cold temperatures, high altitudes, unpressurized aircraft.

V. BLEEDING DISORDERS

A. Usually bruising and bleeding are a part of active childhood. Bruises on the knees and shins and nose bleeds can simply be a fact of life. They become a health problem when the bleeding is hard to control or the bruising is in areas of the body that one does not normally hit, for example, the back or stomach. Also, in adolescence, heavy menses could be the norm for many girls, or it could signal a bleeding problem. The provider needs to decide when further studies would differentiate pathological or nonpathological causes of the bleeding and bruising. Normal clotting involves some 20 clotting factors that work together along with some other chemicals to form a substance called fibrin that leads to a clot.

B. Etiology.
1. Platelets or clotting factors do not work in the right way.
2. Supply of specified clotting factors is deficient.
3. Physical abuse.
4. Vitamin K deficiency.
C. Occurrence.
1. Congenital.
   a. Hemophilia A or B—about 400 newborns a year are diagnosed in the U.S.
      • X-linked recessive pattern of inheritance.
      • Deficiencies in factor VIII (hemophilia A) and factor IX (hemophilia B).
      • Males exclusively affected; some very rare cases of females with hemophilia.
   b. von Willebrand—affects 1:100 or 1% of the population.
      • Autosomal inheritance with variable phenotypic expression.
      • Common in both men and women.
      • Deficiency in the von Willebrand clotting factor.
        o Blood protein that affects platelet function.
        o Is a critical link between platelets and exposed vascular subendothelium.
        o Binds and stabilizes coagulation factor VIII.
2. Acquired.
   a. Acquired hemophilia.
      • Rare condition with no genetic inheritance.
      • Autoimmune etiology that results in development of autoantibodies to coagulation factors.
   b. Disseminated intravascular coagulation.
      • Acquired syndrome that activates the coagulation pathway.
      • Results in intravascular thrombi and depletion of platelets and coagulation factors.
   c. Idiopathic thrombocytopenic purpura.
      • Characterized by thrombocytopenia (platelet count less than 150,000/mcL) in the absence of other causes.
      • Thought to be secondary to an autoimmune phenomenon.
   d. Henoch-Schönlein purpura.
      • Results from autoimmune reaction where the body attacks its own tissues.
      • Small, bluish purple spots on feet, legs, arms, and buttocks.

- Usually develops after respiratory infection but can occur after immunization, insect bite, or allergic reaction to drugs or food.
- Rate at which disease develops and its duration vary.

D. Clinical manifestations.
   1. Excessive bruising or bleeding.
   2. Bleeding history.
      a. Location, duration, frequency, precipitating factors.
      b. What does it take to stop the bleeding?
      c. Reactions to injections, lacerations, toothbrushing, menstruation (as applicable).
      d. Medications taken that may increase tendency to bleed.
      e. Family history of unexpected or severe bleeding (surgery, childbirth, dental procedures).
      f. Consideration of abuse.

E. Physical findings—dependent upon site of bleeding and age of the child.
   1. Epistaxis—unilateral or bilateral—bleeding longer than 15 minutes.
   2. Menorrhagia—menses longer than 7 days, double pads, lightheadedness.
   3. Ecchymosis—where, clusters or not, especially in areas that are anatomically protected.
   4. Skin and mucous membrane bleeding—generalized petechial rash, subcutaneous hemorrhagic nodules, submucosal hemorrhages of the mouth.
   5. Spontaneous hemarthrosis—joints affected, amount of swelling/pain, limited range of motion.
   6. Intracranial bleeding in absence of elicited history of trauma—headache, nausea.
   7. Hepatosplenomegaly.
   8. Hematuria.
   9. GI cramping/pain.

F. Diagnostic tests.
   1. Initial lab screening.
      a. CBC with differential and platelets.
      b. Prothrombin time (PT).
      c. Activated partial thromboplastin time (aPTT; see **Table 33-4**).
   2. Secondary lab screening.
      a. PT/aPTT mixing studies.
      b. von Willebrand panel with vW antigen, vW ristocetin cofactor, and Factor VIII activity. Multimeres needed for differentiation of type of vWD.
      c. Platelet function testing may include a PFA-100.
      d. Platelet aggregation studies.

Table 33-4 Causes of Prolonged Prothrombin Time and Activated Partial Thromboplastin Time

Prolonged PT	Prolonged aPTT	Prolonged PT and aPTT
Inherited		
Factor VII deficiency	vWF, factor VIII, IX, XI, or XII deficiency	Prothrombin, fibrinogen, factor V, X, or combined factor deficiency
Acquired		
Vitamin K deficiency	Heparin use	Liver disease
Liver disease	Inhibitor of vWF, factors VIII, IX, XI, or XII	DIC
Warfarin use	Antiphospholipid antibodies	Supratherapeutic heparin or warfarin
Factor VII inhibitor		• Combined heparin or warfarin use • Inhibitor of prothrombin, fibrinogen, factor V or X • Direct thrombin inhibitor

Abbreviations: aPTT, activated partial thromboplastin time; DIC, disseminated intravascular coagulopathy; PT, prothrombin time; vWD, von Willebrand disease.
Source: Reproduced with permission of the Cleveland Clinic Center for Continuing Education. Baz R, Mekhail T. Bleeding disorders: disease management project. http://www.clevelandclinicmeded.com /medicalpubs/diseasemanagement/hematology-oncology/bleeding-disorders/. Published November 2013. Accessed June 15, 2015. © 2000-2015 The Cleveland Clinic Foundation. All rights reserved.

G. Differential diagnosis.
  1. Child abuse.
  2. Leukemia.
  3. Hemophilia.
  4. von Willebrand's disease.
  5. Autoimmune thrombocytopenia purpura.
  6. Thrombocytopenia.
  7. Henoch-Schönlein purpura.
  8. Acquired hemophilia—presence of inhibitory antibodies.
  9. Scurvy.
  10. Fabry disease.
  11. Ehlers-Danlos syndrome.
  12. Deficiency of other coagulation factors (V, VII, X, XI, or fibrinogen).

H. Treatment.
1. Dependent upon cause of bleeding or bruising and the site of the bleeding.
2. Referral to hematologist if deficient factors or platelet deficiency—chronic illness that needs to have specialist involved and be enrolled in a hemophilia treatment center.
   a. Treatment is prevention of bleeding by replacement therapy.
   b. Long-term management of joint and muscle damage.
   c. Management of complications from treatment.
3. Corticosteroids if Henoch-Schönlein purpura.
4. Child protective services if suspected child abuse.

I. Follow-up.
1. WCCs and immunizations as recommended.
2. Good communication between specialist and primary care.
3. Action plan for family—see Education section that follows.
4. Regular dental care.
5. Support groups.

J. Complications.
1. School absence.
2. Joint deformities.
3. Intracranial hemorrhage.
4. Complications from therapies like corticosteroids.

K. Education.
1. Importance of finding and knowing correct diagnosis.
   a. Untreated bleeding disorder leads to dangerous bleeding after childbirth, miscarriage, dental work, minor surgery, and injury.
2. Epistaxis.
   a. Know procedure to control nosebleeds: Sit up, lean forward, pinch nares.
   b. Know when to seek medical help.
   c. Vaseline around and in the nares at bedtime.
   d. Humidifier in bedroom to provide moisture.
3. Safety precautions with bleeding disorders to minimize long-term permanent damage to joints and muscles and the brain.
4. Importance of keeping regular checkups with primary care provider and the hematology provider if congenital/acquired bleeding disorder.
5. Avoiding platelet-impairing medications such as aspirin and ibuprofen.
6. Limit alcohol as excessive intake can adversely affect blood clotting.
7. Exercise regularly.
8. Medic alert bracelet—if hemophilia, von Willebrand, platelet dysfunction.

VI. CLOTTING DISORDERS (THROMBOPHILIA)

Other thrombophilia, D68.6	Primary thrombophilia, D68.5

A. Thrombophilia refers to the increased ability to form blood clots. There may be acquired or inherited risk factors. Thrombotic events are increasingly recognized in tertiary centers. These events are extremely rare in healthy children, affecting 0.07 children in every 100,000 born.

B. Testing for inherited thrombophilia includes:
1. Factor V leiden.
2. Prothrombin 20210 gene mutation.
3. Antithrombin III deficiency.
4. Protein C deficiency.
5. Protein S deficiency.

C. The most common risk factors for developing a clot include central indwelling venous catheters, trauma, use of oral contraceptives, immobilization, infection, systemic lupus erythematosus, structural venous anomalies, and cancer.

D. Screening testing should be limited to those children with a strong family history of thrombophilia (first-degree relative with thrombotic event at < 40 years of age). Those children will benefit from counseling regarding use of oral hormone therapies, targeted thromboprophylaxis in high-risk situations, and education regarding signs and symptoms of deep vein thrombosis.

E. Counseling will also include direction to avoid smoking and a sedentary lifestyle, and to maintain a healthy weight to avoid obesity.

BIBLIOGRAPHY

Abelsohn AR, Sanborn M. Lead and children: clinical management for family physicians. *Can Fam Physician.* 2010;56(6):531-535.

Abrams SA. Iron requirements and iron deficiency in adolescents. UpToDate. http://www.uptodate.com /contents/iron-requirements-and-iron-deficiency-in-adolescents. Updated December 8, 2014. Accessed March 4, 2015.

American Academy of Pediatrics Committee on Environmental Health. Lead exposure in children: prevention, detection, and management. Revision of June 1998 statement. *Pediatrics.* 2005;116(4):1036-1046.

American Society of Hematology. *2011 Clinical Practice Guidelines on the Evaluation and Management of Immune Thrombocytopenia (ITP).* Washington, DC: American Society of Hematology; 2011.

Baker RD, Greer FR; Committee on Nutrition American Academy of Pediatrics. Diagnosis and prevention of iron deficiency and iron-deficiency anemia in infants and young children (0–3 years of age), *Pediatrics.* 2010;126(5):1040-1050.

Baz R, Mekhail T. Bleeding disorders: disease management project. http://www.clevelandclinicmeded.com /medicalpubs/diseasemanagement/hematology-oncology/bleeding-disorders/. Published November 2013. Accessed June 15, 2015.

Benz EJ. Clinical manifestations and diagnosis of the thalassemias. UpToDate. http://www.uptodate.com /contents/clinical-manifestations-and-diagnosis-of-the-thalassemias. Updated December 17, 2014. Accessed March 4, 2015.

Berkowitz CD. *Berkowitz's Pediatrics: A Primary Care Approach.* 5th ed. Elk Grove Village, IL: American Academy of Pediatrics; 2015.

Burns CE, Dunn AM, Brady MA, Starr NB, Blosser CG. *Pediatric Primary Care.* 5th ed. Philadelphia, PA: Saunders; 2013.

Centers for Disease Control and Prevention. Recommendations to prevent and control iron deficiency in the United States. *MMWR Recomm Rep.* 1998;47(RR-3):1-29.

Centers for Disease Control and Prevention. *Low Level Lead Exposure Harms Children: A Renewed Call for Primary Prevention.* Atlanta, GA: Centers for Disease Control and Prevention; 2012. http://www.cdc.gov /nceh/lead/acclpp/final_document_030712.pdf

Centers for Disease Control and Prevention. Lead: prevention tips. http://www.cdc.gov/nceh/lead/tips.htm. Updated June 19, 2014. Accessed April 2, 2015.

Chan AK, Monagle P. Updates in thrombosis in pediatrics: where are we after 20 years? *Hematology Am Soc Hematol Educ Program.* 2012;2012:439-443.

Cohen, S. Lead poisoning: a summary of treatment and prevention. *Pediatr Nurs.* 2001;27(2):125-126, 129-130.

Environmental Protection Agency. Lead. http://epa.gov/lead/pubs/leadinfo.htm#facts. Updated July 7, 2015. Accessed July 9, 2015.

Hurwitz RL, Lee DA. Childhood lead poisoning: clinical manifestations and diagnosis. UpToDate. http://www .uptodate.com/contents/childhood-lead-poisoning-clinical-manifestations-and-diagnosis. Updated July 15, 2014. Accessed July 20, 2015.

Hurwitz RL, Lee DA. Childhood lead poisoning: management. UpToDate. http://www.uptodate.com /contents/childhood-lead-poisoning-management. Updated November 17, 2014. Accessed March 4, 2015.

Kuter, DJ. Thrombocytopenia (ITP, TTP). *The Merck Manual Consumer Edition.* http://www.merckmanuals .com/home/blood-disorders/platelet-disorders/thrombocytopenia-itp-ttp. Accessed June 15, 2015.

Mahoney DH. Iron deficiency in infants and young children: treatment. UpToDate. http://www.uptodate .com/contents/iron-deficiency-in-infants-and-young-children-treatment. Updated February 2, 2015. Accessed March 4, 2015.

Marcdante KJ, Kliegman RM, Jenson HB, Berhman RE. *Nelson Essentials of Pediatrics.* 6th ed. Philadelphia, PA: Saunders; 2011.

Monagle P, Chan AK, Goldenberg NA, et al. Antithrombotic therapy in neonates and children: Antithrombotic Therapy and Prevention of Thrombosis, 9th ed: American College of Chest Physicians Evidence-Based Clinical Practice Guidelines. *Chest.* 2012;141(2 suppl):e737S-e801S.

Montgomery RR, Scott JP. von Willebrand disease. In: Kliegman RM, Stanton BF, St. Geme JW III, Schor NF, Berhman RE, eds. *Nelson Textbook of Pediatrics.* 19th ed. Philadelphia, PA: Saunders; 2011:1704-1706.

National Heart, Lung, and Blood Institute. *The Diagnosis, Evaluation and Management of von Willebrand Disease.* Bethesda, MD: National Institutes of Health; 2007.

National Heart, Lung, and Blood Institute. What are thalassemias? http://www.nhlbi.nih.gov/health/dci /Diseases/Thalassemia/Thalassemia_WhatIs.html. Updated July 3, 2012. Accessed April 2, 2015.

National Heart, Lung, and Blood Institute. What is iron deficiency anemia? http://www.nhlbi.nih.gov/health /dci/Diseases/ida/ida_whatis.html. Updated March 26, 2014. Accessed April 2, 2015.

National Heart, Lung, and Blood Institute. What is sickle cell disease? http://www.nhlbi.nih.gov/health/dci /Diseases/Sca/SCA_WhatIs.html. Updated September 28, 2012. Accessed April 2, 2015.

National Hemophilia Foundation. MASAC recommendations concerning products licensed for the treatment of hemophilia and other bleeding disorders. http://www.hemophilia.org/Researchers -Healthcare-Providers/Medical-and-Scientific-Advisory-Council-MASAC/MASAC-Recommendations /MASAC-Recommendations-Concerning-Products-Licensed-for-the-Treatment-of-Hemophilia-and -Other-Bleeding-Disorders. Published June 4, 2015. Accessed June 15, 2015.

Neunert C, Lim W, Crowther M, et al. The American Society of Hematology 2011 evidence-based practice guidelines for immune thrombocytopenia. *Blood.* 2011;117(16):4190-4207.

Provan D, Stasi R, Newland AC, et al. International consensus report on the investigation and management of primary immune thrombocytopenia. *Blood.* 2010;115(2):168-186.

Raffini L. Screening for inherited thrombophilia in children. UpToDate. http://www.uptodate.com/contents /screening-for-inherited-thrombophilia-in-children. Updated February 27, 2015. Accessed March 4, 2015.

Raffini LJ, Scott JP. Hereditary predisposition to thrombosis. In: Kliegman R, Behrman R, Jenson HB, et al, eds. *Nelson Textbook of Pediatrics.* 19th ed. Philadelphia, PA: Saunders; 2011:1707-1708.

Rogers ZR. Routine comprehensive care for children with sickle cell disease. UpToDate. http://www.uptodate .com/contents/routine-comprehensive-care-for-children-with-sickle-cell-disease. Updated May 2, 2014. Accessed July 7, 2014.

Savage W, Takemoto C. (2009). Bleeding and bruising. *Contemp Pediatr.* 2009;26(6):60-68.

Srivastava A, Brewer AK, Mauser-Bunschoten EP, et al. *Guidelines for the Management of Hemophilia.* 2nd ed. Hoboken, NJ: Wiley-Blackwell; 2012.

Van Vranken M. Evaluation of microcytosis. *Am Fam Physician.* 2010;82(9):1118.

Vichinsky E, Levine L, Bhatia S, et al. *Standards of Care Guidelines for Thalassemia.* Oakland, CA: Children's Hospital and Research Center Oakland; 2012.

Yee DL. Approach to the child with bleeding symptoms. UpToDate. http://www.uptodate.com/contents /approach-to-the-child-with-bleeding-symptoms. Updated December 29, 2014. Accessed March 4, 2015.

Yee DL. Clinical manifestations and evaluation of thrombocytopenia in children. UpToDate. http://www .uptodate.com/contents/clinical-manifestations-and-evaluation-of-thrombocytopenia-in-children. Updated August 12, 2013. Accessed March 4, 2015.

Pediatric Obesity

Julie LaMothe

I. INTRODUCTION

Obesity (body mass index [BMI] above the 95th percentile for age and gender) is increasing among children and adolescents. Prevalence of pediatric obesity has tripled over the past 3 decades; an increase has also been reported in obesity prevalence overall, with the rate of obesity in adolescents quadrupling. An obese child, especially one with an obese parent, has a high likelihood of being an obese adult. There are several factors that play a role in etiology of pediatric obesity, including inappropriate caloric intake and sedentary lifestyle. Obesity is associated with higher blood pressure, abnormal lipid profile, insulin resistance, impaired glucose tolerance, and subsequent increased risks for several chronic diseases of adulthood, including diabetes, hypertension, dyslipidemia, sleep apnea, cardiovascular disease (CVD), fatty liver, metabolic syndrome, hepatic stenosis, orthopedic complications, pseudotumor cerebri, and some cancers. In addition, obesity in childhood can have psychosocial implications, including low self-esteem, impaired quality of life, and depression.

II. OBESITY ASSESSMENT

A. Vital signs and BMI calculation and blood pressure.
   1. Obesity is a chronic condition involving an excess of body fat. BMI is used as a screening tool to identify possible weight issues for children and teens. Recommended BMI screening by the Centers for Disease Control (CDC) and the American Academy of Pediatrics (AAP) should take place for children beginning at 2 years of age through 19 years of age. BMI is calculated from the child's weight and height and correlates with direct measures of body fat. BMI for children and teens is age and sex specific

and plotted on the CDC BMI for age and sex growth charts to obtain a percentile ranking (**Table 34-1**). The standard formula for BMI is weight in kg divided by height in meters squared (kg/m^2).

a. Measure height accurately by having the child remove his/her shoes, and stand straight with his/her feet together and looking straight ahead. Measure to nearest ⅛ inch or 0.1 cm.

b. Measure weight accurately by having the child remove his/her shoes and heavy clothing. Record to nearest decimal fraction.

c. Calculate BMI and plot on gender-specific growth chart.

d. BMI should be tracked at each well child visit beginning at age 2 years through 19 years of age. The amount of body fat changes with age and differs between girls and boys.

e. The CDC has a BMI calculator for children and teenagers, available on its website: http://nccd.cdc.gov/dnpabmi/Calculator.aspx.

f. Waist circumference and skin fold measurements may be added as screening tools for obesity.

g. Blood pressure is measured correctly by using a cuff that covers ⅔ of upper arm or thigh and is then documented and compared to norms based on age, sex, and height on at least three separate occasions (**Table 34-2**).

Table 34-1 BMI for Age-Weight Status Categories and Corresponding Percentiles

Underweight	Less than 5th percentile
Healthy weight	Between 5th percentile and 85th percentile
Overweight	85th percentile to less than 95th percentile
Obese	Equal or greater than 95th percentile

Table 34-2 Definitions of Normal Blood Pressure

Normal blood pressure	Less than 90th percentile
High-normal blood pressure	Between 90th and 95th percentiles
Hypertension	Greater than or equal to 95th percentile (on 3 separate occasions)

B. Patient history of current habits.
   1. Nutrition.
      a. 24-hour recall of food types, amounts and frequency of food and beverages.
      b. Fruits and vegetables per day.
      c. Sugar-sweetened beverages.
      d. Milk—type and quantity.
      e. No caloric beverages.
      f. Snacking—types and quantity.
      g. Portion size.
      h. Eat at home or eat out in sit-down restaurants or fast food—how often?
      i. Eat breakfast, lunch, and dinner or skip meals.
      j. Eat at table or in front of TV; eat alone or with other family members.
      k. Binge eating.
      l. Barriers to healthy eating such as access to fresh fruits and vegetables, knowledge of healthy foods, and financial barriers.
   2. Physical activity.
      a. Assess family's physical activity habits and barriers.
         • Type and quantity of physical activity and sedentary activity.
         • Access to gym, playground, boys or girls club.
      b. Physical education in schools.
         • Organized sports participation, access and barriers.
         • Sleep patterns and barriers to restful sleep.
         • Breathing difficulties with activity.
         • Assess for joint pain, knee, hip, feet, and type of footwear, any use of orthotics.
   3. Screen time.
      a. Type and quantity.
      b. TV/computer in room.
      c. Video games and texting.
C. Review of systems.
   1. Perform a thorough review including:
      a. Constitutional: Sleep habits, fatigue, and lethargy.
      b. Respiratory: Snoring, wheezing, coughing, difficulty breathing.
      c. Cardiovascular: Chest pain, hypertension.
      d. Gastrointestinal: Abdominal, pain, vomiting, constipation.
      e. Skin: Striae, polycystic acne, hirsutism.
      f. Neurologic: Developmental delay, headache.
      g. Genitourinary: Menarche, oligomenorrhea, amenorrhea.

    h. Urology: urinary tract infection (UTI), bedwetting, buried penis.

    i. Orthopedic: Hip, thigh, knee pain, limping or bowing, flat feet.

    j. Endocrinology: Excessive thirst, fatigue, menarche, and menstruations.

    k. Psychological: Stress, depression, ADHD, learning disorder, bullying, or other psychological disorders.

D. Detailed family health history, including the following:

    1. Overweight/obesity.

    2. Diabetes mellitus.

    3. Gestational diabetes.

    4. CVD before 55 years in men and 65 years in women.

    5. Smoking and passive smoke exposure.

    6. Polycystic ovarian syndrome.

    7. Hypertension.

    8. Hypothyroidism or hyperthyroidism.

    9. Depression.

E. Social history.

    1. School/daycare includes a typical history:

        a. Who lives at home?

        b. Who helps the parent?

        c. Are there multiple caregivers?

        d. Parents' education levels.

        e. Demographic factors, including urban versus rural, single parent, socioeconomic status, non-English-speaking home, and race.

F. Birth and past medical history.

    1. Birth weight and gestational age.

    2. Complications at birth, immunizations, allergies.

    3. Mental health.

        a. Anxiety, school avoidance, social isolation.

        b. Sleepiness/restful sleep.

        c. Recent stressors.

    4. Surgeries.

    5. Illnesses.

    6. Past hospitalizations.

G. Medications.

    1. Neuropsychiatric medications may affect weight gain.

    2. Dietary supplements, including vitamin D.

H. Physical exam.

    1. Skin.

        a. Acanthosis nigricans indicates increased risk of insulin resistance.

        b. Hirsutism, acne may indicate polycystic ovary syndrome.

      c. Irritation and inflammation—a complication of severe obesity.
      d. Violaceous striae indicate possible Cushing's syndrome.
      e. Striae/stretch marks.
  2. Eyes.
      a. Papilledema, cranial nerve V1 paralysis—possible pseudotumor cerebri.
  3. Throat.
      a. Hypertrophy of tonsil and adenoid tissue—possible obstructive sleep apnea (OSA) or sleep disordered breathing (SBD).
  4. Neck.
      a. Goiter may indicate hypothyroidism.
  5. Chest.
      a. Wheezing—possible asthma and exercise intolerance.
  6. Abdomen.
      a. Tenderness may indicate gastroesophageal reflux disorder, gall bladder disease, nonalcoholic fatty liver disease (NAFLD), and constipation.
  7. Reproductive.
      a. Sexual maturity rating (Tanner staging) annually—premature puberty age < 7 years in Caucasian girls, < 6 years in African American girls, and < 9 years in boys.
      b. Micropenis—may be normal penis buried in fat.
      c. Undescended testis/micropenis—may be buried in fat.
  8. Extremities.
      a. Abnormal gait, limp, limited hip range of motion—possible slipped capital femoral epiphysis.
      b. Bowing of tibia—possible Blount's disease.
      c. Small hands and feet, polydactyl—possible Prader-Willi syndrome, Bardet-Biedl syndrome.

I. Laboratory tests.
  1. Complete blood count (CBC).
  2. Comprehensive metabolic panel (CMP).
  3. Fasting lipid profile.
  4. GGT.
  5. Hemoglobin A1C.
  6. T4, TSH.
  7. Sleep study if signs of snoring, napping, headaches, and daytime sleepiness, restless sleep, and unrefreshed sleep.
  8. Additional testing as clinically indicated.

J. Plan.
  1. Assess family's readiness to make changes.
      a. Educate parents and child/teen about growth status and risks for overweight and obesity.

    b. Identify strengths and barriers.

    c. Assess parent's attitudes, beliefs, and spirituality about body size, nutrition, and physical activity.

    d. Use motivational interviewing (MI) skills—patient-centered method for enhancing intrinsic motivation.

    e. Elicit patients' and families' motivation to change.

    f. Encourage patients to take responsibility for their behavior.

    g. Ambivalence needs to be resolved for change to occur.

2. Goal setting.

    a. Create a partnership with family, child, and adolescent.

    b. Set measurable and achievable goals, focusing on strengths.

    c. Take small steps for a gradual change.

    d. Aim for long-term healthy behaviors/lifestyle change with slow weight loss (1–2 pounds per week).

    e. Focus on success, what has worked in the past.

    f. Expect periods of relapse. Be ready to help guide patient and family, as well as troubleshoot situations and support return to plan in nonjudgmental way.

    g. Parents serve as role models and can share food shopping and physical activity with children and adolescents.

    h. Engage extended family members involved in care of child/adolescent such as grandparents, stepparents, siblings, and other relatives who influence the child and adolescent.

    i. Engage the child's/adolescent's school for support and encouragement.

3. Logging of food intake.

    a. Provide a journal to log the diet, with beverages, meal time, food, portion size, and snacks on a daily basis. This will increase awareness of intake and has proven to show weight loss if done consistently.

    b. Several apps are available to log food on smartphones and computers; use of technology is preferred by adolescents.

4. Nutritional goals.

    a. Promote 3 meals a day, not meal skipping, and emphasize that breakfast provides energy for the day.

    b. Eat 5 or more fruit and vegetable servings daily (serving is ½ cup), start small and gradually increase; daily fruit recommendations from www.choosemyplate.gov/.

    c. Water (4–6 glasses/day) and low-fat milk (3–4 glasses/day) as main beverages; eliminate high-calorie, sugar-sweetened beverages; limit 100% fruit juice, diet drinks, and caffeine.

    d. Select whole grain products.

    e. Choose polyunsaturated or monounsaturated fats found in nuts, fish, and vegetable oils.

    f. Avoid distractions during meal time; eat as a family and not alone. This will promote good nutrition practices, increase awareness, and slow down mealtime.

    g. Provide age-appropriate information on portion size. Promote mindfulness.

    h. Limit fast foods.

    i. Limit refined sugars, high-fat foods.

    j. Aim for reasonable daily target for calorie reduction and weight loss (1–2 pounds per week).

    k. Discourage unhealthy weight loss methods such as fasting, eliminating food groups, or skipping meals.

    l. Promote traditional foods of high nutritional quality.

    m. Children up to 10 years of age may need 15 exposures of a food before accepting a new food.

    n. Advocate for nutritious school lunches and nutritious items in vending machines at schools.

    o. Promote breastfeeding.

    p. Eat more fiber, vitamins A and C, calcium, and iron.

5. Physical activity goals.

    a. Assess present activity level of both the individual and the family.

    b. Promote increasing activity on a daily basis, such as increased outside activity—begin slowly, increasing activity as tolerated; goal is 60 minutes or more daily.

    c. Gradually increase vigorous aerobic activity as tolerated; offer a variety of activity choices that are realistic for child/adolescent and family, promote after-school activities.

    d. Limit total screen time to 2 hours or less per day (TV, computer, texting, video games).

    e. Remove TV from the bedroom; keep sleeping area free of distractions.

    f. Provide free pedometers or wristbands with age-appropriate goals for steps; parents may also enjoy walking with children to encourage family activity.

    g. Provide information on community gyms, centers, after-school activity centers that promote increased physical activity. Look for scholarship opportunities or discounts based on family income in these centers. Promote activities provided by schools, sports, clubs, and year-round athletic activities.

   h. Collaboration with schools, communities, and businesses is essential for physical activity programs to be successful.

   i. Promote peer group programs to partner with children and youth with special healthcare needs to increase physical activity like the TOPS soccer program and Special Olympics.

   j. Planned family activities increase opportunities for exercise and enjoyment.

   k. Report daily activity in a journal to be reviewed at health visits.

   l. Active video games may present an opportunity for increased physical activity, with more emphasis on lower extremities than upper extremities.

6. Subspecialist referral for comorbidities.

   a. Provide referrals to orthopedics, physical therapy, or podiatrist for hip/knee pain or flat feet. Consider appropriate X-rays.

   b. Refer for a polysomnography (sleep study) if snoring, unrefreshed sleep, headaches, or daytime sleepiness.

   c. Refer to neurology for headaches; pseudotumor cerebri may present with headaches occurring in the morning.

   d. Pediatric endocrinology for type 2 diabetes, metabolic syndrome, polycystic ovarian syndrome, dyslipidemia.

   e. Pediatric gastroenterology for progressive elevated ALT and AST levels and persistent stomach pain, constipation, and GERD.

   f. Pediatric pulmonary for sleep study and asthma.

   g. Pediatric psychology for depression, anxiety, and low self-esteem, family dysfunction.

   h. Medical genetics for chromosome abnormalities, Prader-Willi syndrome, fragile X, developmental delay.

   i. Cardiology if a family event before age of 55, dizziness, chest pain. Consider stress test.

7. Follow-up.

   a. Appointments with medical provider and patient/family are every 3 weeks. After 3-month visit, the patient/family is seen monthly by health team, with a final visit at 6 months by a medical provider.

   b. Child/adolescents will set and reach healthy weight goals pertaining to physical fitness, activity level, and food choices.

   c. Child/adolescents will develop individualized health plans to encourage increased activity and decreased caloric intake; plan will be revised and updated with each health visit.

   d. Child/adolescent will participate in individual sessions, behavioral modification, and peer group activity sessions.

   e. Child/adolescent will be responsible for keeping a food log, wearing pedometer for 24 hours, and keeping activity log.

f. BMI will be tracked at all clinical visits. Comorbidities will be tracked with referrals to appropriate services.

g. Family members will be involved with child/adolescent goals so they can support the healthy lifestyle plan.

h. Incentives will be offered to encourage program compliance.

i. Participation in school activities, interaction with friends, parents, and families will be promoted and monitored.

j. Monitoring of depression, bullying, sexual victimization, substance abuse, risk of self-harm.

III. CODING FOR OBESITY

A. Many insurance carriers will deny claims submitted with obesity codes. The following is a guide to coding for obesity-related healthcare services, *Obesity and Related Comorbidities Coding Fact Sheet for Primary Care Pediatricians*, from the American Academy of Pediatrics.

B. Healthcare Common Procedure Coding System (HCPCS) education and counseling codes.

1. Patient education individual, S9445.
2. Patient education group, S9446.
3. Weight management class, S9449.
4. Exercise class, S9451.
5. Nutrition class, S9452.
6. Stress management class, S9454.
7. Nutrition counseling, S9470.

C. Common diagnosis codes, ICD-10 codes.

1. Circulatory system.
   a. Essential (primary) hypertension, I10.
   b. Cardiomegaly, I51.7.
   c. Anemia, unspecified, D64.9.
2. Congenital anomalies.
   a. Down syndrome, unspecified, Q90.9.
   b. Congenital malformation syndromes predominantly associated with short stature, Q87.1.
   c. Other specified congenital malformation syndromes, not elsewhere classified, Q87.89.
3. Digestive system.
   a. Gastroesophageal reflux disease without esophagitis, K21.9.
   b. Constipation, K59.0.
   c. Feeding difficulties, R63.3.

    d. Other specified diseases of liver, K76.89.

    e. Hepatomegaly, not elsewhere classified, R16.0.

4. Endocrine, nutritional, metabolic.

    a. Other specified hypothyroidism, E03.8.

    b. Hypothyroidism, unspecified, E03.9.

    c. Diabetes mellitus, E10-E14.

    d. Other disorders of pituitary gland, E23.6.

    e. Other specified disorders of adrenal gland, E27.8.

    f. Polycystic ovarian syndrome, E28.2.

    g. Precocious puberty, E30.1.

    h. Endocrine disorder, unspecified, E34.9.

    i. Pure hypercholesterolemia, E78.0.

    j. Pure hyperglyceridemia, E78.1.

    k. Mixed hyperlipidemia, E78.2.

    l. Hyperlipidemia, unspecified, E78.5

    m. Disorder of lipoprotein metabolism, unspecified, E78.9.

    n. Metabolic syndrome, E88.81.

    o. Obesity, E66.

    p. Morbid (severe) obesity due to excess calories, E66.01.

    q. Overweight, E66.3.

    r. Localized adiposity, E65.

    s. Abnormal weight gain, R63.5.

    t. Disorder of psychological development, unspecified, F89.

    u. Lack of expected normal physiological development in childhood, unspecified, R62.50.

    v. Short stature (child), R62.52.

    w. Polydipsia, R63.1.

    x. Polyphagia, R63.2.

5. Genitourinary system.

    a. Hypertrophy of breast, N62.

    b. Other noninflammatory disorders of ovary, fallopian tube and broad ligament, N83.8.

    c. Irregular menstruation, unspecified, N92.6.

6. Mental disorders.

    a. Generalized anxiety disorder, F41.1.

    b. Eating disorders, F50.

    c. Bulimia nervosa, F50.2.

    d. Other eating disorders, F50.8.

    e. Major depressive disorder, single episode, unspecified, F32.9.

    f. Oppositional defiant disorder, F91.3.

7. Nervous system.
   a. Sleep apnea, G47.3.
   b. Sleep-related hypoventilation in conditions classified elsewhere, G47.36.
   c. Sleep apnea, unspecified, G47.30.
   d. Insomnia, unspecified, G47.00.
   e. Hypersomnia, unspecified, G47.10.
   f. Chronic fatigue, unspecified, R53.82.
   g. Benign intracranial hypertension, G93.2.
   h. Disorder of the skin and subcutaneous tissue, unspecified, L98.9.
   i. Acanthosis nigricans, L83.
8. Respiratory.
   a. Asthma, J45.
   b. Shortness of breath, R06.02.
   c. Sleep disorder, unspecified, G47.9.
9. Orthopedic.
   a. Pain in unspecified hip, M25.559.
   b. Pain in unspecified knee, M25.569.
   c. Juvenile osteochondrosis of tibia and fibula, unspecified leg, M92.50.
   d. Slipped upper femoral epiphysis (nontraumatic), unspecified, unspecified hip, M93.003.
   e. Flat foot [pes planus] (acquired), unspecified foot, M21.40.
   f. Low back pain, M54.5.

BIBLIOGRAPHY

American Academy of Pediatrics. Obesity and relate co-morbidities coding fact sheet for primary care pediatricians. http://www2.aap.org/pubserv/codingforpeds/obesitycodingfactsheet0208.pdf

Barlow SE; Expert Committee. Expert committee recommendations regarding the prevention, assessment, and treatment of child and adolescent overweight and obesity: summary report. *Pediatrics.* 2007;120(suppl 4):S164-S192.

Bleich SN, Ku R, Wang YC. Relative contribution of energy intake and energy expenditure to childhood obesity: a review of the literature and directions for future research. *Int J Obes (Lond).* 2011;35(1):1-15.

Bradlee ML, Singer MR, Qureshi MM, Moore LL. Food group intake and central obesity among children and adolescents in the Third National Health and Nutrition Examination Survey (NHANES III). *Public Health Nutr.* 2010;13(6):797-805.

Chaloupka FJ, Johnston LD. Bridging the gap: research informing practice and policy for healthy youth behavior. *Am J Prev Med.* 2007;33(4 suppl):S147-S161.

Daniels SR, Arnett DK, Eckel RH, et al. Overweight in children and adolescents: pathophysiology, consequences, prevention, and treatment. *Circulation.* 2005;111(15):1999-2012.

Davee AM, Blum JE, Devore RL, et al. The vending and a la carte policy intervention in Maine public high schools. *Prev Chronic Dis.* 2005;2(special issue):A14.

Davis AM, Bennett KJ, Befort C, Nollen N. Obesity and related health behaviors among urban and rural children in the United States: data from the National Health And Nutrition Examination Survey 2003–2004 and 2005–2006. *J Pediatr Psychol.* 2011;36(6):669-676.

Farhat T, Iannotti RJ, Simons-Morton BG. Overweight, obesity, youth, and health-risk behaviors. *Am J Prev Med.* 2010;38(3):258-267.

Fennoy I. Metabolic and respiratory comorbidities of childhood obesity. *Pediatr Ann.* 2010;39(3);140-146.

Foltz JL, Cook SR, Szilagyi PG, et al. U.S. adolescent nutrition, exercise, and screen time baseline levels prior to national recommendations. *Clin Pediatr (Phila).* 2011;50(5):424-433.

Gillis B, Mobley C, Stadler DD, et al. Rational, design and methods of the HEALTHY study nutrition intervention component. *Int J Obes (Lond).* 2009;33(suppl 4):S29-S36.

Hassink SG. *Pediatric Obesity Clinical Decision Support Chart 5210.* Elk Grove Village, IL: American Academy of Pediatrics; 2008.

Hingle MD, O'Connor TM, Dave JM, Baranowski T. Parental involvement in interventions to improve child dietary intake: a systematic review. *Prev Med.* 2010;51(2):103-111.

Kuczmarski RJ, Ogden CL, Guo SS, et al. 2000 CDC growth charts for the United States: methods and development. *Vital Health Stat.* 2002:11(246)1-190. http://www.cdc.gov/nchs/data/series/sr_11/sr11_246.pdf

Melnyk BM, Small L, Morrison-Beedy D, et al. The COPE Healthy Lifestyles TEEN program: feasibility, preliminary efficacy, & lessons learned from an after school group intervention with overweight adolescents. *J Pediatr Health Care.* 2007;21(5):315-322.

Mendoza JA, Watson K, Cullen KW. Change in dietary energy density after implementation of the Texas Public School Nutrition Policy. *J Am Diet Assoc.* 2010;110(3):434-440.

National Heart Lung and Blood Institute. *Expert Panel on Integrated Guidelines for Cardiovascular Health and Risk Reduction in Children and Adolescents: Summary Report.* Bethesda, MD: National Institutes of Health; 2012.

National Institute for Children's Health Quality (NIHCQ) [homepage]. http://www.nichq.org. Accessed June 15, 2015.

Ogden CL, Carroll MD, Kit BK, Flegal KM. Prevalence of childhood and adult obesity in the United States, 2011–2012. *JAMA.* 2014;311(8):806-814.

Parks EP, Kumanyika S, Stettler N. Practical application of the nutrition recommendations for the prevention and treatment of obesity in pediatric primary care. *Pediatr Ann.* 2010;39(3):147-153.

Rhew IC, Richardson LP, Lymp J, McTiernan A, McCauley E, Stoep AV. Measurement matters in the association between early adolescent depressive symptoms and body mass index. *Gen Hosp Psychiatry.* 2008;30(5):458-466.

Riley POWER Program Tool Kit: A comprehensive weight management program designed to improve health of obese children (ages 2–18) Riley Children's Hospital, IU Health Partner.

Schwartz RP. Motivational interviewing (patient-centered counseling) to address childhood obesity. *Pediatr Ann.* 2010;39(3):154-158.

Taber DR, Chriqui JF, Chaloupka FJ. Association and diffusion of nutrition and physical activity policies on the state and district level. *J Sch Health.* 2012;82(5):201-209.

Wang YC, Ludwig DS, Sonneville K, Gortmaker SL. Impact of change in sweetened caloric beverage consumption on energy intake among children and adolescents. *Arch Pediatr Adolesc Med.* 2009;163(4):336-343.

Williams SL, Mummery WK. Associations between adolescent nutrition behaviours and adolescent and parent characteristics. *Nutrition & Dietetics.* 2012;69(2):95-101.

Behavioral Disorders

Donna Hallas

I. BEHAVIORAL ASSESSMENT INSTRUMENTS

A. Various instruments are available for assessment of children with behavioral and emotional disorders in primary care settings. Based on the results of these assessments, referral to a psychiatrist, psychologist, or social worker for completion of additional assessment tools may be indicated. Data from these evaluations will assist in understanding dynamics of family functioning and behavioral management plans (**Box 35-1, Box 35-2,** and **Box 35-3**).

Box 35-1 Behavioral Assessment Rating Scales

Achenbach Child Behavior Checklist System (CBCL)

- Parent form (CBCL)
- Teacher report form (TRF)

Attention Deficit Disorders Evaluation Scales (ADDES)

- Home version
- School version

Behavior Assessment System for Children (BASC)

- Parent rating scale (PRS)
- Teacher rating scale (TRS)
- Connor's Parent/Teacher Rating Scale

Personality Inventory for Children–Revised (PIC–R)
Social Skills Rating Scale (SSRS)
Walker Problem Behavior Identification Checklist (WPBIC)

Box 35-2 Behavioral Assessment: Self-Report Rating Scales

Achenbach Child Behavior Checklist System (CBCL)

Youth Self-Report
Behavior Assessment System for Children (BASC)
Self-Report of Personality

Child Anxiety Scale
Children's Personality Questionnaire (CPQ)
Early School Personality Questionnaire (ESPQ)
High School Personality Questionnaire (HSPQ)
Revised Children's Manifest Anxiety Scale (RCMAS)
Social Skills Rating System (SSRS)–Student Form

Box 35-3 Behavioral Assessment: Protective Measures

Draw a Person: Screening Procedure for Emotional Disturbance (DAP: SPED)
Minnesota Multiphasic Personality Inventory–A (MMPI–A)
Tell-Me-A-Story (TEMAS) Test

II. ATTENTION-DEFICIT/HYPERACTIVITY DISORDER (ADHD)

Attention-deficit hyperactivity disorder, combined type, F90.2

Attention-deficit hyperactivity disorder, predominantly hyperactive type, F90.1

Attention-deficit hyperactivity disorder, predominantly inattentive type, F90.0

Attention-deficit hyperactivity disorder, unspecified type, F90.9

Conduct disorder, unspecified, F91.9

Disorder of adult personality and behavior, unspecified, F69

Disturbance of activity and attention, F90.0

Expressive language disorder, F80.1

Mathematics disorder, F81.2

Other developmental disorders of scholastic skills, F81.89

Specific developmental disorder of motor function, F82

Specific reading disorder, F81.0

A. ADHD is one of the most common chronic conditions of childhood and the most common neurobehavioral disorder in child health. ADHD is characterized by the child presenting with three core behavioral symptoms: Impairing levels of inattention, disorganization, and hyperactivity-impulsivity. Inattention and disorganization refers to the inability of the child to stay on task, appearing not to listen, and losing materials, while hyperactivity-impulsivity refers to overactivity, fidgeting, inability to remain seated, intruding into other individuals' activities, and the inability to wait. All of these symptoms are evaluated to be outside the normal parameters of the psychosocial development for the child's age. Symptoms are displayed by the child before 7 years of age even though diagnosis may not be established until the child enters the school setting. Three presentations for ADHD are now recognized in the *Diagnostic and Statistical Manual of Mental Disorders V* (DSM-V): (1) Combined presentation (behaviors specified in Diagnostic Criterion A1 [inattention] and Criterion A2 [hypersensitivity-impulsivity] for 6 months), (2) predominantly inattentive presentation (behaviors specified in Criterion A1 but not A2 for 6 months), and (3) predominantly hyperactive/impulsive presentation (Criterion A2 is met but not Criterion A1 for the past 6 months).

B. In partial remission: When full criteria were previously met, fewer than the full criteria have been met for the past 6 months, and the symptoms still result in impairment in social, academic, and occupational functioning (DSM-V, p. 60).

C. Severity is specified as mild, moderate, or severe.

D. The American Academy of Pediatrics (AAP) (2015) evidence-based guidelines for diagnosis and management of ADHD now include children 4 to 18 years of age.

E. Etiology.

    1. Specific etiology unknown. It is believed that abnormal dopamine transport and uptake at nerve synapse may account for symptoms displayed.

        a. Other considerations: Combination of genetic, environmental, and cultural factors.

    2. Genetic and physiological.

        a. Incidence elevated if child has a first-degree biological relative with ADHD.

    3. Environmental.

        a. Very low birth weight babies have a two- to three-fold risk for ADHD.

        b. Correlated with intrauterine exposure to maternal smoking behaviors.

        c. Neurotoxin exposures such as lead, infections (encephalitis), and intrauterine alcohol exposure.

4. Cultural.
   a. Cultural variations in attitudes and interpretation of behaviors.
   b. In the U.S., African American and Latino populations tend to have a lower prevalence rate than Caucasian populations, which may be influenced by cultural group of the child and the informants.

F. Occurrence.
   1. The prevalence of ADHD in children is about 5% in most cultures. The prevalence of ADHD is about 2.5% in adults.
   2. Two-thirds of children with ADHD continue to have symptoms in adolescence.
   3. More prevalent in males than females—approximate ratio of 2:1, with females presenting more frequently with primarily inattention.
   4. Prevalence of comorbid conditions ranges from 9–50% depending on specific comorbid condition. Refer to **Table 35-1**.

G. Clinical manifestations.
   1. Child displays and/or parents and teachers report inappropriate degrees of:
      a. Combined hyperactive/impulsive and inattentive behaviors.
      b. Predominantly inattentive behaviors.
      c. Predominantly hyperactive/impulsive behaviors.
   2. DSM-V diagnostic criteria delineate clinical manifestations of ADHD and clarify criteria utilized to make definitive diagnosis.
   3. Identifying at-risk child.
      a. Nurse practitioner plays integral role in identifying children at risk for ADHD by evaluating comprehensive medical history.
      b. Positive family history of one or more of hyperactivity disorder, conduct disorder, learning disorder, substance abuse, psychiatric disorder.

Table 35-1 Prevalence of Comorbid Conditions in Children with ADHD

Comorbid Condition	Prevalence Rate (%)
Conduct disorder, childhood-onset type, F91.1	25
Oppositional defiant disorder, F91.3	33
Major depressive disorder, single episode, unspecified, F32.9	9–38
Generalized anxiety disorder, F41.1	25
Other developmental disorders of scholastic skills, F81.89	12–30

Source: Modified from Green M, Wong M, Atkins D, Taylor J, Feinleib M. *Diagnosis of Attention-Deficit/ Hyperactivity Disorder. Technical Review No. 3.* Rockville, MD: Agency for Health Care Policy and Research; August 1999. AHCPR Publication No. 99-0050.

    c. Intrauterine exposure to smoking and drug/alcohol use, especially during first trimester.

    d. Parent and/or schoolteacher report that child displays impulsive and inattentive behaviors.

- Several symptoms are present before age 12.
  - Adult recall of childhood symptoms may be unreliable; it is important to gather information from other individuals who can provide objective data, such as teachers, counselors, etc.
  - Symptoms occur in more than one setting (i.e., home, school, play activities).
- School-age children tend to steal, tell lies, deliberately destroy property.
- Adolescents display behaviors associated with anger and mood lability: Alcohol/substance abuse, smoking, sexually transmitted infections, early pregnancy, low self-esteem, involvement in motor vehicle accidents.

4. Comprehensive medical history—include questions that elicit details concerning each of following parameters:

    a. Parental concerns.

- Onset and duration of symptoms.
- Parental approaches to displayed symptoms.

    b. Behavioral history.

- Hyperactivity/impulsivity as described by parents, caregivers, teachers.
- Behaviors that display inattentiveness to details.
- Ability to focus on interactive video games.
- Sleep patterns.
- General behavior at home and in school settings.
- Previous results of Denver Developmental Screening Tests and any formal psychological testing.
- School performance.
- Identification of any learning disabilities.
- Behaviors displayed while playing with other children.
- Parenting styles: What works, what does not work with the child.

    c. Significant past medical history.

- Prenatal, birth, neonatal history.
- Evaluation of growth charts.
- Evaluation of previous diagnostic testing, including complete blood count (CBC) results, lead levels, visual and hearing test results.

- Seizures/seizure-like behaviors, including staring episodes, tics, head trauma.
- Medication history (prescribed, OTC, illicit).

d. Developmental history.
- Achievement of developmental milestones.
- Speech and language development.
- Gross motor and fine motor development.
- Coordination.

e. Educational history.
- Type of educational program.
- Early intervention.
- Special education program.
- Participation in mainstream programs.
- One-on-one programs.
- Success/failure in each educational program.
- Mathematical ability.

f. Behaviors at school.
- Reports from teachers, counselors.
- Relationships with children at home and school.
- Relationships with teacher, school nurse, counselor.

g. Family history.
- Parents or siblings diagnosed with ADHD.
- Substance abuse.
- Mental illness.
- Learning disabilities.

h. Psychosocial history.
- Family structure, function.
- Head of family.
- Parents' occupations, employment, levels of education.
- Substance abuse by parents/child.
- Evaluate family–child interactions.
- Family stress level due to child's behavior.

i. Manifestations consistent with comorbid conditions:
- Lack of motor control; clumsiness (developmental coordination disorder [dyspraxia]).
- Preschooler with speech, language delay (learning disability).
- Writes number in reverse order after age 7 (learning disability).
- Poor school performance: Unable to learn to read, write, or do mathematics (learning disability).
- Insomnia.
- Enuresis, encopresis.

- Negative, hostile, defiant behaviors lasting at least 6 months (oppositional defiant disorder [ODD]).
- Violation of home/school rules (conduct disorder).
- Symptoms of depression.
- Inappropriate levels of anxiety.
- Low self-esteem.
- Autism spectrum disorders.
- Tic disorders.

H. Physical findings.
  1. For diagnosis without comorbid conditions, physical examination is usually unremarkable.
  2. Behavior during physical examination is often inappropriate for age: Refuses to cooperate; refuses to respond to questions.
  3. Dysmorphic features may be consistent with comorbid conditions.
  4. Neurocutaneous lesions may be consistent with comorbid conditions.

I. Diagnostic tests.
  1. No specific diagnostic tests for definitive diagnosis.
  2. Diagnostics such as blood tests, brain scans, EEG, and psychological tests are not routinely necessary for children with ADHD without evidence of comorbid conditions.
  3. Laboratory tests that may assist in ruling out or verifying comorbid conditions.
     a. CBC with differential.
     b. Lead level (children 7 years and younger).
     c. Basic metabolic panel.
     d. Liver function panel.
     e. Thyroid studies including thyroid-stimulating hormone (TSH).
     f. ECG: To evaluate heart rate and QT interval (positive family history).
     g. EEG: Recommended for all children who may be placed on medication therapy and have a past medical history of seizures and/or a family history of a seizure disorder.
  4. Diagnosis of ADHD.
     a. For definitive diagnosis, must use DSM-V diagnostic criteria for ADHD.
     b. AAP updated their published evidenced-based guidelines (2015) for primary care diagnosis and clinical evaluation of children suspected of having ADHD. AAP guidelines require that a child meet the DSM-V criteria.
     c. AAP guidelines require evidence directly obtained from the classroom teacher regarding the core symptoms of ADHD, the duration of symptoms, the degree of functional impairment, and coexisting conditions.

    J. Differential diagnosis.
        1. Because diagnosis has several significant comorbid conditions, comprehensive history and physical examination essential to establish definitive diagnosis and formulate treatment plan.
        2. Differential diagnosis included in **Table 35-2**.

Table 35-2 Differential Diagnosis of ADHD

Differential Diagnosis	Characteristic Symptoms or Presentation
Specific learning disorder: Other developmental disorders of scholastic skills, F81.89	Language delay, especially in preschool years
	Persistent reversal of numbers after 7 years of age
	Unsuccessful in achieving reading, writing, and math skills
	Difficulty understanding concept of left and right
Sleep disorders, G47	Insomnia leading to attention deficit in school activities
	Sleeping during class
	Extended daytime naps at home or in school (preschool or kindergarten)
	Frequent episodes of night terrors or nightmares
Mild intellectual disabilities, F70	Children who present with learning difficulties in elementary grades
Tourette's disorder, F95.2	Usually symptoms are evident after 7 years of age
	Reports by parents/caregivers that child has had 2+ motor tics and 1 vocal tic during 1-year interval
Oppositional defiant disorder, F91.3	Negativistic
	Hostile
	Defiant behaviors
	Uncontrolled temper
	Angry
	Refuses to comply with social rules at home, school
	Behaviors are associated with poor school performance because they tend to resist work or school tasks that require self-application as they resist conforming to others' demands

Table 35-2 Differential Diagnosis of ADHD (*continued*)

Differential Diagnosis	Characteristic Symptoms or Presentation
Conduct disorder, unspecified, F91.9	Violates rights of others
	Violates societal norms
	Violates rules at home, school
	Participates in at-risk behaviors: Smoking, substance abuse
	Often suspended from school
Intermittent explosive disorder, F63.81	Displays high levels of impulsive behaviors
	Does not show serious aggressive behavior toward others
Other neurodevelopmental disorders	Increased motor activity that may occur in ADHD is not characterized by repetitive stereotypic movements that are seen in autistic spectrum disorders (ASDs) or Tourette's disorder
Atypical autism, F84.1	Inattention, social dysfunction, difficult-to-manage behavior
	Does not display indifference to facial and tonal communication as is seen in ASDs
Generalized anxiety disorder, F41.1	Inattentive behavior
	ADHD symptoms are not associated with worry or rumination as in anxiety disorder
Other differential diagnosis to consider	Does not display the characteristic symptoms of these major disorders: Reactive attachment disorder, depressive disorders, bipolar disorder, disruptive mood dysregulation disorder, substance abuse disorder, personality disorder, psychotic disorder, medication-induced symptoms of ADHD, neurocognitive disorders

K. Treatment (**Box 35-4**).
1. Both medication and behavior therapy.
2. Evidence suggests that discontinuing treatment leads to reemergence of symptoms.
3. Aimed at alleviating major symptoms child displays and improving child's ability to function within family unit, social and educational environments.
4. In addition, if child also displays symptoms of one or more comorbid conditions, treatment is highly recommended to reduce or alleviate these symptoms.

    5. Mental health referrals for all children suspected of having comorbid psychiatric conditions.

    6. Characteristics of treatment plan.

      a. Parent education.

- Provide education about ADHD and appropriate comorbid condition.
- Identify available resources and support groups for parents (**Box 35-5**).

      b. Preschool-age children (4 to 5 years old).

- Evidence-based parent or teacher behavioral interventions.
- Medication therapy: Methylphenidate if the behavior interventions do not improve.

      c. School-based strategies.

- Behavior therapy plus medication.
- Structured classroom setting.
- Consistent instruction and application of rules of conduct.
- Meets educational needs of child as identified through in-school testing.

      d. Behavior modification.

- Strategies are consistent and followed at home and at school.
- Inform child of rules of acceptable behavior.

Box 35-4 Role of Nurse Practitioner in Managing Children with ADHD

1. Office assessment identifying parental concerns and child's behavior patterns.
2. Establish rapport with psychiatrist or psychologist to identify treatment plan.
3. Include parents, child, and school personnel in the treatment plan.
4. Monitor effects of stimulant medication to ensure desired treatment plan outcomes.
5. Follow-up should include biannual physical examinations and appropriate laboratory studies, including hemoglobin because anemia is a side effect.
6. Emotional support measures for child and parents.
7. Monitor weight, height, and BMI every 3 months. School nurses can assist between the regularly scheduled 6-month office visits. Stimulant therapy may cause weight loss. Gains in height may be slowed.
8. Resources for parents:
   a. Centers for Disease Control and Prevention: Attention-Deficit/Hyperactive Disorder, www.cdc.gov/ncbddd/adhd
   b. National Resource Center on ADHD, www.help4adhd.org
   c. Attention Deficit Disorder Association, www.add.org

Box 35-5 Evidence-Based Treatment Guidelines for Children 4–18 Years of Age

The AAP developed an algorithm to guide the clinical process.

Diagnosis and Evaluation
The primary care clinician should:

1. Initiate an evaluation for ADHD for any child 4 through 18 years old who presents with academic or behavioral problems and symptoms of inattention, hyperactivity, and impulsivity.
2. Determine if the ADHD diagnostic criteria in the DSM-V are met.
3. Determine if comorbid conditions are present.
4. Recognize ADHD as a chronic illness and provide care using chronic care models and principles of medical home care management.

Source: Modified from Centers for Disease Control and Prevention. Attention-deficit /hyperactivity disorder (ADHD): recommendations. http://www.cdc.gov/ncbddd/adhd /guidelines.html. Updated March 18, 2015. Accessed April 27, 2015.

- Rewards for demonstrating positive behaviors (positive reinforcement).
- Consequences for failure to meet the goals (punishment).
- Repetitive application of the rewards and consequences shapes behavioral changes.

   e. Medication therapy.
- Basic principles.
   o Begin with lowest dosage and increase dosage every 5–7 days based on parent and teacher assessment of child's response (changes in behavior) to medication.
   o Once positive response to medication therapy is reported, increase dose at least one more time.
   o Medication administered every 12 hours has been shown to be most effective in controlling symptoms of ADHD.
- Drugs of choice.
   o Evidence strongly supports the use of stimulant medications.
   o The evidence is sufficient but less strong for atomoxetine, extended-release quanfacine, and extended-release clonidine (in that order).
- Potential side effects:
   o Decreased appetite, weight loss.
   o Insomnia.
   o Tachycardia.

- ○ Increased blood pressure.
- ○ Nervousness.
- ○ Headache.
- ○ Dizziness.
- ○ Irritability.
- ○ Rebound moodiness.
- ○ Leukopenia/anemia.
- ○ Skin rash.
- ○ Abnormal liver function tests.
- ○ Exacerbations of tics and Tourette syndrome.
- Management of side effects:
  - ○ Administer dose after meals to improve appetite; frequent high-calorie snacks.
  - ○ Avoid caffeine intake.
  - ○ Modify time of administration if sleep problems.
- For adolescents aged 12 to 18 years, the primary care clinician should prescribe FDA-approved medications for ADHD and behavior therapy. The preferred treatment for adolescents with ADHD includes both medication and behavior therapy.

L. Follow-up.
1. Monitor height, weight, heart rate, blood pressure every 3 months in children younger than 12 years of age. School nurse can play integral role in monitoring these measurements in child every 3 months and report these findings to primary care provider.
2. In children older than 12 years of age, monitor height, weight, heart rate, blood pressure every 6 months.
3. Monitor CBC or hemoglobin every 6 months. Children are at increased risk for leukopenia/anemia while on psychostimulant drug therapy.
4. Perform interval history, physical assessment every 6 months to evaluate child's response to treatment program.
5. Consult with teacher and school psychologist prior to each 6-month healthcare evaluation for continuity of care.
6. Follow up with psychiatric referrals, as appropriate.

M. Complications.

Abnormal weight loss, R63.4	Tic disorder, unspecified,
Essential (primary) hypertension, I10	F95.9
Tachycardia, unspecified, R00.0	Tourette's disorder, F95.2

1. Complications from medication therapy include weight loss, increased heart rate and blood pressure, growth suppression, exacerbations of tics and Tourette syndrome.

2. Once medication is discontinued, symptoms related to complications of medication therapy resolve; however, evidence shows that ADHD symptoms return even with continuous behavior-modification therapy.

N. Education.

1. Parent education is key to successful management.

a. Parents should receive initial and updated education related to behavior modification strategies for successful treatment as child reaches each new developmental stage.

b. Parents need to understand medication management.

c. Know possible side effects of medication therapy.

d. Support groups.

e. Group and family therapy.

f. Internet resources.

- American Academy of Child and Adolescent Psychiatry: www.aacap.org
- American Academy of Pediatrics: www.aap.org
- National Association of Pediatric Nurse Practitioners: www.napnap.org
- Children and Adults with Attention-Deficit/Hyperactivity Disorder (CHADD): www.chadd.org
- National Resource Center on ADHD: www.help4ADHD.org

III. AUTISTIC SPECTRUM DISORDER (ASD)

Asperger's syndrome, F84.5	Other and unspecified symbolic dysfunctions, R48.8
Atypical autism, F84.1	
Expressive language disorder, F80.1	Other childhood disintegrative disorder, F84.3
Intellectual disabilities, unspecified, F79	Other childhood emotional disorders, F93.8
	Rett's syndrome, F84.2

A. ASD is a biologically based neurobiological disorder that includes autistic spectrum disorder; childhood disintegrative disorder; pervasive developmental disorder, not otherwise specified; and Rett syndrome. Characterized by impaired verbal and nonverbal communication, cognitive abilities, and social interactions.

1. Individuals with an established DSM-IV diagnosis of ASD, Asperger's disorder, or pervasive developmental disorder, not otherwise specified,

should be given the diagnosis of ASD. Individuals with significant deficits but whose symptoms do not meet the criteria of ASD should be evaluated for social communication disorders.

2. The first symptoms of ASD involve delayed language development and most often include a lack of social interest or unusual social interactions, odd play patterns, and unusual communication patterns.

B. Etiology.

1. Genetic susceptibility: Children with a diagnosis of tuberous sclerosis, fragile X syndrome, Rett syndrome (identified gene mutation).

2. Genetic susceptibility and environmental factors: *No* single environmental factor identified; however, may be linked to prenatal exposure to thalidomides, valproic acid, and mesoprostol.

3. There is *no* evidence that links the measles-mumps-rubella (MMR) vaccine or any immunizations to the ASDs.

C. Occurrence.

1. Male-to-female ratio is 3:1.

2. In the United States: 1% of the population is affected.

3. Recurrence rate in siblings of affected children is 2–8%.

4. Present in all racial, ethnic, and socioeconomic groups.

D. Clinical manifestations.

1. Red flags.
   a. Significant impairment in social communication and interaction.
   b. Repetitive, restricted, and stereotyped patterns of behavior.

2. Symptoms develop before 30 months of age.
   a. Lack of (or poorly developed) verbal and nonverbal communication skills.
      • Abnormal speech patterns; Echolalia, nonsense rhyming.
      • Bruxism.
   b. Abnormal social play, solitary play, no friendships.
      • No eye contact.
      • No social smile.
      • Regression in language or social skills.
      • Repetitive body movements.
      • Ritualistic behaviors; need for sameness.
      • Preoccupation with an object.
      • Tantrums when ritual is disrupted.
      • Rocking behaviors.
   c. Impaired intellectual functioning.
      • Mental retardation (IQ < 70 in 40–62% of the children).
      • Occasionally child has particular talent (e.g., art, music).

E. Physical findings.
   1. Physical examination is most often normal.
   2. May have dysmorphic features.
      a. Long face and large eyes.
      b. Large head size not observed in infancy but observed in preschool years.
      c. May have microcephaly.
   3. Lack of communication skills and psychosocial skills in interactions in the home and during the office exam.
F. Diagnostic tests.
   1. No specific tests.
   2. Lead screening (children under 7 years old) and genetic testing may be indicated for identification of comorbid conditions.
   3. Refer to psychologist for cognitive and psychological testing.
   4. Refer to neurologist for full neurologic diagnostic workup, including blood work, MRI with contrast, CT scan, EEG.
   5. Refer for early intervention services.
   6. Autistic measures (**Box 35-6**).

Box 35-6 Autistic Measures

Autistic Diagnostic Observation Schedule (ADOS)
Childhood Autism Rating Scale (CARS)

G. Differential diagnosis.

Aphasia, R47.01	Fragile X chromosome, Q99.2
Attention-deficit hyperactivity disorder, combined type, F90.2	Hearing loss, unspecified, H91.90
Attention-deficit hyperactivity disorder, predominantly hyperactive type, F90.1	Intellectual disabilities, unspecified, F79
	Obsessive-compulsive disorder, F42
Attention-deficit hyperactivity disorder, predominantly inattentive type, F90.0	Other childhood disintegrative disorder, F84.3
	Pervasive developmental disorders, F84
Attention-deficit hyperactivity disorder, unspecified type, F90.9	Rett's syndrome, F84.2
Conduct disorder, unspecified, F91.9	Stereotyped movement disorders, F98.4
Expressive language disorder, F80.1	Tourette's disorder, F95.2

1. Obsessive-compulsive disorder, Tourette syndrome.
2. Conduct disorder, mental retardation, hearing disorder.
3. Schizophrenia of childhood.
4. Lead poisoning.
5. Fragile X syndrome.
6. Additional pervasive disorders.
7. Childhood disintegrative disorder.
8. Rett syndrome.
   a. Development normal until 1 year of age, at which time language and motor development regress.
   b. Microcephaly is usually evident by 1 year of age.

H. Treatment.
1. No single best evidence-based treatment.
   a. Treatment is individualized to the child.
      - Management of challenging behaviors.
      - Sleep problems.
      - Social skills training.
   b. Medication.
      - For aggressive behaviors and irritability for children and teens with autism: Resperidone and aripiprazole.
      - Stimulants for comorbid symptoms of ADHD.
      - Other comorbid conditions treated as appropriate by psychiatric specialists.
   c. Implement all early intervention services in home and school: Speech therapy, occupational and physical therapy, behavior modification strategies.
2. Diagnosis.
   a. Denver Developmental II screening test: Valuable tool used to assist in early recognition.
   b. Screening Tool for Autism in Toddlers and Young Children.
   c. Autism Spectrum Screening Questionnaire for 6–17 years old.
   d. Refer to developmental neurologist and early intervention services (under age 5) as soon as symptoms are suspected.
3. Comorbidity.
   a. ADHD.
   b. Intellectual disabilities and structured language disorders.
   c. Mood disorders.
   d. Depression.
   e. Anxiety.
   f. Obsessive–compulsive behaviors.
   g. Phobias.

I. Follow-up.
   1. Recognize early signs and symptoms of autism, Asperger's syndrome, childhood disintegrative disorder, Rett syndrome, and make appropriate referrals.
   2. Support for parents, other primary caregivers is essential. Families may benefit from connecting with the Autism Society (www.autism-society.org).
   3. Encourage parents to find respite care for child.
J. Complications.

Pervasive developmental disorders [autism], F84

---

   1. Autism is a chronic disease with no cure.
K. Education.
   1. Families need education about the disorder, which treatments have been proved to be successful, multidisciplinary interventions.
   2. Families need to be careful when investigating treatment programs and determine proven benefits from these programs. Families must consider own safety and that of their child.
   3. Internet resources.
      a. Autism Society: www.autism-society.org
      b. Centers for Disease Control and Prevention: www.cdc.gov
      c. American Academy of Pediatrics: www.aap.org

IV. BREATH HOLDING

Anoxic brain damage, not elsewhere classified, G93.1	Myoclonus, G25.3
Apnea, not elsewhere classified, R06.81	Other abnormalities of breathing, R06.89
Conduct disorder, childhood-onset type, F91.1	Other specified cardiac arrhythmias, I49.8
Cyanosis, R23.0	Pallor, R23.1
Generalized idiopathic epilepsy and epileptic syndromes, not intractable, without status epilepticus, G40.309	Somnolence, R40.0 Stupor, R40.1

A. Characterized by episodes in which infant/young child involuntarily holds breath, leading to cerebral anoxia resulting in limp body and extremities, unresponsiveness. Two types: Cyanotic spells and pallid spells.

B. Etiology.
   1. Unknown.
   2. May occur when child responds to fear, pain, or traumatic event.
   3. Parental history of breath-holding episodes as a child.
C. Occurrence.
   1. Usually begins after 6 months old.
   2. Highest incidence rate at 2 years old.
   3. Usually resolves by 5 years old.
   4. Usually occurs in response to an upsetting, unexpected, or traumatic event.
   5. May occur with genetic conditions such as Rett syndrome.
   6. Associated with iron-deficiency anemia.
D. Clinical manifestations.
   1. Cyanotic spells.
      a. Brief shrill cry followed by forced expiration and apnea.
      b. Onset of cyanosis.
      c. Loss of consciousness.
      d. Generalized clonic jerks.
      e. Bradycardia.
   2. Pallid spells.
      a. Usually follows fall in which child strikes head, causing pain.
      b. Cessation of normal breathing pattern; prolonged apneic episode.
      c. Loses consciousness.
      d. Pallor.
      e. Tonic seizure activity (occasional).
E. Physical findings.
   1. Normal physical exam findings.
F. Diagnostic tests.
   1. EEG, referral to neurologist is recommended.
G. Prognosis.
   1. Most children outgrow the spells by 4 to 8 years of age.
H. Differential diagnosis.

Convulsions, unspecified, R56.9

Iron deficiency anemia, unspecified, D50.9

---

   1. Seizure disorder.
I. Treatment.
   1. No treatment necessary.
   2. Parental support and reassurance.

    3. Avoid situations that provoke the breath-holding episodes.

    4. Treat iron-deficiency anemia if present.

J. Follow-up.

    1. Call within a few days to assess how family is dealing and to answer questions.

    2. Parents' level of comfort with breath-holding episodes determines further follow-up.

K. Complications.

    1. Head injury if child falls during episode.

L. Education.

    1. Discussion of management plan that parents can follow consistently. Parents must feel comfortable with plan.

    2. Provide safe environment for child during and at conclusion of episode.

    3. Avoid reinforcement of these behaviors.

    4. Most children outgrow breath-holding episodes by 4 to 8 years of age.

V. NIGHTMARES AND NIGHT TERRORS

Hyperventilation, R06.4	Sleep terrors [night terrors], F51.4
Mydriasis, H57.04	Tachycardia, unspecified, R00.0
Nightmares, F51.5	

A. Etiology.

    1. Actual cause unknown.

    2. Dysfunctional family relationships should be suspected.

B. Occurrence.

    1. Occurs in 1–3% of children, mostly in boys between 5 and 7 years old.

C. Clinical manifestations.

    1. Night terrors: Sudden, unexpected screams during sleep; usually occurs within 2 hours of the time the child goes to sleep.

    2. Nightmares: Frightening dreams that awake the child and make the child afraid to return to sleep; usually occurs during the last third of the sleep cycle during REM sleep.

    3. Appears frightened; pupils dilated.

    4. Tachycardia, hyperventilation.

    5. Thrashing of extremities.

    6. Inconsolable, not aware of parents' presence.

    7. Panic.

    8. Sleepwalking.

      9. Returns to sleep.

    10. No recall of night terror in morning.

  D. Physical findings.

      1. None.

  E. Diagnostic tests.

      1. None necessary.

  F. Differential diagnosis.

Convulsions, unspecified, R56.9	Mental and behavioral disorders due to psychoactive substance use, F10-F19
Disappearance and death of family member, Z63.4	
Emotional disorders with onset specific to childhood, F93	Narcolepsy and cataplexy, G47.4
	Panic disorder [episodic paroxysmal anxiety], F41.0
Generalized anxiety disorder, F41.1	
Major depressive disorder, single episode, unspecified, F32.9	REM sleep disorder, G47.52
	Sleep terrors [night terrors], F51.4

      1. Rule out emotional disorder; anxiety; depression.

      2. Seizures.

  G. Treatment.

      1. Child should be encouraged to lie down and be helped back to sleep (e.g., talking quietly, rubbing back).

      2. Turn on light or use a nightlight in the bedroom.

      3. Encourage family to wake child before episode for 1–2 weeks to attempt to break cycle.

      4. Protect child from injury.

      5. Prepare babysitter for possible episode.

      6. Leave bedroom door open.

      7. Provide comfort, reassurance to child.

      8. Counseling may be necessary for children who have severe nighttime fears.

  H. Follow-up.

      1. Refer to psychologist or psychiatrist if night terrors or nightmares persist.

      2. Complete family evaluation may be necessary.

  I. Complications.

Sleep terrors [night terrors], F51.4

      1. Injury.

      2. Continued nighttime fears.

J. Education.
   1. Often night terrors are self-limiting.
   2. Family support may be necessary to reduce parental anxiety.

VI. SCHOOL REFUSAL

A. School-refusal behavior refers to any refusal to attend school or difficulty attending classes for an entire day by a child.
B. Occurrence.
   1. 5–28% of youths.
   2. Prevalence: Fairly equivalent among gender, racial, and economic status.
C. Triggers for school refusal.
   1. Dysfunctional family patterns.
   2. Impending school changes.
   3. Illness.
   4. Traumatic experiences.
D. Clinical manifestations.
   1. Range of behaviors.
   2. Depression.
   3. Social anxiety.
   4. Fears.
   5. Fatigue.
   6. Somatic complaints.
   7. Noncompliance.
   8. Aggression.
   9. Clinging.
   10. Temper tantrums.
   11. Run away from home.
E. Physical findings.
   1. No physical exam findings.
   2. Mental health assessment may reveal comorbid mental health problems.
F. Diagnostic tests and assessment tools.
   1. Consider drug and alcohol screening based on presenting history.
   2. Consider pregnancy testing and screening for sexually transmitted disease if history of runaway.
   3. Anxiety Disorders Interview Schedule for DSM-V (Parent and Child versions).
   4. The School Refusal Assessment Scale-Revised (SRAS-R).

G. Treatment.
   1. Determine who will conduct the interventions: Refer to school psychologist, social worker.
   2. Cognitive behavioral therapy.
   3. Relaxation therapy.
   4. Problem-solving skills instruction.
   5. Parent interventions.
   6. Morning and evening routines.
H. Education.
   1. Instructions for parents on effective parenting skills.
I. Follow-up.
   1. Monitor progress weekly and then monthly until problem resolves.

BIBLIOGRAPHY

Adano N, Huo L, Adelsberg S, Petkova E, Castellanos F, Martino A. Response time intra-subject variability: commonalities between children with autism spectrum disorder and children with ADHD. *Eur Child Adolesc Psychiatry*. 2014;23(2):69-79.

American Psychiatric Association. *Diagnostic and Statistical Manual of Mental Disorders*. 5th ed. Washington, DC: American Psychiatric Association; 2013.

Bass PF. Differential Dx: ADHD or sleep deficit? *Contemp Pediatr*. 2014;31(7):21-26.

Brown AB, Elder JH. Communication in autism spectrum disorder: a guide for pediatric nurses. *Pediatr Nurs*. 2014;40(5):219-225.

Burns CE, Dunn AM, Brady MA, Starr NB, Blosser CG. *Pediatric Primary Care*. 5th ed. Philadelphia, PA: Saunders; 2013.

Centers for Disease Control and Prevention. Attention-deficit/hyperactivity disorder (ADHD): recommendations. http://www.cdc.gov/ncbddd/adhd/guidelines.html. Updated March 18, 2015. Accessed April 27, 2015.

D'Elia L, Valeri G, Sonnino F, Fontana I, Mammone A, Vicari S. A longitudinal study of the TEACCH program in different settings: the potential benefits of low intensity intervention in preschool children with autism spectrum disorder. *J Autism Dev Disord*. 2014;44(3):615-626.

Farmer JE, Clark MJ, Mayfield WA, et al. The relationship between the medical home and unmet needs for children with autism spectrum disorders. *Matern Child Health J*. 2014;18(3):672-680.

Garfield LD, Brown DS, Allaire BT, Ross RE, Nicol GE, Raghavan R. Psychotropic drug use among preschool children in the Medicaid program from 36 states. *Am J Public Health*. 2015;105(3):524-529.

Green BC, Johnson KA, Bretherton L. Pragmatic language difficulties in children with hyperactivity and attention problems: an integrated review. *Int J Lang Commun Disord*. 2014;49(1):15-29.

Green M, Wong M, Atkins D, Taylor J, Feinleib M. *Diagnosis of Attention-Deficit/Hyperactivity Disorder. Technical Review No. 3*. Rockville, MD: Agency for Health Care Policy and Research; August 1999. AHCPR Publication No. 99-0050.

Maljaars J, Boonen H, Lambrechts G, Leeuwen K, Noens I. Maternal parenting behavior and child behavior problems in families of children and adolescents with autism spectrum disorder. *J Autism Dev Disord*. 2014;44(3):501-512.

Nunn KP, Lask B, Owen I. Pervasive refusal syndrome (PRS) 21 years on: a re-conceptualisation and a renaming. *Eur Child Adolesc Psychiatry*. 2014;23(3):163-172.

Posserud MB, Ullebo AK, Plessen KJ, Stormark KM, Gillberg C, Lundervold AJ. Influence of assessment instrument on ADHD diagnosis. *Eur Child Adolesc Psychiatry*. 2014;23(4):197-205.

Sugrue D, Bogner R, Ehert MJ. Methyphenidate and dexmethylphenidate formulations for children with attention-deficit/hyperactivity disorder. *Am J Health Syst Pharm*. 2014;71(14):1163-1170.

Tek S, Mesutem L, Fein D, Naigles L. Longitudinal analyses of expressive language development reveal two distinct language profiles among young children with autism spectrum disorders. *J Autism Dev Disord*. 2014;44(1):75-89.

Mental Health Disorders

Kim Walton and Susan J. Kersey

I. ANXIETY DISORDERS

Conduct disorder, unspecified, F91.9	Other childhood emotional disorders, F93.8
Contact dermatitis, unspecified, unspecified cause, L25.9	Other conduct disorders, F91.8
	Other fatigue, R53.83
Cramp and spasm, R25.2	Panic disorder [episodic paroxysmal anxiety] without agoraphobia, F41.0
Diarrhea, unspecified, R19.7	
Dizziness and giddiness, R42	Post-traumatic stress disorder, unspecified, F43.10
Generalized anxiety disorder, F41.1	
Generalized hyperhidrosis, R61	Restlessness and agitation, R45.1
Headache, R51	Separation anxiety disorder of childhood, F93.0
Irritability and anger, R45.4	
Nausea, R11.0	Shortness of breath, R06.02
Obsessive-compulsive disorder, F42	Sleep disorders, G47

A. Presentation of anxiety disorder; includes both physical and emotional characteristics.
B. Etiology.
1. Biochemical changes in brain.
a. Possible genetic vulnerability.
b. Post-traumatic stress disorder (PTSD) present in children who survive severe or terrifying physical or emotional event. Also occurs when witnessing an event that the child perceives as threatening; this includes domestic violence.
c. Separation anxiety, note relative frequency in children of mothers with panic disorder.

C. Occurrence.
  1. Most common mental illness group occurring in children and adolescents.
  2. Estimated prevalence of any anxiety disorder among children and adolescents is 13% in 6-month period.
D. Clinical manifestations.
  1. Generalized anxiety disorder (also known as overanxious disorder in children).
    a. Characterized by at least 6 months of persistent, excessive anxiety/worry over everyday events; difficult to control the worry.
    b. Anxiety and worry are associated with at least one of following:
      • Restlessness.
      • Being easily fatigued.
      • Difficulty concentrating.
      • Irritability.
      • Muscle tension.
      • Sleep disturbance.
    c. Symptoms must cause significant distress or impairment in functioning.
  2. Obsessive compulsive disorder (OCD).
    a. Obsessions: Recurring thoughts or images that are disturbing, intrusive, cannot be controlled through rational reasoning.
      • Common obsessions:
        o Contamination.
        o Fear of harm to self/family member.
        o Worry about acting on aggressive impulses.
        o Concern about order and symmetry.
      • Thoughts or images are not simply excessive worries about real-life problems.
      • Attempts to ignore or suppress such thoughts or images with some other thought/action.
    b. Compulsions: Repetitive behaviors that one feels obliged to complete. Performance of compulsive behavior, at least temporarily, decreases anxiety, thereby reinforcing behavior.
      • Common compulsions:
        o Handwashing.
        o Cleaning rituals.
        o Requesting reassurance.
        o Ordering and arranging.
        o Complex touching habits.
        o Checking, counting, and repetition of routine activities.
      • Behaviors are aimed at preventing or reducing distress.

    c. Obsessions or compulsions must be time-consuming (take > 1 hour a day), cause marked distress, interfere with daily activities.

    d. Often seen with comorbidities.

    e. Strong familial component.

    f. Immune response to streptococcal infections.

3. PTSD.

    a. Must have exposure to traumatic event with *both* of following:

- Actual or threatened death/serious injury or threat to physical integrity of self/others.
- Response involving intense fear, helplessness, horror. May be expressed as disorganized/agitated behavior in children.

    b. Traumatic event is persistently reexperienced in one or more of following ways:

- Recurrent, intrusive, distressing thoughts of event. In young children, may include repetitive play.
- Recurrent distressing dreams. In children, may be frightening dreams without recognizable content.
- Acting or feeling as if trauma were reoccurring. In young children, may include trauma-specific reenactment, often through play.
- Intense psychologic distress on exposure to internal/external cues reminiscent of traumatic event.
- Physiologic reactivity on exposure to internal/external cues reminiscent of traumatic event.

    c. Persistent *avoidance* of stimuli, numbing of general responsiveness with 3 or more of following:

- Efforts to avoid thoughts, feelings, or talking about trauma.
- Efforts to avoid activities, places, people that arouse memories.
- Inability to recall important aspect of event.
- Diminished interest/participation in activities.
- Feelings of detachment/estrangement.
- Restricted range of affect.
- Sense of foreshortened future.

    d. Persistent symptoms of *arousal* with two or more of following:

- Difficulty falling asleep/staying asleep.
- Irritability or outbursts of anger.
- Difficulty concentrating.
- Hypervigilance.
- Exaggerated startle response.

    e. Duration of symptoms for > 1 month.

   f. Disturbance causes significant distress or impairment in functioning.

   g. Diagnosis may be acute (symptoms < 3 months), chronic (symptoms ≥ 3 months), or delayed (onset of symptoms at least 6 months after stressor).

  4. Separation anxiety.

   a. Onset of excessive anxiety on separation from home/major attachment figure *beyond what is expected* for developmental level as evidenced by 3 or more of following:

- Recurrent excessive distress on separation from home or major attachment figure.
- Persistent/excessive worry about losing or harm coming to major attachment figure.
- Worry that untoward event will lead to separation (e.g., getting lost or kidnapped).
- Reluctance or refusal to go to school.
- Fearful or reluctant to be alone.
- Reluctance or refusal to go to sleep without being near attachment figure or to sleep away from home.
- Repeated nightmares with themes of separation.
- Repeated physical complaints when separation occurs or is anticipated.

   b. Symptoms must be present for at least 4 weeks and must begin before age 18.

   c. Symptoms must cause significant distress/impairment at home, school, with friends.

 E. Physical findings.

  1. May present with symptoms of sleep disturbance, tiredness, school problems, restlessness, irritability, somatic complaints (sweating, nausea, diarrhea, shortness of breath, dizziness, headaches).

  2. For OCD, parents generally bring children in due to increase in temper tantrums, decline in school performance, food restriction, dermatitis. Children rarely request help; may be secretive about thoughts, behaviors.

 F. Diagnostic tests.

  1. None. Requires interview with child and parent/caregiver.

  2. Consider collateral contact with school personnel, especially with separation anxiety.

  3. Assess recent life stressors (family move, death, divorce, new school setting, etc.).

G. Differential diagnosis.

Acute stress reaction, F43.0	Post-traumatic stress disorder, unspecified, F43.10
Disturbance of activity and attention, F90.0	
Generalized anxiety disorder, F41.1	Separation anxiety disorder of childhood, F93.0
Obsessive-compulsive disorder, F42	

1. Attention-deficit/hyperactivity disorder (ADHD).
2. Differentiate among anxiety disorders such as PTSD, separation anxiety, generalized anxiety disorder, OCD.
3. Consider acute stress reaction if exposed to traumatic event, symptoms present < 1 month.

H. Treatment.
1. May require use of medications to reduce anxiety symptoms. Consider use of selective serotonin reuptake inhibitors (SSRIs). These may include:
   a. Fluoxetine (Prozac): Starting dose of 5 mg/day; increase to 15–30 mg/day for children; 10–40 mg/day for teens.
   b. Fluvoxamine (Luvox): Starting dose of 25 mg/day; increase to 50–200 mg/day for children; 150–300 mg/day for teens.
   c. Sertraline (Zoloft): Starting dose of 25 mg/day; increase to 50–100 mg/day for children; 50–200 mg/day for teens.
2. May also consider a tricyclic medication, such as clomipramine (Anafranil): Starting dose of 10 mg/day; increase to 75–100 mg/day for children; 100–200 mg/day for teens.
3. Cognitive behavioral therapy (CBT) to help identify anxiety triggers, awareness of physiologic responses to anxiety. Develop plan for coping, evaluation of success of strategies.
4. Family therapy to address ways family can support the child. Must allow 6–8 weeks before full benefit will be obtained. Follow black box warning regarding increased monitoring of suicide ideation (SI).

I. Follow-up.
1. Follow-up appointment to monitor effectiveness of medications, address side effects of medications, compliance issues.
2. Collaboration with family, mental health treatment provider, school personnel to assess success of treatment approaches and medications.

J. Complications.
1. Poor school performance.
2. Poor self-esteem, social skills, avoidance of peers.
3. Potential for family stress and conflict.
4. Development of comorbid diagnosis of substance abuse or major depression.

K. Education.
   1. Parent/caregiver and child need education about nature of anxiety, ways to identify, evaluate, change anxious thoughts.
   2. Child needs to learn to recognize physiologic symptoms of anxiety, use of positive "self-talk."
   3. Relaxation training may be beneficial.

II. EATING DISORDERS

Abdominal and pelvic pain, R10	Hypothermia, not associated with low environmental temperature, R68.0
Abnormal weight loss, R63.4	
Acidosis, E87.2	
Agranulocytosis, D70	Insomnia, unspecified, G47.00
Alkalosis, E87.3	Nausea, R11.0
Alopecia areata, L63	Other disorders of electrolyte and fluid balance, not elsewhere classified, E87.8
Anemia, unspecified, D64.9	
Anorexia nervosa, unspecified, F50.00	Other fatigue, R53.83
Cardiac arrhythmia, unspecified, I49.9	Other nail disorders, L60.8
Constipation, K59.0	Other specified cardiac arrhythmias, I49.8
Dental caries, K02	
Eating disorders, F50	Polyphagia, R63.2
Erosion of teeth, K03.2	Scar conditions and fibrosis of skin, L90.5
Failure to thrive (child), R62.51	Volume depletion, E86
Hypotension, unspecified, I95.9	Vomiting, unspecified, R11.10

A. Serious, sometimes life threatening; tend to be chronic, usually arise in adolescence.
B. Etiology.
   1. Combination of genetic, neurochemical, psychodevelopmental, socio-cultural factors.
      a. Increased risk among first-degree biological relatives of individuals with disorder. Often co-occurs with other mental health problems such as depression, anxiety, substance abuse, personality disorders.
C. Occurrence.
   1. > 90% of all eating disorders occur in females.
   2. Estimated 0.5% of adolescent females have anorexia nervosa; 1–5% meet criteria for bulimia nervosa.

      3. Rarely begins before puberty, most common in ages 14–18 years.

      4. Onset may be associated with stressful life event.

D. Clinical manifestations.

    1. Anorexia nervosa.

      a. Most severe consequence with mortality rate from starvation, suicide, electrolyte imbalance.

      b. Characterized by refusal to maintain minimally normal body weight for age and height (< 85% of expected weight).

      c. Intense fear of gaining weight or becoming fat.

      d. Significant disturbance in perception of shape or size of body; sees self as overweight even when dangerously thin.

      e. In postmenarchal females, presence of amenorrhea.

    2. Bulimia nervosa.

      a. Repeated episodes of binge eating characterized by:

        • Eating in discrete period of time (e.g., within 2 hours), amount of food larger than most people would eat during same period of time and under similar circumstances.

        • Sense of lack of control over eating during episode.

      b. Recurrent inappropriate compensatory behaviors to prevent weight gain such as self-induced vomiting, misuse of laxatives, diuretics, enemas, other medications, fasting, excessive exercise.

      c. Occurrence of *both* of the previously listed behaviors, on average at least twice a week for 3 months. Individuals place excessive emphasis on body shape, weight in self-evaluation.

E. Physical findings.

    1. Anorexia nervosa.

      a. Reported by family members, individual presents with weight loss or failure to make expected weight gains.

      b. Leukopenia, mild anemia are common.

      c. May present with signs/symptoms of dehydration, sinus bradycardia, arrhythmias.

      d. May present with constipation, abdominal pain, cold intolerance, lethargy, hypotension, hypothermia, dry skin, dental enamel erosion.

    2. Bulimia nervosa.

      a. Typically presents within normal weight range to slightly overweight.

      b. May present with complaints of abdominal pain, nausea, hair loss, brittle nails, fatigue, insomnia, or weakness.

      c. Fluid and electrolyte imbalances: Metabolic alkalosis from vomiting or metabolic acidosis from laxative abuse.

      d. Loss of dental enamel, increased frequency of dental caries.

    e. Enlarged parotid glands.

    f. Possible calluses/scars on dorsal surface of hand from repeated self-induced vomiting.

F. Diagnostic tests.

    1. Ask all preteens, adolescents screening questions about eating patterns, satisfaction with body appearance.

    2. Monitor height, weight, body mass index (BMI) on all visits.

    3. Laboratory studies: Complete blood count (CBC), electrolyte measurement, liver function tests, urinalysis, thyroid-stimulating hormone (TSH) test.

    4. Electrocardiogram.

G. Differential diagnosis.

Abnormal weight gain, R63.5	Generalized anxiety disorder, F41.1
Abnormal weight loss, R63.4	Human immunodeficiency virus [HIV] disease, B20-B24
Adverse effect of drug or medicament, unspecified, T88.7	Major depressive disorder, single episode, unspecified, F32.9
Disease of intestine, unspecified, K63.9	Other disorders of brain, G93

    1. Rule out other possible medical causes for significant weight loss/failure to gain weight (GI disease, brain tumors, malignancies, AIDS, etc.), although these do not present with distorted body image.

    2. Comorbid diagnosis of substance abuse, major depression, anxiety disorder.

H. Treatment.

    1. Anorexia nervosa.

        a. Requires comprehensive treatment plan, including medical care, monitoring, psychotherapy, nutritional counseling, medication (when appropriate). Involves three phases:

- Restoring weight loss due to severe dieting, purging.
- Treating psychologic disturbances such as distorted body image, low self-esteem, interpersonal conflicts.
- Achieving long-term remission, rehabilitation.

        b. Treatment with medication, such as SSRIs; consider *only* after weight gain established.

        c. Acute inpatient hospitalization may be required to restore weight, address fluid and electrolyte imbalance or cardiac disturbances. May require nutrition via nasogastric tube/IV therapy.

        d. Intensive treatment may be needed in specialized day treatment program or intensive outpatient program.

        e. Refer for CBT and family therapy.

2. Bulimia nervosa.
   a. Requires comprehensive treatment plan, including medical care, monitoring, psychotherapy, nutritional counseling, medication (when appropriate).
   b. Primary goal: Reduce/eliminate binge eating, purging behavior.
      - Establish pattern of regular, nonbinging eating.
      - Improve attitudes related to eating disorder.
      - Encourage healthy, not excessive exercise.
      - Resolution of co-occurring disorders such as depression, anxiety.
   c. Treatment approaches may include individual, group/family therapy.
   d. CBT: Useful to address cognitive distortions related to body image and to develop adaptive coping skills.
   e. Antidepressant medications, especially SSRIs, have been found to be effective.
I. Follow-up.
   1. May need weekly visits to monitor weight, lab work.
   2. To achieve long-term remission and rehabilitation, treatment must include ongoing behavioral therapy, continued assessment of weight, and physical health status.
   3. Ongoing assessment of anxiety/depressive symptoms.
   4. Collaboration between family and mental health provider to assess effectiveness of treatment approaches.
   5. Pharmacologic support has found conflicting evidence as benefit.
J. Complications.

Acute kidney failure, unspecified, N17.9	Other diseases of stomach and duodenum, K31.89
Anorexia nervosa, unspecified, F50.00	
Cardiac arrhythmia, unspecified, I49.9	Other disorders of electrolyte and fluid balance, not elsewhere classified, E87.8
Dental caries, K02	
Dysthymic disorder, F34.1	Polyphagia, R63.2
Erosion of teeth, K03.2	Starvation, initial encounter, T73.0XXA
Esophagitis, unspecified, K20.9	State of emotional shock and stress, unspecified, R45.7
Heart disease, unspecified, I51.9	
Major depressive disorder, single episode, unspecified, F32.9	Ulcer of esophagus without bleeding, K22.10
Mental disorder, not otherwise specified, F99	Volume depletion, E86
	Vomiting, unspecified, R11.10

    1. Anorexia nervosa.
       a. Starvation, fluid and electrolyte imbalances, dehydration.
       b. Cardiac complications.
       c. Renal failure.
       d. Potential for suicide.
       e. Development of anxiety/depression.
       f. Potential for family stress and conflict.
    2. Bulimia nervosa.
       a. Dental caries, loss of dental enamel.
       b. Potential for development of depression, substance abuse.
       c. Gastric rupture from acute gastric dilatation secondary to vomiting.
       d. Esophagitis and ulceration of esophagus.
       e. Potential for cardiac arrhythmias.
K. Education.
    1. Educate family on potential complications of disorder, as well as how to best support adolescent in treatment.
    2. Adolescent and family may benefit from nutritional counseling.

III. MOOD DISORDERS

Abdominal and pelvic pain, R10	Major depressive disorder, single episode, unspecified, F32.9
Anorexia, R63.0	
Attention-deficit hyperactivity disorder, combined type, F90.2	Mental disorder, not otherwise specified, F99
Attention-deficit hyperactivity disorder, predominantly hyperactive type, F90.1	Oppositional defiant disorder, F91.3
	Other fatigue, R53.83
Attention-deficit hyperactivity disorder, predominantly inattentive type, F90.0	Other persistent mood [affective] disorders, F34.8
Attention-deficit hyperactivity disorder, unspecified type, F90.9	Sleep disorder not due to a substance or known physiological condition, unspecified, F51.9
Bipolar disorder, unspecified, F31.9	Unspecified mood [affective] disorder, F39
Headache, R51	

A. Etiology.
    1. Close family member with depression or bipolar disorder may be single largest contributor to likelihood of disorder in child.

B. Occurrence.
   1. For depression, prevalence is 2% in children, 6% in adolescents, with life-time prevalence in adolescents estimated to be 20%.
   2. 1% of adolescents 14–18 years of age meet criteria for bipolar disorder. Recent reports indicate a 40-fold increase in the diagnosis of bipolar disorder in children and teens.
C. Clinical manifestations.
   1. Major depression.
      a. Characterized by five or more of the following symptoms present daily for at least 2 weeks:
         • Persistent sadness or irritable mood.
         • Loss of interest in activities once enjoyed.
         • Significant change in appetite or body weight.
         • Difficulty sleeping or oversleeping.
         • Psychomotor agitation or slowing.
         • Loss of energy.
         • Feelings of worthlessness or inappropriate guilt.
         • Difficulty concentrating.
         • Recurrent thoughts of death or suicide.
      b. Other signs associated with depression include:
         • Frequent, vague, nonspecific physical complaints such as stomachaches, headaches, muscle aches, tiredness.
         • Frequent absences from school or poor school performance.
         • Talk of or efforts toward running away from home.
         • Outbursts of shouting, complaining, unexplained irritability or crying.
         • Being bored or lack of interest in playing with friends.
         • Alcohol or substance abuse.
         • Social isolation, poor communication, difficulty with relationships.
         • Fear of death.
         • Extreme sensitivity to rejection/failure.
         • Increased irritability, anger, hostility.
         • Reckless behavior.
   2. Bipolar disorder.
      a. Bipolar I: Experiences alternating episodes of intense mania and depression.
      b. Bipolar II: Experiences episodes of hypomania (markedly elevated or irritable mood with increased physical and mental energy) between recurrent periods of depression.

    c. Bipolar not otherwise specified (NOS): Being used more to describe bipolar spectrum symptoms.

    d. Manic symptoms include:
- Severe or rapid changes in mood: Extremely irritable or overly silly, elated mood.
- Overly inflated self-esteem, grandiosity.
- Exaggerated beliefs about personal talents/abilities.
- Increased energy, decreased need for sleep; able to go with very little/no sleep for days without tiring.
- Talks too much, too fast, changes subjects too quickly.
- Distractibility, hyperactivity: Attention shifts from one thing to another quickly.
- Increased sexual thoughts, feelings, behaviors, or use of explicit sexual language.
- Increased goal-directed activity or physical agitation.
- Excessive involvement in risky, daredevil behaviors/activities.

    e. Depressive symptoms include:
- Pervasive/overwhelming sadness, crying spells.
- Sleeping too much or inability to sleep.
- Agitation, irritability.
- Withdrawal from activities formerly enjoyed.
- Drop in grades, inability to concentrate.
- Thoughts of death and suicide.
- Low energy.
- Significant loss of appetite.

    f. May also present with: Explosive/destructive rages, separation anxiety, defiance of authority, bedwetting, night terrors, strong and frequent cravings, impaired judgment, impulsivity.

    g. Presents with depressive symptoms and also exhibits ADHD-like symptoms that are very severe: Refer to mental health professional for further evaluation, particularly if family history of bipolar disorder.

D. Physical findings.
1. Specifically ask about thoughts of suicide or self-harm: Suicide is third leading cause of death among 10- to 24-year-olds.
2. Major depression may present with multiple, vague somatic complaints (e.g., headache, stomachache, fatigue, sleep, appetite changes).
3. Bipolar disorder may present with symptoms of ADHD, depression, mania, oppositional behavior.

4. Disruptive mood dysregulation disorder.
   a. Severe recurrent temper outbursts, verbal and/or behavioral, that are grossly out of proportion in intensity or duration to the situation or provocation.
      - The temper outbursts are inconsistent with developmental level.
      - The temper outbursts occur, on average, 3 or more times per week.
      - The mood between temper outbursts is persistently irritable or angry.
   b. Symptoms have been present for 12 or more months. Throughout that time, the individual has not had a period lasting 3 or more consecutive months without all of the symptoms.
   c. Symptoms are present in at least two of three settings and are severe in at least one of these.
   d. The behaviors do not occur during an episode of major depressive disorder, mania, or hypomania and are not better explained by another mental disorder.
E. Diagnostic tests.
   1. Several screening tools useful for children/adolescents, including Children's Depression Inventory for ages 7–17 and Beck Depression Inventory for adolescents. Positive screens indicate need for comprehensive diagnostic evaluation by mental health professional.
   2. Requires intensive interview with child/adolescent and family as well as detailed family history.
F. Differential diagnosis.

Adjustment disorder, unspecified, F43.20	Attention-deficit hyperactivity disorder, predominantly inattentive type, F90.0
Attention-deficit hyperactivity disorder, combined type, F90.2	Attention-deficit hyperactivity disorder, unspecified type, F90.9
Attention-deficit hyperactivity disorder, predominantly hyperactive type, F90.1	Intermittent explosive disorder, F63.81
	Oppositional defiant disorder, F91.3

   1. Adjustment disorder.
   2. ADHD.
   3. Intermittent explosive disorder.
   4. Oppositional defiant disorder.
G. Treatment.
   1. Major depression.
      a. Antidepressant medication may be indicated.
         - Consider SSRI medications:

- o Fluoxetine (Prozac): Starting dose of 5 mg/day; increase to 15–40 mg/day for children, 10–60 mg/day for teens.
- o Fluvoxamine (Luvox): Starting dose of 25 mg/day; increase to 50–200 mg/day for children, 100–300 mg/day for teens.
- o Sertraline (Zoloft): Starting dose of 25 mg/day; increase to 50–150 mg/day for children, 50–200 mg/day for teens.
- o Escitalopram (Lexapro): Indicated for 12- to 17-year-olds, start at 10 mg/day, may increase dose after 3 weeks, max dose is 20 mg/day, titrate gradually to discontinue.
- Following remission of symptoms, continue medications *with* therapy for at least several months given high rate of relapse, recurrence of depression. Gradually discontinue medications over 6 weeks or longer.
  b. Short-term psychotherapy, such as CBT.
  - CBT based on premise that young people with depression have distorted view of themselves, world, future. CBT focuses on changing distortions through time-limited therapy.
  - Continued therapy for several months after remission of symptoms may help consolidate skills learned, cope with aftereffects of depression, address environmental stressors, understand how young person's thoughts and behaviors could contribute to relapse.
2. Bipolar disorder.
  a. Use of mood-stabilizing medications such as lithium (Eskalith, Lithobid, lithium carbonate), valproic acid (Depakote), aripiprazole (Abilify), risperidone (Risperdal), quetiapine (Seroquel).
  - Dose lithium at 15–40 mg/kg/day, use IR form for initial titration, adjust dose based on tx response and serum levels, check serum level every 4–7 days until serum level reaches therapeutic range of 0.6–1.2 mEq/L.
    - o Monitoring parameters include pregnancy test at baseline, Ca, Cr, CBC, urinalysis, TSH at baseline, then at least q 6–12 months, EKG at baseline then q 12 months, lithium level q 6–12 months.
  - Dose valproic acid at 15 mg/kg/day, increase by 5 mg/kg/day q 7 days, adjust dose based on tx response and serum levels. Check serum level every 7 days until it reaches therapeutic range of 50–125 mcg/mL, give with food.
    - o Monitoring parameters include LFTs at baseline, then frequently, CBC with diff, coagulation tests at baseline, then periodically, ammonia.

- Dose aripiprazole at 10 mg q day, start at 2 mg q day x 2 days, then 5 mg q day, maximum dose is 30 mg/day.
  - ○ Monitoring parameters include CBC, fasting glucose, lipids, weight, or BMI and stiff or sore muscles.
- Dose risperidone at 0.5–6 mg/day; start at 0.5 mg q day, then increase by 0.5 mg/day no more frequently than q 24 hours to target 2.5 mg/day, doses < 2.5 mg/day rarely more effective.
  - ○ Monitoring parameters include fasting glucose, lipids, prolactin, CBC, weight or BMI, and stiff or sore muscles.
- Dose quetiapine at 400–600 mg/day divided bid–tid, start 25 mg bid x 1 day, then increase by 100 mg/day up to 200 mg bid by day 5.
  - ○ Monitoring parameters include lipids, fasting glucose, CBC, weight, or BMI.
  b. Do not use antidepressant medication alone; may lead to mania or rapid cycling.
  c. Psychostimulant medications frequently used to treat ADHD may worsen manic symptoms.
  d. CBT, interpersonal therapy, multifamily support groups essential part of overall treatment plan.
H. Follow-up.
  1. Monitor effectiveness of medications; address side effects, compliance issues.
  2. Monitor closely for suicidal thoughts and/or behaviors. *Note*: FDA black box warning on use of SSRI antidepressants in children and teens.
  3. Monitor blood levels to assess appropriate medication dosing.
  4. Collaborate with family, mental health treatment provider, school personnel to assess success of treatment approaches.
I. Complications.

Adverse effect of drug or medicament, unspecified, T88.7	Encounter for observation for other suspected diseases and conditions ruled out, Z03.89
Conduct disorder, unspecified, F91.9	Mental disorder, not otherwise specified, F99

  1. Increased risk for suicidal behavior: Attempts may rise, particularly among adolescent males, if depression accompanied by conduct disorder or substance abuse.
  2. Increased risk for poor psychosocial functioning.

    3. School truancy or poor academic performance.

    4. Substance abuse.

J. Education.

    1. Monitor effectiveness of medications.

    2. Educate families on signs/symptoms of both depression and mania and signs/symptoms of suicidal ideation.

BIBLIOGRAPHY

American Psychiatric Association. *Diagnostic and Statistical Manual of Mental Disorders.* 4th ed. Washington, DC: American Psychiatric Association; 2000.

American Psychiatric Association. *Diagnostic and Statistical Manual of Mental Disorders.* 5th ed. Washington, DC: American Psychiatric Association; 2013.

McGuinness TM, Keltner NL. Child and adolescent psychiatric nursing. In: Keltner NL, Bostrom CE, McGuinness TM, eds. *Psychiatric Nursing.* 6th ed. St. Louis: Mosby; 2011:459-468.

National Institute of Mental Health. Brief notes on the mental health of children and adolescents. Bethesda, MD: National Institutes of Mental Health; 2002.

National Institute of Mental Health. Child and adolescent bipolar disorder. NIH Publication No. 00-4778. Bethesda, MD: National Institute of Mental Health; 2000. http://www.nimh.nih.gov/health/topics/bipolar-disorder/index.shtml

National Institute of Mental Health. Depression in children and adolescents: A fact sheet for physicians. NIH Publication No. 00-4744. Bethesda, MD: National Institute of Mental Health; 2002.

National Institute of Mental Health. Eating disorders: about more than food. NIH Publication No. TR 14-4901. Bethesda, MD: National Institute of Mental Health; 2014.

Recommended Immunization Schedule

Figure 1. Recommended immunization schedule for persons aged 0 through 18 years – United States, 2015.

(FOR THOSE WHO FALL BEHIND OR START LATE, SEE THE CATCH-UP SCHEDULE [FIGURE 2]).

These recommendations must be read with the footnotes that follow. For those who fall behind or start late, provide catch-up vaccination at the earliest opportunity as indicated by the green bars in Figure 1. To determine minimum intervals between doses, see the catch-up schedule (Figure 2). School entry and adolescent vaccine age groups are shaded.

Vaccine	Birth	1 mo	2 mos	4 mos	6 mos	9 mos	12 mos	15 mos	18 mos	19–23 mos	2-3 yrs	4-6 yrs	7-10 yrs	11-12 yrs	13-15 yrs	16-18 yrs
Hepatitis B[1] (HepB)	1st dose	2nd dose			3rd dose											
Rotavirus[2] (RV) RV1 (2-dose series); RV5 (3-dose series)			1st dose	2nd dose	See footnote 2											
Diphtheria, tetanus, & acellular pertussis[3] (DTaP: <7 yrs)			1st dose	2nd dose	3rd dose			4th dose				5th dose				
Tetanus, diphtheria, & acellular pertussis[3] (Tdap: ≥7 yrs)														(Tdap)		
Haemophilus influenzae type b[4] (Hib)			1st dose	2nd dose	See footnote 5		3rd or 4th dose, See footnote 5									
Pneumococcal conjugate[5] (PCV13)			1st dose	2nd dose	3rd dose		4th dose									
Pneumococcal polysaccharide[5] (PPSV23)																
Inactivated poliovirus[6] (IPV: <18 yrs)			1st dose	2nd dose	3rd dose							4th dose				
Influenza[7] (IIV; LAIV) 2 doses for some: See footnote 8					Annual vaccination (IIV only) 1 or 2 doses						Annual vaccination (LAIV or IIV) 1 or 2 doses				Annual vaccination (LAIV or IIV) 1 dose only	
Measles, mumps, rubella[8] (MMR)					See footnote 9		1st dose					2nd dose				
Varicella[9] (VAR)							1st dose					2nd dose				
Hepatitis A[10] (HepA)							2-dose series, See footnote 11									
Human papillomavirus[11] (HPV2: females only; HPV4: males and females)											See footnote 13			(3-dose series)		
Meningococcal[12] (Hib-MenCY ≥ 6 weeks; MenACWY-D ≥9 mos; MenACWY-CRM ≥ 2 mos)														1st dose		Booster

Legend:
- Range of recommended ages for all children
- Range of recommended ages for catch-up immunization
- Range of recommended ages for certain high-risk groups
- Range of recommended ages during which catch-up is encouraged and for certain high-risk groups
- Not routinely recommended

This schedule includes recommendations in effect as of January 1, 2015. Any dose not administered at the recommended age should be administered at a subsequent visit, when indicated and feasible. The use of a combination vaccine generally is preferred over separate injections of its equivalent component vaccines. Vaccination providers should consult the relevant Advisory Committee on Immunization Practices (ACIP) statement for detailed recommendations, available online at http://www.cdc.gov/vaccines/hcp/acip-recs/index.html. Clinically significant adverse events that follow vaccination should be reported to the Vaccine Adverse Event Reporting System (VAERS) online (http://www.vaers.hhs.gov) or by telephone (800-822-7967). Suspected cases of vaccine-preventable diseases should be reported to the state or local health department. Additional information, including precautions and contraindications for vaccination, is available from CDC online (http://www.cdc.gov/vaccines/recs/vac-admin/contraindications.htm) or by telephone (800-CDC-INFO [800-232-4636]).

This schedule is approved by the Advisory Committee on Immunization Practices (http://www.cdc.gov/vaccines/acip), the American Academy of Pediatrics (http://www.aap.org), the American Academy of Family Physicians (http://www.aafp.org), and the American College of Obstetricians and Gynecologists (http://www.acog.org).

NOTE: The above recommendations must be read along with the footnotes of this schedule.

FIGURE 2. Catch-up immunization schedule for persons aged 4 months through 18 years who start late or who are more than 1 month behind —United States, 2015.

The figure below provides catch-up schedules and minimum intervals between doses for children whose vaccinations have been delayed. A vaccine series does not need to be restarted, regardless of the time that has elapsed between doses. Use the section appropriate for the child's age. Always use this table in conjunction with Figure 1 and the footnotes that follow.

Vaccine	Minimum Age for Dose 1	Dose 1 to Dose 2	Dose 2 to Dose 3	Dose 3 to Dose 4	Dose 4 to Dose 5
		Children age 4 months through 6 years			
			Minimum Interval Between Doses		
Hepatitis B[1]	Birth	4 weeks	8 weeks and at least 16 weeks after first dose. Minimum age for the final dose is 24 weeks.		
Rotavirus[2]	6 weeks	4 weeks	4 weeks[2]		6 months[3]
Diphtheria, tetanus, and acellular pertussis[3]	6 weeks	4 weeks	4 weeks	6 months	
Haemophilus influenzae type b[4]	6 weeks	4 weeks if first dose was administered before the 1st birthday. 8 weeks (as final dose) if first dose was administered at age 12 through 14 months. No further doses needed if first dose was administered at age 15 months or older.	4 weeks[4] if current age is younger than 12 months and first dose was administered at younger than age 7 months, and at least 1 previous dose was PRP-T (ActHib, Pentacel) or unknown. 8 weeks (as final dose)[4] and age 12 months through 59 months (as final dose)[4] · if current age is younger than 12 months and first dose was administered at age 7 through 11 months; OR · if current age is 12 through 59 months and first dose was administered before the 1st birthday, and second dose administered at younger than 15 months; OR · If both doses were PRP-OMP (PedvaxHIB, Comvax) and were administered before the 1st birthday. No further doses needed if previous dose was administered at age 15 months or older.	8 weeks (as final dose) This dose only necessary for children age 12 through 59 months who received 3 doses before the 1st birthday.	
Pneumococcal[5]	6 weeks	4 weeks if first dose administered before the 1st birthday. 8 weeks (as final dose for healthy children) if first dose was administered at the 1st birthday or after. No further doses needed for healthy children if first dose administered at age 24 months or older.	4 weeks if current age is younger than 12 months and previous dose given at <7months old. 8 weeks (as final dose for healthy children) if previous dose given between 7-11 months (wait until at least 12 months old); OR if current age is 12 months or older and at least 1 dose was given before age 12 months. No further doses needed for healthy children if previous dose administered at age 24 months or older.	8 weeks (as final dose) This dose only necessary for children aged 12 through 59 months who received 3 doses before age 12 months or for children at high risk who received 3 doses at any age.	
Inactivated poliovirus[6]	6 weeks	4 weeks[6]	4 weeks[6]	6 months[6] (minimum age 4 years for final dose).	
Meningococcal[7]	6 weeks	8 weeks[7]	See footnote 13	See footnote 13	
Measles, mumps, rubella[8]	12 months	4 weeks			
Varicella[9]	12 months	3 months			
Hepatitis A[10]	12 months	6 months			
		Children and adolescents age 7 through 18 years			
Tetanus, diphtheria, tetanus, diphtheria, and acellular pertussis[11]	7 years[11]	4 weeks	4 weeks if first dose of DTaP/DT was administered before the 1st birthday. 6 months (as final dose) if first dose of DTaP/DT was administered at or after the 1st birthday.	6 months if first dose of DTaP/DT was administered before the 1st birthday.	
Human papillomavirus[12]	9 years	Routine dosing intervals are recommended.[12]			
Hepatitis A[10]	Not applicable (N/A)	6 months			
Hepatitis B[1]	N/A	4 weeks	8 weeks and at least 16 weeks after first dose.		
Inactivated poliovirus[6]	N/A	4 weeks	4 weeks[6]	6 months[6]	
Meningococcal[7]	N/A	8 weeks[13]	See footnote 13		
Measles, mumps, rubella[8]	N/A	4 weeks			
Varicella[9]	N/A	3 months if younger than age 13 years. 4 weeks if age 13 years or older.			

NOTE: The above recommendations must be read along with the footnotes of this schedule.

Footnotes — Recommended immunization schedule for persons aged 0 through 18 years—United States, 2015

For further guidance on the use of the vaccines mentioned below, see: http://www.cdc.gov/vaccines/hcp/acip-recs/index.html.

For vaccine recommendations for persons 19 years of age and older, see the Adult Immunization Schedule.

Additional information

- For contraindications and precautions to use of a vaccine and for additional information regarding that vaccine, vaccination providers should consult the relevant ACIP statement available online at http://www.cdc.gov/vaccines/hcp/acip-recs/index.html.
- For purposes of calculating intervals between doses, 4 weeks = 28 days. Intervals of 4 months or greater are determined by calendar months.
- Vaccine doses administered 4 days or less before the minimum interval are considered valid. Doses of any vaccine administered ≥5 days earlier than the minimum interval or minimum age should not be counted as valid doses and should be repeated as age-appropriate. The repeat dose should be spaced after the invalid dose by the recommended minimum interval. For further details, see MMWR, *General Recommendations on Immunization and Reports / Vol. 60 / No. 2; Table 1. Recommended and minimum ages and intervals between vaccine doses available online at* http://www.cdc.gov/mmwr/pdf/rr/rr6002.pdf.
- Information on travel vaccine requirements and recommendations is available at http://wwwnc.cdc.gov/travel/destinations/list.
- For vaccination of persons with primary and secondary immunodeficiencies, see Table 13. "Vaccination of persons with primary and secondary immunodeficiencies," in *General Recommendations on Immunization* (ACIP), available at http://www.cdc.gov/mmwr/pdf/rr/rr6002.pdf; and American Academy of Pediatrics. "Immunization in Special Clinical Circumstances," in Pickering LK, Baker CJ, Kimberlin DW, Long SS eds. *Red Book: 2012 report of the Committee on Infectious Diseases. 29th ed.* Elk Grove Village, IL: American Academy of Pediatrics.

1. Hepatitis B (HepB) vaccine. (Minimum age: birth)

Routine vaccination:

At birth:

- Administer monovalent HepB vaccine to all newborns before hospital discharge.
- For infants born to hepatitis B surface antigen (HBsAg)-positive mothers, administer HepB vaccine and 0.5 mL of hepatitis B immune globulin (HBIG) within 12 hours of birth. These infants should be tested for HBsAg and antibody to HBsAg (anti-HBs) 1 to 2 months after completion of the HepB series at age 9 through 18 months (preferably at the next well-child visit).
- If mother's HBsAg status is unknown, within 12 hours of birth administer HepB vaccine regardless of birth weight. For infants weighing less than 2,000 grams, administer HBIG in addition to HepB vaccine within 12 hours of birth. Determine mother's HBsAg status as soon as possible and, if mother is HBsAg-positive, also administer HBIG for infants weighing 2,000 grams or more as soon as possible, but no later than age 7 days.

Doses following the birth dose:

- The second dose should be administered at age 1 or 2 months. Monovalent HepB vaccine should be used for doses administered before age 6 weeks.
- Infants who did not receive a birth dose should receive 3 doses of a HepB-containing vaccine on a schedule of 0, 1 to 2 months, and 6 months starting as soon as feasible. See Figure 2.
- Administer the second dose 1 to 2 months after the first dose (minimum interval of 4 weeks), administer the third dose at least 8 weeks after the second dose AND at least 16 weeks after the first dose. The final (third or fourth) dose in the HepB vaccine series should be administered no earlier than age 24 weeks.
- Administration of a total of 4 doses of HepB vaccine is permitted when a combination vaccine containing HepB is administered after the birth dose.

Catch-up vaccination:

- Unvaccinated persons should complete a 3-dose series.
- A 2-dose series (doses separated by at least 4 months) of adult formulation Recombivax HB is licensed for use in children aged 11 through 15 years.
- For other catch-up guidance, see Figure 2.

2. Rotavirus (RV) vaccines. (Minimum age: 6 weeks for both RV1 [Rotarix] and RV5 [RotaTeq])

Routine vaccination:

Administer a series of RV vaccine to all infants as follows:

1. If Rotarix is used, administer a 2-dose series at 2 and 4 months of age.
2. If RotaTeq is used, administer a 3-dose series at ages 2, 4, and 6 months.
3. If any dose in the series was RotaTeq or vaccine product is unknown for any dose in the series, a total of 3 doses of RV vaccine should be administered.

Catch-up vaccination:

- The maximum age for the first dose in the series is 14 weeks, 6 days; vaccination should not be initiated for infants aged 15 weeks, 0 days or older.
- The maximum age for the final dose in the series is 8 months, 0 days.
- For other catch-up guidance, see Figure 2.

3. Diphtheria and tetanus toxoids and acellular pertussis (DTaP) vaccine. (Minimum age: 6 weeks. Exception: DTaP-IPV [Kinrix]; 4 years)

Routine vaccination:

- Administer a 5-dose series of DTaP vaccine at ages 2, 4, 6, 15 through 18 months, and 4 through 6 years. The fourth dose may be administered as early as age 12 months, provided at least 6 months have elapsed since the third dose. However, the fourth dose of DTaP need not be repeated if it was administered at least 4 months after the third dose of DTaP.

3. Diphtheria and tetanus toxoids and acellular pertussis (DTaP) vaccine (cont'd)

Catch-up vaccination:

- The fifth dose of DTaP vaccine is not necessary if the fourth dose was administered at age 4 years or older.
- For other catch-up guidance, see Figure 2.

4. Tetanus and diphtheria toxoids and acellular pertussis (Tdap) vaccine. (Minimum age: 10 years for both Boostrix and Adacel)

Routine vaccination:

- Administer 1 dose of Tdap vaccine to all adolescents aged 11 through 12 years.
- Tdap may be administered regardless of the interval since the last tetanus and diphtheria toxoid-containing vaccine.
- Administer 1 dose of Tdap vaccine to pregnant adolescents during each pregnancy (preferably during 27 through 36 weeks gestation) regardless of time since prior Td or Tdap vaccination.

Catch-up vaccination:

- Persons aged 7 years and older who are not fully immunized with DTaP vaccine should receive Tdap vaccine as 1 dose (preferably the first) in the catch-up series; if additional doses are needed, use Td vaccine. For children 7 through 10 years who receive a dose of Tdap as part of the catch-up series, an adolescent Tdap vaccine dose at age 11 through 12 years should NOT be administered. Td should be administered instead 10 years after the Tdap dose.
- Persons aged 11 through 18 years who have not received Tdap vaccine should receive a dose followed by tetanus and diphtheria toxoid (Td) booster doses every 10 years thereafter.
- Inadvertent doses of DTaP vaccine:
  - If administered inadvertently to a child aged 7 through 10 years may count as part of the catch-up series. This dose may count as the adolescent Tdap dose, or the child can later receive a Tdap booster dose at age 11 through 12 years.
  - If administered inadvertently to an adolescent aged 11 through 18 years, the dose should be counted as the adolescent Tdap booster.
- For other catch-up guidance, see Figure 2.

5. Haemophilus influenzae type b (Hib) conjugate vaccine. (Minimum age: 6 weeks for PRP-T [ACTHIB, DTaP-IPV/Hib (Pentacel) and Hib-MenCY (MenHibrix)], PRP-OMP [PedvaxHIB or COMVAX], 12 months for PRP-T [Hiberix])

Routine vaccination:

- Administer a 2- or 3-dose Hib vaccine primary series and a booster dose (dose 3 or 4 depending on vaccine used in primary series) at age 12 through 15 months to complete a full Hib vaccine series.
- The primary series with ActHIB, MenHibrix, or Pentacel consists of 3 doses and should be administered at 2, 4, and 6 months of age. The primary series with Pedvaxhib or COMVAX consists of 2 doses and should be administered at 2 and 4 months of age; a dose at age 6 months is not indicated.
- One booster dose (dose 3 or 4 depending on vaccine used in primary series) of any Hib vaccine should be used for the booster dose at age 12 through 15 months. An exception is Hiberix vaccine. Hiberix should only be used for the booster (final) dose in children aged 12 months through 4 years who have received at least 1 prior dose of Hib-containing vaccine.
- For recommendations on the use of MenHibrix in patients at increased risk for meningococcal disease, please refer to the meningococcal vaccine footnotes and also to MMWR February 28, 2014 / 63(RR01):1-13, available at http://www.cdc.gov/mmwr/PDF/rr/rr6301.pdf.

For further guidance on the use of the vaccines mentioned below, see: http://www.cdc.gov/vaccines/hcp/acip-recs/index.html.

5. _Haemophilus influenzae_ type b (Hib) conjugate vaccine (cont'd)

Catch-up vaccination:

- If dose 1 was administered at ages 12 through 14 months, administer a second (final) dose at least 8 weeks after dose 1, regardless of Hib vaccine used in the primary series.
- If both doses were PRP-OMP (PedvaxHIB or COMVAX), and were administered before the first birthday, the third (and final) dose should be administered at age 12 through 59 months and at least 8 weeks after the second dose.
- If the first dose was administered at age 7 through 11 months, administer the second dose at least 4 weeks later and a third (and final) dose at age 12 through 15 months or 8 weeks after second dose, whichever is later.
- If first dose is administered before the first birthday and second dose administered at younger than 15 months, a third (and final) dose should be given 8 weeks later.
- For unvaccinated children aged 15 months or older, administer only 1 dose.
- For other catch-up guidance, see Figure 2. For catch-up guidance related to MenHibrix, please see the meningococcal vaccine footnotes and also MMWR February 28, 2014 / 63;(RR01);1-13, available at http://www.cdc.gov/mmwr/PDF/rr/rr6301.pdf.

Vaccination of persons with high-risk conditions:

- Children aged 12 through 59 months who are at increased risk for Hib disease, including chemotherapy recipients and those with anatomic or functional asplenia (including sickle cell disease), human immunodeficiency virus (HIV) infection, immunoglobulin deficiency, or early component complement deficiency, who have received either no doses or only 1 dose of Hib vaccine before 12 months of age, should receive 2 additional doses of Hib vaccine 8 weeks apart; children who received 2 or more doses of Hib vaccine before 12 months of age should receive 1 additional dose.
- For patients younger than 5 years of age undergoing chemotherapy or radiation treatment who received a Hib vaccine dose(s) within 14 days of starting therapy or during therapy, repeat the dose(s) at least 3 months following therapy completion.
- Recipients of hematopoietic stem cell transplant (HSCT) should be revaccinated with a 3-dose regimen of Hib vaccine starting 6 to 12 months after successful transplant, regardless of vaccination history; doses should be administered at least 4 weeks apart.
- A single dose of any Hib-containing vaccine should be administered to unimmunized* children and adolescents 15 months of age and older undergoing an elective splenectomy; if possible, vaccine should be administered at least 14 days before procedure.
- Hib vaccine is not routinely recommended for patients 5 years or older. However, 1 dose of Hib vaccine should be administered to unimmunized* persons aged 5 years or older who have anatomic or functional asplenia (including sickle cell disease) and unvaccinated persons 5 through 18 years of age with human immunodeficiency virus (HIV) infection.

  Patients who have not received a primary series and booster dose or at least 1 dose of Hib vaccine after 14 months of age are considered unimmunized.

6. Pneumococcal vaccines. (Minimum age: 6 weeks for PCV13, 2 years for PPSV23)

Routine vaccination with PCV13:

- Administer a 4-dose series of PCV13 vaccine at ages 2, 4, and 6 months and at age 12 through 15 months.
- For children aged 14 through 59 months who have received an age-appropriate series of 7-valent PCV (PCV7), administer a single supplemental dose of 13-valent PCV (PCV13).

Catch-up vaccination with PCV13:

- Administer 1 dose of PCV13 to all healthy children aged 24 through 59 months who are not completely vaccinated for their age.
- For other catch-up guidance, see Figure 2.

Vaccination of persons with high-risk conditions with PCV13 and PPSV23:

- All recommended PCV13 doses should be administered prior to PPSV23 vaccination if possible.
- For children 2 through 5 years of age with any of the following conditions: chronic heart disease (particularly cyanotic congenital heart disease and cardiac failure); chronic lung disease (including asthma if treated with high-dose oral corticosteroid therapy); diabetes mellitus; cerebrospinal fluid leak; cochlear implant; sickle cell disease and other hemoglobinopathies; anatomic or functional asplenia; HIV infection; chronic renal failure; nephrotic syndrome; diseases associated with immunosuppressive drugs or radiation therapy, including malignant neoplasms, leukemias, lymphomas, and Hodgkin's disease; solid organ transplantation; or congenital immunodeficiency:
  1. Administer 1 dose of PCV13 if any incomplete schedule of 3 doses of PCV (PCV7 and/or PCV13) were received previously.
  2. Administer 2 doses of PCV13 at least 8 weeks apart if unvaccinated or any incomplete schedule of fewer than 3 doses of PCV (PCV7 and/or PCV13) were received previously.
  3. Administer 1 supplemental dose of PCV13 if 4 doses of PCV7 or other age-appropriate complete PCV7 series was received previously.
  4. The minimum interval between doses of PCV (PCV7 or PCV13) is 8 weeks.
  5. For children with no history of PPSV23 vaccination, administer PPSV23 at least 8 weeks after the most recent dose of PCV13.

6. Pneumococcal vaccines (cont'd)

- For children aged 6 through 18 years who have cerebrospinal fluid leak; cochlear implant; sickle cell disease and other hemoglobinopathies; anatomic or functional asplenia; congenital or acquired immunodeficiencies; HIV infection; chronic renal failure; nephrotic syndrome; diseases associated with treatment with immunosuppressive drugs or radiation therapy, including malignant neoplasms, leukemias, lymphomas, and Hodgkin's disease; generalized malignancy; solid organ transplantation; or multiple myeloma:
  1. If neither PCV13 nor PPSV23 has been received previously, administer 1 dose of PCV13 now and 1 dose of PPSV23 at least 8 weeks later.
  2. If PCV13 has been received previously but PPSV23 has not, administer 1 dose of PPSV23 at least 8 weeks after the most recent dose of PCV13.
  3. If PPSV23 has been received but PCV13 has not, administer 1 dose of PCV13 at least 8 weeks after the most recent dose of PPSV23.

- For children aged 6 through 18 years with chronic heart disease (particularly cyanotic congenital heart disease and cardiac failure), chronic lung disease (including asthma if treated with high-dose oral corticosteroid therapy), diabetes mellitus, alcoholism, or chronic liver disease, who have not received PPSV23, administer 1 dose of PPSV23. If PCV13 has been received previously, then PPSV23 should be administered at least 8 weeks after any prior PCV13 dose.

- A single revaccination with PPSV23 should be administered 5 years after the first dose to children with sickle cell disease or other hemoglobinopathies; anatomic or functional asplenia; congenital or acquired immunodeficiencies; HIV infection; chronic renal failure; nephrotic syndrome; diseases associated with treatment with immunosuppressive drugs or radiation therapy, including malignant neoplasms, leukemias, lymphomas, and Hodgkin's disease; generalized malignancy; solid organ transplantation; or multiple myeloma.

7. Inactivated poliovirus vaccine (IPV). (Minimum age: 6 weeks)

Routine vaccination:

- Administer a 4-dose series of IPV at ages 2, 4, 6 through 18 months, and 4 through 6 years. The final dose in the series should be administered on or after the fourth birthday and at least 6 months after the previous dose.

Catch-up vaccination:

- In the first 6 months of life, minimum age and minimum intervals are only recommended if the person is at risk of imminent exposure to circulating poliovirus (i.e. travel to a polio-endemic region or during an outbreak).
- If 4 or more doses are administered before age 4 years, an additional dose should be administered at age 4 through 6 years and at least 6 months after the previous dose.
- A fourth dose is not necessary if the third dose was administered at age 4 years or older and at least 6 months after the previous dose.
- If both OPV and IPV were administered as part of a series, a total of 4 doses should be administered, regardless of the child's current age. IPV is not routinely recommended for U.S. residents aged 18 years or older.
- For other catch-up guidance, see Figure 2.

8. Influenza vaccines. (Minimum age: 6 months for inactivated influenza vaccine [IIV], 2 years for live, attenuated influenza vaccine [LAIV])

Routine vaccination:

- Administer influenza vaccine annually to all children beginning at age 6 months. For most healthy, nonpregnant persons aged 2 through 49 years, either LAIV or IIV may be used. However, LAIV should NOT be administered to some persons, including 1) persons who have experienced severe allergic reactions to LAIV, any of its components, or to a previous dose of any other influenza vaccine; 2) children 2 through 17 years who are receiving aspirin or aspirin-containing products; 3) persons who are allergic to eggs; 4) pregnant women; 5) immunosuppressed persons; 6) children 2 through 4 years of age with asthma or who had wheezing in the past 12 months; or 7) persons who have taken influenza antiviral medications in the previous 48 hours. For all other contraindications and precautions to use of LAIV, see MMWR August 15, 2014 / 63(32);691-697 [40 pages] available at http://www.cdc.gov/mmwr/pdf/wk/mm6332.pdf.

For children aged 6 months through 8 years:

- For the 2014–15 season, administer 2 doses (separated by at least 4 weeks) to children who are receiving influenza vaccine for the first time. Some children in this age group who have been vaccinated previously will also need 2 doses. For additional guidance, follow dosing guidelines in the 2014–15 ACIP influenza vaccine recommendations, MMWR August 15, 2014 / 63(32);691-697 [40 pages] available at http://www.cdc.gov/mmwr/pdf/wk/mm6332.pdf.
- For the 2015–16 season, follow dosing guidelines in the 2015 ACIP influenza vaccine recommendations.

For persons aged 9 years and older:

- Administer 1 dose.

For further guidance on the use of the vaccines mentioned below, see: http://www.cdc.gov/vaccines/hcp/acip-recs/index.html.

9. **Measles, mumps, and rubella (MMR) vaccine. (Minimum age: 12 months for routine vaccination)**

Routine vaccination:
- Administer a 2-dose series of MMR vaccine at ages 12 through 15 months and 4 through 6 years. The second dose may be administered before age 4 years, provided at least 4 weeks have elapsed since the first dose.
- Administer 1 dose of MMR vaccine to infants aged 6 through 11 months before departure from the United States for international travel. These children should be revaccinated with 2 doses of MMR vaccine, the first at age 12 through 15 months (12 months if the child remains in an area where disease risk is high), and the second dose at least 4 weeks later.
- Administer 2 doses of MMR vaccine to children aged 12 months and older before departure from the United States for international travel. The first dose should be administered on or after age 12 months and the second dose at least 4 weeks later.

Catch-up vaccination:
- Ensure that all school-aged children and adolescents have had 2 doses of MMR vaccine; the minimum interval between the 2 doses is 4 weeks.

10. **Varicella (VAR) vaccine. (Minimum age: 12 months)**

Routine vaccination:
- Administer a 2-dose series of VAR vaccine at ages 12 through 15 months and 4 through 6 years. The second dose may be administered before age 4 years, provided at least 3 months have elapsed since the first dose. If the second dose was administered at least 4 weeks after the first dose, it can be accepted as valid.

Catch-up vaccination:
- Ensure that all persons aged 7 through 18 years without evidence of immunity (see MMWR 2007 / 56 [No. RR-4], available at http://www.cdc.gov/mmwr/pdf/rr/rr5604.pdf) have 2 doses of varicella vaccine. For children aged 7 through 12 years, the recommended minimum interval between doses is 3 months (if the second dose was administered at least 4 weeks after the first dose, it can be accepted as valid); for persons aged 13 years and older, the minimum interval between doses is 4 weeks.

11. **Hepatitis A (HepA) vaccine. (Minimum age: 12 months)**

Routine vaccination:
- Initiate the 2-dose HepA vaccine series at 12 through 23 months; separate the 2 doses by 6 to 18 months.
- Children who have received 1 dose of HepA vaccine before age 24 months should receive a second dose 6 to 18 months after the first dose.
- For any person aged 2 years and older who has not already received the HepA vaccine series, 2 doses of HepA vaccine, separated by 6 to 18 months, may be administered if immunity against hepatitis A virus infection is desired.

Catch-up vaccination:
- The minimum interval between the two doses is 6 months.

Special populations:
- Administer 2 doses of HepA vaccine at least 6 months apart to previously unvaccinated persons who live in areas where vaccination programs target older children, or who are at increased risk for infection. This includes persons traveling to or working in countries that have high or intermediate endemicity of infection; men having sex with men; users of injection and non-injection illicit drugs; persons who work with HAV-infected primates or with HAV in a research laboratory; persons with chronic liver disease; and persons who anticipate close personal contact (e.g., household or regular babysitting) with an international adoptee during the first 60 days after arrival in the United States from a country with high or intermediate endemicity. The first dose should be administered as soon as the adoption is planned, ideally 2 or more weeks before the arrival of the adoptee.

12. **Human papillomavirus (HPV) vaccines. (Minimum age: 9 years for HPV2 [Cervarix] and HPV4 [Gardasil])**

Routine vaccination:
- Administer a 3-dose series of HPV vaccine on a schedule of 0, 1–2, and 6 months to all adolescents aged 11 through 12 years. Either HPV4 or HPV2 may be used for females, and only HPV4 may be used for males.
- The vaccine series may be started at age 9 years.
- Administer the second dose 1 to 2 months after the first dose (minimum interval of 4 weeks); administer the third dose 24 weeks after the first dose and 16 weeks after the second dose (minimum interval of 12 weeks).

Catch-up vaccination:
- Administer the vaccine series to females (either HPV2 or HPV4) and males (HPV4) at age 13 through 18 years if not previously vaccinated.
- Use recommended routine dosing intervals (see Routine vaccination above) for vaccine series catch-up.

13. **Meningococcal conjugate vaccines. (Minimum age: 6 weeks for Hib-MenCY [MenHibrix], 9 months for MenACWY-D [Menactra], 2 months for MenACWY-CRM [Menveo])**

Routine vaccination:
- Administer a single dose of Menactra or Menveo vaccine at age 11 through 12 years, with a booster dose at age 16 years.
- Adolescents aged 11 through 18 years with human immunodeficiency virus (HIV) infection should receive a 2-dose primary series of Menactra or Menveo with at least 8 weeks between doses.
- For children aged 2 months through 18 years with high-risk conditions, see below.

Catch-up vaccination:
- Administer Menactra or Menveo vaccine at age 13 through 18 years if not previously vaccinated.
- If the first dose is administered at age 13 through 15 years, a booster dose should be administered at age 16 through 18 years with a minimum interval of at least 8 weeks between doses.
- If the first dose is administered at age 16 years or older, a booster dose is not needed.
- For other catch-up guidance, see Figure 2.

Vaccination of persons with high-risk conditions and other persons at increased risk of disease:
- Children with anatomic or functional asplenia (including sickle cell disease):
  1. Menveo
     o Children who initiate vaccination at 8 weeks through 6 months: Administer doses at 2, 4, 6, and 12 months of age.
     o Unvaccinated children 7 through 23 months: Administer 2 doses, with the second dose at least 12 weeks after the first dose AND after the first birthday.
     o Children 24 months and older who have not received a complete series: Administer 2 primary doses at least 8 weeks apart.
  2. MenHibrix
     o Children 6 weeks through 18 months: Administer doses at 2, 4, 6, and 12 through 15 months of age.
     o If the first dose of MenHibrix is given at or after 12 months of age, a total of 2 doses should be given at least 8 weeks apart to ensure protection against serogroups C and Y meningococcal disease.
  3. Menactra
     o Children 24 months and older who have not received a complete series: Administer 2 primary doses at least 8 weeks apart. If Menactra is administered to a child with asplenia (including sickle cell disease), do not administer Menactra until 2 years of age and at least 4 weeks after the completion of all PCV13 doses.
- Children with persistent complement component deficiency:
  1. Menveo
     o Children who initiate vaccination at 8 weeks through 6 months: Administer doses at 2, 4, 6, and 12 months of age.
     o Unvaccinated children 7 through 23 months: Administer 2 doses, with the second dose at least 12 weeks after the first dose AND after the first birthday.
     o Children 24 months and older who have not received a complete series: Administer 2 primary doses at least 8 weeks apart.
  2. MenHibrix
     o Children 6 weeks through 18 months: Administer doses at 2, 4, 6, and 12 through 15 months of age.
     o If the first dose of MenHibrix is given at or after 12 months of age, a total of 2 doses should be given at least 8 weeks apart to ensure protection against serogroups C and Y meningococcal disease.
  3. Menactra
     o Children 9 through 23 months: Administer 2 primary doses at least 12 weeks apart.
     o Children 24 months and older who have not received a complete series: Administer 2 primary doses at least 8 weeks apart.
- For children who travel to or reside in countries in which meningococcal disease is hyperendemic or epidemic, including countries in the African meningitis belt or the Hajj, administer an age-appropriate formulation and series of Menactra or Menveo for protection against serogroups A and W meningococcal disease. Prior receipt of MenHibrix is not sufficient for children traveling to the meningitis belt or the Hajj because it does not contain serogroups A or W.
- For children at risk during a community outbreak attributable to a vaccine serogroup, administer or complete an age- and formulation-appropriate series of MenHibrix, Menactra, or Menveo.
- For booster doses among persons with high-risk conditions, refer to MMWR 2013 / 62(RR02):1–22, available at http://www.cdc.gov/mmwr/preview/mmwrhtml/rr6202a1.htm.

For other catch-up recommendations for these persons, and complete information on use of meningococcal vaccines, including guidance related to vaccination of persons at increased risk of infection, see MMWR March 22, 2013 / 62(RR02):1–22, available at http://www.cdc.gov/mmwr/pdf/rr/rr6202.pdf.

CS 244083-B

Source: Centers for Disease Control and Prevention. Recommended immunization schedules for persons aged 0 through 18 years—United States, 2015. http://www.cdc.gov/vaccines/schedules/downloads/child/0-18yrs-child-combined-schedule.pdf

Recommended Dietary Fluoride Supplement Schedule

FLUORIDE SUPPLEMENT DOSAGE SCHEDULE—2010

Approved by the American Dental Association Council on Scientific Affairs

Age	Fluoride Ion Level in Drinking Water (ppm)[a]		
	0.3	0.3–0.6	> 0.6
Birth–6 months	None	None	None
6 months–3 years	0.25 mg/day[b]	None	None
3–6 years	0.50 mg/day	0.25 mg/day	None
6–16 years	1.0 mg/day	0.50 mg/day	None

[a] 1.0 part per million (ppm) = 1 milligram per liter (mg/L)
[b] 2.2 mg sodium fluoride contains 1 mg fluoride ion
Source: Reprinted from Rozier RG, Adair S, Graham F, et al. Evidence-based clinical recommendations on the prescription of dietary fluoride supplements for caries prevention: a report of the American Dental Association Council on Scientific Affairs. *J Am Dent Assoc.* 2010;141(12):1480-1489. Copyright (2010), with permission from Elsevier.

Children's Growth Charts

Birth to 36 months: Boys
Length-for-age and Weight-for-age percentiles

NAME _____

RECORD # _____

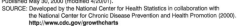

Published May 30, 2000 (modified 4/20/01).
SOURCE: Developed by the National Center for Health Statistics in collaboration with
the National Center for Chronic Disease Prevention and Health Promotion (2000).
http://www.cdc.gov/growthcharts

SAFER · HEALTHIER · PEOPLE™

639

Birth to 36 months: Boys
Head circumference-for-age and
Weight-for-length percentiles

NAME _____

RECORD # _____

Date	Age	Weight	Length	Head Circ.	Comment

Published May 30, 2000 (modified 10/16/00).
SOURCE: Developed by the National Center for Health Statistics in collaboration with
the National Center for Chronic Disease Prevention and Health Promotion (2000).
http://www.cdc.gov/growthcharts

SAFER·HEALTHIER·PEOPLE™

Birth to 36 months: Girls
Length-for-age and Weight-for-age percentiles

NAME _____

RECORD # _____

Published May 30, 2000 (modified 4/20/01).
SOURCE: Developed by the National Center for Health Statistics in collaboration with
the National Center for Chronic Disease Prevention and Health Promotion (2000).
http://www.cdc.gov/growthcharts

SAFER·HEALTHIER·PEOPLE™

Birth to 36 months: Girls
Head circumference-for-age and
Weight-for-length percentiles

NAME _____

RECORD # _____

Published May 30, 2000 (modified 10/16/00).
SOURCE: Developed by the National Center for Health Statistics in collaboration with
the National Center for Chronic Disease Prevention and Health Promotion (2000).
http://www.cdc.gov/growthcharts

SAFER·HEALTHIER·PEOPLE™

2 to 20 years: Boys
Stature-for-age and Weight-for-age percentiles

NAME _____

RECORD # _____

| Mother's Stature _____ Father's Stature _____ |||||
| Date | Age | Weight | Stature | BMI* |

*To Calculate BMI: Weight (kg) ÷ Stature (cm) ÷ Stature (cm) x 10,000
or Weight (lb) ÷ Stature (in) ÷ Stature (in) x 703

AGE (YEARS)

STATURE

WEIGHT

Published May 30, 2000 (modified 11/21/00).
SOURCE: Developed by the National Center for Health Statistics in collaboration with
the National Center for Chronic Disease Prevention and Health Promotion (2000).
http://www.cdc.gov/growthcharts

CDC
SAFER·HEALTHIER·PEOPLE™

2 to 20 years: Boys
Body mass index-for-age percentiles

NAME _____

RECORD # _____

Date	Age	Weight	Stature	BMI*	Comments

*To Calculate BMI: Weight (kg) ÷ Stature (cm) ÷ Stature (cm) x 10,000
or Weight (lb) ÷ Stature (in) ÷ Stature (in) x 703

AGE (YEARS)

Published May 30, 2000 (modified 10/16/00).
SOURCE: Developed by the National Center for Health Statistics in collaboration with
the National Center for Chronic Disease Prevention and Health Promotion (2000).
http://www.cdc.gov/growthcharts

SAFER · HEALTHIER · PEOPLE™

2 to 20 years: Girls
Stature-for-age and Weight-for-age percentiles

NAME _____

RECORD # _____

Mother's Stature _____ Father's Stature _____

Date	Age	Weight	Stature	BMI*

*To Calculate BMI: Weight (kg) ÷ Stature (cm) ÷ Stature (cm) x 10,000
or Weight (lb) ÷ Stature (in) ÷ Stature (in) x 703

Published May 30, 2000 (modified 11/21/00).
SOURCE: Developed by the National Center for Health Statistics in collaboration with
the National Center for Chronic Disease Prevention and Health Promotion (2000).
http://www.cdc.gov/growthcharts

SAFER·HEALTHIER·PEOPLE™

2 to 20 years: Girls
Body mass index-for-age percentiles

NAME _____

RECORD # _____

Date	Age	Weight	Stature	BMI*	Comments

*To Calculate BMI: Weight (kg) ÷ Stature (cm) ÷ Stature (cm) x 10,000
or Weight (lb) ÷ Stature (in) ÷ Stature (in) x 703

AGE (YEARS)

Published May 30, 2000 (modified 10/16/00).
SOURCE: Developed by the National Center for Health Statistics in collaboration with
the National Center for Chronic Disease Prevention and Health Promotion (2000).
http://www.cdc.gov/growthcharts

SAFER · HEALTHIER · PEOPLE™

BMI Table

Height (inches)	BMI	19	20	21	22	23	24	25	26	27	28	29	30	31	32	33	34	35	36	37	38	39	40	41	42	43	44	45	46	47	48	49	50	51	52	53	54
		Normal						Overweight					Obese										Extreme Obesity															
													Body Weight (pounds)																								
58		91	96	100	105	110	115	119	124	129	134	138	143	148	153	158	162	167	172	177	181	186	191	196	201	205	210	215	220	224	229	234	239	244	248	253	258
59		94	99	104	109	114	119	124	128	133	138	143	148	153	158	163	168	173	178	183	188	193	198	203	208	212	217	222	227	232	237	242	247	252	257	262	267
60		97	102	107	112	118	123	128	133	138	143	148	153	158	163	168	174	179	184	189	194	199	204	209	215	220	225	230	235	240	245	250	255	261	266	271	276
61		100	106	111	116	122	127	132	137	143	148	153	158	164	169	174	180	185	190	195	201	206	211	217	222	227	232	238	243	248	254	259	264	269	275	280	285
62		104	109	115	120	126	131	136	142	147	153	158	164	169	175	180	186	191	196	202	207	213	218	224	229	235	240	246	251	256	262	267	273	278	284	289	295
63		107	113	118	124	130	135	141	146	152	158	163	169	175	180	186	191	197	203	208	214	220	225	231	237	242	248	254	259	265	270	278	282	287	293	299	304
64		110	116	122	128	134	140	145	151	157	163	169	174	180	186	192	197	204	209	215	221	227	232	238	244	250	256	262	267	273	279	285	291	296	302	308	314
65		114	120	126	132	138	144	150	156	162	168	174	180	186	192	198	204	210	216	222	228	234	240	246	252	258	264	270	276	282	288	294	300	306	312	318	324
66		118	124	130	136	142	148	155	161	167	173	179	186	192	198	204	210	216	223	229	235	241	247	253	260	266	272	278	284	291	297	303	309	315	322	328	334
67		121	127	134	140	146	153	159	166	172	178	185	191	198	204	211	217	223	230	236	242	249	255	261	268	274	280	287	293	299	306	312	319	325	331	338	344
68		125	131	138	144	151	158	164	171	177	184	190	197	203	210	216	223	230	236	243	249	256	262	269	276	282	289	295	302	308	315	322	328	335	341	348	354
69		128	135	142	149	155	162	169	176	182	189	196	203	209	216	223	230	236	243	250	257	263	270	277	284	291	297	304	311	318	324	331	338	345	351	358	365
70		132	139	146	153	160	167	174	181	188	195	202	209	216	222	229	236	243	250	257	264	271	278	285	292	299	306	313	320	327	334	341	348	355	362	369	376
71		136	143	150	157	165	172	179	186	193	200	208	215	222	229	236	243	250	257	265	272	279	286	293	301	308	315	322	329	338	343	351	358	365	372	379	386
72		140	147	154	162	169	177	184	191	199	206	213	221	228	235	242	250	258	265	272	279	287	294	302	309	316	324	331	338	346	353	361	368	375	383	390	397
73		144	151	159	166	174	182	189	197	204	212	219	227	235	242	250	257	265	272	280	288	295	302	310	318	325	333	340	348	355	363	371	378	386	393	401	408
74		148	155	163	171	179	186	194	202	210	218	225	233	241	249	256	264	272	280	287	295	303	311	319	326	334	342	350	358	365	373	381	389	396	404	412	420
75		152	160	168	176	184	192	200	208	216	224	232	240	248	256	264	272	279	287	295	303	311	319	327	335	343	351	359	367	375	383	391	399	407	415	423	431
76		156	164	172	180	189	197	205	213	221	230	238	246	254	263	271	279	287	295	304	312	320	328	336	344	353	361	369	377	385	394	402	410	418	426	435	443

Source: Reprinted from National Heart, Lung, and Blood Institute. Body mass index table. http://www.nhlbi.nih.gov/health/educational/lose_wt/BMI/bmi_tbl.pdf

MyPlate

Source: Reproduced from the USDA Center for Nutrition Policy and Promotion's ChooseMyPlate.gov website.

Predicted Peak Flow Measurements

MaineHealth
AH! Asthma Health

Predicted Peak Flow Measurements
(based on Personal Best® peak flow meter)

Normal Children and Adolescents

Height (in)	(cm)	Males & Females
43	109	147
44	112	160
45	114	173
46	117	187
47	119	200
48	122	214
49	124	227
50	127	240
51	130	254
52	132	267
53	135	280
54	137	293
55	140	307
56	142	320
57	145	334
58	147	347
59	150	360
60	152	373
61	155	387
62	157	400
63	160	413
64	163	427
65	165	440
66	168	454

Normal Adult Males

Age (Yrs)	(in) 60 (cm)152	65 165	70 178	75 191	80 203
20	554	575	594	611	626
25	580	603	622	640	656
30	594	617	637	655	672
35	599	622	643	661	677
40	597	620	641	659	675
45	591	613	633	651	668
50	580	602	622	640	656
55	566	588	608	625	640
60	551	572	591	607	622
65	533	554	572	588	603
70	515	535	552	568	582
75	496	515	532	547	560

Normal Adult Females

Age (Yrs)	(in) 55 (cm)140	60 152	65 165	70 178	75 191
20	444	460	474	486	497
25	455	471	485	497	509
30	458	475	489	502	513
35	458	474	488	501	512
40	453	469	483	496	507
45	446	462	476	488	499
50	437	453	466	478	489
55	427	442	455	467	477
60	415	430	443	454	464
65	403	417	430	441	451
70	390	404	416	427	436
75	377	391	402	413	422

Source: Courtesy of Philips Respironics, Murrysville, PA. All rights reserved.

Asthma Management Plan

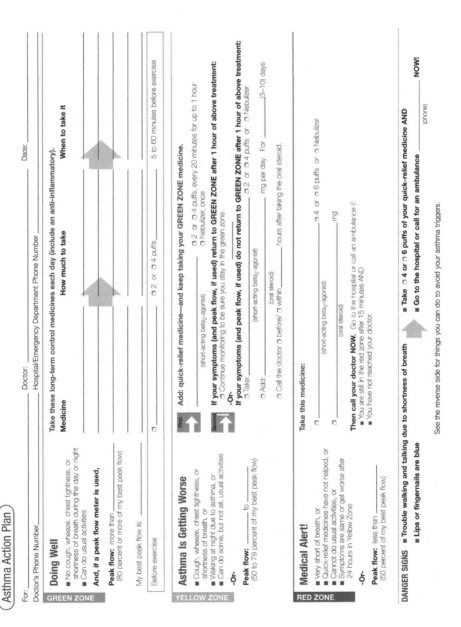

Asthma Action Plan

For: _____ Doctor: _____ Date: _____

Doctor's Phone Number _____ Hospital/Emergency Department Phone Number _____

GREEN ZONE

Doing Well

- No cough, wheeze, chest tightness, or shortness of breath during the day or night
- Can do usual activities

And, if a peak flow meter is used,

Peak flow: more than _____
(80 percent or more of my best peak flow)

My best peak flow is: _____

Take these long-term control medicines each day (include an anti-inflammatory).

Medicine	How much to take	When to take it
Before exercise	□ 2 or □ 4 puffs	5 to 60 minutes before exercise

YELLOW ZONE

Asthma Is Getting Worse

- Cough, wheeze, chest tightness, or shortness of breath, or
- Waking at night due to asthma, or
- Can do some, but not all, usual activities

-Or-

Peak flow: _____ to _____
(50 to 79 percent of my best peak flow)

First Add: quick-relief medicine—and keep taking your GREEN ZONE medicine.

_____ (short-acting beta₂-agonist)   □ 2 or □ 4 puffs, every 20 minutes for up to 1 hour   □ Nebulizer, once

Second If your symptoms (and peak flow, if used) return to GREEN ZONE after 1 hour of above treatment:
□ Continue monitoring to be sure you stay in the green zone.

-Or-

If your symptoms (and peak flow, if used) do not return to GREEN ZONE after 1 hour of above treatment:
□ Take: _____ (short-acting beta₂-agonist) □ 2 or □ 4 puffs or □ Nebulizer
□ Add: _____ (oral steroid) _____ mg per day For _____ (3–10) days
□ Call the doctor □ before/ □ within _____ hours after taking the oral steroid.

RED ZONE

Medical Alert!

- Very short of breath, or
- Quick-relief medicines have not helped, or
- Cannot do usual activities, or
- Symptoms are same or get worse after 24 hours in Yellow Zone

-Or-

Peak flow: less than _____
(50 percent of my best peak flow)

Take this medicine:

□ _____ (short-acting beta₂-agonist) □ 4 or □ 6 puffs or □ Nebulizer
□ _____ (oral steroid) _____ mg

Then call your doctor NOW. Go to the hospital or call an ambulance if:
- You are still in the red zone after 15 minutes AND
- You have not reached your doctor.

DANGER SIGNS ■ Trouble walking and talking due to shortness of breath   ■ Take □ 4 or □ 6 puffs of your quick-relief medicine AND
■ Lips or fingernails are blue   ■ Go to the hospital or call for an ambulance _____ (phone) NOW!

See the reverse side for things you can do to avoid your asthma triggers.

How To Control Things That Make Your Asthma Worse

This guide suggests things you can do to avoid your asthma triggers. Put a check next to the triggers that you know make your asthma worse and ask your doctor to help you find out if you have other triggers as well. Then decide with your doctor what steps you will take.

Allergens

☐ **Animal Dander**

Some people are allergic to the flakes of skin or dried saliva from animals with fur or feathers.

The best thing to do:
- Keep furred or feathered pets out of your home.

If you can't keep the pet outdoors, then:
- Keep the pet out of your bedroom and other sleeping areas at all times, and keep the door closed.
- Remove carpets and furniture covered with cloth from your home. If that is not possible, keep the pet away from fabric-covered furniture and carpets.

☐ **Dust Mites**

Many people with asthma are allergic to dust mites. Dust mites are tiny bugs that are found in every home—in mattresses, pillows, carpets, upholstered furniture, bedcovers, clothes, stuffed toys, and fabric or other fabric-covered items.

Things that can help:
- Encase your mattress in a special dust-proof cover.
- Encase your pillow in a special dust-proof cover or wash the pillow each week in hot water. Water must be hotter than 130° F to kill the mites. Cold or warm water used with detergent and bleach can also be effective.
- Wash the sheets and blankets on your bed each week in hot water.
- Reduce indoor humidity to below 60 percent (ideally between 30—50 percent). Dehumidifiers or central air conditioners can do this.
- Try not to sleep or lie on cloth-covered cushions.
- Remove carpets from your bedroom and those laid on concrete, if you can.
- Keep stuffed toys out of the bed or wash the toys weekly in hot water or cooler water with detergent and bleach.

☐ **Cockroaches**

Many people with asthma are allergic to the dried droppings and remains of cockroaches.

The best thing to do:
- Keep food and garbage in closed containers. Never leave food out.
- Use poison baits, powders, gels, or paste (for example, boric acid). You can also use traps.
- If a spray is used to kill roaches, stay out of the room until the odor goes away.

☐ **Indoor Mold**
- Fix leaky faucets, pipes, or other sources of water that have mold around them.
- Clean moldy surfaces with a cleaner that has bleach in it.

☐ **Pollen and Outdoor Mold**

What to do during your allergy season (when pollen or mold spore counts are high):
- Try to keep your windows closed.
- Stay indoors with windows closed from late morning to afternoon, if you can. Pollen and some mold spore counts are highest at that time.
- Ask your doctor whether you need to take or increase anti-inflammatory medicine before your allergy season starts.

Irritants

☐ **Tobacco Smoke**
- If you smoke, ask your doctor for ways to help you quit. Ask family members to quit smoking, too.
- Do not allow smoking in your home or car.

☐ **Smoke, Strong Odors, and Sprays**
- If possible, do not use a wood-burning stove, kerosene heater, or fireplace.
- Try to stay away from strong odors and sprays, such as perfume, talcum powder, hair spray, and paints.

Other things that bring on asthma symptoms in some people include:

☐ **Vacuum Cleaning**
- Try to get someone else to vacuum for you once or twice a week, if you can. Stay out of rooms while they are being vacuumed and for a short while afterward.
- If you vacuum, use a dust mask (from a hardware store), a double-layered or microfilter vacuum cleaner bag, or a vacuum cleaner with a HEPA filter.

☐ **Other Things That Can Make Asthma Worse**
- Sulfites in foods and beverages: Do not drink beer or wine or eat dried fruit, processed potatoes, or shrimp if they cause asthma symptoms.
- Cold air: Cover your nose and mouth with a scarf on cold or windy days.
- Other medicines: Tell your doctor about all the medicines you take. Include cold medicines, aspirin, vitamins and other supplements, and nonselective beta-blockers (including those in eye drops).

For More Information, go to: www.nhlbi.nih.gov

NIH Publication No. 07-5251
April 2007

U.S. Department of Health and Human Services
National Institutes of Health

National Heart
Lung and Blood Institute

Source: Reproduced from U.S. Department of Health and Human Services, National Heart, Lung, and Blood Institute. Asthma action plan.

Pediatric Dosage Schedules

		Fever 102.5°F (39.2°C) or below 5 mg/kg		Fever 102.5°F (39.2°C) or below 10 mg/kg	
IBUPROFEN SUSPENSION (ADVIL, MOTRIN) every 6 hours					
Age	**Weight (lb)**	**mg**	**tsp**	**mg**	**tsp**
6–11 months	12–17	25	¼	50	½
12–23 months	18–23	50	½	100	1
2–3 years	24–35	75	¾	150	1½
4–5 years	36–47	100	1	200	2
6–8 years	48–59	125	1¼	250	2½
9–10 years	60–71	150	1½	300	3
11–12 years	72–95	200	2	400	4

Source: Data from Motrin. Dosing charts for children & infants. http://www.motrin.com/children-infants/dosing-charts

		Dose	
ACETAMINOPHEN (TYLENOL) every 4–6 hours			
Age	**Weight (lb)**	**Tylenol Oral Suspension (160 mg/5 mL)**	**Tylenol Extra Strength (500-mg tablet)**
0–3 months	6–11	1.25 mL	–
4–11 months	12–17	2.5 mL	–
12–23 months	18–23	3.75 mL	–
24–36 months	24–35	5 mL	–
4–5 years	36–47	7.5 mL	–
6–8 years	48–59	10 mL	–
9–10 years	60–71	12.5 mL	–
11 years	72–95	15 mL	1 tablet
12 years	≥ 96	–	1 tablet

Source: Courtesy of McNeil Consumer Healthcare.

Pediatric Medications

ACYCLOVIR — ANTIVIRAL

Brand Name

Zovirax, Avirax.

Uses

Antiviral, used to treat initial and recurrent episodes of mucocutaneous herpes simplex virus (HSV-1 and HSV-2) infections in immunocompromised patients; varicella (chickenpox) infections in immunocompromised patients; acute herpes zoster infection in immunocompetent patients; herpes simplex encephalitis.

Availability

- Suspension: 200 mg/5 mL.
- Tablets: 400 mg, 800 mg.
- Capsules: 200 mg.
- Injection: 500 mg/vial, 1 g/vial.
- Cream, ointment.

Indications/Routes/Dosage

- Varicella infection in immunocompromised patients: Children age 12 years or older: 800 mg PO q4h (5 times/day while awake) for 5 days. Children age 2 years or older and weighing < 40 kg: 20 mg/kg (max: 800 mg/dose) PO qid for 5 days.
- Acute herpes zoster: Children age 12 years or older: 800 mg PO q4h (5 times/day) for 7–10 days.
- Genital herpes (initial episode): Adults: 200 mg q4h (5 times/day) for 10 days.
- Genital herpes (recurrent episode): Adults: 200 mg q4h (5 times/day) for 5 days. Usual topical dosage: Adults: 3–6 times/day for 7 days.
- Labial herpes: Apply cream to affected area 4–6 times/day for 10 days; apply ointment q3h 6 times/day for 7 days—use glove or applicator stick to apply.

Adverse Reactions

Malaise, headache, encephalopathic changes, nausea, vomiting, diarrhea hematuria, acute renal failure, thrombocytopenia, leukopenia, rash, itching, urticaria, inflammation, or phlebitis at injection site.

Implications

- May increase blood urea nitrogen (BUN) and creatinine levels. May decrease white blood count (WBC) and increase or decrease platelet count.
- Use cautiously in patients with neurologic problems, renal disease, or dehydration. Drink adequate fluids, and monitor renal function.
- Do not touch lesions with fingers to prevent spreading infection to new site, use finger cot or rubber glove to apply topical ointment.
- Avoid sexual intercourse while lesions present to prevent spread to partner.

ALBUTEROL — BRONCHODILATOR

Brand Name

Ventolin, Proventil.

Uses

Relaxes bronchial, uterine, and vascular smooth muscle to prevent or treat bronchospasm.

Availability

- Aerosol inhaler: 90 mcg/metered spray, 100 mcg/metered spray.
- Albuterol sulfate: Capsules for inhalation: 200 mcg.
- Solution for inhalation: 0.083% mg/mL, 0.5% mg/mL, 0.63 mg/mL, 1.25 mg/3 mL.
- Syrup: 2 mg/5 mL.
- Tablets: 2 mg, 4 mg.
- Tablets, extended-release: 4 mg, 8 mg.

Indications/Routes/Dosage

- Prevention/treatment of bronchospasm in patients with reversible obstructive airway disease: Aerosol inhalation: Children 4 years old or older: 1 or 2 inhalations q4–6h. Capsules for inhalation: Children 4 years old or older: 200 mcg inhaled q4–6h.

Solution for inhalation: Children 12 years old or older: 2.5 mg tid or qid by nebulizer; Children 2–12 years old: Initially, 0.1–0.15 mg/kg by nebulizer, with subsequent dosing titrated to response, not to exceed 2.5 mg tid or qid by nebulization. To prevent exercise-induced bronchospasm: 2 aerosol inhalations 15–30 min before exercise.

- Syrup or oral tablets: Children 2–6 years: Initially, 0.1 mg/kg PO tid. Starting dose should not exceed 2 mg (1 tsp) tid. Do not exceed 4 mg tid; Children 6–14 years: 2 mg PO tid or qid. Do not exceed 24 mg daily; Adults, children 14 years old or older: 2–4 mg PO tid or qid. Do not exceed 8 mg qid.
- Extended-release tablets: Children 6–12 years old: 4 mg PO q12h; Adults, children older than 12 years: 4–8 mg PO q12h.

Adverse Reactions

Nervousness, dizziness, headache, weakness, insomnia, nasal congestion, hoarseness, tachycardia, hypertension, nausea, vomiting, heartburn, increased appetite, hypokalemia, muscle cramps, bronchospasm, cough, increased sputum.

Implications

- Use caution in patients with diabetes mellitus, hypertension, or hyperthyroidism.
- Teach family how to use inhaler properly.
- Increase fluid intake.
- Do not take more than 2 inhalations at any one time to prevent paradoxical bronchoconstriction.
- Rinse mouth after inhalation.

AMOXICILLIN—ANTIBIOTIC

Brand Name

Amoxil (generic also available).

Uses

Treat otitis media, upper and lower respiratory tract, soft tissue, skin, GI, GU, and gonorrhea infections. Used to treat: Gram-positive cocci: *Staphylococcus aureus, Streptococcus pyogenes, Streptococcus faecalis, Streptococcus pneumoniae.* Gram-negative cocci: *Neisseria gonorrhoeae, Neisseria meningitidis.* Gram-positive bacillus:

Corynebacterium diphtheriae, Listeria monocytogenes. Gram-negative bacillus: *Haemophilus influenzae, Escherichia coli, Proteus mirabilis, Salmonella*; also used in bacterial endocarditis prophylaxis.

Availability

- Suspension: 125/5 mL, 200/5 mL, 250/5 mL, 400/5 mL.
- Tablets: 500 mg, 875 mg.
- Pediatric drops: 50 mg/mL.
- Tablets, chewable: 125 mg, 200 mg, 250 mg, 400 mg.
- Capsules: 250 mg, 500 mg.

Indications/Routes/Dosage

- Ear, nose, throat, GU, skin/structure infections: Children < 20 kg: 20–40 mg/kg/day divided q8–12h. Children, adults > 20 kg: 250–500 mg q8h or 500–875 mg 2 times/day.
- Lower respiratory tract infections: Children < 20 kg: 40 mg/kg/day divided q8–12h. Children, adults > 20 kg: 500 mg q8h or 875 mg tablets 2 times/day.
- Acute uncomplicated gonorrhea, epididymitis orchitis: Adults: 3 g once with 1 g probenecid PO follow with tetracycline or erythromycin.
- Acute otitis media: Children: 80–90 mg/kg/day divided bid for those at high risk.

Adverse Reactions

Mild diarrhea, rash, oral/vaginal candidiasis; superinfection, colitis, allergic reaction–anaphylaxis.

Implications

- Take all of medication.
- Report rash or severe diarrhea.
- Discard suspension after 14 days.

AMOXICILLIN CLAVULANATE—POTASSIUM ANTIBIOTIC

Brand Name

Augmentin.

Uses

Treat lower respiratory infections, otitis media, sinusitis, skin infections, urinary tract infections caused by susceptible strains of Gram-positive and Gram-negative organisms.

Availability

- Oral suspension: 125 mg/5 mL, 200 mg/5 mL, 250 mg/5 mL, 400 mg/5mL.
- Tablets: 250 mg, 500 mg, 875 mg.
- Tablets, chewable: 125 mg, 200 mg, 250 mg, 400 mg.

Indications/Routes/Dosage

- Recurrent or persistent otitis media caused by *Streptococcus pneumoniae, Haemophilus influenzae,* or *Moraxella catarrhalis:* Augmentin ES-600. Children older than 3 months: 90 mg/kg/day, based on amoxicillin component, PO q12h for 10 days.
- Lower respiratory infections, otitis media, sinusitis, skin infections, urinary tract infections caused by susceptible strains of Gram-positive and Gram-negative organisms: Adults, children weighing > 40 kg: 250 mg (based on amoxicillin component) PO q8h or 500 mg q12h. May use 500 mg PO q8h OR 875 mg PO q12h for more severe infections. Children weighing < 40 kg: 20 to 45 mg/kg, based on amoxicillin component and severity of infection, PO daily in divided doses q8–12h. Children 3 months of age or older: 30 mg/kg/day PO in divided doses q12h.

Adverse Reactions

Nausea, vomiting, diarrhea, agitation, confusion, dizziness, insomnia, enterocolitis, pseudomembranous colitis, abdominal pain, vaginitis, anemia, thrombocytopenia, hypersensitivity reactions.

Implications

- May decrease effectiveness of hormonal contraceptives.
- Oral suspensions have varying clavulanic acid content.
- Continue antibiotic for full length of treatment, take with meals.

AZITHROMYCIN—MACROLIDE ANTIBIOTIC

Brand Name

Zithromax.

Uses

Treat community-acquired pneumonia, otitis media, pharyngitis, tonsillitis, dental prophylaxis in patients allergic to penicillin, uncomplicated gonococcal infections, chlamydial infections.

Availability

- Powder for oral suspension: 100 mg/5 mL, 200 mg/5 mL, 1000 mg/packet.
- Tablets: 250 mg, 500 mg, 600 mg.
- Injection: 500 mg.

Indications/Routes/Dosage

- Otitis media: Children older than 6 months: 10 mg/kg PO daily for 3 days OR 10 mg/kg PO on day 1, then 5 mg/kg once daily on days 2–5.
- Pharyngitis, tonsillitis: Children older than 2 years: 12 mg/kg (max 500 mg) PO daily for 5 days.
- Dental prophylaxis: Adults: 500 mg PO 1 hour before procedure. Children: 15 mg/kg PO 1 hour before procedure.
- Chlamydial infections: Adults, adolescents older than 16 years: 1 g PO as a single dose.

Adverse Reactions

Dizziness, headache, fatigue, palpitations, chest pain, nausea, vomiting, diarrhea, abdominal pain, cholestatic jaundice, pseudomembranous colitis, candidiasis, vaginitis, rash, photosensitivity, angioedema.

Implications

- Use cautiously with liver impairment.
- Give oral suspension 1 hour before or 2 hours after meals.
- Do not give with antacids.

BENZOCAINE—TOPICAL OTIC ANALGESIC

Brand Name

Auralgan otic solution.

Uses

Topical analgesic to reduce pain associated with acute otitis media.

Availability

- 10-mL bottle.

Indications/Routes/Dosage

- Instill drops until ear canal is full, put wick into ear canal. May repeat every 1–2 hours as needed.

Adverse Reactions

Irritation of ear canal.

Implications

- Do not let dropper touch ear canal, do not rinse ear dropper after use, keep out of the reach of children.
- Have child lie on side and tilt the affected ear upward, pull ear lobe up, and instill medication. Have child lie on side for 5 minutes, then insert wick.
- Do not use on perforated eardrum.

BUDESONIDE—INHALATION CORTICOSTEROID ANTI-INFLAMMATORY

Brand Name

Entocort EC, Pulmicort, Rhinocort.

Uses

Manage symptoms of seasonal or perennial allergic rhinitis.

Availability

- Nasal inhaler: 32 mcg/metered spray (Rhinocort AQ).
- Nasal spray: 50 mcg/dose (Pulmicort).

- Powder for inhalation: 200 mcg/inhalation (Pulmicort Turbuhaler).
- Suspension for oral inhalation: 0.25 mg/2 mL, 0.5 mg/2 mL (Pulmicort Respules).

Indications/Routes/Dosage

- Intranasal: Children older than 6 years, adults: Rhinocort: 2 sprays each nostril 2 times/day or 4 sprays to each nostril in morning. Rhinocort Aqua: 1 spray to each nostril once daily. Children younger than 12 years: 4 sprays/day. Children older than 12 years: 8 sprays/day.
- Nebulization: Children 1–8 years: 0.25–1 mg/day titrated to lowest effective dosage.
- Inhalation: Children older than 6 years, adults: Initially 200–400 mcg 2 times/day to max 400 mcg 2 times/day.
- Rhinitis: Nasal inhalation: Children older than 6 years: Initial, 2 sprays/nostril twice daily. Adult: Initial 2 sprays/nostril bid or 4 sprays/nostril in the morning. Max 4 sprays/nostril per day.
- Nasal spray: Children older than 6 years: Initial, 1 spray/nostril once a day. Max dose 4 sprays/nostril/day. Not recommended for children younger than 6 years. Children older than 12 years: 4 sprays/nostril, once a day. Nasal spray: Initial, 1 spray/nostril once daily, max 4 sprays/nostril once a day.

Adverse Reactions

Mild nasopharyngeal irritation, burning, stinging, headache, throat irritation, epistaxis, Cushing syndrome, cataract, adrenal suppression, glaucoma.

Implications

- Use caution in patients with cataracts, diabetes mellitus, exposure to viral infections, glaucoma, liver cirrhosis, peptic ulcer.
- Do not consume grapefruit juice during oral treatment.
- Reduce dose for hepatic insufficiency.
- May take 3–7 days for full effect.

CEFDINIR — THIRD-GENERATION CEPHALOSPORIN ANTIBIOTIC

Brand Name

Omnicef.

Uses

Treat susceptible infections due to *Streptococcus pyogenes, S. pneumoniae, Haemophilus influenzae, H. parainfluenzae, Moraxella catarrhalis*, acute maxillary sinusitis, chronic bronchitis, community-acquired pneumonia, otitis media, pharyngitis/tonsillitis, skin infections.

Availability

- Suspension: 125 mg/5 mL, 250 mg/5mL.
- Capsule: 300 mg.

Indications/Routes/Dosage

- Children older than 6 months: 7 mg/kg PO q12h for 10 days or 14 mg/kg PO once a day for 10 days, max 600 mg/day.
- Children < 20 lbs: 2.5 mL (0.5 tsp) q12h or 5 mL (1 tsp) q24h.
- Children 20–40 lbs: 5 mL (1 tsp) q12h or 10 mL (2 tsp) q24h.
- Children 41–60 lbs: 7.5 mL (1.5 tsp) q12h or 15 mL (3 tsp) q24h.
- Children 61–80 lbs: 10 mL (2 tsp) q12h or 20 mL (4 tsp) q24h.
- Children 81–85 lbs: 12 mL (2.5 tsp) q12h or 24 mL (5 tsp) q24h.
- Adults: 300 mg PO q12h or 600 mg PO once a day for 10 days.

Adverse Reactions

Diarrhea, nausea, oral and vaginal candidiasis, headache.

Implications

- May take with or without food.
- Take antacids 2 hours before or after taking medication.
- Take for full length of treatment.
- Suspension can be stored at room temperature; discard after 10 days.
- Adjust dose in renal impairment.

CEFPROZIL—SECOND-GENERATION CEPHALOSPORIN ANTIBIOTIC

Brand Name

Cefzil.

Uses

Treat susceptible infections due to *Streptococcus pneumoniae, S. pyogenes, Staphylococcus aureus, Haemophilus influenzae, Moraxella catarrhalis,* acute or chronic bronchitis, secondary bacterial infection, acute sinusitis, otitis media, pharyngitis/tonsillitis, skin infections.

Availability

- Oral suspension: 125 mg/5 mL, 250 mg/5 mL.
- Tablets: 250 mg, 500 mg.

Indications/Routes/Dosage

- Acute sinusitis: Children 6 months–12 years: 7.5–15 mg/kg PO q12h for 10 days. Adults: 500 mg PO q12h for 10 days.
- Otitis media: Children 6 months–12 years: 15 mg/kg PO q12h for 10 days (max 1 g/day).
- Bronchitis: Adult: 500 mg PO q12h for 10 days.
- Pharyngitis/tonsillitis: Children 2–12 years: 7.5 mg/kg PO q12h for 10 days. Adults: 500 mg PO q24h for 10 days.
- Skin infections: Children 2–12 years: 20 mg/kg PO q24h for 10 days. Adults: 250 mg–500 mg PO q12–24h for 10 days.

Adverse Reactions

Diarrhea, nausea, vomiting, diaper rash, oral and vaginal candidiasis, dizziness, elevation of liver enzymes, severe hypersensitivity reactions.

Implications

- Refrigerate suspension; discard after 14 days.
- May take with or without food.
- Adjust dose for renal impairment.

CEFTRIAXONE — THIRD-GENERATION CEPHALOSPORIN ANTIBIOTIC

Brand Name

Rocephin.

Uses

Treat susceptible infections due to Gram-negative bacilli: *Haemophilus influenzae, Escherichia coli, Proteus mirabilis, Klebsiella, Enterobacter, Salmonella, Shigella,* Cefuroxime Sodium, Cefuroxime Axetil, *Neisseria, Serratia*; Gram-positive organisms: *Streptococcus pneumoniae, S. pyogenes, Staphylococcus aureus*; serious lower respiratory tract, urinary tract, gonorrhea, meningitis, septicemia, bone, joint infections.

Availability

- Powder for injection: 500 mg, 1 g, 2 g, 10 g.

Indications/Routes/Dosage

- Children: 50–75 mg/kg/day divided q12h; Adult: 1–2 g daily. Max 2 g q12h.
- Uncomplicated gonorrhea: Adults: 250 mg IM as a single dose.
- Meningitis: Children, adult: 100 mg/kg/day IM divided q12h. Max 4 g/day.

Adverse Reactions

Nausea, vomiting, diarrhea, anorexia, hypersensitivity, nephrotoxicity.

Implications

- Assess sensitivity to penicillin and other cephalosporins (10% crossover).
- Watch for adverse reactions.

CEFUROXIME SODIUM, CEFUROXIME AXETIL — SECOND-GENERATION CEPHALOSPORIN ANTIBIOTICS

Brand Name

Kefurox, Zinacef, Cefuroxime Axetil, Ceftin.

Uses

Treat susceptible infections due to group B streptococci, pneumococci, staphylococci, *Haemophilus influenzae, Escherichia coli, Enterobacter, Klebsiella*, bone and joint infection, gonorrhea, lower respiratory tract infections, meningitis, preoperative prophylaxis, septicemia, urinary tract infections.

Availability

- Suspension: 125 mg/5 mL, 250 mg/5 mL.
- Tablet: 250 mg, 500 mg.
- Infusion: 1.5 g/50 mL, 750 mg/50 mL.
- Injection: 1.5 g, 7.5 g, 750 mg.

Indications/Routes/Dosage

- Pharyngitis/tonsillitis: Tablets: 125 mg PO bid for 10 days. Children 3 months to 12 years: 30 mg/kg/day PO in 2 divided doses for 10 days. Max 500 mg/day.
- Impetigo, otitis media, sinusitis: Children 3 months to 12 years: 30 mg/kg/day PO in 2 divided doses for 10 days. Max 1 g/day. Tablets: 250 mg PO bid for 10 days.
- Susceptible infections: Neonates: 20–100 mg/kg/day IV in divided doses q12h. Children older than 3 months: 50–100 mg/kg/day IV/IM divided q6–8h.
- Bone and joint infections: Children older than 3 months: 150 mg/kg/day IV/IM divided q8h.
- Meningitis: Children 3 months old and older: 200–240 mg/kg/day IV/IM divided q6–8h. Max 9 g/day.
- Bronchitis: Adults: 250 or 500 mg PO bid for 10 days.
- Gonorrhea: Adults: 1 g PO as a single dose; 1.5 g IM as a single dose with 1.5 g probenecid PO.
- Gonococcal infections: Adults: 750 mg IV/IM q8h.
- Pharyngitis/tonsillitis/sinusitis: Adults: 250 mg PO bid for 10 days.
- Skin infections: Adults: 250–500 mg PO bid for 10 days.
- Urinary tract infections: Adults: 125 mg or 250 mg PO bid for 7–10 days.

Adverse Reactions

Local reactions at IV/IM site; diarrhea, abdominal cramping, nausea; oral and vaginal candidiasis.

Implications

- Adjust dose for renal impairment.
- Take antibiotic for full length of treatment.

CEPHALEXIN HYDROCHLORIDE—FIRST-GENERATION CEPHALOSPORIN ANTIBIOTIC

Brand Name

Keftab, Keflex, Biocef.

Uses

Treat infections of respiratory tract, GI tract, skin, soft tissue, bone, joints, and otitis media caused by *Escherichia coli* and other coliform bacteria, group A beta–hemolytic streptococci, *Klebsiella* species, *Proteus mirabilis, Streptococcus pneumoniae,* and staphylococci.

Availability

- Cephalexin hydrochloride: Tablets: 500 mg.
- Cephalexin monohydrate: Oral suspension: 125 mg/5 mL, 250 mg/5 mL.
- Tablets: 250 mg, 500 mg, 1 g.
- Capsules: 250 mg, 500 mg.

Indications/Routes/Dosage

- Children: 25–50 mg/kg/day PO in 2 to 4 equally divided doses.
- Adults: 250 mg–1 g PO q6h or 500 mg q12h. Max 4 g daily. Dose can be doubled in severe infections.

Adverse Reactions

Dizziness, headache, confusion, fatigue, hallucinations, nausea, vomiting, diarrhea, pseudomembranous colitis, oral candidiasis, vaginitis, genital pruritus, interstitial nephritis, neutropenia, anemia, thrombocytopenia, arthritis, joint pain, rash, urticaria, hypersensitivity reactions.

Implications

- Take with food or milk.
- There is a possibility of cross-sensitivity with penicillin and other beta-lactam antibiotics.
- Adjust dose for renal impairment.
- Avoid using with aminoglycosides, increases risk of nephrotoxicity.

CETIRIZINE—ANTIHISTAMINE

Brand Name

Zyrtec.

Uses

Rhinitis, allergic symptoms.

Availability

- Syrup: 5 mg/5 mL.
- Tablets: 5 mg, 10 mg.

Indications/Routes/Dosage

- Child 2–6 years: 2.5 mg daily may increase to 5 mg daily or 2.5 mg bid; child older than 6 years, adult: 5–10 mg daily.
- Zyrtec D (5 mg with 120 mg pseudoephedrine) 1 tablet bid.

Adverse Reactions

Thickening of bronchial secretions, dry mouth, headache, drowsiness.

Implications

- Avoid driving if drowsiness occurs; use sunscreen when in sunlight.
- Notify provider of difficulty voiding.

CIPROFLOXACIN HYDROCHLORIDE— FLUOROQUINOLONE ANTI-INFECTIVE

Brand Name

Cipro.

Uses

Treat conjunctival keratitis, keratoconjunctivitis, corneal ulcers, blepharitis, dacryocystitis, blepharoconjunctivitis.

Availability

- Ophthalmic: 0.03%; Otic (Ciprodex).

Indications/Routes/Dosage

- Conjunctivitis: 1–2 drops q2h for 2 days, then q4h next 5 days.
- Corneal ulcer: 2 drops q15min for 6h, then 2 drops q30min remainder first day; 2 drops q1h second day; then q4h days 3–14.
- Otic: Older than 6 months, 4 drops in ear bid for 7 days.

Adverse Reactions

Ophthalmic: Sensitization may contraindicate later systemic use of ciprofloxacin.

Implications

- Tilt patient's head back, put drops in conjunctival sac.
- Do not use ophthalmic solution as injection.

CLARITHROMYCIN — MACROLIDE ANTIBIOTIC

Brand Name

Biaxin, Biaxin XL.

Uses

Treat bronchitis, otitis media, acute maxillary sinusitis, pharyngitis, tonsillitis, pneumonia, skin infections.

Availability

- Suspension: 125/5 mL, 250/5 mL.
- Tablets: 250 mg, 500 mg.
- Tablets, extended-release: 500 mg.

Indications/Routes/Dosages

- Acute otitis media: Children: 15 mg/kg/day in 2 divided doses for 10 days.
- Respiratory/skin infections: Children: 15 mg/kg/day in 2 divided doses for 10 days. Usual adult dose: 250–500 mg q12h for 7–14 days. Extended release: Two 500-mg tablets daily for 7–14 days.

Adverse Reactions

Antibiotic-associated colitis (severe abdominal pain, fever, watery diarrhea), superinfection, hepatotoxicity, thrombocytopenia.

Implications

- Monitor bowel activity and stool consistency.
- For minor GI effects, take with food.
- Doses should be evenly spaced.
- Take with 8 ounces of water.

CLINDAMYCIN—ANTIBIOTIC

Brand Name

Cleocin.

Uses

Treat infections from staphylococci, streptococci, Rickettsia, *Pneumocystis carinii* pneumonia.

Availability

- Oral solution: 75 mg/mL.
- Capsules: 75 mg, 150 mg, 300 mg.

Indications/Routes/Dosage

- Children younger than 1 month: 15–20 mg/kg/day divided q6–8h.
- Children older than 1 month: 8–25 mg/kg/day divided q6–8h.
- Adult: 150–450 mg q6h. Max 1.8 g/day.

Adverse Reactions

Nausea, vomiting, diarrhea, pseudomembranous colitis (severe diarrhea), urinary frequency, vaginitis.

Implications

- Take with full glass of water.
- Give with food to reduce GI symptoms.
- Antiperistaltic drugs may worsen diarrhea.
- Do not break, crush, or chew capsules.
- Call provider for diarrhea.

CLOMIPRAMINE HYDROCHLORIDE — TRICYCLIC ANTIDEPRESSANT

Brand Name

Anafranil.

Uses

Treat obsessive-compulsive disorder (OCD) manifested as repetitive tasks producing marked distress; off label: Mental depression, panic disorder, neurogenic pain, bulimia.

Availability

- Capsules: 25 mg, 50 mg, 75 mg.

Indications/Routes/Dosage

- Children: Starting dose of 10 mg/day; increase to 75–100 mg/day.
- Teens: Starting dose of 10 mg/day; increase to 100–200 mg/day.

Adverse Reactions

Dry mouth, dizziness, sleepiness, tremors, decreased libido, headache, aggressiveness, high doses may produce cardiovascular effects (severe postural hypotension, dizziness, tachycardia, palpitations, arrhythmias, seizures). Abrupt withdrawal from prolonged therapy may produce headache, malaise, nausea, vomiting.

Implications

- Contraindicated within 14 days of monoamine oxidase inhibitor (MAOI) ingestion.
- Caution with history of seizures, hyperthyroidism, cardiac/hepatic/renal disease, diabetes mellitus.

- May cause dry mouth, blurred vision, constipation, drowsiness.
- Ability to tolerate postural hypotension, sedative, and anticholinergic effects occurs during early therapy.
- Maximum therapeutic effect occurs in 2–4 weeks.
- Do not abruptly stop medication.
- Avoid tasks that require alertness, motor skills until drug response is established.
- Wear sunscreen to prevent photosensitivity.

CROTAMITON—SCABICIDE, ANTIPRURITIC

Brand Name

Eurax.

Uses

Treat parasitic infestation (scabies), pruritus.

Availability

- Topical cream: 10%.
- Topical lotion: 10%.

Indications/Routes/Dosage

- For itching, apply locally, massaging affected area until medication absorbed.

Adverse Reactions

Dermatitis, skin irritation.

Implications

- Patient should wash entire body with soap and water.
- Avoid application to face, eyes, mouth, or mucous membranes; avoid applying to inflamed skin or raw, oozing skin surfaces.
- Remove any crusting and apply a thin layer of cream over entire body from the chin down.
- Apply second coat. Wash medication off 48 hours after second coat applied.
- Repeat treatment in 7–10 days if new lesions develop.

DIPHENHYDRAMINE HYDROCHLORIDE— ANTIHISTAMINE, ANTIPRURITIC, ANTITUSSIVE

Brand Name

Benadryl, Nytol, Allerdryl.

Uses

Treat allergy symptoms, rhinitis, motion sickness, urticaria.

Availability

- Elixir: 125 mg/5 mL.
- Syrup: 12.5 mg/5 mL.
- Tablets: 25 mg, 50 mg.
- Tablets, chewable: 25 mg.
- Capsules: 25 mg, 50 mg.

Indications/Routes/Dosage

- Children younger than 2 years: 2 mg/kg q4–6h. Children 2–6 years: 6.25 mg q4–6h, max 37.5 mg/day. Children 6–12 years: 12.5–25 mg q4–6h, max 150 mg/day. Children older than 12 years, adults: 25–50 mg q4–6h, max 300 mg/day.
- Moderate to severe allergic reaction: Children: 5 mg/kg/day divided q6–8h. Max 300 mg/day. Adults: 25–50 mg q4h. Max 400 mg/day.

Adverse Reactions

Dizziness, drowsiness, dry nose, throat.

Implications

- Avoid tasks that require alertness, motor skills until response to drug is established, avoid alcohol.

ERYTHROMYCIN—ANTIBIOTIC

Brand Name

Erythromycin, EES.

Uses

Treat upper and lower respiratory infections such as pneumonia, bronchitis, pharyngitis, otitis media, pertussis, Legionnaires' disease, prophylaxis for rheumatic fever, oral surgery, intestinal and skin infections, gonorrheal pelvic inflammatory infection (if penicillin is contraindicated), Lyme disease (younger than 9 years).

Availability

- Tablets: 250 mg, 333 mg, 500 mg.
- Tablets, delayed-release: 333 mg.
- Capsules, delayed-release: 250 mg.
- Estolate.
    ◦ Oral suspension: 125 mg/5 mL, 250 mg/5 mL.
    ◦ Tablets: 500 mg.
    ◦ Capsules: 250 mg.
- Ethylsuccinate.
    ◦ Oral suspension: 200 mg/5 mL, 400 mg/5 mL.
    ◦ Tablets: 400 mg.
    ◦ Tablets, chewable: 200 mg.
- Stearate: Tablets: 250 mg, 500 mg.

Indications/Routes/Dosage

- Base and ethylsuccinate: Children: 30–50 mg/kg/day divided q6–8h up to 60–100 mg/kg/day for severe infections for 10 days, not to exceed 2 g/day. Adults: Delayed-release: 333 mg q8h increase up to 4 g/day.
- Ethylsuccinate: Adults: 400–800 mg q6–12h.
- Estolate: Children: 30–50 mg/kg/day divided q6–12h. Do not exceed 2 g/day. Adults: 250–500 mg q6–12h.
- Stearate: Children: 30–50 mg/kg/day divided q6h. Do not exceed 2 g/day. Adults: 250–500 mg q6–12h.
- Pertussis: 40–50 mg/kg/day divided q6h for 14 days.
- Prophylaxis for rheumatic fever: 250 mg bid if penicillin allergy.
- *Chlamydia trachomatis*: 50 mg/kg/day divided q6h for 10–14 days.

Adverse Reactions

Nausea, vomiting, abdominal pain, diarrhea, rash, anaphylaxis.

Implications

- Avoid milk and acidic beverages 1 hour before or after a dose.
- Take with food or snack to decrease GI upset.
- Do not break or chew tablets or capsules.
- Suspension is stable for 14 days at room temperature.

FERROUS SULFATE—IRON PREPARATION

Brand Name

Feosol, Fer-In-Sol.

Uses

Treat iron-deficiency anemia.

Availability

- Feosol: Tablets: 200 mg (65 mg elemental iron).
- Fer-In-Sol: Drops: 75 mg/0.6 mL (15 mg elemental iron/0.6 mL).

Indications/Routes/Dosage

- Mild to moderate iron deficiency: 3 mg elemental iron/kg/day in 1–2 divided doses.
- Severe iron deficiency: 4–6 mg elemental iron/kg/day in 3 divided doses.

Adverse Reactions

Nausea, diarrhea, black stools, constipation, black urine, teeth staining.

Implications

- Interactions: Antacids, tetracycline will reduce absorption. Vitamin C enhances absorption.
- Give between meals with orange juice; do not give with milk. Give with a straw or brush teeth after giving.
- May cause abdominal discomfort; keep out of the reach of small children.

FEXOFENADINE HYDROCHLORIDE—ANTIHISTAMINE

Brand Name

Allegra.

Uses

Treat seasonal allergic rhinitis.

Availability

- Tablets: 30 mg, 60 mg, 180 mg.
- Capsules: 60 mg.
- Capsules, extended-release: 180 mg.

Indications/Routes/Dosage

- Children older than 12 years: 60 mg bid or 180 mg once daily.
- Children 6–11 years: 30 mg bid.

Adverse Reactions

Dry mouth, nose, headache, fatigue, nausea, vomiting.

Implications

- Avoid tasks that require alertness, motor skills until response to drug is known.
- Avoid alcohol, coffee, or tea; may decrease drowsiness.

FLUOXETINE—SELECTIVE SEROTONIN REUPTAKE INHIBITOR (SSRI), ANTIDEPRESSANT

Brand Name

Prozac, Sarafem (Prozac weekly).

Uses

Treat major depression, OCD, bulimia nervosa, premenstrual dysphoric disorder (PMDD).

Availability

- Oral solution: 20 mg/5 mL.
- Tablets: 10 mg, 20 mg.
- Capsules: 10 mg, 20 mg, 40 mg.

Indications/Routes/Dosage

- Anxiety disorders: Starting dose of 5 mg/day, increase to 15–30 mg/day for children and 10–40 mg/day for teens.
- Major depression: Starting dose of 5 mg/day, increase to 15–40 mg per day for children and 10–60 mg/day for teens.

Adverse Reactions

Headache, nervousness, insomnia, drowsiness, anxiety, tremor, dizziness, sedation, poor concentration, abnormal dreams, decreased libido, dry mouth, diarrhea, weight loss.

Implications

- Take with food and milk for GI symptoms.
- Can crush tablet if patient unable to swallow.
- Take at night to decrease oversedation.
- Therapeutic effect may take 1–4 weeks.
- Fluvoxamine—SSRI, antidepressant, antianxiety.
- Use sunscreen to prevent photosensitivity.
- Avoid alcohol and other CNS depressants.
- Notify prescriber if pregnant, plan to become pregnant, or are breastfeeding.
- Change position slowly due to orthostatic hypotension.
- Educate parents about FDA concerns of suicide risk in patients on SSRI antidepressants; monitor suicidal risk closely during course of treatment, especially in the first 30 days of treatment.

FLUVOXAMINE—SSRI, ANTIDEPRESSANT, ANTIANXIETY

Brand Name

Luvox.

Uses

Treat OCD, major depression, anxiety disorders.

Availability

- Tablets: 25 mg, 50 mg, 100 mg.

Indications/Routes/Dosage

- Starting dose of 25 mg/day, increase to 50–200 mg/day for children and 150–300 mg/day for teens.

Adverse Reactions

Headache, drowsiness, dizziness, convulsions, nausea, vomiting, anorexia, constipation, diarrhea, decreased libido, increased effect with St. John's wort. Fatal reactions: MAOI interactions increase action of propranolol, diazepam, lithium, warfarin, carbamazepine, theophylline.

Implications

- Give with food, milk for GI distress.
- Therapeutic effects may take 2–3 weeks. Use caution when driving.
- Do not use with other CNS depressants (e.g., alcohol, barbiturates, benzodiazepines, St. John's wort).
- Educate parents about FDA concerns of suicide risk in patients on SSRI antidepressants; monitor suicidal risk closely during course of treatment, especially in the first 30 days of treatment.

FOLIC ACID—NUTRITION SUPPLEMENT

Brand Name

Folate, Folvite.

Uses

Treat anemia due to folate deficiency, nutritional supplement to prevent neural tube defects.

Availability

- Tablets: 0.4 mg, 0.8 mg, 1.0 mg.

Indications/Routes/Dosage

- Recommended daily intake for children: 6 months to 3 years: 50 mcg (15 mcg/kg/day). 4–6 years: 75 mcg. 7–10 years: 100 mcg. 11–14 years: 150 mcg. Older than 15 years: 200 mcg.
- Dosage: Infants: 15 mcg/kg/daily. Children: 1 mg/day initial dosage.
- Maintenance dose: Children 1–10 years: 0.1–0.4 mg/day. Children older than 11 years, adults: 1 mg/day initial dose; maintenance dose 0.5 mg/day.

Adverse Reactions

Flushing, irritability, difficulty sleeping, malaise, rash, itching, GI upset, hypersensitivity reactions.

Implications

- Take every day.
- Call provider if adverse reactions.

LACTULOSE—HYPEROSMOTIC LAXATIVE

Brand Name

Constilac, Constulose, Enulose.

Uses

Treat constipation.

Availability

- Syrup: 10 mg/15 mL.
- Packets: 10 g, 20 g.

Indications/Routes/Dosage

- Children: 7.5 mL/day after breakfast.
- Adults: 15–30 mL/day up to 60 mL/day.

Adverse Reactions

Cramping, flatulence, increased thirst, abdominal discomfort; diarrhea indicates an overdose.

Implications

- Drink water, juice, milk with each dose.
- Evacuation occurs in 24–48 hours of initial dose.
- Patients should also be on a high-fiber diet and exercise to promote defecation.

LEVALBUTEROL — BRONCHODILATOR

Brand Name

Xopenex.

Uses

Prevention of bronchospasm due to reversible obstructive airway disease.

Availability

- Solution for nebulization: 0.63 mg OR 1.25 mg in 3 mL vials (no dilution necessary).

Indications/Routes/Dosage

- Children older than 12 years: 0.63–1.25 mg q6–8h (tid), with max of 1.25 mg tid.

Adverse Reactions

Tremors, nervousness, headache, throat dryness/irritation, palpitations, chest pain, extrasystole.

Implications

- Monitor rate, depth, rhythm, and type of respiration.
- Increase fluid intake.
- Rinse mouth with water after inhalation.
- Avoid caffeine.

LITHIUM CARBONATE—ANTIMANIC, ANTIDEPRESSANT

Brand Name

Eskalith, Dura-Lith.

Uses

Prophylaxis, treatment of acute mania, manic phase of bipolar disorder.

Availability

- Syrup: 300 mg/5 mL.
- Tablets: 300 mg.
- Tablets, slow-release: 300 mg, 450 mg.
- Capsules: 150 mg, 300 mg, 600 mg.

Indications/Routes/Dosage

- Start at 25 mg/kg/day, gradually increase until serum level reaches therapeutic range of 0.9–1.1 mEq/L.

Adverse Reactions

Headache, drowsiness, dizziness, anorexia, nausea, vomiting, diarrhea, hypotension, dry mouth. May increase effects of antithyroid medication, iodinate glycerol, potassium iodide. Nonsteroidal anti-inflammatory drugs (NSAIDs) and diuretics may increase concentration, toxicity. May decrease absorption of phenothiazines.

Implications

- Give with meals, milk.
- Limit alcohol, caffeine.
- May cause dry mouth.
- Do not crush, chew, or break extended-release or film-coated tablets.
- Assess serum lithium levels q3–4 days during initial phase of therapy, q1–2 months thereafter, and weekly if no improvement.
- Monitor for signs of lithium toxicity: Vomiting, diarrhea, drowsiness, incoordination, hand tremor, muscle twitching, mental confusion, ataxia.

LORATADINE—ANTIHISTAMINE

Brand Name

Claritin.

Uses

Treat seasonal rhinitis.

Availability

- Syrup: 5 mg/5 mL.
- Tablet: 10 mg.

Indications/Routes/Dosage

- Children 2–12 years: 5 mg daily.
- Children older than 12 years, adult: 10 mg daily.

Adverse Reactions

Sedation is more common with larger doses, headache.

Implications

- Use sunscreen (photosensitive).
- Avoid driving if drowsiness occurs.
- Additive CNS effects with alcohol and antidepressants.

MEBENDAZOLE—ANTHELMINTIC

Brand Name

Vermox.

Uses

Treatment of *Enterobius vermicularis* (pinworms), *Ascaris lumbricoides* (roundworm), *Trichuris trichiura* (whipworm), and *Ancylostoma duodenale* (common hookworm).

Availability

- Tablets, chewable: 100 mg.

Indications/Routes/Dosage

- Enterobiasis: Children, adults: 100 mg PO as a single dose.
- Other infestations: Children, adults: 100 mg 2 bid for 3 days.

Adverse Reactions

GI transient abdominal pain. Carbamazepine and phenytoin can increase metabolism of mebendazole.

Implications

- Tablets may be chewed, swallowed, or crushed and mixed with food.
- Do not administer to children younger than 2 years or pregnant and lactating women.
- If patient is not cured in 3 weeks following treatment, retreatment is necessary.
- All family members should be treated at the same time.
- Discuss hygiene, transmission, and reinfection.

MONTELUKAST—ANTIASTHMATIC

Brand Name

Singulair.

Uses

Prophylaxis and chronic treatment of asthma.

Availability

- Tablets: 10 mg.
- Tablets, chewable: 4 mg, 5 mg.
- Oral granules: 4 mg.

Indications/Routes/Dosages

- Children 1–5 years: One 4-mg tablet taken in the evening.
- Children 6–14 years: One 5-mg chewable tablet taken in the evening.
- Children older than 14, adults: 10 mg daily taken in the evening.

Adverse Effects

Headache, abdominal pain, fever, restlessness, irritability.

Implications

- Do not use to reverse bronchospasm as in an acute asthma attack.
- Increase fluid intake.
- Continue other asthma medications while taking this one.
- Chewable table contains phenylalanine.
- Patients sensitive to aspirin should avoid aspirin and NSAIDs while on this medication.

NITROFURANTOIN — ANTIBIOTIC

Brand Name

Furadantin, Macrobid, Macrodantin.

Uses

Treat urinary tract infections caused by *Escherichia coli, Klebsiella, Pseudomonas, Proteus vulgaris, Staphylococcus aureus, Salmonella, Shigella.*

Availability

- Suspension: 25 mg/5 mL.
- Tablets: 50 mg, 100 mg.
- Capsules: 25 mg, 50 mg, 100 mg.

Indications/Routes/Dosage

- Active infections: Children 1 month to 3 years old: 5–7 mg/kg/day divided qid; 1–3 mg/kg/day for long-term treatment. Children older than 12 years, adult: 50–100 mg qid PO or 50–100 mg at bedtime for long-term treatment.
- Chronic suppression: Children: 1 mg/kg/day every night. Adults: 50–100 mg every night.

Adverse Reactions

Dizziness, headache, nausea, vomiting, abdominal pain, diarrhea.

Implications

- Do not use in infants younger than 1 month old.
- Take with food or milk.
- Avoid alcohol.
- Drowsiness may occur; do not drive or operate machinery until response to drug is established.
- Do not crush tabs or open capsules.
- May turn urine rust-yellow to brown.

OFLOXACIN — FLUOROQUINOLONE ANTI-INFECTIVE

Brand Name

Floxin Otic, Floxin Otic Drops, Ocuflox.

Uses

Ophthalmic: Treat bacterial conjunctivitis, corneal ulcers. Otic: Treat otitis externa, acute/chronic otitis media.

Availability

- Ophthalmic solution: 3 mg/mL.
- Otic solution: 0.3%.

Indications/Routes/Dosage

- Bacterial conjunctivitis: 1–2 drops q2–4h for 2 days, then 4 times/day for 5 days.
- Corneal ulcers: Ophthalmic: 1–2 drops q30min while awake for 2 days, then q60min while awake for 5–7 days, then 4 times/day. Otic: Twice daily.

Adverse Reactions

Allergic reaction.

Implications

- Ophthalmic:
  - Tilt patient's head back, place solution in conjunctival sac.
  - Do not use ophthalmic solution for injection.

- Otic:
  - Eardrops should be at room temperature.
  - Instruct patient to lie down with head turned so affected ear is upright.
  - Pull the auricle down and posterior in children, pull up and posterior in older adolescents and adults.
  - Instill toward canal wall.

OMEPRAZOLE—GASTRIC ACID PUMP INHIBITOR

Brand Name

Prilosec.

Uses

Short-term treatment (4–8 weeks) and maintenance of erosive esophagitis, gastro-esophageal reflux disease (GERD), poorly responsive to other treatments. Unlabeled treatment of *Helicobacter pylori*–associated duodenal ulcer.

Availability

- Tablets: 10 mg, 20 mg, 40 mg.

Indications/Routes/Dosage

- Children older than 2 years: 20 mg/day, < 20 kg 10 mg/day.

Adverse Reactions

May increase concentration of oral anticonvulsants, diazepam; phenytoin may increase serum glutamic oxaloacetic transaminase (SGOT), serum glutamic pyruvic transaminase (SGPT), alanine aminotransferase (ALT).

Implications

- Report headache to provider.
- Take before meals.
- Swallow capsule whole; do not crush or chew.

PAROXETINE HYDROCHLORIDE—SSRI, ANTIDEPRESSANT, ANTIPANIC, ANTIANXIETY

Brand Name

Paxil, Paxil CR.

Uses

Treat major depressive disorder, OCD, panic and generalized anxiety disorders.

Availability

- Oral suspension: 10 mg/kg.
- Tablets: 10 mg, 20 mg, 30 mg, 40 mg.
- Tablets, controlled-release (CR): 12.5 mg, 25 mg, 37.5 mg.

Indications/Routes/Dosage

- Children, adolescents: Initial dose 5–10 mg, titrate up to 20 mg and monitor for side effects.
- Paxil CR: Children, adolescents: Initial dose 12 mg titrate up to 25 mg.

Adverse Reactions

Nausea, headache, nervousness, insomnia, sedation, agitation, fatigue, dry mouth, constipation, diarrhea, decreased libido/sexual dysfunction.

Implications

- Dose changes should occur at 1-week intervals for both drugs.
- Do not use with MAOI.
- Use with cimetidine may increase concentrations.
- Use with phenytoin may decrease concentrations.
- Use with risperidone may increase paroxetine concentration enough to cause extrapyramidal symptoms.
- May cause dry mouth; avoid alcohol.
- Therapeutic effect may occur in 1–4 weeks.
- Do not abruptly discontinue medication.
- Avoid tasks that require alertness or motor skills until response to drug is established.

- Give with food or milk if GI symptoms.
- Educate parents about FDA concerns of suicide risk in patients on SSRI antidepressants; monitor suicidal risk closely during course of treatment, especially in the first 30 days of treatment.

PENICILLIN V POTASSIUM — ANTIBIOTIC

Brand Name

Pen VK, V-Cillin K.

Uses

Treatment of mild to moderate infections of respiratory tract, skin/skin structures, otitis media, prophylaxis for rheumatic fever, dental procedures.

Availability

- Oral solution: 125 mg/5 mL, 250 mg/5 mL.
- Tablets: 125 mg, 250 mg, 500 mg.

Indications/Routes/Dosage

- Children younger than 12 years: 25–50 mg/kg/day divided q6–8h. Max 3 g/day. Children older than 12 years, adults: 125–500 mg q6–8h.
- Rheumatic fever prophylaxis: Children, adults: 250 mg 2–3 times/day.

Adverse Reactions

Hypersensitivity reaction, colitis, fever, rash, pruritus.

Implications

- Question history of drug allergies.
- Continue antibiotic for full treatment.
- Notify provider of rash, sensitivity reaction.

PREDNISOLONE — ANTI-INFLAMMATORY

Brand Name

Pediapred, Prelone, Orapred.

Uses

Treat reactive airway disease and asthma flare.

Availability

- Syrup: 5 mg/5 mL, 15 mg/5 mL
- Tablets: 5 mg.

Indications/Routes/Dosage

- 1–2 mg/kg/day in divided doses bid usually for 5 days, although longer may be required.

Adverse Reactions

Insomnia, heartburn, nervousness, abdominal distention, mood swings, increased sweating, and delayed healing. Long term: Hypocalcemia, hypokalemia, muscle wasting, especially the arms and legs, osteoporosis, spontaneous fractures, amenorrhea, cataracts, glaucoma, peptic ulcer disease.

Implications

- Notify healthcare provider of fever, sore throat, muscle aches, swelling, weight gain.
- Avoid alcohol, caffeine.
- Avoid exposure to chickenpox or measles.

RANITIDINE—ANTIULCER AGENT, GASTRIC ACID SECRETION INHIBITOR

Brand Name

Zantac.

Uses

To prevent and treat gastric and duodenal ulcers.

Availability

- Syrup 15 mg/5 mL.
- Tablets 75 mg, 150 mg, 300 mg.
- Effervescent capsules 150 mg, 300 mg.

Indications/Routes/Dosage

- GERD and ulcers: Children 1 month to 16 years: 2–4 mg/kg bid; effervescent tabs 2.5–5 mg/kg bid; adults and adolescents: 150 mg bid.

SERTRALINE—SSRI, ANTIDEPRESSANT, ANTIPANIC AGENT

Brand Name

Zoloft.

Uses

Treat major depression, OCD, post-traumatic stress disorder, panic disorder, PMDD.

Availability

- Oral liquid: 20 mg/mL.
- Tablets: 25 mg, 50 mg, 100 mg.

Indications/Routes/Dosage

- Anxiety: Children: Starting dose of 25 mg/day, increase to 50–100 mg/day; 50–200 mg/day for teens.
- Major depression: Children: Starting dose of 25 mg/day, increase to 50–150 mg/day; 50–200 mg/day for teens.

Adverse Reactions

Headache, nausea, diarrhea, insomnia, drowsiness, fatigue, rash, dry mouth, anxiety, sexual dysfunction.

Implications

- Do not give within 14 days of MAOI.
- Therapeutic effect may take 2–3 weeks.
- Avoid tasks that require alertness, motor skills until response to drug is established.
- Take with food or milk, avoid alcohol.
- Weigh weekly: Appetite may decrease.

- Notify provider if intending to become pregnant, are pregnant, or are breastfeeding.
- Do not use with St. John's wort, SAM-e.
- Avoid CNS depressants.
- Do not stop quickly, need to taper.
- Educate parents about FDA concerns of suicide risk in patients on SSRI antidepressants; monitor suicidal risk closely during course of treatment, especially in the first 30 days of treatment.

SULFAMETHOXAZOLE/TRIMETHOPRIM— ANTI-INFECTIVE

Brand Name

Bactrim, Septra.

Uses

Treat acute/complicated and recurrent urinary tract infections, *Shigella*, enteritis, otitis media, traveler's diarrhea, enteritis, *Pneumocystis carinii* pneumonia.

Availability

- Oral suspension: 40 mg trimethoprim/200 mg, 400 mg sulfamethoxazole/5 mL.
- Tablets: 80 mg trimethoprim/400 mg sulfamethoxazole; 160 mg/800 mg.

Indications/Routes/Dosage

- Urinary tract infection caused by *Escherichia coli, Klebsiella, Proteus mirabilis, Enterobacter*, enteritis, acute otitis media: Children older than 2 months: 7.5–8 mg/kg/day divided q12h for 10 days. Adults: 160 mg q12h for 7–14 days.
- Travelers' diarrhea, bronchitis: Adults: 1 double-strength tablet q12h for 5 days.

Weight: lbs, kg	Suspension	Tablets
22, 10	1 tsp (5 mL)	½
44, 20	2 tsp (10 mL)	1
66, 30	3 tsp (15 mL)	1½
88, 40	4 tsp (20 mL)	2 or 1 DS

Adverse Reactions

Anorexia, nausea, vomiting, urticaria, diarrhea, abdominal pain, rash, fever, sore throat, cough, shortness of breath.

Implications

- Take each dose with one glass water and increase fluid intake.
- Take for full treatment time as prescribed.
- Do not use in children < 2 months.
- Do not use in patients sensitive to sulfa drugs.

Note: All patients weighing > 100 lbs should be dosed according to adult dosage guidelines.

Abbreviations

AAP—American Academy of Pediatrics

ABG—arterial blood gas

ABO—blood types

ABR—auditory brainstem response

AC—air conduction

ACE—angiotensin-converting enzyme

AD—atopic dermatitis

ADD—attention deficit disorder

ADH—antidiuretic hormone

ADHD—attention-deficit/hyperactivity disorder

ADL—activity of daily living

AFP—alpha fetal protein

ANA—antinuclear antibody

AOM—acute otitis media

AOME—acute otitis media with effusion

ASO—antistreptolysin enzyme

AVN—avascular necrosis

BAER—brainstem auditory-evoked response

BC—bone conduction

bid—twice daily

BM—bowel movement

BMI—body mass index

BP—blood pressure

BPM—beats per minute

BUN—blood urea nitrogen

CBC—complete blood count

CBT—cognitive behavioral therapy

CDC—Centers for Disease Control and Prevention

CF—cystic fibrosis

CHF—congestive heart failure

cm—centimeter

CMV—cytomegalovirus

CNS—central nervous system

CP—cerebral palsy

C/S—culture/sensitivity

CSF—cerebrospinal fluid

CT—computed tomography (X-ray exam)

CVA—costal-vertebral angle

CXR—chest X-ray

DDAVP—synthetic vasopressin (posterior pituitary hormone)

DDH—developmental dysplasia of the hip

DRSP—drug-resistant *Streptococcus pneumoniae*

DTaP—diphtheria-tetanus-acellular pertussis (vaccine)

DTP—diphtheria-tetanus-pertussis (vaccine)

EBV—Epstein-Barr virus

EC—emergency contraception

ECG—electrocardiogram
(also known as EKG)
ED—emergency department
EDC—estimated date of confinement
EEG—electroencephalogram
EENT—eye, ear, nose, throat
ENS—enteral nutritional support
ENT—ear, nose, throat
EOAE—evoked otoacoustic emissions
ESR—erythrocyte sedimentation rate
ETD—eustachian tube dysfunction
ETOH—alcohol
FEV—forced expiratory volume
g—gram
GABHS—group A beta-hemolytic
streptococcus
GD—gestational diabetes
GER—gastroesophageal reflux
GI—gastrointestinal
GU—genitourinary
h—hour
H. flu—*Haemophilus influenzae* b (bacteria)
HAB—hepatitis A virus
HBsAg—hepatitis B surface antigen
HBV—hepatitis B virus
HCG—human chorionic gonadotropin
Hct—hematocrit
HCV—hepatitis C virus
HDL—high-density lipoprotein
HEENT—head, eyes, ear, nose, throat
Hep—hepatitis
Hep B—hepatitis B vaccine
Hgb—hemoglobin
Hib—*Haemophilus influenzae* b
(vaccine)

HIV—human immunodeficiency virus
HPV—human papillomavirus
HR—heart rate
HS—at bedtime
HSV—herpes simplex virus
IBD—inflammatory bowel disease
IBS—irritable bowel syndrome
ICP—intracranial pressure
Ig—immunoglobulin
IgC—immunoglobulin C
IgE—immunoglobulin E
IgM—immunoglobulin M
IM—intramuscular
I&O—intake and output
IPV—inactivated poliovirus vaccine
IV—intravenous
JRA—juvenile rheumatoid arthritis
kcal—kilocalorie
kg—kilogram
KOH—potassium chloride
KUB—kidneys, ureters bladder
(X-ray examination)
lbs—pounds
LDLs—low-density lipoproteins
LES—lower esophageal sphincter
LFT(s)—liver function test(s)
LMP—last menstrual period
LOC—level of consciousness
LP—lumbar puncture
LRI—lower respiratory infection
LTB—laryngotracheobronchitis
LTBP—laryngotracheobronchopneumonia
MAO(I)—monoamine oxidase (inhibitor)
MCV—mean corpuscular volume
mg—milligram

min—minute

mL—milliliter

mm—millimeter

MMR—measles-mumps-rubella (vaccine)

MMWR—*Morbidity and Mortality Weekly Report* (www.cdc.gov)

mo(s)—month(s)

MRI—magnetic resonance imaging (X-ray examination)

NCHS—National Center for Health Statistics

NPO—nothing by mouth

NSAID(s)—nonsteroidal anti-inflammatory drug(s)

N/V—nausea and vomiting

OD—right eye

OFC—occipital frontal circumference

OM—otitis media

O&P—ova and parasites

OS—left eye

OTC—over the counter

OU—both eyes

Pap—Papanicolaou

PCOS—polycystic ovary syndrome

PCV—Prevnar or pneumococcal vaccine

PID—pelvic inflammatory disease

PIH—pregnancy-induced hypertension

PMNs—polymorphonucleotides

PnC—pneumococcal conjugate

PO—by mouth

Postop—postoperative

PPD—purified protein derivative

PPI—proton pump inhibitors

Preop—preoperative

PRN—as required

PS—pyloric stenosis

PT—prothrombin time

PTT—partial thromboplastin time

PUD—peptic ulcer disease

q—every

qd—every day

qh—every hour

q2h—every 2 hours

q3h—every 3 hours

q4h—every 4 hours

q6h—every 6 hours

q12h—every 12 hours

qid—four times daily

RAP—recurrent abdominal pain syndrome

RBC—red blood cell

Rh—blood group on surface of erythrocytes

R/O—rule out

ROM—range of motion

RSV—respiratory syncytial virus

SBE—subacute bacterial endocarditis

SD—standard deviation

SGOT—serum glutamic-oxaloacetic transaminase

SGPT—serum glutamic-pyruvic transaminase

SIADH—syndrome of inappropriate antidiuretic hormone

SIDS—sudden infant death syndrome

SMR—sexual maturity rating

SSRI—selective serotonin reuptake inhibitor

STI—sexually transmitted infection

TB—tuberculosis

TBSA—total body surface area

Tbsp—tablespoon

Td—tetanus toxoid

TD—tetanus and diphtheria vaccine

Temp—temperature

TIBC—total iron-binding capacity

tid—three times daily

TM—tympanic membrane

TMJ—temporomandibular joint dysfunction

TMP-SMX—trimethoprim-sulfamethoxazole

TSH—thyroid-simulating hormone

tsp—teaspoon

UA—urinalysis

UCG—urine chorionic gonadotropin (pregnancy test)

URI—upper respiratory infection

UTI—urinary tract infection

VBAC—vaginal birth after cesarean

VCUG—voiding cystourethrogram

WBC—white blood count

wk(s)—week(s)

WNL—within normal limits

wt—weight

yr(s)—year(s)

$>$ — greater than

$<$ — less than

$\geq$ — greater than or equal to

$\leq$ — less than or equal to

Index

Note: Page numbers followed by *b*, *f*, and *t* indicate material in boxes, figures, and tables respectively.

Figure 1 Acne vulgaris of the forehead. © F.C.G./Fotolia.com

Figure 2 Acne vulgaris of the lower face. © Olga Sapegina/Fotolia.com

Figure 3 Atopic dermatitis. Minute excoriations with lichenification in the antecubital fossa seen. © iStockphoto/Thinkstock

Figure 4 Impetiginized atopic dermatitis. © Dr. P. Marazzi/Science Source

Figure 5 Flexural involvement of popliteal fossa in atopic dermatitis. © Jingling Water/Fotolia.com

Figure 6 Urticaria. © Rob Byron/ Shutterstock

Figure 7 Scabies. Courtesy of CDC.

Figure 8 Irritant diaper dermatitis. © Biophoto Associates/Science Source

Figure 9 Chafing type of diaper dermatitis. © Mediscan/Alamy

Figure 10 Candidiasis in the diaper area. A positive culture for *Candida* can be obtained from satellite pustules. © Dr. P. Marazzi/Science Source

Figure 11 Inflammatory superficial fungal infection. Courtesy of K. Mae Lennon, Tulane Medical School/ Clement Benjamin/CDC.

Figure 12 Recurrent herpes simplex. Courtesy of Dr. Herrmann/CDC.

Figure 13 Impetigo infection of a 7-year-old girl. © Dr. P. Marazzi/ Science Source

Figure 14 Infant with primary herpes gingivostomatitis. © Dr. P. Marazzi/Science Source

Figure 15 Erosion of the tongue in a child with hand-foot-and-mouth syndrome. © Dr. P. Marazzi/Science Source

Figure 16 Common wart on child's finger. © leschnyhan/Fotolia.com

Figure 17 Slapped-cheek appearance of a child with parvovirus B19 infection (erythema infectiosum). Courtesy of Dr. Philip S. Brachman/CDC.

Figure 18 Lacy pink eruption over dorsal surfaces in erythema infectiosum. Courtesy of CDC.

Figure 19 Lacy pink eruption of erythema infectiosum on chest and upper abdomen. Courtesy of Dr. Gary P. Williams, MD.

Figure 20 Rocky Mountain spotted fever (RMSF), acral dusky oval purpuric lesions. Courtesy of CDC.

Figure 21 Pityriasis alba. In some atopic patients, subtle inflammation may result in poorly demarcated areas of hypopigmentation, known as pityriasis alba. Lesions are most prominent in darkly pigmented individuals. © Mediscan/Alamy

Figure 22 Pityriasis rosea. The large herald patch on the chest of this 10-year old girl shows central clearing, which mimics tinea corporis. Courtesy of Dr. Sellars/CDC.

Figure 23 Pityriasis rosea. Numerous oval lesions on the chest of a Caucasian teenager. Courtesy of CDC.

Figure 24 Tinea versicolor. The well-demarcated, scaly papules appear darker than surrounding skin on the back of a Caucasian adolescent. Courtesy of Dr. Lucille K. Georg/CDC.

Figure 25 Roseaola/exanthema subitum. A generalized, pink, maculopapular rash suddenly appeared on this infant after 3 days of high fever. Courtesy of Arthur E. Kaye/CDC.

Figure 26 Scarlet fever. A generalized, bright red, sandpaper-like papular rash developed in a 7-year-old boy with a streptococcal pharyngitis. Courtesy of CDC.

Figure 27 Scarlet fever. A white strawberry tongue precedes red strawberry tongue. Courtesy of Jere J. Mammino, DO, FAOCD.

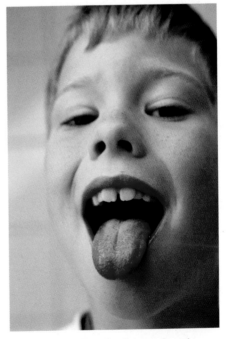

Figure 28 Scarlet fever. A red strawberry tongue as the erythrotoxin-mediated enanthema evolves. © imageBROKER/Alamy Stock Photo

Figure 29 Kawasaki syndrome. A generalized, morbilliform erythema-multiforme-like rash is a characteristic clinical finding. Courtesy of CDC.

Figure 30 Kawasaki syndrome. Palmar and plantar erythema with edema of the hands and feet is a characteristic clinical finding. © Ralph Hutchings/Visuals Unlimited, Inc.

Figure 31 Reaction to bedbug bites. © Joel Carillet/E+/Getty

Figure 32 Molluscum contagiosum. Individual lesions are 2- to 5-mm, flesh colored, dome-shaped umbilicated papules. © Jarrod Erbe/ Shutterstock

Figure 33 Molluscum contagiosum spreads rapidly in eczematous skin. This patient has atopic dermatitis of the popliteal fossa. © Dr. P. Marazzi/ Science Source